AF718789

THE PRAEGER HANDBOOK OF SOCIAL JUSTICE AND PSYCHOLOGY

THE PRAEGER HANDBOOK OF SOCIAL JUSTICE AND PSYCHOLOGY

Volume 2

Well-Being and Professional Issues

Chad V. Johnson and Harris L. Friedman, Set Editors
Jeannette Diaz, Zeno Franco, and Bonnie K. Nastasi, Volume Editors

Foreword by Mary A. Fukuyama

Social Justice and Psychology

PRAEGER

AN IMPRINT OF ABC-CLIO, LLC
Santa Barbara, California • Denver, Colorado • Oxford, England

Copyright 2014 by Chad V. Johnson and Harris L. Friedman

All rights reserved. No part of this publication may be reproduced, stored in a retrieval system, or transmitted, in any form or by any means, electronic, mechanical, photocopying, recording, or otherwise, except for the inclusion of brief quotations in a review, without prior permission in writing from the publisher.

Library of Congress Cataloging-in-Publication Data

The Praeger handbook of social justice and psychology / Chad V. Johnson [and five others].
volumes cm. — (Social justice and psychology)
Includes index.
Contents: volume 1. Fundamental issues and special populations
ISBN 978-1-4408-0378-9 (hardcopy : alk. paper) — ISBN 978-1-4408-0379-6 (ebook)
1. Social psychiatry. 2. Social justice—Psychological aspects. 3. Psychology, Pathological—Social aspects. I. Johnson, Chad (Chad Vernon) II. Title: Handbook of social justice and psychology.
RC455.P6962 2014
616.89'071—dc23 2014000218

ISBN: 978-1-4408-0378-9
EISBN: 978-1-4408-0379-6

18 17 16 15 14 1 2 3 4 5

This book is also available on the World Wide Web as an eBook.
Visit www.abc-clio.com for details.

Praeger
An Imprint of ABC-CLIO, LLC

ABC-CLIO, LLC
130 Cremona Drive, P.O. Box 1911
Santa Barbara, California 93116-1911

This book is printed on acid-free paper ∞

Manufactured in the United States of America

Dedicated to the Memory of George Albee (1921–2006)

George was a pioneering psychologist whose path was to envision "a world free from exploitation and domination of one group by another, a world in which each person has the freedom and the resources to develop her or his potential to the fullest, a world in which the highest goal would be one person's concern and regard for others" (Kessler, Goldston, & Joffe, 1992, p. 19). And he worked ceaselessly toward these ends. When I first met him in the late 1990s, he and I were keynote speakers at a conference on psychology and juvenile justice. Having my attitudes and values toward professional psychology profoundly shaped by reading many of his contributions, I excitedly blurted out, "you are my hero." Unabashedly George responded, "We all must be heroes."—Harris L. Friedman

Kessler, M., Goldston, S., & Joffe, J. (1992). George Albee: An appreciation. In M. Kessler, S. Goldston, & J. Joffe (Eds.), *The present and future of prevention: In honor of George W. Albee* (pp. 3–32). Newbury Park, CA: Sage.

Contents

Acknowledgments

We would like to thank the contributing authors for their highly informative chapters, diligence, and responsive to requests for revision. We are deeply indebted to our editorial assistant, Lindsay Plott-Buckner, who worked tirelessly, superbly, and without complaint throughout the editing process. We are also grateful for additional editorial assistance provided by Heather Threadgill and Eamon Slattery. Finally, we acknowledge all those, both within psychology and without, who struggle with oppression and injustice and work toward social justice and peace.

Introduction to Volume 2

Zeno Franco

Volume 2 of the *Praeger Handbook of Social Justice and Psychology* addresses an impressive array of concerns related to promoting health and well-being as well as integrating social justice activities into one's psychological practice. This overview introduces the chapters in the volume and provides a brief comment on their import. Part 1 examines many different topics related to the promotion of health and well-being and alleviation of suffering. These informative chapters include topics such as the ecology of social justice, environmental justice, dignity, disasters, neuroscience, and spirituality. Part 2 explores professional issues such as approaches for integrating social justice into teaching, training, and research.

WELL-BEING AND SUFFERING

Prilleltensky and Huygens set the tone for this part by presenting an ecological notion of social justice and well-being in Chapter 1, describing social justice as a complex, multifaceted construct with at least eight aspects (rather than the usually described dimensions)—distributive, procedural, intrapersonal, developmental, relational, informational, retributive, and cultural justice. The authors argue that these ideas relate not just to individuals as psychology often does, but also to broader units of analysis, including organizations and societies. The authors suggest that justice is directly tied to well-being and that a society's orientation toward justice sets the stage for thriving, coping, resisting, or suffering at both the individual and population levels. Overall, mental and physical well-being may center on social action and organizing designed to liberate entire groups of people from social injustice.

Prilleltensky and Huygens enumerate several types of organizing viewed as central to moving toward more just societies, which include organizing for economic prosperity, for health promotion, for effective functioning, for freedom, for equality, and organizing for participation, inclusion, and dignity. They articulate specific linkages between organizing approaches and the eight social justice domains. Prilletensky and Huygens's chapter sets forth a wide reaching framework for the entire volume providing a more nuanced view of social justice and how these distinctions relate to overall well-being within individuals, communities, and societies. Their conceptualization of the overlap between social justice and well-being also underscores the need for interdisciplinary approaches to mental health training, therapeutic interventions, and governance and public policy in this arena.

In Chapter 2, Williams, Dhami, and Moody explore the intersection between race, gender, and class oppressions, and related socially sanctioned injustices that increase instances of stress and its resultant mental and physical health consequences. The authors apply Collins's Intersectionality Analysis and Injustice Stress Theory to contextualize the lives of Black/African descendants and Latina girls in urban contexts, describing the relationship between intersecting oppressions, societal injustice, and optimal mental health and wellness. These concepts are extended to examine the global citizenship of Black/African descents and Latina American and Brazilian adolescent girls reared in urban environments. Exploration of the ways gender, race/ethnicity, and class intersect to shape their experience of stress, health, and well-being is discussed, and the importance of community-based intervention programming for addressing the risk concerns of these populations is highlighted. The authors point to two such programs as exemplars for future work designed to address these intersecting social justice concerns, and preliminary findings from a U.S. sample are presented. Their work illustrates the profound importance of developing a better understanding of intersecting injustices, showing real-world examples of the overlaps of the various facets of injustice offered by Prilletensky and Huygens. The chapter also illustrates how what the society describes as negative behaviors in individuals often points to societal ills as described by Robbins and Friedman (Chapter 4) and Williams and Arrigo (Chapter 9).

Riemer and Voorhees, in Chapter 3, note that over the past 60 years human activities have changed the biosystem more rapidly and extensively than in any comparable period of history. They argue that there is little doubt that global climate change and environmental degradation should be on the top of the priority list for any discipline, with psychology being no exception. There are many important psychological questions that bridge psychological and environmental issues, such as how to create a culture of sustainability and how to deal with the severe impacts of global climate changes, some of which will likely have significant psychological implications. In this chapter, the authors explore the connection of psychology to environmental justice and sustainability in particular. They begin by contemplating the relationship of humans to nature followed by introducing the issues of environmental justice and sustainability. Then, important psychological questions and existing psychological research on environmental issues are discussed. For example, the authors pose the question of why societies tolerate the suffering of certain peoples from negative environmental impacts while others live in comfort, with much lower environmental exposures to potentially harmful agents.

The authors describe both the negative psychological impacts of environmental degradation and the positive effects of access to nature using an environmental justice lens. This is followed by an exploration of environmental action and how environmental justice can serve as an important motivator to engage people in environmental change. Finally, the authors conclude with some thoughts for practice and future research. This chapter underscores the need for collective social action as a way to achieve environmentally transformative social justice goals. This call toward collective action extends the remarks on this subject offered by Prilleltensky and Huygens (Chapter 1), Robbins and Friedman (Chapter 4) and Williams and Arrigo (Chapter 9) to a specific problem domain with wide-reaching impact on personal and community health outcomes.

In Chapter 4, Robbins and Friedman offer a resounding critique of current trends toward the biological reductionism of mental illness. The authors note important gaps in understanding about relationship between social justice and mental illness for many frontline providers (i.e., mental health providers). The chapter also centers on existential-personalist ethics as a potential antidote to these problems, bringing the idea of human dignity to the fore to effectively treat and diagnose mental health consumers. Robbins and Friedman contend the medical system is victimizing the very people it says it intends to treat through initial social disenfranchisement, to medical labeling, to long-term disability. Personalist-existential ethical approaches were the foundation for the Third Force or humanistic psychology movement, and the authors suggest that this approach sets a framework for addressing human dignity as a foundational issue in mental health. From this perspective dignity and stigma can be conceptualized as in polar opposition to each other, with stigma ultimately threatening to dehumanize the individual at the most basic level, taking away from what is intrinsically valuable about that person.

The authors offer a powerful warning to therapists to not be complicit in social oppression by trying to treat only symptoms, without understanding the underlying societal causes of psychiatric suffering. In its call to therapists to avoid being part of subtle forms of social oppression, the chapter sets the stage for specific pedagogical tools for psychology (Adams, Perry-Jenkins, and Tropp, Chapter 13) and doctoral training (Goodman, Liang, Tummala-Nara, Borges, and Claudius, Chapter 14). The chapter also suggests a role for much broader interdisciplinary training and interpretations of personal dignity as a form of interpersonal justice (Prilleltensky and Huygens, Chapter 1). The ideas around creative maladjustment as a form of social critique closely echo the thoughts of Williams and Arrigo (Chapter 9), and call us to explore where best in the cycle of injustice we can intervene as individuals and professionals.

In Chapter 5, Oberoi and Islam propose that the term organizational justice was originally applied specifically to workplace contexts, but has gradually been applied in a wider area of situations, including law, politics, business, and at the societal level as a whole. The perception of unjust organizations has been empirically linked to legal action and antisocial behavior, while just actions on the part of those in charge of organizations typically lead to increased acceptance of decisions and greater conformity with employer expectations. The authors discuss organizational justice as it relates to the four domains of overall social justice typically agreed on by researchers in this arena, while also providing some background on empirical arguments about the factorial nature of the social justice construct. The authors also explore how individuals judge and respond to actions that speak to an organizations level of justness, exploring process theories and integrative theories that can be used to explain these individual assessments of social justice in the workplace. Oberoi and Islam go on to point out that the multilevel nature of organizations also complicates the social justice questions involved, and they argue that researchers must deliberately recontextualize the four main dimensions of social justice for each level of the organization they are examining.

The authors also offer that the overlap between societal issues in social justice and organizational justice is underexplored and potentially fruitful, as developing a better understanding of how organizations interact with wider social phenomena will be key to ultimately understanding the structural determinants of well-being. Within organizations, Oberoi and Islam note the importance of team environments, cross-cultural considerations within organizations and between organizational units (e.g., multinational corporations), and the role of power and how it impacts which types of social justice considerations are important in a given organization. The authors conclude with some practical wisdom for managers trying to create more just work environments, but they also critique a reactive stance that looks to reduce existing injustices without proactively seeking to create socially just organizational structures from their foundation. The authors note that recent changes in the structure of employment can reduce human solidarity, community, and dignity. This chapter's focus on considerations of how organizations interact with wider society suggests the potential for fruitful interdisciplinary work at the nexus of social justice, environmental justice (Riemer and Voorhees, Chapter 3), and organizational justice. The multilevel considerations of how power dynamic change address issues raised by Possamai-Inesedy (Chapter 15) in her considerations of the politics of evidence. The chapter also provides deeper empirical exploration of some of the broad dimensions of social justice provided by Prilleltensky and Huygens in Chapter 1 of this volume.

In Chapter 6, Tucker et al. describe empowerment as a process by which people, organizations, and communities gain control or power over their lives and health. The authors state that to accomplish this often requires balancing power differences between large and small organizations, assisting organizations to identify community health needs, and to deliver health promotion programming in culturally appropriate ways. The authors note that both national and international groups that focus on health outcomes (e.g., AHRQ in the United States) increasingly hold these community-enhancing processes as priorities. Moreover, they enumerate significant health disparities, increasing health care costs particularly for health issues where substantial disparities exist, limited health literacy in marginalized communities as fundamental reasons why health promotion is inextricably linked to social justice. The chapter advances the notion that within the broader social justice frameworks, psychologists must also consider the specific health care justice equal distribution of health care resources, fair health care policies, and equal rights for those receiving and those delivering health care service.

Tucker et al. review the history of psychology's role in highlighting the need for deeper inclusion of communities in their collective and individual health outcomes, including input from positive, critical, community, and health psychology domains. Next, the authors describe the evolution in thought in this arena from the socioecologic model to social cognitive theory, health self-empowerment theory, to the patient-centered culturally sensitive health care model. The authors also summarize a number of instruments that can be used to assess individual provider and systems' cultural sensitivity and readiness to provide care in ways that appropriately address social justice concerns. Finally, the chapter summarizes the major elements of community-based participatory research (CBPR) from a health promotion perspective. This chapter's focus on the application of social justice considerations to the specific domain of health care extends the theoretical discussions about social justice offered by Prilleltensky and Huygens, Williams and Arrigo, and Possamai-Inesedy to the applied setting of health and health care. The chapter also sets the stage for the underpinnings of community applications of psychology and CBPR that are illustrated in the context of a community-academic partnership for health in Chapter 7 by Franco, Flower, Curry, Berte, and Whittle.

Franco, Flower, Curry, Berte, and Whittle explore the social justice issues surrounding military service. The chapter points to a number significant mental health outcome disparities for veterans, including higher incidence of posttraumatic stress disorders, family discord, unemployment, substance abuse, homelessness, interpersonal violence, and suicide. The authors argue for greater use of community-based, veteran-led peer-to-peer services as part of the continuum of care for supporting the overall notion of restorative justice for this group. To attempt to more deeply interconnect veteran-led peer mentoring with traditional mental health care, the authors formed a community-academic partnership between DryHootch of America (a veterans group in Milwaukee, Wisconsin), the Milwaukee VA Healthcare System, and the Medical College of Wisconsin. The chapter chronicles some of the difficulties in trying to maintain this partnership, with its vision of transformative improvement in access to mental health care for veterans, while attending to the unique perspectives and constraints of each of the constituent partner organizations. Deep tensions arose early in the partnership between the large health care system representatives and the small community-based organization that were worked through across a series of difficult conversations regarding where DryHootch should center its activities (on the VA campus or in the community), what types of services it should offer (professional counseling or only peer services), and how the partnership would approach research priorities. This deepening dialogue allowed for mutual exploration about the assumptions of therapeutic intervention; differences in views between professional providers and peer mentors about the value, meaning, and impact of therapeutic boundaries on veterans with the greatest psychological and social difficulty; and deeper understanding in the professional providers about their own roles in assisting to nurture DryHootch as an organization, while fundamentally allowing it to take its own course—a process of democratizing expertise.

The authors note that early in the partnership, members of DryHootch often vigorously pointed out that systems of care (both VA and non-VA) have "rules that hurt" veterans, but gradually DryHootch also learned to appreciate that it is possible to negotiate about these rules, barriers, and other issues that diminish care for veterans in ways that catalyze change rather than threaten institutions and those who must practice within professional health provider roles. The authors suggest that accommodations that met all of the needs within the partnership were the foundation of equitable, just, and restorative interpersonal practice and governance, setting an example for how large and small entities can inclusively work together toward a commonly held goal for improved mental health access.

This chapter reflects the ideas of profound inclusion suggested later in this volume by Williams and Arrigo's (Chapter 9) interpretation of social justice as jurisprudential psychology and their consideration that macro-level social injustice is often perpetuated in micro-level interactions, while grounding this view in the realities of actual collaborative practice between organizational partners operating at very different scales and with very different constraints, but toward a unified vision of improved well-being for a group that experiences significant health and mental health disparities. The chapter also illustrates a slightly different example of Prilleltensky and Huygens' ideas (Chapter 1) concerning developmental justice—in this case as it relates to young organizations trying to enter a complex service provision environment and ways experienced professional providers can assist such organizations, while refraining from using the mantle of expertise to block innovation.

Bretherton and Ride explore the relationship between community resilience for disasters and social justice in Chapter 8. Psychologists usually view their role in disasters as designing programming for those who have experienced trauma. The authors suggest that the heightened emotional aspects of the immediacy of disaster impel people to act, when they should really be asking what the best action would be, and that acting impetuously (and wrongly) often violates the principle of nonmaleficence. The authors suggest that society needs to begin shifting how we see disasters, typically from the perspective of first responders to the perspective of the impacted communities. With this lens comes less emphasis on the disaster event's scale, and instead on how communities are impacted in real terms through damage to people and property. The authors also note that for major disasters, often the only acute response available comes from the community itself as declarations of emergency mobilizing outside resources come hours or days later. The term *natural disaster* obscures the fact that most disasters involve differential exposure to hazards that represent structural decisions taken by leaders.

Bretherton and Ride sought to create a deeper understanding of the linkages between disaster and community resilience through a comparative case study process examining the 2004 tsunami in Aceh, Indonesia, the 2005 earthquake in Pakistan, the 2007 tsunami in the Solomon Islands, 2008 cyclone in Myanmar, and the drought in Kenya. Results suggested that contrary to disaster victim portrayal in the media, the local residents saw themselves as self-organizing (e.g., to form ad hoc rescue teams, gather tools, and identify those with special skills or assets needed for road reconstruction) and efficacious in rallying their own response to the disaster event. International disaster response teams were typically flown in after the most critical period was over, were often specialized in a very particular type of disaster issue while the community needs general practitioners, often lacked the language and cultural skills necessary, and if they viewed themselves as superior to the *ad hoc* local response network, problems arose.

The authors point to a number of relief efforts that were culturally inappropriate, underscoring the potential for unintentional social injustice because of ignorance about those one is trying to help, as well as the opportunity costs associated with those forms of "help" at the expense of other activities that would have truly made a difference. The authors offer a warning that psychologists typically try to use what they know, rather than what is actually needed in a given situation. For example, it may not be possible to provide individual therapy or intervention because of physical constraints, collectivist approach of the community impacted, or the need for a much broader intervention to assist an entire population with recovery. This chapter's focus on socially just research methods extends the theoretical offerings of Possamai-Inesedy (Chapter 15) to an applied setting.

Next, in Chapter 9, Williams and Arrigo advance the notion that the forces of captivity and risk management create a society of captives and that society itself is trapped by its own rules and lack of ability to imagine a different set of circumstances. The authors argue that despite what are taken as advanced toward social justice, these are at best half-measures and that notions of self and other, citizenship and social justice, freedom and responsibility, community and society are no more than shadows of what they could be. Williams and Arrigo offer the idea of psychological jurisprudence as novel and experimental theory, which they describe as emerging from cultural criticism and designed to identify and marshal inherent, but underexplored individual and societal potential. The authors link psychological jurisprudence to Aristotelian virtue, noting that it is based on the ideals of transformation, compassion, and human flourishing—the achievement of eudaimonic states for individuals, communities, and society as a whole.

Williams and Arrigo challenge the idea that that social injustice is largely a macro-level issue, pointedly noting that ultimately injustices are manifested in the most personal ways at the intra- and interpersonal levels. The authors argue that to achieve social justice, change agents must radically accept the profound interdependency of individual goods. From this perspective they suggest that "the virtue of compassion may very well be the most foundational of humanistic goods regarding communal and other forms of social health" and that this virtue is actually a *generative force* that produces social justice. Of particular concern to the authors are preventable harms that are perpetuated by both commission and omission, or failure to act. To overcome these ultimately personal shortcomings (i.e., one's own personal involvement in daily social injustices), the authors continue to point to Aristotle, noting that nurturing one's own compassion as a virtue requires taking others' injuries seriously, understanding that the injury is undeserved, and that our own fate is wrapped up in others' suffering. This stance allows for, and in some sense forces us, to be present with others who are experiencing injustice and this presence creates the required change in vantage point needed to adjudicating the self, other, and society in ways that are more profoundly socially just.

Psychological jurisprudence draws attention to the politics of discourse and the contested areas of meaning-making where the authors suggest intention, choice, and action reside. The authors remind us that these are not remote, but are in fact the banal expression of our professional lives, legal documents, psychiatric records, release and discharge plans, treatment manuals, and professional codes of conduct are all texts that must be examined through the lens of social justice. Williams and Arrigo argue that by using psychological jurisprudence as a framework for how we encounter our practice, we can better evaluate how and for whom justice is symbolized, narrated, practiced, and disseminated. The theoretical aspects of this chapter—and the deep challenges it offers to reconsider how psychologists apply social justice thought at multiple levels of society, but most particularly in how it is manifested in interpersonal relationships and through collective action—relate it directly to the other theoretical chapters in this volume, including those by Prilleltensky and Huygens (Chapter 1), Robbins and Friedman (Chapter 4), and Possamai-Inesedy (Chapter 15).

In Chapter 10, Zalaquett and Ivey address the recent explosion of cutting-edge neuroscience research as it pertains to social justice and psychology. They review key neuroscience findings and their implications for psychotherapy and social justice action. They argue that this research has resulted in a veritable paradigm shift in psychology and social justice as it has revealed how social conditions literally affect brain formation and functioning. Zalaquett and Ivey argue that oppression, such as from hostile regimes or social discrimination, and other stressful injustices, such as poverty or domestic violence, result in deleterious consequences for brain development and performance. These effects occur not only in brain processing but in its literal structure and architecture as well. Therefore, they posit that it is incumbent upon psychologists to both advocate for increased justice and intervene and prevent injustice to target suffering at its source—that is, the social and environmental conditions that shape the brain. They propose several recommendations for today's psychologists: first, become educated regarding the neuroscience and psychology literature. Second, teach colleagues and students about this research and its implications. Third, extend psychology's practice beyond individual therapy and intervention to include systems, policies, and communities.

Fourth, intervene and prevent problems from arising as early as possible in the course of human development. Fifth, utilize empirically supported interventions for social action. Sixth, conduct and support research that supports social justice and psychology practices. Finally, engage in professional activities that reduce social and environmental inequalities and stigmatization, increase access and opportunities for all people, and develop and promote innovative wellness programs that support health and prevent malaise.

Coder, DeYoung, and Friedman in Chapter 11 explore ways that spirituality may serve to promote, and in some cases oppose, social justice. They challenge the trend toward secularization of social justice work within religion and spirituality and review spiritual foundations for advocacy. They propose an approach termed *socially engaged spiritual psychology* to bridge this divide and encourage spiritually informed and supported social justice. They argue that personal transformation of consciousness, like that encouraged in many spiritual practices, is necessary for far-reaching and lasting social justice. This is required to manage the increasing complexities of life and the world and possess the ability to hold multiple perspectives for understanding and working effectively in such a world. They also maintain that religion and spirituality, while occasionally the instigators of oppression, have quite often heralded compassion, equality, generosity, love, and justice. Indeed, many of the current icons of social justice such as Gandhi and Martin Luther King Jr., emerged from deep spiritual traditions. Finally, they review several major models of socially engaged spirituality and empirical research that supports such practices. This chapter serves as a reminder of the need for heart and soul in social justice work, and how the various religions and spiritualities may serve as allies in the march toward peace and justice.

In Chapter 12, Bryant-Davis, Counts, and Gray revisit the United Nation's 1948 declaration on human rights, noting that the document protects the ideals of equality, dignity, and freedom for all people. The Geneva Convention also sets forth specific protections within the context of armed combat for wartime rights of prisoners, protections for the wounded, and protections for the civilians in and around a war zone. The authors emphasize that psychologists have undertaken a growing number of interdisciplinary projects designed to address psychologists' human rights violations, human trafficking, mistreatment of immigrants/refugees, torture, sexual violence, political oppression, genocide, and denial of resources in war contexts. The chapter reviews a number of evidence-based, trauma-informed interventions for refugees and other victims of war-related psychological and physical injury, and it highlights the importance of cultural tailoring, including careful attention to religious, spiritual, and language considerations when operating outside the United States. It also underscores the fact that those experiencing war-related trauma have often been relocated, either forcibly or by choice, to new locations where they are outsiders, unable to communicate their needs, and likely to suffer from discrimination in addition to the initial traumas they already faced in their country of origin. The authors also note the unique role of psychologists in these context, a role that necessitates the ability to seamlessly work with international policymakers, local community officials, medical personnel, and the impacted individuals themselves, ultimately working not only in primary treatment but also in educational and advocacy roles. This chapter's focus on the importance of careful cultural tailoring of intervention efforts as a method for embodying a social justice perspective mirrors the ideas offered by Possamai-Inesedy (Chapter 15) in international disaster research efforts. Additionally, Robbins and Friedman (Chapter 4) expand on this chapter's discussion of the fundamental ideals found in social justice, including human dignity.

PROFESSIONAL ISSUES

In "Pedagogical Tools for Social Justice and Psychology," Adams, Perry-Jenkins, and Tropp provide a much-needed and highly applicable tools for integrating social justice into academic instruction and training. They utilize their personal experiences combined with their academic training to propose useful principles for integrating social justice concepts and practices into pedagogical practice. While submitting that social justice practice pertains to recognizing and establishing greater equity in the allocation and opportunity for resources, they also propose that it attempts to make explicit the implicit assumptions, systems, and processes that perpetuate advantages and disadvantages based on social status. Their six principles for social justice education (SJE) are (1) balancing emotional and cognitive components of classroom learning; (2) focusing on both personal/individual and systemic levels of experience and understanding; (3) attending to social relations/dynamics in classroom and how they may reflect oppressive processes from the world at large; (4) emphasizing student-centered learning through integrating reflection and experience as tools; (5) valuing awareness, personal growth, change as outcomes of learning process; and (6) recognizing and changing ways oppression manifests in classroom and everyday contexts.

They each provide a personal account of how they integrate these pedagogical principles in the classroom. Adams begins by examining students' first and last names for their social, cultural, and historical meanings. She also highlights the distinction between comfort and safety in social justice discussions. Finally, she stresses the normalcy and importance of risk-taking and making mistakes for optimal learning. Perry-Jenkins emphasizes the importance of social/environmental contexts in individual development with her students. She attempts to integrate both experiential learning of social justice concepts, such as racial identity, and the theoretical and empirical literature that informs such concepts. Finally, Tropp promotes three core values in SJE: namely, rigorous research to address social justice, translation of research to practitioners and policymakers, and training/mentoring younger generations of scholars for social justice work.

In Chapter 14, Goodman, Liang, Tummala-Nara, Borges, and Claudius propose an innovative three-pronged model for integrating social justice into graduate training in psychology, using counseling psychology as a case example. They emphasize the need for integrating social justice principles across all disciplines in psychology, while acknowledging there is no consensus in the field for whether this should be done or what this should look like. Their training model includes three important components. First, increasing students' awareness regarding their own and others' social identities and positions (i.e., related to power, privilege, and oppression) through teaching experiences. As many can testify, people often learn most effectively and transformatively through instructing others. Second, students learn to integrate traditional clinical practices with social justice–oriented ones (i.e., advocacy focused on systemic, contextual changes). Here students learn how mental health is inextricably intertwined with social factors and strategies for empowering clients to change such conditions where appropriate. Finally, students learn tactics for changing communities and systems themselves through service learning. While their chapter focuses on counseling psychology, their approach could be applied to any subdiscipline in psychology. For example, students in more research-oriented fields such as experimental or social psychology could certainly benefit from increased awareness of their social identities (like race or gender privilege), how they may influence the research process (e.g., selection of research topics and questions, recruitment strategies and racial/ethnic composition, culturally sensitive research methods such as community-based participatory research, dissemination of results to communities), and ways to integrate social justice–oriented research approaches and projects that may simultaneously demonstrate cultural sensitivity and potentially change social policies and community well-being.

Both chapters on training have implications for undergraduate, graduate, and professional training within psychology, but also across many other social and applied science domains that interface with individuals and communities seeking more equitable interactions with society as a whole.

In the final chapter of this volume (Chapter 15), Possamai-Inesedy reminds us of the vision offered in Mills's *Sociological Imagination*, advancing the idea of social justice at the core of both methodology and method itself. The author emphasizes that research questions should be the central focus, rather than what method researchers plan to use, precisely because the imposition of a set method increases the likelihood of reinforcing social injustice through the research process, and ultimately, its findings. The author notes that psychologists face a crisis of imagination and a reemergence of scientism that threatens to dilute the phenomenological reality of what researchers are trying to observe and understand. Possamai-Inesedy argues that in maintaining its role as a challenge to the status quo, social justice research necessarily must engage in methodological creativity. Moreover, the author worries that discussions that seek to cross the quantitative-qualitative divide often represent superficial tolerance without exploring deeper, more interesting distinctions and discontinuities in methodological frameworks. She summarizes Denzin and Lincoln's seven moments of qualitative research, exploring the progression from the privileged role of observer challenged during the blurred genres period between 1970 and 1986 and the "crisis of representation" period from 1986 through 1990, which critiqued the premise of objective ethnography.

Possamai-Inesedy notes that the final periods, postmodern and future, are considered to move toward the radical inclusion of other (non-expert) voices and use of fictional ethnographies, ethnographic poetry, and multimedia texts that seek to connect the academic more directly to the needs of a society looking for avenues to address its democratic, moral, and spiritual needs. Possamai-Inesedy highlights problems in the dissemination of qualitative research, particularly where it is indigenous and nonpositivistic that prevent these voices from entering the scholarly dialogue. She argues that ultimately real knowledge is not as clean as positivist would like to believe, that it is praxis-based and democratizing. From this perspective, research is most effective and insightful when it is viewed as an interactive and collaborative endeavor toward social justice. The author summarizes a number of postmodern qualitative approaches, including visual arts–based inquiry, autoethnography, and performance ethnography. Importantly, she provides a balanced view of these approaches, noting their strengths and weaknesses. The author writes that the culture wars and neoconservatism in Australian and U.S. government have undermined the power and reach of postmodern qualitative research and that pressure on universities to adopt more commercial, entrepreneurial models is adversely impacting the adoptability of these approaches because of the politics of funded research that are now reemphasizing quantitative measurement. The theoretical aspects of this chapter, and its emphasis on socially just construction of knowledge and dissemination of this information, bring together thoughts offered elsewhere in this volume by Williams and Arrigo (Chapter 9), Prilleltensky and Huygens (Chapter 1), and Robbins and Friedman (Chapter 4).

Part 1

Well-Being and Suffering

Chapter 1

Well-Being, Justice, and Social Change

Isaac Prilleltensky and Ingrid Huygens

Recall a situation in which you felt excluded from a group. Now think of a situation in which you were the victim of an injustice, such as unfair treatment by your boss. If you are a member of a minority group, remember a situation in which you may have been the subject of discrimination. In all these cases, your well-being would have been affected by these instances of injustice—you feel upset, angry, or depressed. Now multiply these experiences a million fold and you get a picture of how injustice can affect society as a whole. Furthermore, imagine the impact of not just individuals acting unjustly, but entire systems acting unfairly toward some groups or communities. Experiences of injustice affect your sense of well-being, your integrity, and your overall health. In this chapter we explore the connections among justice, well-being, and social change.

Although much has been written about psychological well-being and many strategies have been devised to foster it (Hupert & Linley, 2011a), less has been said about the ecological nature of well-being and the need to address it through the promotion of justice (Commission on Social Determinants of Health, 2008; Corning, 2011; Powers & Faden, 2006). Well-being, justice, and social change are interdisciplinary constructs that require interdisciplinary analyses. In this chapter we try to realize the much-avowed call for psychologists to interpret psychosocial phenomena in multidisciplinary ways. Our hope is to integrate diverse bodies of scholarship in coherent ways that will facilitate further research and action on the connections among well-being, justice, and transformative change.

Well-being is an ecological construct. As such, we can talk about the well-being of persons, relationships, teams, organizations, communities, nations, and the earth (Prilleltensky & Prilleltensky, 2006). This follows systems thinking propagated in psychology by Bronfenbrenner (1977, 1979). To assess the respective well-being of various systems, we can use a variety of objective and subjective measures (Diener, Diener, & Diener, 1995; Diener, Helliwell, & Kahneman, 2010; Diener, Lucas, Schimmack, & Helliwell, 2009; Kahneman & Riis, 2005; Prilleltensky, 2011; Rath & Harter, 2010; Veenhoven, 2007). In this chapter we concentrate on the impact of diverse types of justice and injustice on the well-being of individuals in relationships, organizations, and communities. Although environmental well-being is very important, on its own accord and because of its impact on people, it is beyond the scope of this chapter. If well-being is predicated on justice, as we will try to show, then society should strive to improve conditions of justice. To achieve that, people need to engage in social change: not just any kind of social change, but change that specifically addresses diverse types of justice. Thus, our chapter is concerned with the relationships among well-being, justice, and social change.

Our argument unfolds as follows: first, we identify how well-being in the interpersonal, communal, occupational, physical, psychological, and economic domains contributes to the well-being of people as individuals, in their relationships, organizations, and societies. Next, we explore the impact of eight types of justice on these systems. Specifically, we review the role of distributive, procedural, developmental, relational, informational, retributive, and cultural justice on personal, interpersonal, organizational, and community systems. Our assumption is that the healthier the system is, the healthier the people who inhabit it. Following that we will argue that prevalent conditions of justice or injustice predispose people to experience particular states of well-being: thriving, coping, resisting, or suffering. By thriving we mean the highest level of well-being (Buettner, 2010; Seligman, 2011); by coping we mean efforts to deal effectively with suboptimal conditions of justice (Lyubomirsky, 2011); by resisting we mean the struggle to overcome conditions of injustice (Prilleltensky, 2011); and by suffering we mean the hopelessness and misery that result from persisting conditions of injustice. We dedicate the last portion of the chapter to social change strategies to promote justice and well-being.

WELL-BEING

Our construction of well-being is both ecological and multidimensional (Bronfenbrenner, 1977, 1979). We define well-being as a positive state of affairs in individuals, relationships, organizations, and communities, brought about by the satisfaction of objective and subjective needs in multiple domains of life. By objective needs we refer to material goods such as money and housing, and physical needs such as food. By subjective needs we mean positive emotions, cognitive stimulation, affection, love, and psychological nurturance (Diener et al., 1995; Prilleltensky, 2011; Prilleltensky & Prilleltensky, 2006). These needs are met to the extent that conditions of justice prevail in the lives of individuals, relationships, institutions, and societies. To reiterate, we believe that systems such as organizations and communities can enjoy various levels of well-being, and that the health and wellness of systems will impact the health and wellness of the people affected by said systems. The ecological nature of well-being is justified on two counts. First, we can legitimately talk about the well-being of single individuals, relationships, organizations, and communities. In other words, these entities can be described in terms of specific objective and subjective criteria on diverse measures of well-being. Second, the well-being of a single unit, such as the individual, is influenced by the level of well-being of other ecological units, pointing to their interdependence (Hupert & Linley, 2011b). Thus, our conceptualization of well-being rests on two well-established principles of ecology: multiplicity of levels and interdependence among levels (Kelly, 2006).

The multidimensional nature of our conceptualization rests on empirical evidence that the overall well-being of humans and communities depend on satisfaction of complex needs (Maslow, 1968, 1971). For instance, Rath and Harter (2010) relied on extensive international data to compile expressions of well-being in five domains which they call social, career, financial, physical and community well-being. Similarly, I (Isaac) have clustered complex needs into six domains: interpersonal, communal, occupational, physical, psychological, and economic (ICOPPE; Prilleltensky, 2012) based on a review of existing research (Buettner, 2010; Graham, 2009; Hupert & Linley, 2011b; Nelson & Prilleltensky, 2010; Prilleltensky & Prilleltensky, 2006; Rath & Harter, 2010; Seligman, 2011; Totikidis & Prilleltensky, 2006). Upon close examination of the vast well-being literature, it turns out that most domains of well-being have subjective or psychological expressions associated with them. For example, the dimension of community well-being can be ascertained by one's sense of community and acceptance. Similarly, physical well-being can be gauged by a person's feelings of vitality and energy. Interpersonal well-being, in turn, can be assessed by a person's feelings of being supported emotionally by friends and relatives. We present here illustrations of how conditions at the personal, interpersonal, organizational, and community levels influence each other and affect psychological well-being.

Personal Well-Being

The well-being of an individual is highly affected by the quality of relationships. The *interpersonal* domain of well-being requires the satisfaction of specific needs having to do with feeling supported, heard, appreciated, valued, and treated with respect. These feelings and perceptions correlate highly with reports of well-being and with physical health (Berkman & Glass, 2000). Social support has long been correlated with physical and emotional health and wellness (Cohen, 2004). The availability of friends and relatives for support as well as the frequency of interpersonal conflict condition the quality of interpersonal well-being (Cacioppo, Reis, & Zauta, 2011).

The *community* dimension of personal well-being is reflected in the need to belong to a community and feel part of a group (Baumeister & Leary, 1995). Feeling valued by community members, along with pride in one's community, is a protective factor that enhances the chances of positive outcomes for adults and children (McKnight & Block, 2010). The "psychological sense of community" construct measures people's place in a community (Fisher, Sonn, & Bishop, 2002). The quantity and quality of social capital, along with access to needed educational, recreational, and health services, influence the psychological sense of belonging (Black & Hughes, 2001).

In our view, the *occupational* dimension of personal well-being encompasses more than a paid job. By occupation we mean vocation and avocation and not just paid employment. Engagement in passionate pursuits in which people occupy themselves is an important part of meaning-making (Rath & Harter, 2010; Seligman, 2011). Growth opportunities through study or apprenticeship stimulate the brain and foster cognitive and skill development. The need to learn has long been recognized as a universal requisite for growth. Meaning-making, engagement, flow, and working in a climate of support and stimulation are psychological expressions of this domain of well-being (Buettner, 2010; Fullan, 2008; Seligman, 2011). Working conditions such as a supportive climate, effective communication, and clarity of roles enhance occupational well-being (Elovainio, Kivimaki, Steen, & Vahtera, 2004; Lawson, Noblett, & Rodwell, 2009; Prilleltensky & Prilleltensky, 2006; Tepper, 2001).

Physical needs find psychological expression in self-evaluations of health and reports of vitality and energy. Without physical health people often report lethargy and impediments in fulfilling activities of daily living. Access to healthy foods and opportunities for physical activity enhances the subjective experience of physical health and vitality (Edlin & Golanty, 2010, Ornish, 2007).

Psychological needs associated with personal well-being have to do with perceptions of self-determination, self-efficacy, self-esteem, self-actualization, sense of control, life satisfaction, spirituality, and mastery (Baumgardner & Crothers, 2009; Maslow, 1968, 1971; Ryan & Deci, 2000; Ryff & Keyes, 1995). The more a person feels competent and in control, the better his or her overall well-being (Marmot, 2004; Peterson, 1999; Rodin, 1986; Rodin & Langer, 1977). A nurturing, humor-filled environment fosters positive emotions (Fredrickson, 2009).

Subjective indicators of *economic* well-being include feeling financially secure and enjoying the purchase of experiences as opposed to consumer goods. The research demonstrates that acquiring experiences such as walks in nature and fun trips provide satisfaction that outlasts the pleasure of buying clothes or fashionable items (Rath & Harter, 2010; Van Boven & Gilovich, 2003). All types of purchases require sufficient funds for basic needs and recreation. Job opportunities and adequate safety nets are prerequisites for feeling economically secure. In addition, the literature demonstrates that spending money on other people enhances personal well-being more than spending money on oneself (Dunn, Ankin, & Norton, 2008).

Interpersonal Well-Being

The healthier the relationships, the stronger the personal well-being. In relationships, people need to feel affirmed and validated, not just in times of need, but also in times of celebration (Gable, Gonzaga, & Strachman, 2006; Gable, Reis, Impett, & Asher, 2004; Gottman, 2001). Couples, friends, and relatives who cherish each other create rituals to mark accomplishments and celebrate each other's accomplishments. Mindful people invest time and effort in listening to each other and in recognizing achievements. They create conditions for the emergence of support and validation. Furthermore, they build a small community in which people feel equal, valued, respected, and not taken for granted. To achieve that sense of community in relationships it is necessary to share burdens and enjoy benefits in fair and equitable ways.

Relationships require that people do things and not just appreciate one another. It is crucial to find meaning in what one does to support his or her family and household, from doing the dishes to earning a paycheck (Rosenberg, 2012). Finding meaning and passion in what one does requires support from loved ones, but also opportunities to practice and develop strengths. Spouses, parents, and friends can either support one's pursuit of hobbies or block one's personal development (Buettner, 2010; Seligman, 2011). To attain a sense of control in interpersonal relationships, people have to afford each other voice and choice. The more one feels heard, the better one feels. Moreover, people have to enable each other to pursue growth opportunities through study, friendships, or recreation. Stress-free, supportive relationships foster physical health. Likewise, associating with people who are healthy enhances the chances that we will adopt healthy habits ourselves. Research demonstrates the social contagion effect of spending time with obese people. The more friends you have who are overweight, the higher the chances that you will become overweight yourself (Christakis & Fowler, 2007). Relatives and associates can be friend or foe when it comes to health habits.

Economic worries feature prominently in the health of relationships. Shared perceptions of what is important and what is not can provide strength in resisting consumerism and avoiding unnecessary debt. Friends and relatives can help one another realize that many consumer goods are not going to improve one's spiritual well-being beyond the transitory excitement of purchasing an item featured in magazines (Kasser & Ryan, 1993).

Organizational Well-Being

Feeling engaged, involved, and appreciated at work is correlated with overall well-being. Occupational climate plays a big role in the success of organizations and the well-being of their people (Fullan, 2008; Harter, Schmidt, & Keyes, 2003; Sisodia, Wolfe, & Sheth, 2007). Institutions that seek input from employees, celebrate their accomplishments, and support them in time of need create a caring space and a sense of community. Perceiving supervisors as fair, transparent, and interested in the opinions of workers promotes the well-being of the workforce. Overall, opportunities for self-determination, control, mastery, and growth in the occupational realm promote meaning and self-respect (Marmot, 2004).

Increasingly, organizations are realizing the connection between body and mind and trying to encourage healthy eating and physical activity (Leka & Houdmont, 2010). To minimize stress and health risk, organizations must have policies regarding exposure to occupational hazards and toxic substances. Realizing that risk minimization is not enough, smart organizations also promote health and wellness among employees. Indeed, research demonstrates that work climate and relationship with one's boss are powerful determinants of health and well-being (Rath & Harter, 2010).

Community Well-Being

Feeling included, respected, and that one's voice matters depends on participatory policies and practices in the community. Citizens who vote on referenda and participate in civic affairs more often report higher levels of well-being than citizens who are not afforded similar opportunities (Frey & Stutzer, 2002). Feeling respected by officials and trusting government institutions enhances the well-being of citizens. On the contrary, perceiving elected officials as corrupt erodes social capital, corrodes public trust, and diminishes subjective well-being (Tavits, 2008). Feeling safe and protected by society's institutions, along with freedom of movement, expression, and association are essential to the health and well-being of citizens and to the sense of community (Ingelhart, 2010; Ingelhart, Foa, Peterson, & Welzel, 2008).

Lack of access to health care is a source of stress in many communities (Levy & Sidel, 2006; Powers & Faden, 2006). Countries without universal health care impose upon their citizens extraordinary burdens. Not only do people have to worry about the physical health of their children, they also have to confront systems that discriminate against the poor and the uninsured, compounding their stress (Deogaonkar, 2004). Many poor communities lack access not only to medical treatment but also to fresh fruits and vegetables, as merchants do not like investing in poor communities. Moreover, many poor communities are beset by drugs and crime, which prevent children and parents from exercising and walking outside (Commission on Social Determinants of Health, 2008). Finally, demonstrations of equality and economic well-being in a community affect citizens as much as the absence of health care or government services (Graham, 2009; Isbister, 2001; Wilkinson & Pickett, 2009). Employment opportunities and safety nets affect how people cope with stress (Lyubomirsky, 2011).

To sum up, we have illustrated how sociocultural conditions regulate the psychological experience of wellness. Next, we argue that these contextual conditions are largely shaped by the relative presence of eight types of justice.

JUSTICE

The extent to which environments respond to human needs is largely determined by configurations of justice. Whereas some modes of justice permeate most environments, some exert particular influence on specific ones. For example, distributive justice is fairly ubiquitous, but developmental justice is particularly relevant in interpersonal contexts. In this section we elaborate on various types of justice and their unique role in creating environments conducive to well-being.

Distributive Justice

This type of justice refers to the fair and equitable allocation of burdens and resources, and duties and opportunities, in society. In essence, distributive justice is about determining what is due a person or group in a particular context. At the core, it is about fairness (Corning, 2011; Isbister, 2001; Jost & Kay, 2010; Sandel, 2009). Based on the fundamental principle of equality, it is fair that all people have access to educational institutions, without discriminating on the basis of race, religion, or skin color. Similarly, it is fair that all people within a certain income bracket pay taxes, and that nobody should be exempt on the basis of privilege. This abstract desideratum for fair and equitable distribution of resources is difficult to achieve in reality (Barry, 2005; Isbister, 2001). Scholars collide on what should be the preferred criterion for sharing burdens and allocating resources (Facione, Scherer, & Attig, 1978; Miller, 1999). Two criteria are often invoked: *merit* and *need*. Thinkers favoring the former contend that if one works hard, or is really smart, one should be entitled to more goods, such as scholarships or job interviews, than one's languid friends. That makes sense for as long as you and your friends have benefited from similar opportunities growing up. But if one person and his or her competitor grew up in diametrically opposed circumstances, such as great privilege and great disadvantage, then it no longer makes sense to think only of merit, for while one person enjoyed great privilege that afforded his or her advantages, his or her competitor was enduring suffering and poverty. Under these contrasting scenarios, merit must be tempered by the context of development (Prilleltensky, 2011). It is because of developmental circumstances that policies such as affirmative action have been put in place. If merit is a deficient criterion under circumstances of great disparity, we ought to consider alternative criteria, such as need.

If all human beings are entitled to the satisfaction of basic needs, such as food, shelter, medical care, and a dignified job, then need should be accorded a role in the distribution of resources. Enlightened societies do not deprive poor children of food or medical care because their parents are incapacitated and cannot work. Hence, they invoke need instead of just merit in helping poor children. Society runs into problems, and injustice, when it allocates basic goods, such as medical care only on the basis of private health insurance, which depends on a good job with benefits. Although the poor are supposedly entitled to government basic care, as in the United States, the reality is that the poor are offered third-, fourth-, and fifth-rate care if at all. Differential access to health care is a prime example of failure in distributive justice in countries where access is conditioned by membership in a private health plan (Powers & Faden, 2006). In industrialized countries without universal health insurance, like the United States, minorities suffer from more cases of HIV/AIDS, more cases of infant mortality, more premature mortality, and poorer treatment options (Clark, 2013; Daniels, 2008; Donohoe, 2013). Even in countries like Canada, with universal health care, indigenous populations suffer from higher rates of suicide, alcohol, and limited access to health care (Segal & Fries, 2011). In developing countries like India, lack of access to basic health services by people in rural areas is well known (Rosenberg, 2012; Venkatapuram, 2011).

Although the argument may be made that providing services on the basis of need might encourage dependency among some people, it does not justify depriving most citizens in need from claiming their health rights. The provision of health services on the basis of need should not be seen to promote lack of motivation to work. To the extent that such reasoning exists, it is the result of ideological tendencies to portray the free provision of social and medical services as antithetical to the development of character and virtue (Beauchamp, 2013; Donohoe, 2013). Advanced countries with universal health care, like Canada and Sweden, do not seem to suffer from educational failure or lack of moral fiber. If the argument for the development of dependency would hold, one would see entire countries, such as Canada and Sweden, suffering from dependent population syndrome!

Access to high-quality schools is another instance in which poor children, due to no fault of their own, grow up receiving a third rate education in ill-equipped schools struggling with drugs and crime (Darling Hammond, 2010). On the other end of the income continuum, many corporations do not pay taxes and avoid carrying their fair share of paying for government services (Dobbin, 2003).

Societies that pay attention to the context in formulating policies balance distributions of goods and burdens between need and merit. Societies that dogmatically support merit and are blind to context perpetuate conditions of social injustice. As a result, children growing up in poverty are many times more likely to suffer than to experience well-being. In Britain, Halpern (2010) found that children growing up in the lowest 5% of the income bracket have as much as 300 times more chances of experiencing any one of 12 risk factors than those growing in the top 50% of the income scale. In summary, distributive justice is crucial for well-being. The more distributive justice there is, the higher the chances that poor and minorities will enjoy favorable conditions. The less distributive justice there is, the higher the chances of deleterious social circumstances leading to suffering (Halpern, 2010).

Procedural Justice

This type of justice refers to impartial decision-making processes, not just in the legal system, as the concept is often used, but also in organizations, families, and communities. Any time that a decision affecting an individual or group is to be made, a fair, transparent, informative, and respectful process ought to take place. If *distributive justice* is about what is shared in society, *procedural justice* is about how decisions are made of justice (Tornblom & Vermunt, 2007). Is favoritism avoided? Do all parties have a say in the decision? Have people followed the rules they created? These are some of the questions impacting decisions in families, organizations, communities, courts, and government. In short, has the explicit or implicit contract established between all parties been respected? These are the fundamental questions of procedural justice. In our view, both kinds of justice, distributive and procedural, play a major role in all levels of the human experience: interpersonal, organizational, communal, and national (Schmitt & Dorfel, 1999).

Intrapersonal Justice

Prilleltensky (2011) has argued that people can be unfair to themselves. Due to complex connections among feelings, thoughts, behaviors, and the unconscious, people often engage in self-injurious behaviors. Self-inflicted pain is an example of intrapersonal injustice. Although these conditions may be labeled pathological, the justice element is relevant nonetheless. In certain circumstances, such as suicide, which may be regarded as a form of intrapersonal injustice, the person may have internalized negative views imposed by others acting unjustly toward them. This raises the possibility that intrapersonal injustice is connected to interpersonal or cultural injustice. It is quite remarkable that no relevant literature has been found on the construct of intrapersonal injustice. Although theories of self-injurious behavior abound, they all account for it in medical or pathological terms, leaving the moral aspects of the behavior to theology. In our view, there is merit in advancing a third position that is neither quite pathological nor religious, but ethical.

Interpersonal Justice

According others the respect and dignity they deserve is a form of justice. Interpersonal justice takes place in families, schoolyards, workplaces, parks, communities, shops, and business offices (De Vogli, Ferrie, Chandola, Kivimaki, &

Marmot, 2007; Fujishiro, & Heaney, 2009; Fuligni, 2007; Hatfield, Rapson, & Aumer-Ryan, 2008; Lareau & Conley, 2008; Olson, DeFrain, & Skogrand, 2008). In just about every human encounter one has the opportunity to treat others with dignity and respect, regardless of demographic attributes. Violations of this type of justice lead to a range of negative outcomes, from micro-aggressions to divisive comparison to psychological, physical, and sexual abuse (Fiske, 2011; Kivimäki et al., 2004).

Developmental Justice

This type of justice deals with developmentally appropriate expectations of children, teens, and seniors. From a distributive and procedural point of view, it is unfair to expect children to assume parental roles. Parentification of children is a case of developmental injustice. Economic abuse of the elderly on the basis of their diminished mental capacities is another. Similarly, it is developmentally unjust to neglect children. This kind of injustice is most prevalent in families.

Taking advantage of individuals on the basis of their developmental stage deserves a category of its own. One might persuasively argue that young adults and adults dominate society. Children and youth are not quite yet competent to lead groups or communities, while elderly people are retiring from public life. As such, adults are more prone to control the fate of children and the elderly, and thus should be prevented from exploiting other groups, consciously or unconsciously, for personal benefit.

Informational Justice

This type of justice originates in the organizational development literature but is applicable to communities and nations alike (Colquitt, 2001; Jost & Kay, 2010). In essence, it is about the right to access information. As such, it is a close relative of procedural justice. Information and communication are preconditions to inclusion or exclusion in decision making in organizations, communities, and countries. Lack of information prevents people from feeling part of a process or an organization. Furthermore, it breeds mistrust. What is it that is hidden from certain groups? What are the motives behind lack of transparency? These are valid questions when decisions and data are hidden from the public eye.

Cultural Justice

This is the societal analog of interpersonal justice. If interpersonal justice is about treating each other with respect in micro settings, *cultural justice* is about treating other groups with dignity (Fuligni, 2007; Nussbaum, 2006). Racial, ethnic, sexual, and disability minorities are often excluded from mainstream institutions. This is about how heterosexuals treat homosexuals and how able-bodied people treat people with disabilities. Communities with high levels of cultural justice facilitate the well-being of minorities and society as a whole (Halpern, 2010).

Retributive Justice

Closely related to procedural justice, *retributive justice* is about holding people accountable for their transgressions. Countries with high levels of corruption erode public trust and diminish social capital. Lack of honesty at the highest levels, in the penal, government, and business systems, putrefies civil society (Ruhl, 2011; Tavits, 2008). The less retributive justice there is, the fewer the chances of a thriving community. Societies with reliable retributive justice give citizens a sense of fairness, transparency, and security.

A type of retributive justice is restorative justice. As Jost and Kay explain, "In restorative justice sentencing, the various parties are encouraged to express their feelings, come to an agreement about the harm that has occurred, and decide together what actions should be taken to reestablish a sense of justice" (2010, p. 1146). This form of justice seeks to foster healing through open dialogue between the parties involved, giving them a sense of ownership over the process and the outcome. We will discuss later instances in which restorative justice has been applied effectively in indigenous communities.

Our claim is that the higher the level of the eight types of justice, the healthier and more conducive an environment is to well-being. If communal well-being depends on cultural and retributive justice, and vibrant communities support individual well-being, the more justice and wellness there is. The same logic applies to relationships and organizations. Thus, to foster well-being in individuals, justice has to be fostered in communities.

FAILURES IN JUSTICE

Very few societies could be considered to enjoy optimal conditions of justice, based on this framework. Even the OECD countries (rated as the wealthiest, fairest, and safest in the world) have, at best, suboptimal conditions of justice (Schraad-Tischler & Azahaf, 2011). Objective, measurable differences in wealth and health among cultural groups, age groups, and socioeconomic classes are signs of a failure in optimal conditions of justice.

Prevailing conditions of justice have a direct and indirect impact on well-being. For instance, interpersonal injustice has a direct impact on well-being, whereas procedural or retributive injustice has an indirect effect on well-being (Jost & Kay, 2010). The indirect effect is mediated through certain settings and environments like educational, court, and taxation systems. If these systems are unjust and corrupt, eventually they will affect people when they come into contact with them. Differences in well-being may stem from former historical oppressions such as colonialism, slavery, and racism, leading to differences in economic advantage, as in the case of African Americans in the United States. Past colonial regimes have often been the basis for ongoing "internal colonialisms" (Feagin & Feagin, 1978, p. 12) whereby alienation of indigenous lands (distributive injustice), institutional racism, slavery (procedural injustice), and differential treatment in criminal justice systems (retributive injustice), all stem from early cultural injustice. Further failures in justice arise from assimilative policies by dominant cultural groups regarding the cultures of indigenous and minority groups. In monocultural societies, procedural justice may be rigidly upheld as being the same process applied to everyone without regard for cultural diversity in belief systems and practices.

U.S. psychologist Sloan (2010) gives a historical overview of the development of capitalism as an economic system, and the ensuing impact of European colonization, imperialism, and modernization worldwide. Although processes such as industrialization, urbanization, public education, literacy, and democratization have delivered technological and human rights progress in many countries, such development has been extremely uneven. It has benefitted mostly the middle classes of urban centers while creating new problems for urban poor and rural agrarian people everywhere. Sloan warns that ideologies held by Western elites, such as uncritical adherence to market economies and free trade, are now leading to major failures in distributive, procedural, and cultural justice worldwide.

Procedural injustice is as important to people as distributive injustice. Consultations carried out around the world by the Poverty Group of the World Bank showed that abuses of basic human rights by police and bureaucrats ranked just as high among citizen concerns as improved economic conditions (Narayan, Chambers, Shah, & Petesch, 2000). Community organizers needed to be able to represent their communities without fear of reprisal from paramilitary groups or corporate security forces.

Failures in retributive justice are also significant. People in one population group may find themselves incarcerated at higher levels (e.g., Maori in Aotearoa, or African Americans in the United States) for the same crimes that other groups commit, implying discrimination in arrest and sentencing (Mauer & King, 2007).

In summary, conditions of injustice in a society typically involve failures in more than one type of justice.

STATES OF WELL-BEING

On the basis of regnant conditions of justice, we identify four states of well-being: thriving, coping, resisting (or confronting), and suffering (Prilleltensky, 2011).

Thriving

Conditions of optimal justice create healthy environments and communities, which, in turn, operate effectively and efficiently, affording the population opportunities for growth and development. In a study of 68 countries Tavits (2008) showed that people report higher levels of subjective well-being when they regarded their government as clean and honest rather than corrupt. Similarly, Frey and Stutzer (2002) demonstrated that citizens in Swiss cantons with frequent referenda also reported higher levels of well-being. People-centered institutions and honest government impact citizen well-being in a positive way. This is accomplished through the experience of control and self-determination, which is a universal component of subjective well-being (Veenhoven, 2012).

Although it is hard to achieve ideal conditions of justice and an ideal government, some countries do a much better job than others, with Scandinavian countries usually topping the charts in terms of clean government and satisfaction with life (Halpern, 2010; Schraad-Tischler & Azahaf, 2011; Wilkinson & Pickett, 2009). There is evidence to support the claim that the cleaner, more effective, inclusive, participatory, and democratic the society is, the higher the levels of well-being (Tavits, 2008), facilitating thriving and flourishing responses. But conditions for thriving exist not just at the macro level. Meso- and micro-level settings such as organizations and families, respectively, can also promote thriving by adhering to as many of the eight types of justice as possible. The more informational, relational, distributive, and procedural justice there is in a workplace, the higher the well-being of its employees (De Vogli et al., 2007; Elovainio, Kivimaki, & Vahtera, 2002). In families and close relationships, the higher the level of interpersonal and distributive justice, the better the well-being of relatives and partners (Jost & Kay, 2010).

We argue that although considerable literature has been devoted to documenting the inner resources of individuals in thriving, external and objective conditions pertaining to justice can help the person in his or her pursuit of happiness and well-being. In short, under optimal conditions of justice it is more likely that a higher percentage of the population will be thriving (Corning, 2011). At the same time, it is important to note that excess material goods can lead to meaningless lives and consumerist behavior. Therefore, abundant material conditions, in our view, are not the same as optimal conditions.

Coping

Coping is a degree down from thriving. Whereas people in the thriving state reach for higher levels of life satisfaction, those in the coping state struggle to cope with less than ideal circumstances. Coping is the act of maintaining a desirable state in the face of obstacles. Suboptimal levels of justice, in any one of the eight types reviewed earlier, can lead people to coping instead of thriving. Whereas people are remarkably resilient and can adapt to less than satisfactory conditions, society's goal should be to enhance all types of justice to bring a greater number of people from coping to thriving. There is no doubt that people have the capacity to cope with untoward circumstances, individually and collectively (Rosenberg, 2012), but this quality should not diminish the determination to improve society as a whole.

Resisting

Yet a notch below coping we find resisting. This is the act of struggling against conditions of injustice. We are no longer talking about suboptimal conditions of justice, but rather about prevailing conditions of injustice. This is a defensible category in that many people around the world know little justice (Eckstein & Wickham-Crowley, 2003). Considering the eight types of justice described earlier, several permutations are possible. Some people may enjoy relational justice at the micro level of family and friends, but suffer from cultural injustice in society at large. Others may live in democratic and safe societies where they enjoy procedural and distributive justice at the macro level, but their private lives may be torn by relational injustice. Therefore, resisting is not just a group phenomenon, but an individual one as well.

Suffering

This state reflects individuals and groups for whom the balance is tipped toward injustice in most spheres of life: interpersonal, organizational, and communal. People in this category suffer helplessness and oppression and cannot see the light at the end of the tunnel. Famine, war, and gender discrimination often go together, subjecting women especially to a life of despair (Sen, 1995, 2010). Although people sometimes heroically survive the most destructive of circumstances, no one should be subjected to the test. What is more, many of those who do survive suffer from posttraumatic stress disorder and its lifelong effects. Again, as in the case of coping, we do not doubt that many people derive meaning from suffering and may even experience growth, but these positive outcomes never justify the perpetuation of unjust conditions.

In our linking of well-being to conditions of justice, we have claimed that there are four distinct states of well-being, differentiated by prevailing norms of justice. Under optimal conditions of justice, people have a higher chance of thriving. Under suboptimal conditions of justice, people merely cope. When it comes to conditions of injustice, people either resist or suffer, depending on the extent of injustice. We can conclude from the foregoing discussion that to promote well-being it is also necessary to improve social conditions and to advocate for optimal conditions of justice for all groups.

SOCIAL CHANGE TO PROMOTE JUSTICE

If the well-being of individuals, organizations, and communities is reliant on conditions of justice pertaining to a society, then strategies to improve well-being must take into account these conditions of justice. In this section we show how, in most societies today, social change efforts are required to achieve optimal conditions of justice. Venezuelan psychologist Maritza Montero (2010) argues that liberation is freedom from conditions of injustice, and that well-being may spring from people's actions for liberation. She concludes that liberation, change, and well-being must operate in concert. Although the phrase *social change* encompasses many forms of change affecting a society, the form of change described here is intentional organizing for social justice: "Organizing is intentional group action against maldistribution of rights, resources and privileges, and the creation of new institutional structures and belief systems" (Crowfoot, Chesler, & Boulet, 1983, p. 237).

First we consider a range of strategies to directly promote well-being and how they link to types of justice, and then we turn to social change efforts to improve conditions of justice, and their impact on well-being.

STRATEGIES TO PROMOTE WELL-BEING

Organizing for Economic Prosperity

The history of every society is replete with schemes to improve prosperity. For instance, women's movements in diverse regions of the world have organized for economic prosperity. The Koran refers to an uprising of women in South Arabia who were protesting against Mohammed's ban on women trading (Molyneux, 1993). The first workers' guilds of Europe were organized by textile craftswomen—newly moved to cities from rural areas. Organizing for economic prosperity is based on improvements to distributive justice, through changes to unequal incomes, taxation, or opportunities. Equally, it may be through improvements to procedural justice by lifting traditional religious restrictions.

Organizing for Health Promotion

Myriad examples can be found around the world of organizing to maintain and improve the health and well-being of populations. For instance, a Physical Welfare and Recreation Act passed in New Zealand in 1937 provided government support for community and youth initiatives in sport, recreation, culture, and youth clubs. In addition, it provided for the building of community halls, which lasted well into the 1960s. As well as improving health and welfare, these facilities gave voice to marginalized groups and communities in the 1970s, prompting calls for social change by women and minority groups (Chile, 2006). Thus, community organizing for well-being and health promotion can simultaneously develop social change practices that change conditions of justice.

Organizing for Effective Functioning

Organizing for effective functioning, such as practicing emancipatory management at national, community, and organizational levels, may increase conditions of justice in multiple spheres. Barros (2010) suggests that organizational learning, when focused on participation, solidarity, and collective well-being, rather than individualism, creates a climate in which internal practices of inequality, manipulation, and exploitation cannot flourish. Thus, emancipatory management practices assist in furthering procedural and retributive justice.

Organizing for Freedom

In 2006–2007, migrant communities in Chicago mobilized to oppose federal immigration bill HR 4437, which harshly criminalized illegal immigration into the United States. The movement was initially carried out by community-based organizations and eventually advanced by direct political action. The learning achieved through the combination of organizational work and mass action substantially developed community capacity to pursue other initiatives around civil liberties, immigrant welfare, and political representation (Betancur & Garcia, 2011).

Organizing for Equality

Efforts to increase respect and equality of the social, cultural, and psychological status of social groups may target the historical antecedents of particular inequalities. For instance, research into historical comparisons between cultural groups in Kyrgyzstan showed that well-being suffered under negative historical comparisons (De la Sablonniere, Auger, Sadykova, & Taylor, 2010). Thus, education efforts may need to revisit history to increase respect for marginalized social groups (Miller, 2001). In New Zealand, a long-standing Treaty Education campaign by activist educators provides accurate information about the settlement treaty signed with indigenous leaders, and highlights the rights and status of the indigenous people (Huygens, 2011).

Organizing for Participation, Inclusion, and Dignity

Organizing may focus on participation, social inclusion, and increased social cohesion in communities. Art classes for poor children in Caracas, Venezuela, encouraged community participation and action, development of the children's identity as citizens, and knowledge of their political history and rights (Montero, 2009). Although there is a revival of interest in civic engagement for youth in Western education systems (Putnam, 2000), researchers warn that the emphasis must be on social, emotional, ethical, political education, and consciousness-raising, rather than uncritical orientation toward existing institutions (Cohen, 2006; Watts & Flanagan, 2007). In summary, organizing for well-being typically achieves gains in many sites of human activity, and may directly or indirectly improve conditions of justice.

SOCIAL CHANGE TO PROMOTE JUSTICE

Efforts at social change are usually a response to suboptimal, vulnerable, or persisting conditions of injustice. Brazilian literacy educator Paulo Freire (2004) believed that a struggle for change should result in "overcoming dehumanizing injustice" (p. 35). Indeed, the appearance of social change efforts points to contexts of injustice (Schutz & Sandy, 2011). For instance, the now centuries-long efforts for change by indigenous peoples in former colonies signal persisting conditions of injustice. In this section, we outline efforts at intentional organizing to make gains in social justice, showing how these often address several types of justice at once and result in improved well-being. We focus on the four types of justice most significant at the societal level: distributive, procedural, cultural, and retributive.

Social Change for Distributive Justice

Marx's critique of the maldistribution of economic benefits in capitalism has helped mobilize working classes and agrarian workers worldwide to establish alternative means of production. Struggles for radical or reformist change in distributive justice include the Landless Peasants movement in Brazil (Freire, 2004), and many others throughout the world.

In countries making transitions to capitalist democracy, it is not necessarily certain that distributive justice will improve. In the Central Asian republics, transition from the bureaucratic-redistributive system of the former Soviet Union to an imperfect market order has been accompanied by a dramatic decline in GDP, a decline in state spending on health, education, and social security benefits, an increase in unemployment and underemployment, the non- and late payment of wages, a decline in the influence of trade unions, and an increase in inequalities, poverty, and malnutrition (Abbott, Wallace, & Sapsford, 2011). In other parts of the world, increased military spending in countries making a transition to democracy undermines the likelihood of distributive justice, owing to decreased spending on welfare and economic growth (Clardie, 2011). Based on the same critical analysis of military spending, long-standing peace movements such as the Women's International League for Peace and Freedom and antinuclear campaigns continue to protest against military allocations in national budgets. These allocations are usually at the expense of spending on health and welfare, which would improve distributive justice.

Within capitalist societies, workers' movements, trades unions, and tax systems achieve a measure of distributive justice so that the wealthy share economic benefits with the poor. However, tax systems are subject to such frequent reform that unjust situations can develop. Contemporary movements such as Occupy Wall Street aim to force global corporations to contribute to alleviating global poverty, hunger, and disease through a Tobin ("Robin Hood") tax or a Financial Transactions Tax on all across-border financial transactions (Consedine, 2011; Cullen, 2011). Similarly, campaigns for a Universal Basic Income aim to give an income to all members of a society, whatever their status, in place of complex welfare entitlements (Carnegie Council, 2005).

Dozens of international NGOs and thousands of local nonprofit organizations work to transform local economies to increase distributive justice. Noncorporatized exchange systems such as green dollar and barter economies, farmers' markets, and fair trade arrangements are all significant actions to improve distributive justice locally and globally. Participatory solutions to distributive injustice and poverty have been developed in many countries. In Kerala, India, and Curitiba, Brazil, a major portion of the budget is set aside for citizens themselves to allocate after reviewing the state's or city's needs, illustrating a form of direct democratic decision making (Sloan, 2010).

Social Change for Procedural Justice

Nobel Prize laureate Amartya Sen (1995) has pointed to the interplay between distributive and procedural justice, arguing that economic development cannot proceed fully unless it is accompanied by civil liberties and freedom of assembly and speech. Second wave feminism is an example of a diverse and long-lived movement for both distributive and procedural justice. In the European and American contexts, feminists campaigned for employment rights and opportunities, equal pay and legal status to men, and equality in social benefits and taxation (Barrett, 1993). Governments that protect human rights for all ensure that the fruits of economic development will be enjoyed beyond urban elites. They also reduce the possibility that corruption will interfere with the efforts of individuals and businesses upholding the law.

Procedural justice may also intersect with retributive justice. For instance, liberal democracies take for granted the right for every citizen to publicly mourn and bury their dead. If the cause of death is neither natural nor accidental, families further expect that an investigation and criminal procedures will follow. In a campaign of state-directed genocide in the 1980s, Guatemalan military and paramilitary forces were responsible for high fatalities in Rabinal. Stewart (2008) reported that human rights activists in Rabinal organized to demand exhumation of mass graves, erection of appropriate memorials, and criminal investigations. Although few of those responsible for the violence have received the punishment required in conditions of retributive justice, the success of local mobilization in achieving procedural justice is restoring a sense of community agency and expectations of human rights. These changes have made vast improvements in community well-being and strengthened the resolve for democratization.

However, democratization toward human rights and procedural justice may violate other conditions of justice, such as cultural justice. In rural China, there has been a struggle over "the rule of law" between rural communities and the state (Brandstadter, 2011). The neo-socialist state followed an agenda to create law-abiding, formally equal citizens through new processes of local government. However, in rural areas peasants have defended themselves against local government infringements on their existing civil and human rights. Their rural activism seeks to redress injustice and hold local governments accountable to the people. They aim to identify themselves as both peasants and citizens, as subjects for new human rights that include their traditional practices. Such transformational citizenship struggles demonstrate the significance of historical and cultural contexts in struggles for social justice.

Social Change for Cultural Justice

Efforts at organizing for cultural justice often target the differential outcomes of national, state and city policies upon different cultural groups. For instance, when assimilative pressures toward English and other majority languages endanger native and minority languages, activism is required to claim resources for language revitalization and maintenance (Macedo, Dendrinos, & Gounari, 2003; Reyhner & Lockard, 2009).

Changes in this area are often aimed simultaneously at cultural justice and other forms of justice. In Aotearoa, New Zealand, Maori protested the loss of cultural institutions as a consequence of colonization, including the loss of traditional forms of restorative justice. Critical reviews of the monocultural justice system and its effects on young Maori men led to reforms that now include a Family Group Conference for all youth offenders (Jackson, 1988). This family decision-making process allows families and communities to apply their own principles for healing and restoring social harmony, thereby supporting cultural justice for Maori. It also achieves links between cultural, procedural, and retributive justice, in that young people have the opportunity to be judged within a familiar cultural framework, and families and communities can influence the consequences (Morris & Maxwell, 1998). Although focused on reducing injustice for Maori youth, this innovation created a transformative change in the treatment of youth offenders that is now heralded as a world leader.

Social Change for Retributive Justice

Researchers have found that people prefer restorative justice over punishment (Okimoto, Wenzel, & Feather, 2009), since restorative justice restores and develops social relationships, thereby maintaining or improving social cohesion. Movements for restorative justice exist in many countries. Indigenous peoples and other cultural groups have worked toward justice systems more in keeping with indigenous values of restoring balance and harmony within social systems (Jackson, 1988).

Public investigation and compensation for past wrongs are often prominent interventions in a society. Around the world, Truth and Reconciliation Commissions investigate and sometimes compensate crimes that occurred during previous regimes. In New Zealand, the Waitangi Tribunal investigates indigenous claims of breaches of the Treaty of Waitangi, and recommends land and monetary compensations. The Simon Wiesenthal Centre investigates crimes committed during the Holocaust and provides evidence for criminal prosecutions. In each case, these processes toward retributive justice help to improve cultural justice, although commentators note that collective reconciliation between social groups generally requires further work (Avruch & Vejarano, 2002; Humphrey, 2005).

Our examples from rural China and New Zealand have shown that conditions of cultural justice intersect strongly with other types of societal justice. Distributive, procedural, and retributive justice cannot progress from a monocultural framework in a culturally diverse society. Interdependence in types of justice shows how one type of justice intersects with others so that effective change efforts must focus on holistic and ecological gains. We turn now to exemplars from Cameroon and India to illustrate the importance of attending to all forms of justice in concert when planning well-being interventions.

Intersections of Forms of Justice: Cameroon and Kerala as Exemplars

Many African countries experience vulnerable or persisting conditions of injustice, but in Cameroon in particular, modern development interventions have exacerbated the situation. Development efforts there and in other parts of Africa have proceeded from a Eurocentric, expert-driven approach that ignores ancient traditions in African communal farming and communitarian social thought. Nsamenang, Fru, and Browne (2007) consider that Eurocentric values and concepts confuse and undermine African community initiatives and worsen many forms of injustice because the imported modernist approach "takes away ownership for the development and progress of Africa's communities from its people" (p. 400). Psychology and the social sciences are implicated in providing a systematized set of values imported to assist modernization. Nsamenang et al. describe how traditional African practices engaged group members in rotational systems of collective self-help work by which they all worked on each member's farm until everyone's work was completed. In Cameroon, these practices gave rise to rotational systems for thrift and loan schemes that offer more dependable finance to ordinary citizens than do conventional banks. Such delivery of distributive and procedural justice is based in the African social thought of being "better together" (p. 404), following principles of collective self-reliance and mutual supportiveness. Nsamenang et al. look forward to change efforts based on a weaving together of African social theory and humane productive values. They exhort psychologists and other well-being interventionists working in situations of cultural diversity to think of themselves first and foremost as learner. The cultural injustice in Cameroon is an example of how uncritical adherence to inappropriate cultural ideologies of Western capitalism and modernism leads to failures in other forms of justice (Sloan, 2010).

In contrast, an example from Kerala in India illustrates a successful use of traditional cultural ideologies to inform changes in conditions of justice. The southern Indian state of Kerala has attained exceptional levels of social development despite high fragmentation of society along religious and caste lines. Beset by poverty, malnutrition, overcrowding, and other health and social problems, Kerala has been a candidate for vulnerable or persisting conditions of injustice. However, a historical analysis of development in Kerala by Singh (2011) challenges the notion that cultural diversity is a negative factor in the public good. Kerala has a long tradition of religious tolerance and cooperation to maintain collective cohesion (N. Narasimhan, personal communication, November, 27, 2011). Over the past century, Kerala instituted a campaign of social policies to ensure a more equitable distribution of existing resources, goods, and services across the population, described as achieving "social justice through transformative policy" (Peirson, 2010, p. 494). Various social movements gained structural reforms to conditions of justice, such as amendments to land tenure and equalization of income (distributive justice), legislation to provide better social security, pensions and working conditions, free primary- and secondary-level education (procedural justice), increased production of high-yield crops and access to price-controlled food, enforcement of child labor laws (retributive justice), and increase in female participation in the workforce (cultural justice). The well-being outcomes of this holistic approach to conditions of justice have been significant. For instance, life expectancy and literacy are now among the highest in India and disease rates are very low. Increased understanding of rights by the poor majority has raised political consciousness to the point where at persistent grassroots activity such as monitoring of schools and clinics forces the government to listen to the poor and respond to their needs (Peirson, 2010).

Kerala has thus managed to significantly improve the quality of life for a broad majority of its citizens through structural changes for equity and participation, based on their own cultural traditions rather than emphasizing aggregate economic prosperity, as do Western capitalist states. Although there are certainly wealthy citizens in Kerala (N. Narasimhan, personal communication, November 27, 2011), social policy promotes responsive conditions of justice rather than focusing on objective diversity. Such responsiveness is achieved through a determination to listen to confrontation (procedural and retributive justice) and a shared commitment to prevent suffering and to cooperate to deliver high levels of public good and prosperity (distributive justice). Singh concludes that the most significant element is a sense of cohesion, or *we-ness* among very diverse communities (cultural justice).

Indeed, other commentators have suggested that cultural diversity should be seen as an advantage rather than a problem, since countries with more immigration and diversity are often doing better than those maintaining White hegemony (Van Dijk, 2007). Both the Cameroon and Kerala examples suggest that a shared sense of *we-ness* and being *better together* have enormous potential to transform social policy and promote a state of thriving well-being.

IMPLICATIONS FOR ACTION

Reviewing the links between well-being and types of justice, it is clear that for a society to consider itself thriving, every social and cultural group needs to experience optimal conditions of justice. Thriving cannot be an exclusive state for a privileged group in a society, but needs to involve a responsive posture of listening to those in the coping, resisting, or suffering states of well-being, and joining them to work for change. De Herdt and Bastiaensen (2008) speak of the "relational character of unfreedom" and suggest that local political processes are the key to the reproduction and reduction of injustices such as poverty. When thriving is a responsive state, a relational ethic opens up the possibility for effective, localized social change. Such a responsive strategy aligns with the ideologies of *we-ness* described in Kerala, and being *better together* in African social thought. Such a relational ethic is now being discussed in Western social thought, partly in response to indigenous philosophies (Hoskins, Martin, & Humphries, 2011). In summary, a responsive, relational stance among groups in society creates necessary links among groups in the suffering, resistant, coping and thriving states to encourage transformative efforts for change.

From these key points, we can draw the following implications for action:

1. Be responsive in listening to voices of confrontation, protest, and pain.
2. Encourage ideologies and practices of responsiveness between social groups in order for those who are thriving to be responsive to those who are coping, struggling, or suffering.
3. Address all types of social justice in an ecological approach. Avoid sacrificing one form of justice to pursue another.
4. Support social movements that directly pursue conditions of justice, such as social policy changes, conscientization work, cultural conflict resolution, and literacy campaigns.
5. Support interventions that aim for modest gains in well-being. Small interventions have the potential to be transformative, and directly or indirectly improve conditions of justice.
6. Consider yourself always a learner. As stated in the Millennium Development Goals, proceed with humility.

CONCLUSION

The link between efforts to improve social justice and states of well-being is often implicit. Our aim in this chapter has been to make these links explicit and to introduce a richer vocabulary for justice and well-being. Accordingly, we introduced domains of well-being (interpersonal, communal, occupational, physical, psychological, and economic) and described eight types of justice (distributive, procedural, intrapersonal, interpersonal, informational, developmental, retributive, and cultural). As noted throughout the chapter, it is possible to experience well-being in some domains but not in others. Similarly, it is possible to experience some types of justice but not others. Optimal well-being, or thriving, is achieved when we experience optimal conditions of justice, and when we feel fulfilled in each domain of life.

Psychology has had a tradition of concentrating on intrapsychic processes to achieve well-being. Our goal has been to suggest means for well-being to thrive through efforts at social change. To maximize justice and well-being, it is not only people who need changing, but also the very societal structures that condition people to behave in certain ways. Thus, we brought examples from various parts of the world to show that social change can indeed improve justice and well-being, as in the case of Kerala. Through our examples we concluded that well-being is achieved through improvements in conditions of justice in society and that the various forms of societal justice intersect. The conditions of justice and well-being of every group in society need attention. Ideologies of collective responsibility—such as *we-ness*, being *better together*, and a relational ethic of responsibility toward all groups in society—encourage change efforts toward a thriving society. It is our hope that readers will explore the links among justice, well-being, and social change more in depth, and consider this triangle an important topic of study, discussion, and practice.

REFERENCES

Abbott, P., Wallace, C., & Sapsford, R. (2011). Surviving the transformation: Social quality in Central Asia and the caucuses. *Journal of Happiness Studies, 12,* 199–223.

Avruch, K., & Vejarano, B. (2002). Truth and reconciliation commissions: A review essay and annotated bibliography. *The Online Journal of Peace and Conflict Resolution, 4*(2), 37–76.

Barrett, M. (1993). Feminism. In W. Outhwaite & T. Bottomore (Eds.), *Dictionary of twentieth century social thought* (pp. 226–228). Oxford, UK: Blackwell.

Barros, M. (2010). Emancipatory management: The contradiction between practice and discourse. *Journal of Management Inquiry, 19*(2), 166–184.

Barry, B. (2005). *Why social justice matters.* Cambridge, UK: Polity Press.

Baumeister, R., & Leary, M. (1995). The need to belong: Desire for interpersonal attachments as a fundamental human motivation. *Psychological Bulletin, 117*(3), 497–529.

Baumgardner, S. R., & Crothers, M. K. (2009). *Positive psychology.* Upper Saddle River, NJ: Prentice Hall.

Beauchamp, D. (2013). Public health as social justice. In M. Donohoe (Ed). *Public health and social justice* (pp. 11–20). San Francisco, CA: Jossey-Bass.

Berkman, L., & Glass, T. (2000). Social integration, social networks, social support and health. In L. Berkman & I. Kawachi (Eds.), *Social epidemiology* (pp. 137–173). Oxford, UK: Oxford University Press.

Betancur, J. J., & Garcia, M. (2011). The 2006–2007 immigration mobilizations and community capacity: The experience of Chicago. *Latino Studies, 9*(1), 10–37.

Black, A., & Hughes, P. (2001). *The identification and analysis of indicators of community strength and outcomes.* Occasional Paper No. 3. Canberra, Australia: Department of Family and Community Services.

Brandtstadter, S. (2011). The law cuts both ways: Rural legal activism and citizenship struggles in neosocialist China. *Economy & Society, 40*(2), 266–288.

Bronfenbrenner, U. (1977). Toward an experimental ecology of human development. *American Psychologist, 32,* 513–531.

Bronfenbrenner, U. (1979). *The ecology of human development*. Cambridge, MA: Harvard University Press.

Buettner, D. (2010). *Thrive*. Washington, DC: National Geographic.

Cacioppo, J., Reis, H., & Zautra, A. (2011). Social resilience: The value of social fitness with an application to the military. *American Psychologist, 66*(1), 43–51.

Carnegie Council. (2005). Financing equity: The campaign for a basic income grant. In *Policy* Innovations for a fairer globalisation. Retrieved from http://www.policyinnovations.org/ideas/briefings/data/000015

Chile, L. (2006). The historical context of community development in Aotearoa New Zealand. *Community Development Journal, 41*(4), 407–425.

Christakis, N., & Fowler, J. (2007). The spread of obesity in a large social network over 32 years. *New England Journal of Medicine, 357*, 370–379.

Clardie, J. (2011). The impact of military spending on the likelihood of democratic transition failure: Testing two competing theories. *Armed Forces and Society, 37*(1), 163–179.

Clark, P. (2013). Prejudice and the medical profession: A five-year update. In M. Donohoe (Ed.), Public health and social justice (pp. 123–152). San Francisco: Jossey-Bass.

Cohen, J. (2006). Social, emotional, ethical, and academic education: Creating a climate for learning, participation in democracy, and well-being. *Harvard Educational Review, 76*(2), 201–237.

Cohen, S. (2004). Social relationships and health. *American Psychologist, 59*, 676–684.

Colquitt, J. (2001). On the dimensionality of organizational justice: A construct validation of a measure. *Journal of Applied Psychology, 86*, 386–400.

Commission on social determinants of health. (2008). *Closing the gap in a generation: Health equity through action on the social determinants of health.* Geneva: World Health Organization.

Consedine, J. (2011). Vatican endorses "Robin Hood" tax. *The Common Good, 59*, 1.

Corning, P. (2011). *The fair society: The science of human nature and the pursuit of social justice.* Chicago, IL: University of Chicago Press.

Crowfoot, J., Chesler, M. A., & Boulet, J. (1983). Organizing for social justice. In E. Seidman (Ed.), *Handbook of social intervention* (pp. 237–267). Beverly Hills, CA: Sage.

Cullen, S. C. S. (2011). The Occupation Movement. *The Common Good, 59*, 5.

Daniels, N. (2008). *Just health: Meeting health needs fairly.* New York, NY: Cambridge University Press.

Darling-Hammond, L. (2010). *The flat world and education: How America's commitment to equity will determine our future.* New York, NY: Teachers College Press.

De Herdt, T., & Bastiaensen, J. (2008). The circumstances of agency: A relational view of poverty. *International Development Planning Review, 30*(4), 339–357.

De la Sablonnière, R., Auger, É., Sadykova, N., & Taylor, D. M. (2010). When the "We" impacts how "I" feel about myself: Effect of temporal collective relative deprivation on personal well-being in the context of dramatic social change in Kyrgyzstan. *European Psychologist, 15*(4), 271–282.

De Vogli, R., Brunner, E., & Marmot, M. (2007). Unfairness and the social gradient of metabolic syndrome in the Whitehall II study. *Journal of Psychosomatic Research, 63*(4), 413–419.

De Vogli, R., Ferrie, J., Chandola, T., Kivimäki, M., & Marmot, M. (2007). Unfairness and health: Evidence from the Whitehall II study. *Journal of Epidemiology and Community Health, 61*, 513–518.

Deogaonkar, M. (2004). Socio-economic inequality and its effect on healthcare delivery in India: Inequality and healthcare. Electronic Journal of Sociology. Retrieved from http://www.sociology.org/content/vol8.1/deogaonkar.html

Diener, E., Diener, M., & Diener, C. (1995). Factors predicting the subjective well-being of nations. *Journal of Personality and Social Psychology, 69*(5), 851–864.

Diener, E., Helliwell, J., & Kahneman, D. (Eds.). (2010). *International differences in well-being.* New York, NY: Oxford University Press.

Diener, E., Lucas, R., Schimmack, U., & Helliwell, J. (2009). *Well-being for public policy.* New York, NY: Oxford University Press.

Dunn, E. W., Ankin, L. B., & Norton, M. I. (2008). Spending money on others promotes happiness. *Science, 319*(5870), 1678–1688.

Dobbin, M. (2003). *The myth of the good corporate citizen* (2nd ed.). Toronto, Canada: Lorimer.

Donohoe, M. (Ed.). (2013). *Public health and social justice.* San Francisco: Jossey-Bass.

Eckstein, S., & Wickham-Crowley, T. (Eds.). (2003). *What justice? Whose justice? Fighting for fairness in Latin America.* Los Angeles: University of California Press.

Edlin, G., & Golanty, E. (2010). *Health & wellness* (10th ed.). Sudbury, MA: Jones and Bartlett Publishers.

Elovainio, M., Kivimäki, M., & Vahtera, J. (2002). Organizational justice: Evidence of a new psychosocial predictor of health. *American Journal of Public Health, 92*(1), 105–108.

Elovainio, M., Kivimäki, M., Steen, N., & Vahtera, J. (2004). Job decision latitude, organizational justice and health: Multilevel covariance structural analysis. *Social Science and Medicine, 58,* 1659–1669.

Facione, P. A., Scherer, D., & Attig, T. (1978). *Values and society: An introduction to ethics and social philosophy.* Englewood Cliffs, NJ: Prentice-Hall.

Feagin, J. R., & Feagin, C. B. (1978). *Discrimination American style: Institutional racism and sexism.* Englewood Cliff, NJ: Prentice-Hall.

Fiske, S. (2011). *Envy up, scorn down: How status divides us.* New York, NY: Russell Sage Foundation.

Fisher, A. T., Sonn, C. C., & Bishop, B. J. (2002). *Psychological sense of community: Research, applications, and implications.* New York, NY: Kluwer Academic/Plenum Publishers.

Fredrickson, B. (2009). *Positivity.* New York, NY: Crown Publishers.

Freire, P. (2004). *Pedagogy of indignation.* Boulder, CO: Paradigm Publishers.

Frey, B. S., & Stutzer, A. (2002). *Happiness and economics: How the economy and institutions affect well-being.* Princeton, NJ: Princeton University Press.

Fujishiro, K., & Heaney, C. (2009). Justice at work, job stress, and employee health. *Health Education and Behavior, 36*(3), 487–504.

Fuligni, A. J. (2007). *Contesting stereotypes and creating identities: Social categories, social identities, and educational participation.* New York, NY: Russell Sage Foundation.

Fullan, M. (2008). *The six secrets of change: What the best leaders do to help their organizations survive and thrive* (1st ed.). San Francisco, CA: Jossey-Bass.

Gable, S., Gonzaga, G., Strachman, A. (2006). Will you be there for me when things go right? Supportive responses to positive events disclosures. *Journal of Personality and Social Psychology, 90,* 904–917.

Gable, S., Reis, H., Impett, E., & Asher, R. (2004). What to do when things go right? The intrapersonal and interpersonal benefits of sharing good events. *Journal of Personality and Social Psychology, 87,* 228–245.

Graham, C. (2009). *Happiness around the world: The paradox of happy peasants and miserable millionaires*. New York, NY: Oxford University Press.

Halpern, D. (2010). *The hidden wealth of nations*. Cambridge, UK: Polity Press.

Harter, J., Schmidt, F., & Keyes, C. (2003). Well-being in the workplace and its relationship to business outcomes. In C. H. Keyes, J. (Ed.), *Flourishing: The positive person and the good life*. (pp. 205–224). Washington, DC: American Psychological Association.

Hatfield, E., Rapson, R., & Aumer-Ryan, K. (2008). Social justice in love relationships: Recent developments. *Social Justice Research, 21*, 413–431.

Hoskins, Te K., Martin, B., & Humphries, M. (2011). The power of relational responsibility. *EJBO Electronic Journal of Business Ethics and Organization Studies, 16*(2), 22–27.

Humphrey, M. (2005). Reconciliation and the therapeutic state. *Journal of Intercultural Studies, 26*(3), 203–220.

Huppert, F. A., & Linley, P. A. (2011a). *Happiness and well-being: Critical concepts in psychology; Vol IV: The impacts and enhancement of happiness and well-being: consequences, interventions and public policy*. New York, NY: Routledge.

Huppert, F. A., & Linley, P. A. (2011b). *Happiness and well-being: Critical concepts in psychology; Vol III: Causes and correlates of happiness and well-being: What makes us happy*. New York, NY: Routledge.

Huygens, I. (2011). Developing a decolonisation practice for settler-colonisers: A case study from Aotearoa New Zealand. *Settler Colonial Studies, 1*(2), 53–81.

Inglehart, R. (2010). Faith and freedom: Traditional and modern ways to happiness. In E. Diener, J. Helliwell, & D. Kahneman (Eds.), *International differences in well-being* (pp. 351–397). New York, NY: Oxford University Press.

Inglehart, R., Foa, R., Peterson, C., & Welzel, C. (2008). Development, freedom, and rising happiness. *Perspectives on Psychological Science, 3*(4), 264–285.

Isbister, J. (2001). *Capitalism and justice: Envisioning social and economic fairness*. Bloomfield, CT: Kumarian Press.

Jackson, M. (1988). *The Maori and the criminal justice system: He Whaipaanga Hou—A new perspective*. Wellington: New Zealand Department of Justice.

Jost, J. T., & Kay, A. C. (2010). Social justice: History, theory, and research. In S. Fiske, D. Gilbert, & G. Lindzey (Eds.), *Handbook of social psychology* (pp. 1122–1165). Hoboken, NJ: Wiley.

Kahneman, D., & Riis, J. (2005). Living, and thinking about it: Two perspectives on life. In F. Huppert, N. Baylis, & B. Keverne (Eds.), *The science of well-being* (pp. 285–306). New York, NY: Oxford University Press.

Kasser, T., & Ryan, R. (1993). A dark side of the American dream: Correlates of financial success as a central life aspiration. *Journal of Personality and Social Psychology, 65* (2), 410–422.

Kelly, J. (2006). *Becoming ecological*. New York, NY: Oxford University Press.

Kivimäki, M., Ferrie, J., Head, J., Shipley, M., Vahtera, J., & Marmot, M. (2004). Organizational justice and change in justice as predictors of employee health: The Whitehall II study. *Journal of Epidemiology and Community Health, 58*, 931–937.

Lareau, A., & Conley, D. (Eds.). (2008). *Social class: How does it work?* New York, NY: Russel Sage Foundation.

Lawson, K., Noblett, A., & Rodwell, J. (2009). Promoting employee well-being: The relevance of work characteristics and organizational justice. *Health Promotion International, 24*(3), 223–233.

Leka, S., & Houdmont, J. (Eds). (2010). *Occupational health psychology.* West Sussex, UK: Wiley-Blackwell.

Levy, B., & Sidel, V. (Eds.). (2006). *Social injustice and public health.* New York, NY: Oxford University Press.

Lyubomirsky, S. (2011). Hedonic adaptation to positive and negative experiences. In S. Folkman (Ed.), *The Oxford handbook of stress, health, and coping* (pp. 200–224). New York, NY: Oxford University Press.

Macedo, D., Dendrinos, B., & Gounari, P. (2003). *The hegemony of English.* Boulder, CO: Paradigm.

Marmot, M. G. (2004). *The status syndrome: How social standing affects our health and longevity* (1st American ed.). New York, NY: Times Books.

Mauer, M., & King, R. (2007). *Uneven justice: State rates of incarceration by race and ethnicity.* Washington, DC: The Sentencing Project.

Maslow, A. H. (1968). *Toward a psychology of being* (2nd ed.). New York, NY: Van Nostrand.

Maslow, A. H. (1971). *The farther reaches of human nature.* New York, NY: Penguin.

McKnight, J., & Block, P. (2010). *The abundant community.* San Francisco, CA: Berret-Koehler.

Miller, D. T. (2001). Disrespect and the experience of injustice. *Annual Review of Psychology, 52,* 527–553.

Miller, D. (1999). *Principles of social justice.* Cambridge, MA: Harvard University Press.

Molyneux, M. (1993). Women's movement. In W. Outhwaite & T. Bottomore (Eds.), *Dictionary of twentieth century social thought* (pp. 712–715). Oxford, UK: Blackwell.

Montero, M. (2009). Community action and research as citizenship construction. *American Journal of Community Psychology, 43,* 149–161.

Montero, M. (2010). Between person and society: Community psychology's voyage into complexity. In G. Nelson & I. Prilleltensky (Eds.), *Community psychology: In pursuit of liberation and well-being* (pp. 519–532). New York, NY: Palgrave Macmillan.

Morris, A., & Maxwell, G. (1998). Restorative justice in New Zealand: Family group conferences as a case study. *Western Criminology Review, 1*(1).

Narayan, D., Chambers, R., Shah, M., & Petesch, P. (2000). *Voices of the poor: Crying out for change.* New York, NY: Oxford University Press.

Nelson, G. B., & Prilleltensky, I. (2010). *Community psychology: In pursuit of liberation and well-being* (2nd ed.). New York, NY: Palgrave Macmillan.

Nsamenang, B., A., Fru, F. N., & Browne, M. A. (2007). The roots of community psychology in Cameroon. In S. Reich, M. Riemer, I. Prilleltensky, & M. Montero (Eds.), *International community psychology history and theories* (pp. 394–408). New York, NY: Springer.

Nussbaum, M. (2006). *Frontiers of justice: Disability, nationality, and species membership.* Cambridge, MA: Harvard University Press.

Okimoto, T., Wenzel, M., & Feather, N. (2009). Beyond retribution: Conceptualizing restorative justice and exploring its determinants. *Social Justice Research, 22*(1), 156–180.

Olson, D., DeFrain, J., & Skogrand, L. (2008). *Marriages and families: Intimacy, diversity, and strengths* (6th ed.). New York, NY: McGraw-Hill.

Ornish, D., & Smith, A. (2007). *The spectrum: A scientifically proven program to feel better, live longer, lose weight, and gain health* (1st ed.). New York, NY: Ballantine Books.

Peirson, L. (2010). Disadvantaged children and families. In G. Nelson & I. Prilleltensky (Eds.), *Community psychology: In pursuit of liberation and well-being* (pp. 477–497). New York, NY: Palgrave MacMillan.

Peterson, C. (1999). Personal control and well-being. In D. Kahneman, E. Diener, & N. Schwartz (Eds.), *Well-being: The foundations of hedonic psychology* (pp. 288–301). New York, NY: Russell Sage Foundation.

Powers, M., & Faden, F. (2006). *Social justice: The moral foundations of public health and health policy.* New York, NY: Oxford University Press.

Prilleltensky, I. (2011). Wellness as fairness. *American Journal of Community Psychology, 49,* 1–21. doi: 10.1007/s10464-011-9448-8

Prilleltensky, I. (2012). The what, why, who and how of globalization: What is psychology to do? *Journal of Social Issues, 68*(3), 612–629.

Prilleltensky, I., & Prilleltensky, O. (2006). *Promoting well-being: Linking personal, organizational, and community change.* Hoboken, NJ: John Wiley.

Putnam, R. D. (2000). *Bowling Alone: The collapse and revival of American community.* New York, NY: Simon & Schuster

Rath, T., & Harter, J. (2010). *Well being: The five essential elements.* New York, NY: Gallup Press.

Reyhner, J., & Lockard, L. (Eds.). (2009). *Indigenous language revitalization: Encouragement, guidance & lessons learned.* Flagstaff, AZ: Northern Arizona University.

Rodin, J. (1986). Aging and health: Effects of sense of control. *Science, 233*(4770), 1271–1276.

Rodin, J. & Langer, E. (1977). Long-term effects of a control-relevant intervention with the institutionalized aged. *Journal of Personality and Social Psychology, 35,* 897–902.

Rosenberg, Y. (2012). *Join the club: How peer pressure can transform the world.* New York: Norton.

Ruhl, J. (2011). Political corruption in Central America: Assessment and explanation. *Latin American Politics and Society, 53*(1), 33–58.

Ryan, R., & Deci, E. (2000). Self-determination theory and the facilitation of intrinsic motivation, social development, and well-being. *American Psychologist, 55,* 68–78.

Ryff, C., & Keyes, C. (1995). The structure of psychological well-being revisited. *Journal of Personality and Social Psychology, 57,* 1069–1081.

Sandel, M. (2009). *Justice: What's the right thing to do.* New York, NY: Farrar, Straus and Giroux.

Schmitt, M., & Dorfel, M. (1999). Procedural injustice at work, justice sensitivity, job satisfaction and psychosomatic well-being. *European Journal of Social Psychology, 29,* 443–453.

Schraad-Tischler, D., & Azahaf, N. (2011). *Social justice in the OECD—How do the member states compare?* Güthersloh, Germany: Bertelsmann Stiftung.

Schutz, A., & Sandy, M. (2011). *Collective action for social change.* New York, NY: Palgrave.

Segal, A., & Fries, C. (2011). *Pursuing health and wellness: Healthy societies, healthy people.* Toronto, Canada: Oxford University Press.

Seligman, M. E. P. (2011). *Flourish.* New York, NY: Free Press.

Sen, A. (1995). *Development as freedom.* New York, NY: Anchor Books.

Sen, A. (2010). *The idea of justice.* Cambridge, MA: Harvard University Press.

Singh, P. (2011). We-ness and welfare: A longitudinal analysis of social development in Kerala, India. *World Development, 39*(2), 282–293

Sisodia, R., Wolfe, D., & Sheth, J. (2007). *Firms of endearment: How world-class companies profit from passion and purpose.* Upper Saddle River, NJ: Wharton.

Sloan, T. (2010). Globalisation, poverty and social justice. In G. Nelson & I. Prilleltensky (Eds.), *Community psychology: In pursuit of liberation and well-being* (pp. 331–352). New York, NY: Palgrave Macmillan.

Stewart, J. (2008). A measure of justice: The Rabinal Human Rights Movement in post-war Guatemala. *Qualitative Sociology, 31*(3), 231–250.

Tavits, M. (2008). Representation, corruption, and subjective well-being. *Comparative Political Studies, 41*(12), 1607–1630.

Tepper, B. (2001). Health consequences of organizational injustice: Tests of main and interactive effects. *Organizational Behavior and Human Decision Processes, 86*(2), 197–215.

Tornblom, K., & Vermunt, R. (Eds.). (2007). *Distributive and procedural justice: Research and social applications*. Burlington, VT: Ashgate.

Totikidis, V., & Prilleltensky, I. (2006). Engaging community through a cycle of praxis: Multicultural perspectives on personal, relational, and collective wellness. *Community, Work, and Family, 9(1)*, 47–67.

Van Boven, L. & Gilovich, T. (2003). To do or to have? That is the question. *Journal of Personality and Social Psychology, 85*(6), 1193–1202.

Van Dijk, T. (2007). Racism, the press and freedom of expression: A summary of ten theses. Retrieved from http://www.discourses.org/UnpublishedArticles/ECRI-Theses.pdf

Veenhoven, R. (2007). Subjective measures of well-being. In M. McGillivray (Ed.), *Human well-being: Concept and measurement* (pp. 214–239). New York, NY: Palgrave Macmillan.

Veenhoven, R. (2012). Does happiness differ across cultures? In H. Selin & G. Davey (Eds.), *Happiness across cultures* (pp. 451–472). New York, NY: Springer.

Venkatapuram, S. (2011). *Health justice*. Cambridge, UK: Polity Press.

Watts, R. J., & Flanagan, C. (2007, August 6). Pushing the envelope on youth civic engagement: A developmental and liberation psychology perspective [Special issue]. *Journal of Community Psychology, 35*, 779–792.

Wilkinson, R., & Pickett, K. (2009). *The spirit level: Why more equal societies almost always do better*. London, UK: Penguin.

Chapter 2

The Social Injustice of Stress: Identity Intersectionality and Well-Being among Urban Black/African and Latina Adolescent Girls

Wendi S. Williams, Amarpreet K. Dhami, and Anissa L. Moody

Social ills such as racism, sexism, and classism negatively impact the ability of a society and its members to function in socially just and healthy ways. For individuals belonging to marginalized racial, gender, or class groups, the effect of societal injustice is localized in their psychological and physical stress responses (Carter, 2007; Vermunt & Steensma, 2003). Recent developments in the health and psychological literature have pointed to the specific relationship between race (Carter, 2007), gender (Shih & Eberhart, 2010; Soffer, 2010), and social class (Thoit, 2010) on stress levels. Furthermore, although the experiences of adults have been primary (APA, 2012), the coping needs of children and adolescents are extremely important as early experience with stressors suggest potential for chronicity and potential long-term harm (Thoit, 2010).

Adolescence has been conceived as a time of emotional and physical growth and instability (Somerville, Jones, & Casey, 2010). Faced with many new life challenges and experiences for which they are not always fully prepared, adolescents are at risk for increased stress and negative health consequences. Furthermore, lacking adequate coping supports and resources, adolescents are likely to employ underdeveloped problem-solving skills that may place them at risk. As their ability to healthfully respond to the challenges of their environments develops with time, and varies in type and across gender and situation (Seiffge-Krenke, Aunola, & Nurmi, 2009; Sontag & Graber, 2010), adolescents are in need of supports to buttress challenges to optimal development. Moreover, developing within a context of interlocking gendered, racialized, and class-based systems of oppression necessitates the development of culturally responsive intervention programming to promote health and minimize stress experiences among adolescent Black/African and Latina girls in low-income urban communities.

This chapter examines the experiences of adolescent Black/African and Latina girls in an urban community. An intersectionality analysis (Collins, 2000) of their identities is viewed through the lens of injustice stress theory (Vermunt, Peeters, & Berggren, 2007; Vermunt & Steensma, 2003). U.S. Black/African descent and Latina girls' global citizenship is considered in light of the dynamics of globalism, imperialism, and economic distress drawing parallels with their international counterparts, Afro-Brazilian adolescent girls, with whom they share racial/ethnic and gender overlap. The importance of community-based intervention programming for this population is discussed with the presentation of two exemplar programs: one implemented in Salvador da Bahia, Brazil, and the other in Brooklyn, New York, the United States. Preliminary data from a U.S. sample are presented. The discussion begins with a presentation of the theoretical frames that guide our analysis.

COMPREHENSIVE COVERAGE OF THE TOPIC

Theoretical Frames

Intersectionality

Many scholars trace the roots of intersectionality to abolitionist Sojourner Truth's "Ain't I a Woman" address at the 1851 Women's Rights Convention where she personally identified with the complex and varied impact of patriarchy to gender, race, and class (Brah & Phoenix, 2004; Collins, 1998; Crenshaw, 1989; Goff, Thomas, & Jackson, 2008). The subjective impact of oppression identified by Truth continues to be challenged by modern-day Black feminists who often use the term *intersectionality* to describe how multiple identities such as religion, race, class, gender, citizenship status, sexual orientation, geographic location, and disability status shape and reflect unique individual responses to privilege and oppression (Collins, 2000; Combahee River Collective, 1986; Mann & Huffman, 2005). Though the intersectionality perspective was first coined and located in feminist legal studies and critical race theory nomenclature, feminist scholar and sociologist Patricia Hill Collins broadened the theoretical framework by including the "matrix of domination," or identifying the overall organization of power in a society, allowing for a more sophisticated analysis of the "interconnectedness" of social identities to macro-level structures (Collins, 2000; Weber & Parra-Medina, 2003). In opposition to reductionist perspectives wherein injustice is seen as the result of singular "isms," an intersectional analysis conveys the understanding that oppressions work together to create different types of injustices with specific effects on life experiences.

Consistent in the intersectionality literature are the constructs of identity, social category, and power, which are assumed to be interrelated and moderated by micro-level determinants, such as experience, age, education (van Mens-Verhulst & Radtke, 2008). This framework allows an identification of relationships on a systematic level, on a personal level, as well as the ability to identify connections within or between systems of power or between individuals. By placing emphasis on the construction of social inequality, this framework is uniquely suited to examine the complex overlay of interlocking systems of oppression due to race, gender, nation, age, and socioeconomic status (SES) that socially sanction injustice and cause stressful life circumstances. In this chapter, we explore the specific effect on the mental and physical health of urban Black/African and Latina adolescent girls.

The main purpose for using intersectionality as the guiding framework is to explore urban culture, social identity, and SES as salient determinants of urban adolescents' emotional and biological development and its impact on their stress reactivity and health outcomes (Kelly et al., 2010; Mason, 2010; Pinto, 2004). An analysis of multiple factors is fundamental to the theoretical framework of focus; however, as stated by Collins (2000), "All systems of power are always in every situation, but the salience of any given system of power varies across time and space" (p. 74). It is established that race and class are operative in the daily lives of individuals; however, geographic locations, in this case poor urban environments, are less understood as significant macro-level oppressive systems (Lee, 2005; Mason, 2010; Miller, 2008).

Given that adolescence is a time for defining one's identity (Erikson, 1966), adolescents are sensitive to environmental factors and have yet to develop an understanding of, or appropriate responses to cope with, oppressive systems and resultant stress. Girls' role socialization to be compliant and relational may also contribute to how they experience oppression and manage stressors (Gilligan, 1982; Valaitis, 2002). The pressures to be a "good girl" may mean acceptance at the individual level with peers, educators, parents, family, community, and at the macro-level with schools, community cultural norms and expectations, and media. Thus, the intersecting matrix of a Black/African or Latina girl living in an under-resourced urban community is illuminated using the intersectionality framework.

Injustice Stress Theory (IST)

The conceptual framework presented in Figure 2.1 illustrates how social injustices can lead to health outcomes in adolescent girls. The injustice stress theory (IST) was devised by Vermunt and Steensma (2001) to explain worker stress as

Figure 2.1
Graphic Representing Macro- and Micro-Level Systems and Injustices Impact on Cognitive Processing and Stress Responses.

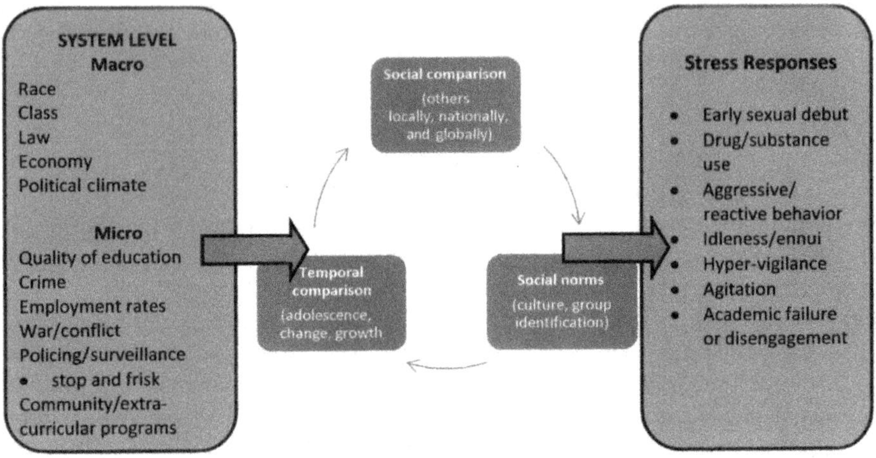

a function of inequities in the form of external factors, such as allocation of resources, on the micro-level (e.g., supervisor) or macro-level (e.g., organizational procedures), which are mitigated by an employee's perceptions of fairness and may influence the employee's experience of stress with potential for impacting health behaviors and outcomes (Vermunt & Steensma, 2001, 2003; Vermunt et al., 2007). The current discussion builds upon the IST model and incorporates the intersectional framework by acknowledging that injustices are interlocking, are multiple, and operate at the institutional level (e.g., governmental, economic, and political). These injustices affect individuals (e.g., mental/physical health) by influencing resource allocation and are attenuated by perceptions of fairness, or lack thereof, due to the matrix of social injustice, thus imposing stress and influencing physical, mental, and behavioral health.

IST locates stress in external factors such as individual actions or institutional resources that impose on individuals to cause stress responses (Vermunt & Steensma, 2003), and distinguishes itself from other stress models that focus on individual reactions to stress. This perspective not only allows for a more justice-oriented analysis of stressors by not blaming the victim but also for environmental interventions to ameliorate the negative impact of stress and support coping (e.g., Vermunt et al., 2007).

The proposed model elucidates the dynamic pathways between social constructs and individual health behavior by acknowledging that social location determines the allocation of psychosocial and material resources (see Figure 2.1).

This in turn makes it possible to operationalize the impact of environmental conditions on one's perception of fair or just treatment and how one manages and experiences stress. As adolescent girls have yet to develop the understanding and coping skills to negotiate their subordinate locations with regard to social, political, and economic inequities, and rely on environmental cues (i.e., underresourced urban environments) and expectations for information about their status and access (Somerville et al., 2010), acquisition of coping skills and resources may alleviate feelings of low self-worth or low self-esteem (Mason, 2010; Vermunt, et al., 2007) and consequent risk behaviors (Bachanas et al., 2002). Likewise, the stressors inherent in inner-city living means that urban girls may expend energy dealing with multiple stressors and rely on overly simplistic or maladaptive coping skills imitated or initiated within the same overburdened community (e.g., aggressive responses, early sexual initiation, drug/alcohol use, over-eating). As underdeveloped stress coping may lead to health risk, intervention programming with a focus on positive stress coping is imperative to diminish risk.

GLOBAL/INTERNATIONAL CONSIDERATIONS

Viewing American youth, particularly poor youth of color outside of a global perspective, is limiting when attempting to consider how systems of oppression overlay and restrict the life experiences and healthy psychological development of all persons. U.S. Black/African and Latina adolescent girls' global citizenship is discussed and their shared experiences with Afro-Brazilian adolescent girls in the urban community of Salvador da Bahia is presented to demonstrate parallels and the need for a global approach to address health and wellness concerns with attention to intersecting identities and economic and other sociopolitical oppressions associated with injustice.

Over the course of U.S. history, the archetype of the American citizen has been shaped along with the attributed qualities that capture the ideals of meritocracy and the potential for upward economic mobility (Kwate & Myer, 2010). Geronimus and Thompson (2004; as cited by Kwate & Myer, 2010) suggest that these concepts are so ingrained in the collective psyche of the populace and reflected back through various mediums that to argue otherwise may likely draw political and patriotic ire. The collective perceived status of American economic power and advantage has come at a cost to some of its citizens—those who deal with the intersections of race, class, and gender discrimination (Kwate & Myer, 2010, p. 1832). Poor, under, and uneducated people of color are held to standards of citizenship that are arguably unrealistic and nonexistent (Kwate & Myer, 2010, p. 1832).

Macro-level influences such as urban culture, globalization, imperialism, and present-day economic distress (Turner, Kaplan, & Badger, 2006) are localized in the day-to-day life experiences of Black, African, Caribbean, and Latina descent adolescent girls and their families. These influences shape the disparity between the myth of meritocracy and the reality of disenfranchisement via discriminatory action, which impact the girls' meso- and micro-level experiences of their immediate environments as well as their sense of identity and worth. As noted by Kwate and Myer (2010), meritocratic idealism has been seen as a panacea to social injustices that create inequitable access to opportunity. It has been espoused as a solution to be applied to the social problems of racism, classism, immigration, and resultant discrimination in that the onus of overcoming social injustice is conceptualized as the responsibility of the individual. Consequently, systemic practices that endorse institutionalized sexism, racism, and classism work to disenfranchise some citizens while granting access and opportunity to others under the guise that all have an equal opportunity to access and live out their rights. Under this belief system, adolescent Black/African and Latina girls reared in poor, under-resourced urban communities are charged to create their own equality. They are asked to change their own access to opportunities within circumstances in which they have limited power and within a rubric that, by definition, denies them access and opportunity. Furthermore, their failure to achieve within these circumstances is deemed an inherent flaw and testament to their lack of virtue and motivation. This context is unfair, and urban youth are not immune to the effects of this disparity or the consequent physical and psychological stress responses (Neblett, Terzian, & Harriott, 2010).

The cascade effect that results from the overlap of racism, poverty, and sexism is felt no more acutely than in the home of the Black/Latina adolescent girl. Low- and minimum-wage earnings force domestic and household care onto the female children in the home as a survival strategy to account for parental absence due to work demands and insufficient income (Dodson & Dickert, 2004). According to Hassler, Mora, and Zeira (2007), an essential part of upward mobility across generations is the ability for children to move from being unskilled to skilled as a result of education. The ability for the parent to allocate resources to education is vital in a child's opportunity to becoming skilled (Hassler et al., 2007). The resultant effects of economic marginalization are the inability for poor urban mothers to devote the resources necessary to allow the opportunity for their daughters to move upward in education and job opportunity. Poor urban families tax their daughters to assist in their own economically challenged household in order to cope financially—at a cost to their daughters in the form of their educational and economic advancement and future opportunity. According to Dodson and Dickert (2004), this results in the intergenerational cycle of poverty that passes from mother to daughter. In essence, poor urban mothers are forced to withdraw from focusing on the future of their daughters in order to pay for the debt of the present.

The meritocratic myth has the unfortunate consequence of clouding the reality of the immigration experience and has in part allowed U.S. low-income urban girls to recede into the background of poverty and disenfranchisement. Providing a context that reconstructs the immigrant experience to match the contemporary economic reality and its consequences re-conceptualizes the notion of what it means to be a global citizen and provides a pathway by which to consider the international citizenship of all girls. Furthermore, re-conceptualization of citizenship, and the macro-level forces that impact meso- and micro-level experiences, contributes to a fuller appreciation of the stressors that lead to suboptimal mental and physical wellness among adolescent Black/African and Latina girls living in low-income communities such as Brooklyn, New York, and their counterparts, Afro-Brazilian adolescent girls, in Salvador da Bahia (Bahia), Brazil, further justifying the need for effective intervention programming informed by a global perspective.

Parallels: Brooklyn and Bahia

Rapid urbanization and economic growth in Bahia, Brazil, has created social disparities similar to those in the United States (Sherman, Duarte, & Verdelli, 2011). In their review of the extant literature, Sherman et al. (2011) found that mental and physical health concerns among poor adolescents in Bahia were associated with sociodemographic risk factors. The racial demographic of Bahia consists of mostly poor, Black, and mulatto residents, and research has indicated a positive correlation between racial discrimination and major depression among Brazilian adolescents (Santana, Almeida-Filho, Roberts, & Cooper, 2007). Urban, poor, adolescent girls in Bahia face similar circumstances to adolescent girls in low-income communities such as Brooklyn, New York, with one glaring exception. Globalization and imperialistic ideology have shaped the American worldview to permit view of Bahian adolescents as disenfranchised and in need of aid, while negating the global citizenry and responsibility to poor Black/African and Latin descent girls within its borders. The mission statement of the U.S. Agency for International Development (USAID) captures this sentiment:

> The US has a long history of extending a helping hand to people overseas struggling to make a better life. It is a history that both reflects the American people's compassion and support of human dignity as well as advances U.S. foreign policy interests. (USAID, 2013)

This dichotomy is entirely representative of the concept of the "other," which defines the space outside of Western ideals, in which other countries and societies may exist, and the way in which American imperialistic ideology views them. According to Fukuyama (1989; as cited by Keyman 1995), "There is an increasing awareness in the domain of International Political Economy (IPE) of how the appropriation of the 'Other' as an empirical/cultural object has led to the justification of Western universalism as global modernity" (p. 71). The United States has been able to justify creating interventions for, and assisting on a global scale, the adolescent girls outside its borders because they are viewed as not having the advantage of American privilege, even if their circumstances are similar to poor and Black/

African or Latina girls in the United States. Since the American citizenry is considered to abound with privilege and opportunity, American citizens are not considered in need of intervention on a domestic or international scale, but rather are relegated to austerity measures, which threaten programs and funding that would benefit them. This worldview pits the needs of U.S. Black/African and Latina girls against their international counterparts by assuming advantage and privilege that does not exist, as both groups require intervention programming to cope with stress related to the social injustice associated with their racial, gender, and socioeconomic status.

Intervention

The increased level of health risk among Black/African and Latina adolescent girls in underresourced urban communities necessitates development of socioculturally relevant interventions. Common characteristics of underresourced urban communities, such as exposure to illicit substances and coercion to use or sell them (Miller, Webster, & McIntosh, 2002), financial concerns (Buzi, Weinman, & Smith, 2000), rising housing costs, issues of community and individual-level violence (Fredland, Campbell, & Han, 2008), and overcrowding have the potential to leave residents in these communities feeling hopeless (Bolland, 2003) and disconnected—with detrimental consequences for their mental health and well-being (Harris & Hawton, 2011; Ivory, Collings, Blakely, & Dew, 2011). Consequently, instances of posttraumatic stress disorder (PTSD; Horowitz, Weine, & Jekel, 1995; Schwartz, Bradley, Sexton, Sherry, & Ressler, 2005), depression, emotional and conduct problems, hyperactivity and self-harm (Fernandez, Kramer, Fong, Doig, & Garrralda, 2009) have been identified among adolescents coping with the dynamics of urban environments, necessitating intervention to support optimal development. Furthermore, significantly more instances of PTSD have been reported among Black/African and Latin descent persons, with Black/African persons more likely to experience PTSD than their White counterparts, despite fewer experiences of trauma and Latin descent persons reporting higher rates of PTSD than any other ethnic groups (Capodilupo & Sue, 2010). Furthermore, youth exposed to the stressors of the urban environment reported increases of stress up to 35% more compared to nonurban youth who have experienced trauma.

As is typical for anyone experiencing the degree of challenge faced in urban contexts, adolescents seek refuge from the strain of their environments. Encouraging findings suggest safe spaces and supportive networks (e.g., homes of their friends and family) are sought to balance stress (Lindsey, Barksdale, Lambert, & Ialongo, 2010). However, young people whose home environments are deemed unsupportive or unsafe are at increased risk (Fredland et al., 2008; Mason & Korpela, 2009). Adolescents reared in urban context are likely to engage in unhealthy coping, unsafe sexual practices (e.g., early sexual debut, increased sexual activity, with multiple partners and under the influence of controlled substances and/or without a condom; Bachanas et al., 2002; Bolland, 2003; Boyer, Tschann, & Shafter, 1999; Brook et al., 2004) and externalizing behaviors (Bannon & McKay, 2007), such as drug/alcohol abuse (Schwinn, Schinke, & Trent, 2010), violence (Caminis, Henrich, Ruchkin, Schwab-Stone, & Martin, 2007), and attention-seeking behaviors (Fredland et al., 2008).

Researchers have advocated for the development of early adolescent interventions to address the composite (i.e., sexual, drug/alcohol and violence) risks associated with being reared in underresourced urban communities (Bachanas et al., 2002). A brief discussion of two programs, Didá and Project SisterCircle (PSC), are briefly described as examples of community-based culturally relevant intervention programs for adolescent Black/African and Latina girls. Didá is a nonprofit organization serving the city of Salavador da Bahia in Brazil, providing educational and cultural programming (Arsenault, 2007). Founded in 1993 by musician Neguinho do Samba of the famed group Olodum, Didá, a Yoruba word for "power of creation," was created to provide girls and women with access to learn how to play the drums. In his work, do Samba sought to capitalize on the traditional and cultural significance of the drum and the empowerment it evokes. His work was to share this with girls and women, along with a host of African-centered community-based educational and arts programming, to improve on health, educational, and vocational outcomes among urban Afro-Brazilians. Examples of the types of programming offered include a carnival drumming and dancing group, technical courses in Afro-Brazilian beauty and hairstyling, a merchandise store, vocational training, and the Sódomo Project, which partners with schools and families to support students (Arsenault, 2007).

Project SisterCircle (PSC) is a psychosocial, spiritual intervention developed to address sexual risk vulnerability (SRV), the likelihood of placing oneself at risk for the negative consequences of sexual activity, among adolescent Black/African and Latina girls in middle school settings in Brooklyn, New York (Williams, Karlin & Wallace, in press). The program identified the girls' gender, racial, and leadership identities as the foundation for a stable and healthy self-concept by which healthy decisions related to risk behaviors are made. Rates of sexually transmitted infections (STIs) and teenage pregnancy among New York City adolescents were higher among Black/African descent and Latina girls (Karpati et al., 2004) and have necessitated intervention programming that addresses issues of stress and unhealthy coping in the form of risk behaviors among this population. PSC provided girls with information and therapeutic processing to build positive stress coping through programming that emphasized positive notions of the girls' gender and racial/ethnic identity and leadership esteem. The program sought to subvert the need for risk behaviors used to cope with urban environmental stressors. Preliminary findings relative to some of these variables are discussed.

Preliminary Findings

Within the PSC framework, health and wellness outcomes for adolescent Black/African descent and Latina girls in urban environments were assessed by examining alternative factors that may likely minimize their vulnerability for risk. The girls' racial, gender, and leadership identities were considered predictors of academic attitudes, health and wellness, and risk vulnerability. Utilization of these indicators of health and wellness for adolescent girls was intended to assess the girls' inherent resources toward resilience upon which the intervention could build. Cursory analysis of baseline data yielded useful information for practitioners interested in working with this population.

An internal study assessment tool was developed to explore key concepts (see Williams et al., 2012). A correlation analysis of all relationships was performed. Self-leadership, health and wellness, and racial esteem; racial esteem, general self-esteem, and self-leadership; and academic attitudes, leadership, and self-esteem were significantly related. Additionally, a regression analysis found racial esteem and self-leadership were predictive of health and wellness scores. Thus, aspects of the girls' identity (racial esteem) and abilities (leadership and academic attitudes) are related and have the potential to influence health and wellness promoting attitudes. These preliminary findings support the rationale for culturally relevant arts and educational programming, similar to Didá and PSC, to minimize risk among Black/African and Latina girls.

IMPLICATIONS AND CONCLUSION

This chapter explicated the intersection of interlocking systems of oppression, such as race, gender, class, and nation, and their effect on the lives of adolescent Black/African and Latina girls in low-income, urban communities. Through a focus on girls in the United States, a re-conceptualization of global citizenry was offered to highlight the effect of the macro-level social and political forces that are more descriptive of contemporary economies and policies that impact the day-to-day lives and development of girls across the globe. Based on the work with girls in Brooklyn, we explained the need to consider vulnerability, risk, and resilience in the context of the global economy, and the political motives that have shaped the immigration circumstances of them and their families. The following theoretical and practical implications for work with Black/African and Latina adolescent girls hold this conceptualization as the guiding principle for working in socially just ways toward youth health and wellness empowerment.

The preliminary findings from the PSC program suggest that a wellness, rather than risk, perspective may be most effective for work toward health and wellness among Black/African and Latina adolescent girls. As positive relationships and predictions were found for girls' self-directed leadership and racial esteem for the health/wellness scale, conceptualization of girls as empowered agents of wellness, rather than victims of environmental and circumstantial risks, would likely contribute to relevant theorization and development of intervention programming that addresses the promotion of health and wellness.

As the injustices of the privileged are revealed to the public over and again, more and more people are aware of the ways they lose advantage at the hands of those who have amassed wealth and power at their expense. Specifically, the impact on those who are poor, non-White, female, and young is intensely felt, underscoring the importance of an intersectional analysis with a focus on justice and parity among all persons. As it has been proven that stress reactions to experiences of injustice negatively impact the health of individuals (Carter, 2007; Shih & Ebert, 2010; Soffer, 2010; Thoit, 2010), interventions within communities that utilize a group approach have the potential to reshape the social and cultural meaning applied to the conditions in which people live. Intervention programming of this type also has the potential to create opportunities for individual growth and group-level consciousness-raising toward achieving social change, rather than self-blame and internalization of oppressive circumstances.

Finally, as the results from the preliminary findings indicate that a focus on wellness and leadership may be a fruitful pathway toward the promotion of healthy attitudes and behaviors, the development of intervention programming that takes a stance of guiding girls toward their development as empowered self-leaders for their health and wellness may be most relevant. Curricula with a pedagogical stance toward healthy decision making in a health averse context, and providing girls with positive stress coping and leadership skills with utility across various social and risk contexts, has the potential to support their health and wellness while also priming them for positive socio-emotional and academic attitudes and achievement outcomes. Although girlhood esteem did not prove a strong relationship or predictor of health outcomes, it is likely a flaw relative to the assessment tool, rather than evidence that a strong girlhood self-concept is unrelated to health outcomes. Black/African and Latina adolescent girls in urban communities have a specific standpoint with regard to health and risk as their gender, class, and racial identities overlay to be sexualized and socialized as dangerous and vulnerable for their health and safety (Gallegos-Castillo, 2006; Miller, 2008). Thus, cultivating a sense of pride and strength for Black/African and Latina girlhood and womanhood is essential for development and implementation of health promotion behaviors, especially those related to sexual health and violence, as these affect girls in gender-specific ways. The example provided by programs such as Didá speaks to the importance of highlighting girls' and women's roles in society. As the program's cultural director declared in describing the decision to choose their carnival theme, "Samba of the Washer Woman," to honor the collection of women along the "banks of lakes and rivers to work, talk and sing," "The focus is always to appreciate women and their achievement" (Aresenault, 2007, p. 41). Intervention programs for Black/African and Latina girls, localized in their social and cultural context, like Didá and Project SisterCircle, encourage them to "work, talk, and sing" and have the potential to be the pathway toward their collective social parity, health, and healing.

REFERENCES

APA (2012). *Stress in America: Our health at risk.* Washington, DC: Author.

Arsenault, N. (2007). Didá: Empowering Afro-Brazilian women through the arts. *LLILAS Portal, 2,* 40–41.

Bachanas, P. J., Morris, M. K., Lewis-Gess, J. K., Sarett-Cuasay, E. J., Sirl, K., Ries, J. K., & Sawyer, M. K. (2002). Predictors of risky sexual behavior in African American adolescent girls: Implications for prevention interventions. *Journal of Pediatric Psychology, 27*(6), 519–530.

Bannon, W. M., & McKay, M. M. (2007). Addressing urban African American youth externalizing and social problem behavioral difficulties in a family-oriented prevention project. *Social Work in Mental Health, 5*(1/2), 221–240.

Bolland, J. M. (2003). Hopelessness and risk behavior among adolescents living in high poverty inner city neighborhoods. *Journal of Adolescence, 26,* 145–158.

Boyer, C. B., Tschann, J. M., & Shafter, M. (1999). Predictors of risk for sexually transmitted diseases in 9th grade urban high school students. *Journal of Adolescent Research, 14*(4), 448–465.

Brah, A., & Phoenix, A. (2004). Ain't I A Woman? Revisiting Intersectionality. *Journal of International Women's Studies, 5*(3), 75–86.

Brook, J. S., Adams, R. E., Balka, E. B., Whiteman, M., Zhang, C., & Sugerman, R. (2004). Illicit drug use and risky sexual behavior among African American and Puerto Rican urban adolescents: The longitudinal links. *The Journal of Genetic Psychology, 165*(2), 203–220.

Buzi, R., Weinman, M. L., & Smith, P. (2000). Mental health problems and symptoms among adolescents attending a family planning clinic. *North American Journal of Psychology, 2*(2), 337–346.

Caminis, A., Henrich, C., Ruchkin, V., Schwab-Stone, M., & Martin, A. (2007). Psychosocial predictors of sexual initiation and high risk sexual behavior in early adolescence. *Child and Adolescent Psychiatry and Mental Health, 1*(14), 1–12. doi: 10.1186/1753-2000-1-14

Capodilupo, C. M., & Sue, D. W. (2010). Cultural perspectives on trauma. In C. Claus-Ehlers (Ed.), *Encyclopedia of cross-cultural school psychology* (pp. 318–320). New York, NY: Springer.

Carter, R. T. (2007). Racism and psychological and emotional injury: Recognizing and assessing race-based traumatic stress *The Counseling Psychologist, 35,* 1–93.

Collins, P. (1998). Searching for Sojourner Truth: Toward an epistemology of empowerment. In Patricia H. Collins (Ed.), *Fighting words: Black women and the search for justice (contradictions of modernity)* (pp. 229–251). Minneapolis: University of Minnesota.

Collins, P. H. (2000). *Black feminist thought: Knowledge, consciousness and the politics of empowerment.* New York, NY: Routledge.

Combahee River Collective. A Black Feminist Statement 1977. (1986). Combahee River Collective Statement. In L. Smith (Ed.), *Black feminist organizing in the seventies and eighties. Freedom Organizing Series.* New York, NY: Kitchen Table-Women of Color.

Crenshaw, K. W. (1989). Demarginalizing the intersection of race and sex: A Black feminist critique of antidiscrimination doctrine, feminist theory, and antiracist politics. *The University of Chicago Legal Forum,* 139–167.

Dodson, L., & Dickert, J. (2004). Girls' family labor in low income households: A decade of qualitative research. *Journal of Marriage and Family, 66*(2), 318–332.

Erikson, E. (1966). Eight stages of man. *Journal of Psychiatry, 2*(3), 281–300.

Fernandez, V., Kramer, T., Fong, G., Doig, A., & Garralda, M. E. (2009). Depressive symptoms and behavioral health risks in young women attending an urban sexual health clinic. *Child Care, 35*(6), 799–806.

Fredland, N. M., Campbell, J. C., & Han, H. (2008). Effects of violence exposure on health outcomes among young urban adolescents. *Nursing Research, 57*(3), 157–165.

Fukuyama, F. (1989). *Have we reached the end of history*. Santa Monica, CA: Rand.

Gallegos-Castillo, A. (2006). La casa: Negotiating family cultural practices, constructing identities. In J. Denner & B. L. Guzman (Eds.), *Latina girls: Voices of adolescent strength in the United States* (pp. 44–58). New York, NY: New York University.

Geronimus A. T., & Thompson J. P. (2004). To denigrate, ignore or disrupt: Racial inequality in health and the impact of a policy-induced breakdown of African American communities. *Du Bois Rev, 1*(2), 247–279.

Gilligan, C. (1982). *In another voice: Psychological theory and women's development.* Cambridge, MA: Harvard University Press.

Goff, P. A., Thomas, M. A., & Jackson, M. C. (2008). "Ain't I a Woman?": Towards an intersectional approach to person perception and group-based harms. *Sex Roles, 59*(5/6), 392–403.

Harris, L., & Hawton, K. (2011). Deliberate self-harm in rural and urban regions: A comparative study of prevalence and patient characteristics. *Social Science & Medicine, 73*, 274–281.

Hassler, J., Rodriguez Mora, J. V., & Zeira, J. (2007). Inequality and mobility. *Journal of Economic Growth, 12*(3), 235–259. doi: 10.1007/s10887-007-9019

Horowitz, K., Weine, S., & Jekel, J. (1995). PTSD symptoms in urban adolescent girls: Compounded community trauma. *Journal of the American Academy of Child & Adolescent Psychiatry, 34*, 1353–1361.

Ivory, V. C., Collings, S. C., Blakely, T., & Dew, K. (2011). When does neighborhood matter? Multilevel relationships between neighborhood fragmentation and mental health. *Social Science and Medicine, 72*, 1993–2002.

Karpati, A., Kerker, B., Mostashari, F., Singh T., Hajat, A., Thorpe, L., . . . Frieden, T. (2004). *Health disparities in New York City*. New York, NY: New York City Department of Health and Mental Hygiene.

Kelly, E. B., Parra-Medina, D., Pfeiffer, K. A., Dowda, M., Conway, T. L., Webber, L. S., . . . Pate, R. R. (2010). Correlates of physical activity in black, Hispanic, and white middle school girls. *Journal of Physical Activity and Health, 7*(2), 184–193.

Keyman, F. (1995). Articulating difference: The problem of the other in international political economy. *Review of International Political Economy, 2*(1), 70–95.

Kwate, N. A., & Myer, I. H. (2010). The myth of meritocracy and African American health. *American Journal of Public Health, 100*(10), 1831–1834.

Lee, C. C. (2005). Urban school counselors: Context, characteristics and competencies. *Professional School Counseling, 8*, 184–188.

Lindsey, M. A., Barksdale, C. L., Lambert, S. F., & Ialong, N. S. (2010). Social network influences on service use among urban, African American youth with mental health problems. *Journal of Adolescent Health, 47*, 367–373.

Mann, S. A., & Huffman, D. J. (2005). The decentering of second wave feminism and the rise of the third wave. *Science and Society, 69*(1), 56–91.

Mason, M. J. (2010). Mental health, school problems and social networks: Modeling urban adolescent use. *Journal of Primary Prevention, 31,* 321–331. doi: 10/1007/s10935-010-0227-3

Mason, M. J., & Korpela, K. (2009). Activity spaces and urban adolescent substance use and emotional health. *Journal of Adolescence, 32,* 925–939. doi: 10.1016/j.adolescence.2008.08.004

Miller, D. B., Webster, S. E., & MacIntosh, R. (2002). What's there and what's not: Measuring daily hassles in urban African American adolescents. *Research on Social Work Practice, 12*(3), 375–388.

Miller, J. (2008). *Getting played: African American girls, urban inequality, and gendered violence.* New York, NY: New York University Press.

Neblett, Jr., E. W., Terzian, M., & Harriot, V. (2010). From racial discrimination to substance abuse: The buffering effects of racial socialization. *Child Development Perspectives, 4*(2), 131–137. doi: 10.1111/.1750-8606.2010.00131.x

Pinto, K. C. (2004). Intersections of gender and age in health care: Adapting autonomy and confidentiality for the adolescent girl. *Qualitative Health Research, 14*(1), 78–99.

Santana, V., Almeida-Filho, N., Roberts, R., & Cooper, S. P. (2007). Skin colour, perception of racism and depression among adolescents in urban Brazil. *Child and Adolescent Mental Health, 12*(3), 125–131.

Schwartz, A. C., Bradley, R. L., Sexton, M., Sherry, A., & Ressler, K. J. (2005). Posttraumatic stress disorder among African Americans in an inner city mental health clinic. *Psychiatric Services, 56*(2), 212–215. doi: 10.1176/appi.ps.56.2.212

Schwinn, T. M., Schinke, S. P., & Trent, D. N. (2010). Substance use among late adolescent urban youths: Mental health and gender influences. *Addictive Behaviors, 35,* 30–34. doi: 10.1016/j.addbeh.2009.08.005

Seiffge-Krenke, I., Aunola, K., & Numi, J. (2009). Changes in stress perception and coping during adolescence: The role of situational and personal factors. *Child Development, 80*(1), 259–279.

Sherman, B. J., Duarte, C. S., & Verdeli, H. (2011). Internalizing and externalizing problems in adolescents from Bahia, Brazil. *International Journal of Mental Health, 40*(3), 55–76.

Shih, J. H., & Eberhart, N. K. (2010). Gender difference in the associations between interpersonal behaviors and stress generation. *Journal of Social and Clinical Psychology, 29*(3), 243–255.

Soffer, M. (2010). The role of stress in the relationships between gender and health-promoting behaviors. *Scandinavian Journal of Caring Services, 24*(3), 572–580.

Somerville, L. H., Jones, R. M., & Casey, B. J. (2010). A time of change: Behavioral and neural correlates of adolescent sensitivity to appetitive and aversive environmental cues. *Brain and Cognition,* 124–133. doi: 10.1016/j.bandc.2009.07.003

Sontag, L. M., & Graber, J. A. (2010). Coping with perceived peer stress: Gender-specific and common pathways to symptoms of psychopathology. *Developmental Psychology, 46*(6), 1605–1620. doi: 10.1037/a0020617

Thoit, P. A. (2010). Stress and health: Major findings and policy implications. *Journal of Health and Social Behavior, 51*(1), S41–S53.

Turner, S. G., Kaplan, C. P., & Badger, L. W. (2006). Adolescent Latinas' adaptive functioning and sense of well-being. *Journal of Women and Social Work, 21*(3), 272–281.

USAID (2013). *Who we are.* Retrieved from http://www.usaid.gov/who-we-are.

Valaitis, R. (2002). "They don't trust us: we're just kids." Views about community from predominantly female inner-city youth. *Health Care for Women International, 23,* 248–266.

van Mens-Verhulst, J., & Radtke, L. (2008). Intersectionality and mental health: A case study. *IST-travelling,* Retrieved from http://www.vanmens.info/verhulst/en/wp-content/INTERSECTIONALITY%20AND%20MENTAL%20HEALTH2.pdf

Vermunt, R., Peeters, Y., & Berggren, K. (2007). How fair treatment affects saliva cortisol release in stressed low and high type-A behavior individuals. *Scandinavian Journal of Psychology, 48,* 547–555. doi: 10.1111/j.1467-9450.2007.00593.x

Vermunt, R., & Steensma, H. (2001). Stress and justice in organizations. In R. Cropanzo (Ed.), *Justice in the workplace* (Vol. 2, pp. 34–43). Hillsdale, NJ: Lawrence Erlbaum.

Vermunt, R., & Steensma, H. (2003). Physiological relaxation: Stress reduction through fair treatment. *Social Justice Research, 16*(2), 135–149.

Weber, L., & Parra-Medina, D. (2003). Intersectionality and women's health: Charting a path to eliminating health disparities. *Advances in Gender Research, 7*(1), 181–230.

Williams, W. S., Karlin, T. K. & Wallace, D. (2012). Project SisterCircle: Risk, intersectionality and intervening in urban schools. *Journal of School Counseling, 10*(17). Retrieved from http://www.jsc.montana.edu/articles/v10n17.pdf

Chapter 3

Psychology, Sustainability, and Environmental Justice

Manuel Riemer and Courte Van Voorhees

SUSTAINABILITY AND ENVIRONMENTAL JUSTICE

We live in an era where environmental dilemmas are increasingly prominent in our psychological experience. Over the past 60 years human activities have changed our biosystem more rapidly and extensively than in any comparable period of history (IPCC, 2007; MEA, 2005). Daily realities increasingly force us to see the connections between environmental issues (e.g., pollution, climate change, energy crises, response to natural disasters, and urban planning) and psychological well-being. Our ability to cope with the results of global climate change, natural disasters, and other environmental issues is becoming increasingly important to psychological researchers and practitioners. James Gustave Speth, a former White House environmental advisor to U.S. president Jimmy Carter and distinguished leader in the environmental movement, rightly points out: "Today's environmental reality is linked powerfully with other realities, including growing social inequality and neglect and the erosion of democratic governance and popular control" (Speth, 2008, p. xi). Thus, in determining the right path to action, and for psychologists to contribute to this in a meaningful way, it is critical to fully explore the connections between these realities and find solutions that consider these complex interactions (Riemer & Schweizer-Ries, 2012).

In this chapter we explore the connection of psychology to environmental justice. We begin by contemplating the relationship of humans to nature followed by introducing the issues of environmental justice and sustainability. Then, we discuss important psychological questions and existing psychological research on environmental issues. We describe both the negative psychological impacts of environmental degradation and the positive effects of access to nature using an environmental justice lens. This is followed with an exploration of environmental action and how environmental justice can serve as an important motivator to engage people in environmental change. We conclude with suggestions for practice and future research.

Humans' Relationship to Nature

Koger and Winter (2010) argue that part of the reason we are approaching the limits of the earth's ability to sustain humans is that the dominant worldview of the industrialized societies "provides a set of beliefs that encourages people to use and abuse natural resources" (p. 36). These beliefs hold that people see themselves as separate from nature, which consists of inert, physical elements that humans can and should control and exploit for their personal gain. This differs drastically from most ancient and contemporary indigenous and some Eastern belief systems, which see humans as being embedded in nature in a complex and spiritual web of interconnections and unity (Agyeman, Cole, Haluza-DeLay, & O-Riley, 2009; Koger & Winter, 2010). In addition, this worldview has fostered an ideology of limitless economic growth that, in the last century, has been fueled and exacerbated by the dominance of capitalism, globalization, and more recently, the neoliberal policies of deregulation, privatization, and individualization of risk (Beck, 1992; Hossay, 2006; Kovel, 2007).

This ideology of limitless economic growth is accompanied by an increased urbanization that is further weakening the relationships between people and nature. Furthermore, increased individualization has eroded a sense of interdependency and left a spiritual void that many try to fill with increased consumption of material goods—an approach that is intentionally fueled by marketing for profit-driven global companies (Leonard, 2007; Putnam, 2000). By decreasing the sense of community and emphasizing the need for independence, more resources are needed because people are less likely to share their belongings (Putnam, 2000). The combination of the dominant worldview and the rise of individualism and materialism have created a world in peril that will not be able to sustain future generations. Human actions have created an unprecedented level of pollution and led to a changing climate that has the potential to create catastrophic consequences and human suffering far beyond what we are already observing today. This includes water shortages, starvation, mass migration, community interruptions, wars, and economic crises—to just name a few. These consequences are not equally distributed, however. What links environmental pollution and degradation to issues of social justice is that those who have already been marginalized by society suffer the most.

Environmental Justice

The links between environmental degradation and oppression are evidenced in unjust and uneven access to utilities and amenities, exposure to toxic and radioactive waste, responses to natural disasters, and more. Empirical literature displays widespread disparities in exposure to environmental hazards by race and class (Bullard, Mohai, Saha, & Wright, 2007). Experiences of these disparities have led to the emergence of the environmental justice (EJ) movement—although local movements predate the EJ movement and exist in many nations outside of the United States.

The U.S. EJ movement began in 1982 when communities in Warren County, North Carolina, began protesting the illegal dumping of toxic compounds along roadways (Agyeman, 2005). The polluted dirt was placed in an insufficiently built landfill surrounded by communities populated predominantly (69%) by people of color. The protests lasted for over 20 years without resolution until the landfill was finally designated a Superfund site by the EPA (North Carolina Department of Environmental and Natural Resources, 2004).

EJ literature often contrasts Warren County's toxic legacy with the Love Canal disaster in Niagara Falls, New York (see Agyeman, 2005; Bullard, 2005; Taylor, 2000). According to the U.S. EPA (2009) the Love Canal neighborhood was built over a waste site containing 21,000 tons of chemical waste that began to enter the water supply after heavy rains. This disaster resulted in birth defects and other health problems, eventually leading to the relocation of residents out of the neighborhood and President Carter's establishment of the Superfund program (U.S. EPA, 2009). The government reaction in this case came earlier and was more significant compared to the Warren County case. According to EJ proponents, the difference in reactions to Love Canal and Warren county can be attributed to class and race differences—although class differences are less pronounced in this comparison (Love Canal was predominantly working class) than in others. Although multiple factors make direct comparisons problematic, this disparity in response has had sufficient traction to propel EJ advocates to seek out other instances of environmental injustice.

EJ has evolved beyond activism—now encompassing its own research, action, theories, and methods. The EJ movement has gained federal recognition, resulting in Clinton's Environmental Justice Executive Order in 1994, which encouraged federal and state environmental agencies to take race and class into account when creating policies and granting permits for potential sources of pollution. Additionally, the U.S. EPA (2007) has adopted a definition of EJ as: "fair treatment for people of all races, cultures, and incomes, regarding the development of environmental laws, regulations, and policies" (p. 1).

In the 1970s, the mainstream environmental movement grew out of the more widespread acceptance of environmental degradation as a threat to human survival (Miller, 2006). Mainstream environmental groups that have since emerged have been slow in broadening their member base to include people of color and poor or working-class White people (Camacho, 1998). This lack of diversity may emerge from the different environmental issues faced by marginalized groups when compared to the affluent White people who traditionally populate environmental organizations. Springing from these differences, the EJ movement integrated mainstream environmental concerns (e.g., natural resource conservation) with related issues for people of color and those in poverty (e.g., health, local economy, education, housing, and urban land use) to form a more comprehensive vision of the human environment (Camacho, 1998). However, the mainstream environmental movement in North America has not adopted environmental justice issues significantly into its work (Haluza-DeLay & Fernhout, 2011). Ecofeminists have also pointed out specific environmental injustices experienced by women and have linked environmental problems to the patriarchal power structure of society (Mies & Vandana, 1993).

National studies of EJ in the United States reveal consistent disparities in exposure to environmental hazards by race and class (as separate, significant variables; Downey & Hawkins, 2008). Ringquist and Clark (1999) found that although there are notable exceptions, the vast majority of EJ studies show a clear relationship between toxic pollution sites and residents' race and income. The landmark 1987 *Toxic Wastes and Race in the United* States report and its 20th anniversary update determined that racial disparities in hazardous waste distribution are significant and growing (Bullard et al., & Wright, 2007, pp. x–xi). For example:

(1) More than 9 million people (9,222,000) live in circular host neighborhoods within three kilometers of the nation's 413 commercial hazardous waste facilities.
(2) Host neighborhoods of commercial hazardous waste facilities are composed of 56% people of color, whereas nonhost areas are composed of 30% people of color.
(3) Poverty rates in host neighborhoods are 1.5 times greater than nonhost neighborhoods (18% vs. 12%).

Defur et al. (2007) also demonstrate that cumulative risks from several environmental hazards over time may significantly increase vulnerability to future risk from environmental hazards. Additionally, vulnerability effects on wildlife and ecosystems are even less predictable.

EJ considerations have also been applied on an international scale to global climate change. In reviewing the empirical evidence on the likely consequences of global climate change, Rejendra K. Pauchauri, the chairman of the International Panel on Climate Change (IPCC), concludes that "it's the poorest of the poor in the world, and this includes poor people even in the prosperous societies, who are going to be the worst hit. . . . People who are poor are least-equipped to be able to adapt to the impact of climate change" (cited in Kanter & Revkin, 2007). In the 1980s and 1990s, a person in the developing world was 25 times more likely to be affected by a climate-related disaster than a person in a developed country; in the last decade that figure doubled to at least 50 times (World Bank, 2008). This stands in stark contrast to the fact that industrialized countries are responsible for 60 percent of the worldwide greenhouse gas emissions (Roberts & Park, 2007). Within industrialized countries, it is also lower-income groups who will be most affected, such as people living in substandard housing, small farmers, and people experiencing homelessness (Klein & Riemer, 2011). People who live on the street or in tents, for example, are more likely to be exposed to extreme weather situations—especially if there are sudden changes—such as a rainstorm or blizzard, and have less means to cope with the consequences (Wandel et al., 2010). It is exactly these extreme and sudden weather situations that are expected to become more likely with global climate change (IPCC, 2007).

Sustainability

With the growing realization of the threat of environmental destruction and global climate change, people have begun wondering about the ability of the biosystem to provide us with the resources needed to live a comfortable and satisfying life. Starting in the 1970s (e.g., United Nations Environment Programme, 1972) international efforts emerged to address these looming environmental threats and identify alternative lifestyles, societal structures (e.g., smart cities), and economic production that are less harmful to nature (Münger & Riemer, 2012). These local and international efforts comprise what is generally referred to as the sustainability movement.

Although there is no commonly agreed-upon definition of sustainability, the Brundtland Report's wording of " development that meets the needs of the present without compromising the ability of future generations to meet their own needs" (United Nations, 1987) seems to be the most popular guiding principle for the sustainability movement. It highlights the intra- and intergenerational justice aspect of sustainability, which generally include economic and social considerations. However, parties disagree on what type of change is needed and how much. On one end of the spectrum, the "technocentric" orientation advocates for adjustments to the existing system primarily through technological changes and individual behavior changes. On the other end of the spectrum are the advocates of a new environmental paradigm (Milbrath, 1989), who believe that a more radical cultural shift is needed, " one which represents fundamental rethinking of most patterns of human activity, which integrates ecological sustainability with social justice, and which sees sustainability as a promising metaphor for a historic and necessary structural and personal transformation" (Sterling, 1996, pp. 18–19; see also Münger & Riemer, 2012).

Within the context of the sustainability movement, psychology, as an academic and applied discipline, has primarily focused on developing approaches to pro-environmental behavior changes (e.g., recycling), such as community-based social marketing (McKenzie-Mohr, 2000). In a recent article Riemer and Schweizer-Ries (2012) argue that psychology could contribute a lot more to the emerging field of sustainability science but may be limited in doing so by disciplinary expectations and methodologies. This may be important to address as there is no shortage of relevant psychological questions in sustainability (as we will discuss next).

PSYCHOLOGY AND THE ENVIRONMENT

The issues of global climate change, environmental justice, and sustainability certainly have many psychological dimensions. Why do people tolerate the suffering of certain peoples from negative environmental impacts so that some can live a luxurious and comfortable life? What do people experience when the government decides to place a toxic waste site in their neighborhood? Why do some people conserve energy while others do not? These are just a few of many examples of questions that have psychological applications. Most types of psychological questions can be organized in the following categories: causes, impacts, and reactions to environmental change and injustice.

Regarding causes of environmental change and injustice, scholars have argued from very early on that the environmental crisis is a crisis of maladaptive behavior (Syme, Kals, Nacarrow, & Montada, 2000). This includes both individual behavior and political decision making. An example of a relevant psychological question about behavioral causes is: Why are humans continuing to pollute the environment at current levels even though the negative impacts of that behavior have been well established? Another example is: Why do people believe that it is acceptable to allow significant increases in pollution in an area that already experiences a high level of industrial pollution? In answering these questions it is useful to consider both the primary (e.g., the desire to consume) and secondary causes (e.g., capitalistic interests to link happiness to consumption).

Impacts of ecologically relevant behaviors and decisions can either be direct and immediate (e.g., the emotional reaction to a political decision perceived as unfair) or indirect and delayed (e.g., the loss of a loved one due to cancer caused by prolonged exposure to toxins). They can also be either positive (e.g., gaining public access to a forest area that was previously private) or negative (e.g., stress related to a prolonged drought). Relevant questions for psychologists include: What are the effects on mental well-being of feeling powerless about important environmental decisions? How do people cope when they become environmental refugees?

There are two main reactions to negative environmental impacts: one can either adapt to the situation or try to mitigate the causes of the problem. Of course, people can also do both. The following are examples of relevant psychological questions: Why do some people deny the negative impacts whereas others become environmental activists and fight the causes of the problem? What is the most effective way of motivating people to work collaboratively on mitigating the causes of global climate change? Is it more effective to motivate people to change by using marketing techniques or through consciousness raising? Only a small fraction of these and other relevant questions have been empirically investigated by psychologists.

Psychological Research on Environmental Issues

There has been a long tradition within psychology of exploring behavioral issues related to environmental degradation—especially since the foundation of the subfield of environmental psychology (Gifford, 2008). According to Gifford (2008), some psychological studies on energy conservation and other environmental issues date back over 40 years. There are several specialized journals (such as *The Journal of Environmental Psychology*, *Environment and Behavior*, *Umweltpsychologie*, and *Ecopsychology*), hundreds of individual journal articles in related journals, and many books on psychology and the environment. Most of this work focuses on using psychological research and theory to develop effective strategies aimed at individual, organizational, and community changes. There are many helpful reviews of this literature (see Harré, 2011; Koger & Winter, 2010; Moser & Dilling, 2007; Riemer, 2010; Schmuck & Schultz, 2002; Stern, 2000). Some of this research addresses the human causes of environmental degradation such as consumerism, lack of conservation, and the *tragedy of the commons*. This refers to a social dilemma made prominent by Hardin in 1968, wherein individuals acting independently and rationally according to their own short-term self-interest deplete a shared resource—despite their understanding that this is contrary to their long-term best interests.

Another area of research focuses on how people understand, perceive, and assess the risk of environmental issues such as global climate change. This research has contributed significantly to the understanding of how to communicate and frame environmental issues (Moser & Dilling, 2007). Another area of focus is the psychological impacts of pollution and environmental degradation and how people cope with them. The psychological benefits of nature are another area of psychological research. The majority of environmentally focused psychological research, however, has been aimed at finding effective ways of getting people to behave and act in pro-environmental and sustainable ways. This includes multiple theories of behavior change, research on changing attitudes, and investigation of specific behavior change strategies.

McKenzie-Mohr (2000) has developed an accessible and practical approach to encouraging pro-environmental behaviors called community-based social marketing (CBSM), which applies much of this research. CBSM is probably the most widely used application of psychology in environmental change practice. Some critics have noted that many of these psychology-informed behavior change strategies focus primarily on simple individual behaviors and appeal to the self-interest of the person (e.g., financial and social status gains) rather than challenging them to seek more complex and transformative methods of change (Dittmer & Riemer, 2013; Harré, 2011; Riemer, 2010; World Wildlife Fund, 2008). With some exceptions, connections to environmental justice are rare in this body of literature. This may be a significant limitation since some research suggests that people who are able to make connections between environmental issues and social justice are more likely to care for the environment and act sustainably. They are also more likely to go beyond simple individual behavior changes, as we will discuss later in this chapter.

PSYCHOLOGICAL IMPACTS OF ENVIRONMENTAL DEGRADATION

Psychologists have been studying stress and its impact on psychological and physical well-being for a long time. Stress is considered to be a " negative emotional experience accompanied by biochemical, physiological, cognitive, and behavioral changes that are directed toward altering the stressful event or accommodating to its effect" (Taylor & Sirois, 2009, p. 151). The negative emotional experience is typically connected to a stressor, that is, a stressful event, situation, or circumstance for the individual (e.g., loss of a loved one, violence of a partner, surgery, or an earthquake). Some stressors primarily affect individuals (e.g., surgery), whereas community stressors affect whole communities (e.g., an earthquake). Environmental stressors include forces or events in the human or natural environment that can cause a person to experience stress, such as excessive noise, air pollution, natural disasters, and overcrowding.

The most widely accepted stress models today are interactional models first proposed by Lazarus and further developed by Lazarus and Folkman (1984). In these models, stress is conceptualized as an interaction between characteristics of the stressor and characteristics of the individual. People's assessment of risk and their ability to cope is linked to social factors such as income and minority status. This is the case because these social factors are related to resources and social power, which are important in effectively coping with environmental threats (e.g., get the government to respond to a toxic accident).

The psychological consequences of stress have been described at four levels: the physiological level, the emotional level, the cognitive level, and the behavioral level (Vingerhoets, 2004). Examples of physiological impacts that have been linked to environmental stressors are headaches, neurological changes, somatization (i.e., physical symptoms such as pain and aches that are caused by mental and emotional stress and for which there is no other medical explanation) and fatigue. Examples of emotional impacts are anxiety, depression, fear, health worries, hopelessness, despair, and hostility. Behavioral consequences include stress behaviors such as smoking and alcohol consumption as well as sleeping problems. At the cognitive level, exposure to environmental stressors can significantly shift a person's normal life assumptions, causing long-term consequences for a person's well-being. Edelstein (2004) describes five important life assumptions for which that shift can occur: (1) a shift from health optimism to health pessimism, (2) a breakdown of the belief in a controllable and predictable world, (3) the association of home with feelings of fear and insecurity instead of a place of safety, (4) a shift from perceiving the environment as an abstract concept to it being a prominent and malevolent force, and (5) a loss of trust for others (e.g., the government).

Not all psychological consequences of environmental stressors result directly from the appraisal process described earlier. Even people who do not perceive the event, situation, or circumstance as stressful can still experience negative psychological consequences. For example, exposure to toxins and ongoing pollution can have significant negative impact on physical health, such as causing cancer (Brown, 2007). Similarly, extreme weather conditions connected with the changing climate can cause negative health impacts either through direct exposure or indirectly through reduced access to natural resources and nutrition (Smit & Wandel, 2006). Many of these negative health impacts can cause significant levels of stress. Environmental stressors can also cause collective consequences for families and communities that have been disrupted by dislocation or other resultant issues (Edelstein, 2004).

It has been a key mission of the EJ movement to demonstrate that these negative consequences are not evenly distributed. In the North American context, groups who are marginalized because of their income level or race are much more likely to live close to environmental stressors such as toxic waste disposal sites, heavily industrialized areas, and heavy traffic areas (as we have discussed earlier). Black children, for example, are five times more likely than White children to have lead poisoning, which is a significant environmental health threat to children in the United States (Bullard et al., 2007). The reasons for these developments are complex but can be linked to the fact that neighborhoods close to polluted areas are often more affordable to people with low incomes and these groups have less social power to advocate for their rights.

In the context of global climate change, Doherty and Clayton (2011) suggest that there are three classes of psychological impacts: direct (e.g., acute or traumatic effects of extreme weather events and a changed environment), indirect (e.g., threats to emotional well-being based on observation of impacts and concern or uncertainty about future risks);,and psychosocial (e.g., chronic social and community effects of heat, drought, migrations, and climate-related conflicts, and postdisaster adjustment). Responses, according to these authors, "include providing psychological interventions in the wake of acute impacts and reducing the vulnerabilities contributing to their severity; promoting emotional resiliency and empowerment in the context of indirect impacts; and acting at systems and policy levels to address broad psychosocial impacts" (p. 265). As we pointed out earlier, the impacts of global climate change, including these psychological ones, are not evenly distributed across and within countries, pointing to another link between psychology and environmental justice. It is important to note, however, that not only are the negative impacts of environmental degradation unequally distributed but also are the positive impacts of having access to nature.

PSYCHOLOGICAL BENEFITS OF ACCESS TO NATURE

There is a long tradition in Western and other cultures emphasizing the psychological and physical benefits of being close to nature. According to Kuo (2001) reports of the rejuvenating effects of spending time in natural settings have been found in the writings of philosophers (e.g., Thoreau), naturalists (e.g., Leopold), and landscape architects (e.g., Olmsted). Being in nature, and in some cases just viewing images of nature, has been found to have several positive psychological benefits, including reduced stress (Bell, Greene, Fisher, & Baum, 2001; Kaplan, 1995; Ulrich, Dimberg, & Driver, 1991), improved cognitive functioning (Bell et al., 2001; Kaplan, 1995), increased ability to manage life issues (Kaplan, 1995; Kaplan & Kaplan, 1989), and increased sense of community (Kuo, Sullivan, Coley, & Brunson, 1998). The stress reduction theory explains some of these effects from a functional evolutionary perspective, suggesting that humanity should have a " biologically prepared affiliation for certain restorative natural settings, but no such prepared response to urban environments since they have generally affected only a few generations of human experience" (Bell et al., 2001, p. 48). Another prominent theory, attention restoration theory, holds that the fascination experienced by restorative environments renews humanity's ability to consciously direct attention to the challenges of life (Kaplan, 1995; Kaplan & Kaplan, 1989).

If contact with nature has clear psychological (and physical) benefits, then an important ethical question is whether everybody has equal access to those benefits. In this context, it is useful to differentiate between access to public and private green space, since some research suggests that the benefits of public green space tend to be most pronounced in those areas where people have no or only little access to private green space, such as in dense urban areas (Mitchell & Popham, 2007). Within urban settings, higher-income and majority groups are more likely to own larger homes with private green space in their front- and backyards (Lefebvre, 2002). This picture might change, however, with the increased development of high-end condominiums in the inner-city core. People of color and people who live in poverty are more likely to live in substandard housing with less access to green spaces, and youth from these families have relatively limited access to greenways, sports fields, and trails (Strife & Downey, 2009). Traffic volume and air pollution are also more likely to be higher in low-income and minority neighborhoods, making it less attractive to spend time outdoors and lessening the positive impact on health (Houston, Wu, Ong, & Winer, 2004; Pastor, Sadd, & Morello-Frosch, 2002).

In conclusion, both the negative psychological impacts of environmental pollution and degradation and the benefits of access to nature are unequally distributed to the disadvantage of low-income and minority groups. For some, this injustice, as well as the intergenerational injustice of depleting natural resources and destroying the environment beyond sustainable levels, is a reason to act.

ENVIRONMENTAL ACTION

Clearly, significant action is needed to address these environmental issues. These actions can take on many different forms, such as government policies, technological advances, and lifestyle changes. At the individual level, Stern (2000) distinguishes among three types of environmentally significant behavior. Most psychological research has been focused on *private-sphere behaviors* such as recycling, household energy or water conservation, and transportation and food choices. These behaviors primarily reflect personal lifestyle choices and their impact is limited to the individual's environmental footprint. Although these behaviors may be motivated by environmental concerns, other motivators, such as saving money or gaining social status, can also drive them. *Non-activist behaviors in the public sphere*, however, are directly influenced by environmental concerns and include those environmental actions that take place in a public domain, but are not group-based. This includes support for public policies (e.g., financially contributing to an environmental organization) and active environmental citizenship actions such as writing letters to officials or signing petitions. Finally, *environmental activism* typically involves active involvement in organizations or groups that have an environmental focus and include activities such as lobbying the government and organizing a boycott. These types of actions and activities typically require significant effort and personal commitment and are targeted at transformative change at a systems level. Activities at this level have the capacity to impact the behavior and actions of many individuals, or the policy system as a whole (Stern, Dietz, Abel, Guagnano, & Kalof, 1999). Recently, Alisat and Riemer (2013) developed a psychometric scale to assess which of these types of environmental actions people engage in and how that may change over time, for example, after they attend an environmental workshop. Kenis and Mathijs (2012) point out that researchers who focus on the latter two types of actions (e.g., Clover 2002, 2003; Courtenay-Hall & Rogers 2002; Dittmer & Riemer, 2013; Harré, 2011; Hickman, Riemer, & Sayal, 2012; Jensen, 2002; Jensen & Schnack, 2006) often have different conceptions of power, appropriate goals for change, knowledge required for realizing change, and the root causes of the problem. A common criticism, according to Kenis and Mathijs (2012), is that traditional psychological behavior change strategies seem to consider people as passive objects to be conditioned and manipulated rather than taking them seriously as active agents of change, which is not surprising given the criticism of mainstream psychology more generally (e.g., Fox & Prilleltensky, 1997).

An important psychological question to ask in changing environmental behaviors is why people choose one type of behavior and action over another. The answer to this question is complex and is related to motivation, comprehension, action competence, self- and collective efficacy, and opportunity, among others (Hickman et al., 2012). People who are motivated to act because of their concern for harm, fairness, and social justice, and those with a more progressive political orientation seem to be more likely to favor stronger responses and engage in collective environmental action compared to those who are mostly driven by their own self-interests (Dawson & Thysen, 2012; Kenis & Mathijs, 2012; Koger & Winter, 2010). Also, people who have a more comprehensive understanding of the nature of the problem and its effects and root causes are more likely to engage in transformative action (Clover, 2002; Dittmer & Riemer, 2013; Montada & Kals, 2000). There is another important aspect to this transformative action, however, and that is having a vision and understanding of what an alternative to the status quo might be (Jensen, 2004; Kenis & Mathijs, 2012). Furthermore, most people lack the knowledge and skills to engage in effective collective actions (i.e., action competence), which becomes a significant deterrent to engage in those actions even if they are considered necessary (Jensen & Schnack, 2006). In contrast, many private-sphere behavior changes (e.g., starting to recycle) require relatively little knowledge and specialized skills and are primarily a matter of awareness, motivation, and available resources. The belief that a group or community can make a difference together and that one can personally contribute to that collective action (i.e., collective efficacy) is another determinant of what types of action people take (Lubell, 2002). Finally, concrete opportunities to connect with others who also engage in environmental action appear to be another factor in this complex decision-making process (Hickman et al., 2012; Quimby & Angelique, 2011). In our own multinational research, we are finding that using environmental justice as a guiding framework in combination with fostering system thinking, personal reflection, and action competence (as well as providing opportunities for sustained engagement) is a promising approach to engage young people in collective environmental action (Riemer, 2011).

In addition to the factors mentioned earlier, experiences of direct exposure to environmental harm or threat and experiences of environmental injustice can, by themselves, be significant motivators to take environmental action as a way of action-focused coping with the environmental stressor (Edelstein, 2004). In this context it is useful to consider the concept of empowerment. Empowerment is a process wherein people gain control over their lives and the processes of governance and decision making (Zimmerman & Rappaport, 1988). This is both a psychological and instrumental process that is necessary for citizen control toward social and environmental justice. Psychological empowerment refers to the belief in one's agency and is a critical factor in the motivation to take action whereas instrumental empowerment describes tangible gains in social power such as control over resources and key decisions. Rich, Edelstein, Hallman, and Wandersman (1995) modeled the process of empowerment as a reaction to environmental threats faced by communities.

IMPLICATIONS FOR FUTURE RESEARCH, PRACTICE, AND ACTION

The current global environmental crisis illustrates how environmental problems cannot be solved without understanding and addressing the complex interconnections with other societal realities such as social justice and civic participation. As we embark on developing strategies to move toward sustainability, it is critical to consider important psychological questions and link these to considerations of social justice as we have done in this chapter. Social change agents who want to apply psychological knowledge for their cause need to carefully evaluate what the underlying assumptions of that knowledge are. Are these psychological strategies following the same path as those that created the environmental problems in the first place (e.g., marketing focused on people's self-interests), which are likely to sustain the status quo, or are the strategies raising consciousness about the root causes of the problems and empowering individuals to take transformative collective actions?

Several important areas for future psychological research emerge. Many people struggle to take action because they are overwhelmed by the complexity of the issue and feel they have no control over the factors that are the primary causes of the problem. More research is needed to understand how to help people deal with this complexity and how to foster systems thinking. Theoretical frameworks such as the ecological model popular in developmental and community psychology (see Dittmer & Riemer, 2013, for an application to environmental engagement) as well as the development of action competence (Jensen & Schnack, 2006) are helpful in this context. Also, a narrative approach to understanding environmental justice (i.e., the personal account by somebody who has experienced environmental injustice firsthand) may be a powerful way to engage with this topic not only at a cognitive but also at an emotional level (Stovold, 2013). Furthermore, although the environmental education literature has produced an impressive body of knowledge on how to engage young people in formal education settings, much less is known about environmental engagement programs outside of that context (Riemer, Lynes, & Hickman, 2012). More research is also needed on how to create a shared vision that presents a joined orientation toward a true alternative to current societal models that are not sustainable and just (Jensen, 2004; Kenis & Mathijs, 2012; Kovel, 2007). A particular challenge here is to create a vision that is truly global, inclusive, and respectful to unique cultural contexts. In general, it is important to not look at environmental issues in isolation, but to make social justice an integral part of any solution or intervention that is considered. Psychologists need to carefully reflect on their role in addressing the environmental crisis and what role psychology may have played in creating it (e.g., by fostering consumerism through marketing). As a discipline that is heavily based on individualistic thinking, psychologists may have to reconsider the very ontological and epistemological foundation of the field. The root causes of environmental problems go deep into the social fabric of society and they are not going to be resolved with a few clever behavior change strategies. If psychologists can make this shift, then the field can make a major contribution to dealing with this crisis, because ultimately, the critical questions are inherently psychological.

REFERENCES

Agyeman, J. (2005). *Sustainable communities and the challenge of environmental justice.* New York, NY: New York University Press.

Agyeman, J., Cole, P., Haluza-Delay, R., & O-Riley, P. (Eds.) (2009). *Speaking for ourselves: Environmental justice in Canada.* Vancouver, CA: The University of British Columbia Press.

Alisat, S., & Riemer, M. (2013, submitted). *The environmental activities and actions scale: Development and psychometric evaluation.* Waterloo, ON: Wilfrid Laurier University.

Beck, U. (1992). *Risk society: Towards a new modernity.* New Delhi, India: Sage.

Bell, P. A., Greene, T. C., Fisher, J. D., & Baum, A. (2001). *Environmental psychology* (5th ed.). Fort Worth, TX: Harcourt College.

Brown, P. (2007). *Toxic exposures: Contested illnesses and the environmental health movement.* New York, NY: Columbia University Press.

Bullard, R. (2005). *The quest for environmental justice: Human rights and the politics of pollution.* San Francisco, CA: Sierra Club.

Bullard, R. D., Mohai, P., Saha, R., & Wright, B. (2007). *Toxic wastes and race at twenty 1987–2007: A report prepared for the United Church of Christ Justice & Witness Ministries.* Cleveland, OH: Justice and Witness Ministries, United Church of Christ.

Camacho, D. E. (1998). The environmental justice movement: A political framework. In D. E. Camacho (Ed.), *Environmental injustices, political struggles: Race, class, and the environment* (pp. 11–30). Durham, NC: Duke University Press.

Clover, D. (2002). Traversing the gap: Concientización, educative-activism in environmental adult education. *Environmental Education Research, 8*(3), 315–23.

Clover, D. (2003). Environmental adult education: Critique and creativity in a globalizing world. *New Directions for Adult and Continuing Education, 99,* 5–16.

Courtenay-Hall, P., & Rogers, L. (2002). Gaps in mind: Problems in environmental knowledge-behaviour modelling research. *Environmental Education Research, 8*(3), 283–297.

Dawson, S. L., & Tyson, G. A. (2012). Will morality or political ideology determine attitudes to climate change? *Australian Community Psychologist, 24*(2), 8–25.

Defur, P. L., Evans, G. W., Cohen Hubal, E. A., Kyle, A. D., Morello-Frosch, R. A., & Williams, D. R. (2007). Vulnerability as a function of individual and group resources in cumulative risk assessment. *Environmental Health Perspectives, 115,* 817–824.

Dittmer, L. D., & Riemer, M. (2013). Fostering critical thinking about climate change: Applying community psychology to an environmental education project with youth. *Global Journal of Community Psychology Practice, 4*(1). Available electronically at http://www.gjcpp.org/en/

Doherty, T. J., & Clayton, S. (2011). The psychological impacts of global climate change. *American Psychologist, 66*(4), 265–276. doi: 10.1037/a0023141

Downey, L., & Hawkins, B. (2008). Inequality in the United States. *Sociological Perspectives, 51,* 759–781.

Edelstein, M. R. (2004). *Contaminated communities: Coping with residential toxic exposure* (2nd ed.). Boulder, CO: Westview Press.

Fox, D., & Prilleltensky, I. (1997). *Critical psychology: An introduction*. London, UK: Sage.

Gifford, R. (2008). Psychology's essential role in alleviating the impacts of climate change. *Canadian Psychology/Psychologie Canadienne, 49*(4), 273–280.

Haluza-Delay, R., & Fernhout, H. (2011). Sustainability and social inclusion? Examining the frames of Canadian English-speaking environmental movement organizations. *Local Environment, 16*(7), 727–745.

Hardin, G. (1968). The tragedy of the commons. *Science, 162,* 1234–1248.

Harré, N. (2011). *Psychology for a better world*. Auckland, New Zealand: Department of Psychology, University of Auckland.

Hickman, G. M., Riemer, M., & Sayal, R. (2012). *Youth leading environmental change: Facilitator manual*. Waterloo, CA: Laurier Centre for Community Research, Learning and Action.

Hossay, P. (2006). *Unsustainable: A primer for global environmental and social justice*. London, UK: Zed Books.

Houston, D., Wu, J., Ong, P., & Winer, A. (2004). Structural disparities of urban traffic in Southern California: Implications for vehicle-related air pollution exposure in minority and high-poverty neighborhoods. *Journal of Urban Affairs, 26,* 565–592.

Intergovernmental Panel on Climate Change [IPCC]. (2007). *Summary for policymakers. In Climate change 2007: The physical science basis. Contribution of Working Group I to the Fourth Assessment Report of the Intergovernmental Panel on Climate Change.* S. Solomon, D. Qin, M. Manning, Z. Chen, M. Marquis, K. B. Averyt, M. Tignor, & H. L. Miller (Eds.), New York, NY: Cambridge University Press.

Jensen, B. B. (2002). Knowledge, action and pro-environmental behaviour. *Environmental Education Research, 8*(3), 325–34.

Jensen, B. B. (2004). Environmental and health education viewed from an action-oriented perspective: A case from Denmark. *Journal of Curriculum Studies, 36*(4), 405–425.

Jensen, B. B., & Schnack, K. (2006). The action competence approach in environmental education. *Environmental Education Research, 12*(3–4), 471–486.

Kanter, J., & Revkin, A. C. (2007, April 7). Scientists detail climate changes, poles to tropics. *The New York Times,* p. A1.

Kaplan, R., & Kaplan, S. (1989). *The experience of nature: A psychological perspective*. New York, NY: Cambridge University Press.

Kaplan, S. (1995). The restorative benefits of nature: Toward an integrative framework. *Journal of Environmental Psychology, 15,* 169–182.

Kenis, A., & Mathijs, E. (2012). Beyond individual behavior change: The role of power, knowledge and strategy in tackling climate change. *Environmental Education Research, 18*(1), 45–65.

Klein, K., & Riemer, M. (2011). Experiences of environmental justice and injustice in communities of people experiencing homelessness. *Ecopsychology, 3*(3), 195–204.

Koger, S. M., & Winter, D. D. (2010). *The psychology of environmental problems* (3rd ed.). New York, NY: Taylor & Francis, Psychology Press.

Kovel, J. (2007). *The enemy of nature: The end of capitalism or the end of the world?* Blackpoint, NS: Fernwood.

Kuo, F. E. (2001). Coping with poverty: Impacts of environment and attention in the inner city. *Environment and Behavior, 33*(1), 5–34.

Kuo, F. E., Sullivan, W. C., Coley, R. L., & Brunson, L. (1998). Fertile ground for community: Inner-city neighborhood common spaces. *American Journal of Community Psychology, 26*(6), 823–851.

Lazarus, R. S., & Folkman, S. (1984). *Stress, appraisal, and coping.* New York, NY: Springer.

Lefebvre, S. (2002). Housing: An income issue. *Perspectives on Labour and Income: The online edition, 3*(6). Retrieved from http://www.statcan.gc.ca/pub/75-001-x/00602/8442-eng.html

Leonard, A. (2007). *Story of stuff, referenced and annotated script.* Retrieved from http://www.storyofstuff.com

Lubell, M. (2002). Environmental activism as collective action. *Environment and Behavior, 34*(4), 431–454.

McKenzie-Mohr, D. (2000). Promoting sustainable behavior: An introduction to community-based social marketing. *Journal of Social Issues, 56,* 543–554.

Mies, M., & Vandana S. (1993). *Ecofeminism.* Halifax, CA: Fernwood.

Milbrath, L. (1989). *Envisioning a sustainable society: Learning our way out.* Albany, NY: SUNY Press.

Millennium Ecosystems Assessment [MEA]. (2005). *Ecosystems and human well-being: Current state and trends: Findings of the condition and trends working group of the millennium ecosystem assessment* (Vol. 2). Washington, DC: Island Press.

Miller, G. T. Jr. (2006). *Sustaining the earth: An integrated approach* (8th ed.). London, UK: Brooks/Cole.

Mirabelli, M. C., Wing, S., Marshall, S. W., & Wilcosky, T. C. (2006). Race, poverty, and potential exposure of middle-school students to air emissions from confined swine feeding operations. *Environmental Health Perspectives, 114,* 591–596.

Mitchell, R., & Popham, F. (2007). Greenspace, urbanity and health: Relationships in England. *Journal of Epidemiological Community Health, 61,* 681–683. doi: 10.1136/jech.2006.053553

Montada, L., & Kals, E. (2000). Political implications of psychological research on ecological justice and proenvironmental behaviour. *International Journal of Psychology, 35*(2), 168–176.

Moser, S. C., & Dilling, L. (Eds.) (2007). *Creating a climate for change: Communicating climate change and facilitating social change.* New York, NY: Cambridge University Press.

Münger, F., & Riemer, M. (2013). Sustainability. *Encyclopedia of Critical Psychology.* Retrieved from http://www.springerreference.com/docs/navigation.do?m=Encyclopedia+of+Critical+Psychology+%28Behavioral+Science%29-book162#Encyclopedia+of+Critical+Psychology+%28Behavioral+Science%29-book162-rS

North Carolina Department of Environment and Natural Resources, Division of Waste Management. (2004). *Warren County PCB landfill fact sheet.* Retrieved from http://www.wastenotnc.org/WarrenCo_Fact_Sheet.htm

Pastor, M., Sadd, J. L., & Morello-Frosch, R. (2002). Who's minding the kids? Pollution, public schools, and environmental justice in Los Angeles. *Social Science Quarterly, 83,* 263–280.

Putnam, R. D. (2000). *Bowling alone: The collapse and revival of American community.* New York, NY: Touchstone.

Quimby, C. C., & Angelique, H. (2011). Identifying barriers and catalysts to fostering pro-environmental behavior: Opportunities and challenges for community psychology. *American Journal of Community Psychology, 47,* 388–396.

Rich, R. C., Edelstein, M., Hallman, W. I., & Wandersman, A. H. (1995). Citizen participation and empowerment: The case of local environmental hazards. *American Journal of Community Psychology, 23,* 657–676.

Riemer, M. (2010). Community psychology, the natural environment, and global climate change. In G. Nelson & I. Prilleltensky (Eds.), *Community psychology: In pursuit of liberation and well-being* (2nd ed., pp. 498–516). New York, NY: Palgrave.

Riemer, M. (Chair) (2011). Engaging young people in political and community activism: Opportunities and challenges. Symposium conducted at the biennial conference of the Society for Community, Research, and Action, Chicago, Illinois. June 15–18, 2011.

Riemer, M., Lynes, J., & Hickman, G. (2013). Engaging youth in environmental change. A model for developing and assessing youth-based environmental engagement programmes. *Journal of Environmental Education Research.* Retrieved from http://www.tandfonline.com/eprint/YKX8yiej74riJE382C9k/full. doi: 10.1080/13504622.2013.812721

Riemer, M., & Schweizer-Ries, P. (2012). Complexity, normativity, and transdisciplinarity: Is psychology ready to meet the sustainability challenges? *Umweltpsychologie, 16*(1), 143–165.

Ringquist, E. J., & Clark, D. H. (1999). Local risks, states' rights, and federal mandates: Remedying environmental inequities in the U.S. federal system. *Publius, 29,* 73–93.

Roberts, J. T., & Park, B. C. (2007). *A climate of injustice.* Cambridge, MA: MIT Press.

Schmuck, P., & Schultz, W. P. (Eds.). (2002). *Psychology of sustainable development.* Boston, MA: Kluwer Academic.

Smit, B., & Wandel, J. (2006). Adaptation, adaptive capacity and vulnerability. *Global Environmental Change, 16*(3), 282–292.

Speth, J. G. (2008). *The bridge at the edge of the world: Capitalism, the environment, and crossing from crisis to sustainability.* New Haven, CT: Yale University Press.

Sterling, S. (1996). Education in change. In J. Huckle & S. Sterling (Eds.), *Education for sustainability* (pp. 18–39). London, UK: Earthscan.

Stern, P. C. (2000). Toward a coherent theory of environmentally significant behavior. *Journal of Social Issues, 56*(3), 407–424.

Stern, P. C., Dietz, T., Abel, T., Guagnano, G. A., & Kalof, L. (1999). A value-belief-norm theory of support for social movements: The case of environmental concern. *Human Ecology Review, 6,* 81–97.

Stovol, A. (2013). *The power of the narrative approach in facilitating students' learning about environmental justice.* Unpublished honour thesis. Waterloo, ON: Wilfrid Laurier University.

Strife, S., & Downey, L. (2009). Childhood development and access to nature: A new direction for environmental inequality research. *Organ Environment, 22*(1), 99–122.

Syme, G. J., Kals, E., Nancarrow, B. E., & Montada, L. (2000). Ecological risks and community perceptions of fairness and justice: A cross-cultural model. *Risk Analysis, 20*(6), 905–916.

Taylor, D. (2000). The rise of the environmental justice paradigm. *American Behavioral Scientist, 43,* 508–580.

Taylor, S. E., & Sirois, F. M. (2009). *Health psychology* (Canadian ed.). Toronto, ON: McGraw-Hill.

Ulrich, R. S., Dimberg, U., & Driver, B. L. (1991). Psychophysiological indicators of leisure benefits. In B. L. Driver, P. J. Brown, & G. L. Peterson (Eds.), *Benefits of leisure* (pp. 73–89). State College, PA: Venture.

United Nations. (1987). Our common future, from one earth to one world. Retrieved from http://www.un-documents.net/ocf-ov.htm#1.2

United Nations Environment Programme. (1972). Report of the United Nations conference on the environment. Retrieved from http://www.unep.org/Documents. multilin gual/ Default.asp?DocumentID=97

United States Environmental Protection Agency. (2007). *Definition of environmental justice.* Retrieved from http://www.epa.gov/osw/EJ/

United States Environmental Protection Agency. (2009). *Fact sheet—Love Canal decision.* Retrieved from http://www.epa.gov/history/topics/lovecanal/06.htm

Vingerhoets, A. (2004). Stress. In A. Kaptein & J. Weinman (Eds.), *Health psychology* (pp. 113–140). Malden, MA: Blackwell.

Wandel, J., Riemer, M., de Gómez, W., Klein, K., de Schutter, J., Randall, L., . . . Singleton, C. (2010). *Homelessness and global climate change: Are we ready? A report from the study on the vulnerability to global climate change of people experiencing homelessness in Waterloo Region.* Waterloo, ON.

World Bank. (2008). *Environment.* Retrieved from http://web.worldbank.org/WBSITE/EXTERNAL/TOPICS/ENVIRONMENT/0,contentMDK:20118248~menuPK:4366001~pagePK:210058~piPK:210062~theSitePK:244381,00.html

World Wildlife Fund [WWF]. (2008). *Weathercocks and signposts: The environment movement at crossroads.* Retrieved from http://www.wwf.org.uk/strategiesforchange

Zimmerman, M. A., & Rappaport, J. (1988). Citizen participation, perceived control, and psychological empowerment. *American Journal of Community Psychology, 16,* 725–750.

Chapter 4

Social Justice, Human Dignity, and Mental Illness: A Psychological Perspective Informed by Personalist Ethics

Brent Dean Robbins and Harris L. Friedman

Much of the discipline of psychology focuses on mental illness (e.g., clinical psychology is its largest subdiscipline; Bruno, 2002). Increasingly, however, mental illness is often portrayed in a reductionistic way as being only a brain disease, whereas alternatives to the medical model of mental illness are hardly discussed. Such a biological reductionism privileges some and penalizes others, and it obfuscates the many social justice implications of how mental illness can be best understood and treated. Even psychologists who are on the frontline of mental health service delivery often have little awareness of the important social justice underpinnings related to their profession. Consequently, our chapter addresses some themes related to the interface of social justice and mental illness for psychologists. By drawing upon the insights of existential personalist ethics, we will argue that the concept of human dignity provides an important basis upon which to critically evaluate the ethics of diagnosis and treatment in a way that serves social justice for mental health consumers.

MENTAL ILLNESS IS NOT EQUAL OPPORTUNITY

Mental health problems are widely linked to discrimination due to social class, race, sexual orientation, and other variables that are not biological in nature (e.g., Feinstein, Goldfried, & Danila, 2012; Fuller-Rowell, Evans, & Ong, 2012; Pieterse, Todd, Neville, & Carter, 2012). For example, the poor and disadvantaged are more likely to develop mental illness, a fact supported by numerous studies (e.g., Boe, Overland, Lundervold, & Hysing, 2012; Santigo, Kaltman, & Miranda, 2012; Turney, Kissane, & Edin, 2013; Yoshikawa, Abert, & Beardslee, 2012), whereas decreases in the level of poverty in populations at high risk for developing mental illness, such as African American women and adolescent girls, relate to prevention of mental illness (e.g., Osypuk et al., 2012; Turney et al., 2013). This literature suggests that more than just biological causes are involved in mental illness, and many of these are core social justice issues, such as poverty and discrimination.

One dynamic related to social justice and mental illness involves labeling and its resulting stigmatization. Although anyone given a mental illness label is subject to stigmatization, this is exacerbated for members of disadvantaged groups who already carry the burden of discrimination. The labeling process introduces both social and self-stigmatization, which can further hinder mental health, well-being, and recovery (Ilic et al., 2013; Wahl, 2012). Biological, and even genetic, explanations of mental illness are increasing, which places members of minority groups who are already subject to discrimination at especially high risk of being stigmatized from labeling (Angermeyer, Holzinger, Carta, & Schomerus, 2011; Read, 2007; Read, Haslam, Sayce, & Davies, 2006). Stigma resulting from presumed genetic causes in particular can reinforce negative group stereotypes, as well as exacerbate individual prejudice and discrimination. For example, those labeled as mentally ill are often perceived to be more dangerous, resulting in other people being more likely to distance themselves socially from the labeled person (Wahl, 2012).

In addition, although psychotherapy can be helpful to those suffering from mental distress, even when they are coming from conditions of poverty (Santigo et al., 2012), and neuroleptic forms of medications have been found to reduce various psychiatric symptoms associated with psychosis, a growing body of evidence suggests that long-term and overuse of neuroleptics may create unnecessary risk of long term, iatrogenic disability in clients who might otherwise recover without medical intervention, or with short-term medical interventions (Centorrino et al., 2004; Frances, 2010a, 2010b; Gianfrancesco, Grogg, Mahmoud, Wang, & Nasrallah, 2002; Leung, Barr, Procyshyn, Honer, & Pang, 2012; Robbins, 2012; Robbins, Higgins, Fisher, & Over, 2011; Rummel-Kluge et al., 2010, 2012; Whitaker, 2010, 2012; Wunderink, Nieboer, Wiersma, Syterra, & Nienhuis, 2013). However, poorer individuals, due to the high cost of personalized care involved in psychotherapy, are much more likely to receive medications only for mental health concerns (Stewart, 2009), and they are more likely than others to be placed on anitpsychotics (Crystal, Olfson, Huang, Pincus, & Garhard, 2009; Marrdani, Tu, Austin, & Alter, 2002; Zito, Burcu, Ibe, Safer, & Madger, 2013). The facts laid out thus far paint a picture that suggests a dangerous pattern. Culturally and socially disenfranchised individuals and groups—the poor and victims of discrimination—are at higher risk of mental distress and are more likely to be treated with medications of dubious worth and likely iatrogenic side effects. And, when mental distress is explained in medicalizing terms as if solely caused by internal biological and genetic vulnerabilities, this labeling may serve to increase, rather than mitigate, stigma for these individuals and groups. Worse still, even when social context may best explain the mental distress of the disenfranchised person, medical explanations tend to imply that causal attributions should apply within the individual, which in effect blames the victim for his or her social victimization. Such internalized biological and genetic attributions, in turn, tend to be treated with biological interventions, such as medications, which come with a variety of risks of their own, including potentially debilitating side effects and the possibility of long-term disability. This vicious cycle identified, which involves the shift from social disenfranchisement to medical label to long-term disability, demonstrates how mental health is a social justice issue.

PERSONALIST ETHICS

Science alone is insufficient for addressing these matters; critical thinking within the extra-scientific field of ethics is also required to consider the weighty moral implications of the application of mental health concepts in clinical practice. Although a variety of ethical theories have relevance to the questions raised by these facts, we focus on an approach to ethics that emerges from the field of existential personalism and that is informed by an integration of traditions that include existentialism, phenomenology, and neo-Thomist metaphysics (Dahlstrom, 1987; Williams & Bengtsson, 2009).

Our analysis is particularly indebted to the philosophical foundation for personalist ethics developed by Thomas D. Williams (2005), Karol Wojtyla (Woznicki, 1980), Max Scheler (1973; Frings, 1997) and exemplified in the social activism and writings of Martin Luther King Jr. (Burrow, 2006; Steinkraus, 1973). As the lead author has argued elsewhere, this personalist ethical worldview, from a historical perspective, was especially influential on the emergence of the Third Force, or humanistic psychology, in mid-20th-century American psychology (Robbins, 2013), and is in need of further explicit articulation and refinement. Although a philosophical defense of personalist ethics and its concept of human dignity are beyond the scope of this chapter, those seeking in-depth arguments for this perspective are referred especially to Thomas D. Williams' (2005) book, *Who Is My Neighbor? Personalism and the Foundations of Human Rights* and John F. Crosby's (1996) *The Selfhood of the Human Person*. For the purpose of this chapter, we will provide only a brief sketch of the theory of human dignity, but we do encourage the interested reader to seek these texts for the systematic philosophical arguments that provide the conceptual foundation for this ethical worldview. It should be noted that, when the term *dignity* as a concept is used in this personalist context, the meaning may differ from certain common sense understandings of the word, and therefore it should be appreciated to have a well-defined technical meaning that must be understood primarily within the context of this philosophical tradition with ancient roots.

A central concept of existential personalist ethics is the notion of human dignity. It was in no small part due to the influence of French personalist and neo-Thomist, Jacques Maritain (Maritain, 2012), that the United Nations Declaration of Human Rights founded universal human rights on the cornerstone of human dignity (Glendon, 2002; Joas, 2013). Article I of the Declaration states, "All human beings are born free and equal in dignity and rights. They are endowed with reason and conscience and should act towards one another in a spirit of brotherhood." When the Human Rights Commission founded its declaration on the concept of dignity, it did so knowing that it had yet to flesh out a commonly agreed upon definition of what dignity means and where it comes from (Glendon, 2005). Some have even suggested that the notion of dignity is an outmoded philosophical concept without grounds (Macklin, 2003; McCrudden, 2008)—an attitude that literally risks undermining the very foundations of universal human rights (Robbins, 2013). Personalism provides an answer to the question of human dignity. In one of the most mature expressions of personalism, Williams (2005) defined it as "the inherent value of the person, as 'someone' and not merely 'something.' . . . Every person without exception, therefore, is of inestimable worth, and no one is dispensable or interchangeable" (pp. 118–119).

Psychologically, one way to illustrate the concept of dignity is through the psychology of interpersonal loss. For example, after the death of a child from cancer, researchers identified in families of the victims an "empty space phenomenon" (McClowry, Davies, May, Kulenkamp, & Martinson, 1987). Even seven to nine years after the death of the child, the parents and siblings of the deceased child continued to experience the gravity of the loss, and this center of gravity was felt as the vacuum left by the deceased child's death. A similar phenomenon has been identified in love relationships (Kadlac, 2012; Robbins, 2013). When another person is loved, it has been suggested, the love is not for the person's characteristics, but for the irreplacebility of the person him- or herself (Kadlac, 2012).

These powerful examples of human experiences demonstrate concretely how a particular person's dignity is given through relationships of love and attachments to others, who bear witness to the revelation that the beloved person is indispensable and irreplaceable, and therefore a person who is of inestimable worth. It is important to emphasize here that being loved does not result in the dignity of the person, but when a person is loved, the quality of dignity in the other person becomes more salient than it might otherwise be, for example, by contrast, in state of indifference or hatred. In other words, agape love provides a hermeneutic organ of perception by which the dignity of a person can stand forth more clearly than might otherwise be the case (Robbins, 2013). In ways that might anticipate the ethical phenomenology of the French philosopher Emmanuel Levinas (1969), the dignity of the other could literally be said to be infinite in the sense that it is beyond calculation or exchange (Robbins, 2013). This infinite, nonquantifiable, nonreducible, nonexchangeable, irreplaceable quality of the person is what we call that person's dignity.

The etymology of the word dignity is revealing. The word *dignity* comes from the Old French, *dignite*, which means dignity, privilege, honor, which in turn derives from the Latin, *dignitatum*, meaning worthiness or *dignus*, worth. The Latin root is *decus*, or grace (Harper, 2013). Thus dignity is to be graced—literally to be given gratuitously, without merit or without earning it—a value or worth. Thus, a dignitary is one who has special rank or is given honor. Within personalist ethics, in keeping with the most primordial roots of the word, dignity is understood as a blessing that is given to all persons without merit because it is intrinsic to personhood. To emerge into the world as a human being is always to call others to an obligation to witness to one's dignity. This is not to say that a person's dignity cannot be violated; indeed, of course, it can. However, assaults on the dignity of others appear to require that the personhood of the individual is denied or repressed, through dehumanization and objectification of the person, perhaps in order for the victimizer to assuage his or her guilt (Bastian, Jelten, & Radke, 2012; Rudman & Mescher, 2012; Wall & Monahan, 2011).

THE STRUCTURAL POLARITY OF DIGNITY AND STIGMA

The problem of stigma, and its relationship to the labeling of mental illness, can be illuminated through the personalist theory of dignity. The concept of *stigma* was originally developed by sociologist Erving Goffman (1963) to describe attributes of persons that serve to discredit and reduce the person to a tainted and discounted identity. Corrigan (2004) identified stereotyping, prejudice, and discrimination as integral to the definition of stigma. To stigmatize a person is to mark that person in a way that, through stereotyping, associates the person to undesirable characteristics that discredit him or her as a person. Variations in the impact of stigma are linked to dimensions such as the extent to which the stigmatized identity can be concealed, how much the stigmatizing identity disrupts a person's interpersonal relationships, the type of aesthetic reactions (e.g., disgust) aroused in others by the stigmatizing identity, the perceived causes or origins of the stigmatizing identity, the extent to which the course of the stigmatizing identity is seen to be reversible, and the perceived danger or peril associated with the stigmatized identity (Jones et. al., 1984).

It is clear from these definitions that stigma involves a reduction of status or perceived worth or value of the person in the eyes of others and as a result of self-stigmatization, a reduction in the sense of perceived self-worth. Thus, stigma and dignity can be seen to be in polar tension: whereas dignity bears witness to the unconditional and intrinsic worth of the person, stigmatizing identities through stereotyping, prejudice, and discrimination threaten to dehumanize a person by concealing his or her intrinsic dignity.

The process of dehumanization through stigma seems to follow a typical pattern (Link & Phelan, 2001; Link, Yang, Phelan, & Collins, 2004). First, the individual is labeled as different in some way, and then, second, negative stereotypes are associated with the label. By virtue of the label, the person is subject to social distancing by being placed in the category of "other" or as one of "them" over and against "us." The consequence of the stigma and social distancing includes a loss of status (i.e., perceived value and worth; perceived dignity). The victimization by this type of stigmatization is influenced and driven by groups with social, economic, and political power against those without equivalent power (Link & Phelan, 2001). The stigmatization further disempowers the stigmatized groups and individuals.

EUGENICS AS A STIGMATIZING ASSAULT ON HUMAN DIGNITY IN THE HISTORY OF PSYCHIATRY

The link between psychiatric diagnosis and stigmatization of disenfranchised groups is quite evident in the history of psychiatry over the past several centuries. For example, in a dark period of psychiatric history in the early 20th century, psychiatry was very influenced by the eugenics movement (Black, 2003; Robbins, 2012; Whitaker, 2002). Eugenics was a movement that began in the late 1800s. It was influenced by the ideas of Thomas Malthus and Charles Darwin, as well as by selective breeding in the farming of plants and animals (Whitaker, 2002). At that time—the dawn of the Industrial Age—populations within urban areas were swelling at breakneck speed, and it became increasingly difficult to feed these populations. It took government intervention and strategic planning to find ways to innovate farming in order to be able to feed the growing and hungry masses. Selective breeding of crops and farm animals allowed farmers to maximize the potential of the land so that it could feed many more people than had previously been conceived. Selective breeding was so successful, many powers-that-be began to raise the question: if selective breeding can be beneficial with crops and farm animals, why not apply this new technology to shape the genetic future of the human species? This was the birth of eugenics.

Those who began to study eugenics took it that the human population can be separated into two genetic classes—the eugenic, or those who were deemed to have fit genes that should be perpetuated into the future, and the cacogenic, or those who were condemned as having ill-fit genes that were believed to be toxic to the future health of the human species (Whitaker, 2002). Given that rich, White, Anglo-Saxon males were the ones with wealth, power, and influence, it was predictable that, of course, they deemed themselves to be the ones who were fittest, and anyone who threatened their power was conveniently situated on the cacogenic side of the eugenic divide. Those deemed cacogenic at this time included Blacks, immigrants, criminals, the poor, the mad, the disabled, the mentally retarded, those with drug and alcohol addiction, and gays and lesbians, among others (Black, 2003). The eugenic movement viewed individuals in these social classes as persons who were victimized by disease that must be cured by eliminating these people from the population, whether through segregation, sterilization, or extermination.

Few people will be ignorant of the fact that the eugenics project came to its fullest realization with the Final Solution of Hitler and the Nazis in World War II Germany. What many do not realize, however, is that it was in fact America that led the international movement toward eugenics, and it was only because of America's example of putting eugenics successfully into practice that Hitler was able to persuade the Germans that their own eugenics project was the way to go (Black, 2003). The end product of eugenics in Nazi Germany was the death of somewhere between 11 and 17 million human beings—6 million Jews (a quarter of them children under 15), about 270,000 Gypsies, 3.3 million Soviet POWs, 2 million non-Jewish Poles, 250,000 disabled, 15,000 homosexuals, and many others (Whitaker, 2002). Those who were targeted first were those who were considered to be mentally unfit—the mad and the mentally retarded. These unfortunate individuals were corralled into rooms, and succumbed to exhaust fumes (the tail pipes of trucks had been connected by hoses to vents in the room). The result was the first mass killings by the Nazis (Whitaker, 2002). How could this happen?

In America, the eugenics movement was funded by big money: Andrew Carnegie, John D. Rockefeller, and the widow of Edward Harriman (Black, 2003). At this time, for example, Victoria Woodhull stated, "Imbeciles, criminals, paupers, and the otherwise unfit . . . must not be bred," and supported the forced sterilization of American citizens (Whitaker 2010, p. 46). Charles Davenport, a Harvard-trained biologist, was appointed head of the Eugenics Record Office on Long Island, and Davenport and his team of heavily funded researchers began to investigate and maintain files on family lines in the general population who they considered to have defective genes (Black, 2003). Meanwhile, money and influence was used to manipulate politicians and judges in order to make eugenics legal and to put it into practice.

Connecticut has the dubious distinction of being the first state to ban marriage among those deemed unfit. By 1914, more than 20 states had followed in the footsteps of Connecticut, and by 1933, every single state in the union had fallen into line. At this time, those deemed to be disabled or unfit were segregated into populations in order to prevent them from reproducing in the general population. These asylums were later rationalized to be treatment centers rather than the concentration camps they were originally intended to be. Between 1907 and 1927, the United States had victimized over 8,000 people with eugenic sterilization so that they could never again reproduce (Whitaker, 2002).

California took the evil of involuntarily sterilization to the level of an art form. Faced with the problem that involuntarily sterilization is a form of medical intervention that is intended to harm—that is, intended to destroy the ability to procreate—it was in violation of the Hippocratic Oath to "do no harm." To remedy this problem, California medical doctors quickly rationalized their behavior by claiming their eugenics project was actually a form of treatment that would cure patients of their mental illness (Whitaker, 2002). In the case of *Buck v. Bell*, the U.S. Supreme Court upheld the "right" of California to sterilize its own citizens in an 8–1 decision in 1927 (Black, 2003).

The American eugenics project, with the backing of the U.S. Supreme Court and support from the huge pockets of the robber barons, inspired European nations to initiate their own eugenics programs. Soon, Denmark, Norway, Sweden, Finland, and Iceland were sterilizing citizens the elite deemed to be unfit according to their classist, xenophobic, sexist, and racist standards (Whitaker, 2002). It was only later that Hitler came to power and used these movements to initiate Germany's own eugenics program, which took the American eugenics project to its logical conclusion with the extermination of those deemed unfit. No public outcry against the Nazi extermination of the disabled could be heard. In fact, American publications from *The New England Journal of Medicine* to *The New York Times* sang Hitler's praises as "progressive" for his "humane" extermination of "unfortunates" (Black, 2003).

The stigma linking marginalized groups to psychiatric labeling led to a systematic program of segregating those deemed mentally ill from the rest of the population (Whitaker, 2002). The new state hospitals were often justified on the grounds that segregation of the mentally ill from the rest of the population would serve eugenic ends. The horrible conditions and barbaric treatments of the state hospitals were the stuff of nightmares, and eventually led to public outcry for reform. When Walter Freeman introduced the lobotomy to this population, it was seen as a possible solution to this crisis, a potential "cure" in the eyes of the mass media. In reality, as we know, Freeman's lobotomies were little more than targeted brain damage (El-Hai, 2007). Although many of Freeman's colleagues were privately scandalized, no one spoke out against him. The fact that he was allowed to treat patients in mass with an assembly line approach to brain surgery of the mentally ill is a sign of just how stigmatized mental health patients had become. The image of the lobotomist puncturing the brain through the periphery of the eye of the patient, even young children, is perhaps one of the most tragic images of 20th century's assault on the dignity of the psychiatric patient.

After World War II, in the public perception, eugenics became too easily associated with Hitler, and so there was a major retreat from the language and logic of eugenics among elites, politicians, and intellectuals. The language of eugenics shifted to the language of genetics, although often these fields were not too far apart in practice (Black, 2003). Despite the public retreat from a eugenics discourse, the link between disenfranchised groups and psychiatric labeling continued to have strong, lingering effects.

Jonathan Metzl (2011) conducted in-depth research on the records of patients at Iona State Mental Hospital outside of Detroit, Michigan. His investigation unearthed some fascinating results about the patterns of diagnosis in the hospital records of patients and how they shifted over the course of the 20th century. In the early part of the century, peaking at the time of the women's suffrage movement, the label of schizophrenia tended to be applied to women of the hospital, often women involuntarily committed by their husbands who viewed their partners as dysfunctional in their duties as housewives. The criteria for schizophrenia used by clinicians tended to be tailored to this particular population. However, by the 1960s, and peaking during the height of the civil rights movements, especially the emergence of race riots and the Black Power movement, Iona State Hospital saw a massive influx of Black males into the state hospital systems. In results of the data analysis that can only be described as chilling, Metzl (2011) found that not only were Black men arrested and diagnosed with schizophrenia in unprecedented numbers during this time, in fact the diagnostic criteria for schizophrenia shifted to better confirm (and perhaps to justify) the involuntary and indefinite commitment of these Black men to the prison of the state hospital. In the meantime, the female population that would have traditionally been labeled as schizophrenic was suddenly overnight diagnosed instead with depression.

These historical patterns in Iona State Hospital illustrate in a powerful way the vicious cycle of stigmatization discussed at the start of this chapter. First, a disenfranchised group, lacking in power and challenging the status quo, is stigmatized in public perception through stereotypes, prejudice, and discrimination, and then oppressive practices, such as involuntary imprisonment and abusive treatment, are justified under the guise of medical care. A psychiatric label, typically schizophrenia, seemed to be the label of choice to effectively silence a subculture or marginalized group, women, or Black males, for example, who for whatever reason served to threaten the status quo. To this day, a disproportionate number of women diagnosed with depression and a disproportionate number of African Americans labeled with schizophrenia are seen in clinical practice (Barnes, 2004; Beauboeuf-Lafontant, 2007; Brown & Harris, 1978; Lafrance & McKenzie-Mohr, 2013; Neighbors, Trierweiler, Ford, & Muroff, 2003; Stoppard, 2000; Trierweiler, Neighbors, Munday, Thompson, Binion, & Gomez, 2000; Ussher, 2010; Whaley, 2004). Most likely, as expressed by the authors cited, these labels continue to serve, at least in part, oppressive social practices, despite what are surely good intentions of the clinicians who diagnose their patients with these disorders with clear intent to help.

In these cases, the data suggest that gender and racial issues of a deeply cultural and social nature were reframed and treated as medical issues, and in ways that covered over and concealed cultural oppression of these groups. This form of medicalization appears to have primarily served the interests of those in power and those wishing to maintain the status quo. As such, these historical examples serve as profound representations of how biologically reductive and medicalizing approaches to psychiatric diagnosis can often undermine efforts to realize the ends of social justice. By recasting as medical problems behaviors and experiences that represent normal or even healthy forms of maladjustment to a dysfunctional and oppressive society, psychiatry has served to assault the dignity of those struggling to find a voice in a culture that is unwilling to listen.

MARTIN LUTHER KING JR. ON CREATIVE MALADJUSTMENT

An alternative and more liberating approach to psychiatry of the oppressed could follow the example of Martin Luther King Jr.'s appeal to *creative maladjustment* (Kinderman, 2013; King, 1958, 1968; Robbins, 2013; Roysircar, 2011). On September 1, 1967, Dr. King delivered the Invited Distinguished Address to the American Psychological Association, and the concept of creative maladjustment was the centerpiece of this work. The essay was still in galley proofs for publication in *Journal of Social Issues* on the day Dr. King was assassinated.

Dr. King argued that the discourse of "adjustment" and "maladjustment" in the psychiatry and social science literature provided subtle but powerful comfort to forces of oppression in our society (King, 1968). The implication of a discourse of maladjustment is that any person who fails to conform to society is in some way deficient, or less worthy of esteem, as a citizen of that society. King argued, on the contrary, that when a society is sick in some way, it is the duty of the conscientious citizen to refuse and resist conformity to the norms of that sick society. When a society includes racial segregation, when a society perpetuates oppressive wars and advances a philosophy of militarism, and when the suffering poor of society are forgotten or ignored, King argued, it is the duty of citizens to refuse adjustments to these social pathologies. Social justice in society requires that citizens allow themselves to be creatively maladjusted to injustices until justice is won.

Dr. King's argument for creative maladjustment is echoed by Erich Fromm's concept of the *pathology of normalcy* (Fromm, 1990). According to this notion, a society as a whole can be insane, or deemed pathological, to the extent that it fails to meet the fundamental needs of its citizens, including the human need for social justice and for, we might add, a basic sense of dignity and corresponding, universal human rights. Fromm was critical of psychiatrists and psychologists "who refuse to entertain the idea that society as a whole may be lacking in sanity" (p. 6). Within the context of a pathological culture, Fromm argued, the person who suffers is actually the one who is sane. The suffering, activist person, who in King's language remains creatively maladjusted to the norm, is actually the healthiest one, due to his or her refusal to conform to the pathological norm. Thus, an understanding of mental health requires criteria for mental health that "is not one of individual adjustment to a given social order, but a universal one valid for all men, of giving a satisfactory answer to the problems of human existence" (p. 14).

Within the same mind-set as King and Fromm, Felder and Robbins (2011) have argued in favor of a cultural-existential approach to therapy. This approach to therapy aims to pay attention not only to the psychological depth of the client's issues but also understands these dynamics within the breadth of the cultural-historical context within which the therapist and client are situated. This approach refuses to identify the individual as the sole source of the client's suffering, nor as the sole locus of psychological meaning; in addition, the therapist working within this perspective must pay attention to the ways that language and social-cultural influences frame the issues with which the client is struggling. At times, clients may come to recognize that their liberation from suffering may not be a merely individual project, but must be a process of social activism in which an individual joins with others to change the conditions of his or her community in a positive direction, including toward the ends of a more loving, inclusive, and peaceful community.

In addition, this cultural-existential approach can shift therapist attitudes toward those labeled with mental illness. Rather than merely stigmatized as the victim of a medical disease, symptoms can be understood to be revelatory of social meanings that can point to social and cultural problems in need of remedy (see for example the cultural-existential analysis of the case of Schreber by Robbins, 2000, or Romanyshyn's, 1989, cultural analysis of the hysteric and anorexic). Rather than viewed as a social outcast with nothing to offer to society, those who most suffer from mental anguish can be appreciated as persons who are especially sensitive barometers of oppressive cultural forces that might otherwise go unnoticed or ignored by those who merely adjust themselves to it. The maladjusted, mentally dysfunctional person, within this context, is not stigmatized but, quite the contrary, appreciated as bearing a gift of wisdom to the culture at large by revealing social meanings that most people have learned to ignore in unhealthy ways that may perpetuate injustice or other forms of social neglect.

Whereas a cultural-existential approach to therapy works to appreciate symptoms and how creatively maladjusted individuals can inform us about ways society and culture can better move in the direction of liberation from oppression, most conventional forms of psychotherapy and psychiatry have the complete opposite effect. Most medications in psychiatry serve an anesthetizing effect, making us "comfortably numb," as one author suggests in homage to the British rock group, Pink Floyd (Barber, 2009). Treatments typically relieve suffering but at the cost of helping the creatively maladjusted to ignore their symptoms and the meaning of those symptoms, including symptoms that inform the person and society about the need for social reform. Cognitive and behavioral treatments, similarly, serve to reduce and eliminate symptoms rather than working to understand their meaning and their social context. Yet history suggests that to ignore symptoms, and to engage in treatments focused merely on adjustment of the individual to social norms, the clinician becomes easily complicit with toxic and oppressive social forces, rather than serving in a process of moving toward productive and liberating social change.

CONFLICTS OF INTEREST IN PSYCHIATRIC RESEARCH AND PRACTICE AS A THREAT TO HUMAN DIGNITY

Not only does psychiatry and clinical psychology often work to adjust individuals to pathological cultural norms, these professions also often unwittingly collude with socioeconomic forces that are overtly exploiting consumers of psychiatry and clinical psychology (Robbins et al., 2011). Namely, corporate agencies, such as the pharmaceutical industry, often use psychiatric patients as a means to the end of profit, even at the expense of the client's ultimate best interests. This type of exploitation is another way that psychiatry and industry, even with good intentions, can make assaults upon human dignity.

Exploitation of clinical patients for the sole means of personal and corporate gain is, according to existential personalism, a violation of human dignity (Williams, 2005; Wojtyla, 1995). To treat a person as only a means to one's own end, rather than also an end in him- or herself is to objectify that person. This is to turn him or her from a "thou" into an "it," as Martin Buber (2000) articulated in his own version of personalist ethics.

To put the pharmaceutical industry in perspective, consider that in 2002 the top 10 drug companies profited more than the rest of the *Fortune 500* companies combined (Angell, 2004). Psychotropic medications, moreover, tend to be among the most profitable of all pharmaceuticals (Barber, 2008). Although there is nothing intrinsically wrong with profiting in business, and in fact making a decent profit on medications is necessary if pharmaceuticals are to survive and thrive, the real issue is one of greed, when corporations beholden to their share holders, place profit above the welfare of the consumers served by the medication products. For example, as various drug industry whistle-blowers have revealed, the marketing of psychiatric drugs is often dishonest and self-serving (Carlat, 2010; Fugh-Berman & Ahari, 2007; Olsen, 2012).

The greed of pharmaceuticals becomes especially dangerous when financial conflicts of interest risk compromising psychiatry's ability to produce research and critical analysis of research that serves the public rather than the interests of industry and the profession (Robbins et al., 2011). Research by Lisa Cosgrove and colleagues (e.g., Cosgrove, Bursztajn, Krimsky, Anaya, & Walker, 2009) has demonstrated that financial conflicts of interests are pervasive in psychiatry, both in the development of clinical practice guidelines (CPGS) and in the *Diagnostic and Statistical Manual of Mental Disorders, Volumes IV and V*. The *DSM-5* Task Force, for example, disclosed that 70% of its task force had ties to the drug industry (Cosgrove et al., 2009). These conflicts of interests are of concern because research demonstrates that empirical findings are, in fact, biased by industry funding (Healy, 2001; Perlis et al., 2005).

One cautionary tale at this time is the pharmaceutical industry's push to expand the market of atypical antipsychotic drugs (Olfman & Robbins, 2012). The off-label marketing of atypical antipsychotic drugs has resulted in some of the largest corporate settlements in legal history (Robbins et al., 2011). Despite the lawsuits, the marketing effort has been tremendously successful at increasing sales to child and elderly markets, despite either lack of evidence or evidence of likely iatrogenic harm to these populations as a result of taking these drugs (Alexander, Gallagher, Mascola, Moloney, & Stafford, 2011; Domino & Swartz, 2009; Robbins et al., 2011). A very fast and alarming increase in prescriptions of atypical antipsychotics in children has, in part, been fueled by a 40-fold increase in the number of children diagnosed with pediatric bipolar disorder (Olson, 2011, June 23). In fact, children between the ages of two and five are the fastest-growing market for these drugs (Olfson, Blanco, Liu, Moreno, & Laje, 2006)—a shocking statistic, to say the least. The DSM-5 Task Force, however, with pharmaceutical conflicts of interest, has introduced into the new *DSM* diagnostic categories that are likely to increase prescriptions of atypical antipsychotic drugs to children, adolescents, and the elderly (Olfman & Robbins, 2012; Robbins et al., 2011).

Any collusion between drug industry and psychiatric medical research is a dangerous mix that threatens the integrity of research findings and ultimately increases risk of iatrogenic illness in consumers served by these industries. When risks that compromise the safety of psychiatric consumers are taken, but which nevertheless serve the financial and professional interests of pharmaceutical companies and psychiatry, it is fair to say the fundamental human dignity of psychiatric consumers is under assault.

CONCLUSION

Our chapter has focused on just a few of the many important topics involving the interface of mental health and social justice from a psychological perspective. Due to space limitations, many important and relevant issues could not be included, so we decided to take more of a depth, rather than breadth, approach, focusing on dignity as a unifying theme. Some of what we could not include involves very concerning trends, such as the growing number of U.S. youth, a vulnerable population, diagnosed as having attentional problems and consequently placed on powerful, and potentially dangerous, psycho-stimulant medications, especially as the likelihood of diagnoses driving such treatment is expected to greatly increase with the new *DSM-V* (Batstra & Frances, 2012). Other trends are more hopeful, such as the growth of self-support movements (Davidson, Rakfeldt, & Strauss, 2010) and resistance against involuntary administration of treatment to those labeled mentally ill (e.g., use of electroconvulsive treatment and forced medication; Kallert, Messich, & Monahan, 2011) coming from activist organizations, such as Mad Pride, which view mental health rights as fundamental civil rights (Friedman, 2004).

Human dignity, understood as an appreciation for the intrinsic and incalculable worth and irreplaceability of each person, is a key concept of existential personalist ethics. This concept seems to have great promise in guiding critical reflection on ethical concerns central to psychiatry and clinical psychological research and practice. Assaults on human dignity in psychiatry and clinical psychology include biologically reductive approaches to conceptualizing mental illness—a rhetoric that frames mental health in terms of mere adjustment to pathological social norms, stigmatization that remains blind to the intrinsic value of persons suffering mental anguish, and the exploitation of psychiatric consumers that results from the collusion of the drug industry and the psychiatric profession. These are social justice issues, because social justice, as articulated, for example, in the United Nations Declaration of Human Rights, is predicated upon the foundation of human dignity. When human dignity is under assault, this substantially increases the risk that those under assault will be stigmatized and their rights will be jeopardized. To protect mental health consumers from human rights violations, it is first and foremost necessary to protect assaults on their dignity.

REFERENCES

Alexander, G. C., Gallagher, S. A., Mascola, A., Moloney, R. M., & Stafford, R. S. (2011). Increasing off-label use of antipsychotic medications in the United States, 1995–2008. *Pharmacoepidimiology & Drug Safety, 20*(2), 177–184.

Angell, M. (2004). *The truth about the drug companies: How they deceive us and what to do about it.* New York, NY: Random House.

Angermeyer, M. C., Holzinger, A., Carta, M. G., & Schomerus, G. (2011). Biogenetic explanations and public acceptance of mental illness: Systematic review of population studies. *British Journal of Psychiatry, 199*, 367–372.

Barber, C. (2009). *Comfortably numb: How psychiatry is medicating a nation.* New York, NY: Vintage.

Barnes, A. (2004). Race, schizophrenia, and admission to state psychiatric hospitals. *Administration and Policy in Mental Health & Mental Health Services Research, 31*(3), 241–257.

Bastian, B., Jelten, J., & Radke, H. R. M. (2012). Cyber-dehumanization: Violent video game play diminishes our humanity. *Journal of Experimental Social Psychology, 48*(2), 486–491.

Batstra, L., & Frances, A. (2012). DSM-5 further inflates attention deficit hyperactivity disorder. *Journal of Nervous & Mental Disease, 200*(6), 486–488.

Beauboeuf-Lafontant, T. (2007). You have to show strength: An exploration of gender, race, and depression. *Gender & Society, 21*(1), 28–51.

Black, E. (2003). *War against the weak: Eugenics and America's campaign to create a master race.* New York, NY: Four Walls Eight Windows.

Boe, J., Overland, S., Lundervold, A., & Hysing, M. (2012). Socioeconomic status and children's mental health: Results from the Bergin Child Study. *Social Psychiatry and Psychiatric Epidemiology, 47*(10), 1557–1566.

Brown, G. W., & Harris, T. (Eds.). (1978). *Social origins of depression: A study of psychiatric disorder in women.* New York, NY: Routledge.

Bruno, F. (2002). *Psychology: A self-teaching* guide. Hoboken, NJ: Wiley.

Buber, M. (2000). *I and thou*. New York, NY: Scribner.

Burrow, R., Jr. (2006). *God and human dignity: The personalism, theology, and ethics of Martin Luther King, Jr.* Notre Dame, IN: University of Notre Dame.

Carlat, D. (2010). *Unhinged: The trouble with psychiatry—a doctor's revelations about a profession in crisis*. New York, NY: Free Press.

Centorrino, F., Goren, J. L., Hennen, J., Salvatore, P., Kelleher, J. P., & Baldessarini, R. J. (2004). Multiple versus single antipsychotic agents for hospitalized psychiatric patients: Case-control study of risks versus benefits. *American Journal of Psychiatry, 161*(4), 700–706.

Corrigan, P. (2004). How stigma interferes with mental health care. *American Psychologist, 59*(7), 611–675.

Cosgrove, L., Bursztajn, H., Krimsky, S., Anaya, M., & Walker, J. (2009). Conflicts of interest and disclosure in the American Psychiatric Association's Clinical Practice Guidelines. *Psychotherapy and Psychosomatics, 78*, 228–232.

Crosby, J. F. (1996). *The selfhood of the human person*. Washington, DC: Catholic University of America Press.

Crystal, S., Olfson, M., Huang, C., Pincus, H., & Gerhard, T. (2009). Broadened use of atypical antipsychotics: Safety, effectiveness, and policy challenges. *Health Affairs, 28*(5), 770–781.

Dahlstrom, D. O. (1987). *Existential personalism*. Charlottesville, VA: American Catholic Philosophical Association.

Davidson, L., Rakfeldt, J., & Strauss, J. (Eds.). (2010). *The roots of the recovery movement in psychiatry: Lessons learned*. Hoboken, NJ: Wiley.

Domino, M. E., & Schwartz, M. (2009). Who are the new users of antipsychotic medications? *Psychiatric Services, 59*(5), 507–514.

El-Hai, J. (2007). *The lobotomist: A maverick medical genius and his tragic quest to rid the world of mental illness*. Hoboken, NJ: John Wiley & Sons.

Feinstein, B. A., Goldfried, M. R., & Danila, J. (2012). The relationship between experiences of discrimination and mental health among lesbians and gay men: An examination of internalized homonegativity and rejection sensitivity as potential mechanisms. *Journal of Consulting and Clinical Psychology, 80*(5), 917–927.

Felder, A. J., & Robbins, B. D. (2011). A cultural-existential approach to therapy: Merleau-Ponty's phenomenology of embodiment and its implications for practice. *Theory & Psychology, 21*(3), 255–276.

Frances, A. (2010a). DSM-5 temper dysregulation—good intentions, bad solution. *Psychology Today*, n.p.

Frances, A. (2010b). DSM-5 "psychosis risk syndrome"—far too risky. *Psychology Today*, n.p.

Friedman, H. (2004). Prescription privileges and abusive mental health systems: Focus on the mad pride movement and the wars on terror and drugs. *Florida Psychologist, 55*(1), 5–8.

Frings, M. S. (1997). *The mind of Max Scheler: The first comprehensive guide based on the complete works*. Milwaukee, WI: Marquette University Press.

Fromm, E, (1990). *The Sane Society*. New York, NY: Holt.

Fugh-Berman, A. & Ahari, S. (2007). Following the script: How drug reps make friends and influence doctors. *PLoS Medicine, 4*(4), e150. doi: 10.1371/journal.pmed.0040150

Fuller-Rowell, T. E., Evans, G. W., & Ong, A. D. (2012). Poverty and health: The mediating role of perceived discrimination. *Psychological Science, 23*(7), 734–739.

Gianfrancesco, F. D., Grogg, A. L., Mahmoud, R. A., Wang, R. H., & Nasrallah, H. A. (2002). Differential effects of risperidone, olanzapine, clozapine, and conventional antipsychotics on type 2 diabetes: Findings from a large health plan database. *The Journal of clinical psychiatry, 63*(10), 920–930.

Glendon, M. A. (2002). *A world made new: Eleanor Roosevelt and the Universal Declaration of Human Rights*. New York, NY: Random House.

Glendon, M. A. (2005). Foreword. In T. D. Williams (Ed.), *Who is my neighbor? Personalism and the foundations of human rights* (pp. vii–xi). Washington, DC: The Catholic University of America Press.

Goffman, E. (1963). *Stigma: Notes on the management of spoiled identity*. Upper Saddle River, NJ: Prentice-Hall.

Harper, D. (2013). Dignity (n.p.). *Online etymological dictionary*. Retrieved from http://www.etymonline.com

Healy, D. (2001). The dilemmas posed by new and fashionable treatments. *Advances in Psychiatric Treatment, 7,* 322–327.

Ilic, M., Reinecke, J., Bohner, G., Rottgers, H. O., Beblo, T., Driessen, M., . . . Corrigan, P. W. (2013). Belittled, avoided, ignored, denied. Assessing forms and consequences of stigma experiences of people with mental illness. *Basic and Applied Social Psychology, 35*(1), 31–40.

Joas, H. (2013). *The sacredness of the person: A new genealogy of human rights*. Washington, DC: Georgetown University Press.

Jones, E. E., Farina, A., Hastorf, A. H., Markus, H., Miller, D. T., & Scott, R. A. (1984). *Social stigma: The psychology of marked relationships*. New York, NY: Freeman.

Kadlac, A. (2012). Irreplaceability and identity. *Social Theory and Practice, 38*(1), 33–54. doi: 10.5840/soctheorpract20123812

Kallert, T., Messich, J., & Monahan, J. (Eds.). (2011). *Coercive treatment in psychiatry: Clinical, legal and ethical aspects*. Hoboken, NJ: Wiley.

Kinderman, P. (2013). The role of the psychologist in social change. *International Journal of Social Psychiatry, 59*(4). doi: 10.1177/0020764013491741

King, M. L., Jr. (1958). The power of nonviolence. *Intercollegian*. Retrieved from http://www.asdk12.org/staff/miller_roger/pages/US_History/Civil%20Rights/The%20Power%20of%20Non.pdf

King, M. L., Jr. (1968). The role of the behavioral scientist in the civil rights movement. *American Psychologist, 23*(3), 180–186.

Lafrance, M. N., & McKenzie-Mohr, S. (2013). The DSM and its lure of legitimacy. *Feminism & Psychology, 23*(1), 119–140.

Leung, J. Y. T., Barr, A. M., Procyshyn, R. M., Honor, W. G., & Pang, C. Y. (2012). Cardiovascular side-effects of anti-psychotic drugs: The role of the autonomic nervous system. *Pharmacology & Therapeutics, 135*(2), 113–122.

Levinas, E. (1969). *Totality and infinity: An essay on exteriority*. Pittsburgh, PA: Duquesne University Press.

Link, B. G., & Phelan, J. C. (2001). Conceptualizing stigma. *Annual Review of Sociology, 27,* 363–385.

Link, B. G., Yang, L. H., Phelan, J. C., & Collins, P. Y. (2004). Measuring mental illness stigma. *Schizophrenia Bulletin, 30*(3), 511–541.

Macklin, R. (2003). Dignity is a useless concept: It means no more than respect for persons or their autonomy. *British Medical Journal, 327*(7429), 1419–1420.

Maritain, J. (2012). *Christianity and democracy, and the rights of man and natural law.* San Francisco, CA: Ignatius Press.

Marrdani, M. M., Tu, K., Austin, P. C., & Alter, D. A. (2002). Influence of socioeconomic status on drug selection for the elderly in Canada. *The Annals of Pharmacotherapy, 36*(5), 804–808.

McClowry, S. G., Davies, E. B., May, K. A., Kulenkamp, E. J., & Martinson, I. M. (1987). The empty space phenomenon: The process of grief in the bereaved family. *Death Studies, 11*(5), 361–374.

McCrudden, C. (2008). Human dignity and judicial interpretation of human rights. *European Journal of International Law, 19*(4), 655–724.

Metzl, J. (2011). *The protest psychosis: How schizophrenia became a black disease.* Boston, MA: Beacon Press.

Neighbors, H. W., Trierweiler, S. J., Ford, B. C., & Muroff, J. R. (2003). Racial differences in DSM diagnosis using a semi-structured instrument: The importance of clinical judgment in the diagnosis of African Americans. *Journal of Health & Social Behavior, 44*(3), 237–256.

Olfman, S., & Robbins, B. D. (Eds.). (2012). *Drugging our children: How profiteers are pushing antipsychotics on our youngest and what we can do to stop it.* Santa Barbara, CA: Praeger.

Olfson, M., Blanco, C., Liu L., Moreno, C., & Laje, G. (2006). National trends in the outpatient treatment of children and adolescents with antipsychotic drugs. *Archives of General Psychiatry, 63*(6), 679–685.

Olsen, G. (2012). The marketing of madness and psychotropic drugs to children (pp. 51–80). In S. Olfman & B. D. Robbins (Eds.), *Drugging our children: How profiteers are pushing antipsychotics on our youngest and what we can do to stop it.* Santa Barbara, CA: Praeger.

Olson, J. (2011, June 23). Bipolar soars among kids. StarTribute, n.p. Retrieved from http://www.startribune.com/lifestyle/wellness/124136764

Osypuk, T., Tchetgen, E. J., Acevedo-Garcia, D., Earls, F. J., Lincoln, A., Schmidt, N. M., & Glymour, M. (2012). Differential mental health effects of neighborhood relocation among youth in vulnerable families: Results from a randomized trial. *Archives of General Psychiatry, 69*(12), 1284–1294.

Perlis, R., Perlis, C., Wu, Y., Hwang, C., Joseph, M., & Nierenberg, A. (2005). Industry sponsorship and financial conflict of interest in the reporting of clinical trials in psychiatry. *American Journal of Psychiatry, 162*(10), 1957–1960.

Pieterse, A. L., Todd, N. R., Neville, H. A., & Carter, R. T. (2012). Perceived racism and mental health among Black American adults: A meta-analytic review. *Journal of Counseling Psychology, 59*(1), 1–9.

Read, J. (2007). Why promoting biological ideology increases prejudice against people labeled "schizophrenic." *Australian Psychologist, 42*(2), 118–128.

Read, J., Haslam, N., Sayce, L., & Davies, E. (2006). Prejudice and schizophrenia: A review of the "mental illness is an illness like any other" approach. *Acta Psychiatrica Scandinavica, 114*(5), 303–318.

Robbins, B. D. (2000). Schreber's soul-voluptuousness: Mysticism, madness and the feminine in Schreber's memoirs. *Journal of Phenomenological Psychology, 31*(2), 117–154.

Robbins, B. D. (2012). From ice pick lobotomies to antipsychotics as sleep aids for children: A historical perspective (pp. 17–34). In S. Olfman & B. D. Robbins (Eds.), *Drugging our children: How profiteers are pushing antipsychotics on our youngest, and what we can do to stop it*. Santa Barbara, CA: Praeger.

Robbins, B. D. (2013). *The problem of human dignity at the heart of humanistic psychology: Retrieving existential personalism and a hermeneutics of love within the humanistic tradition*. Paper presented at the Society for Humanistic Psychology's Annual Conference, Pacifica Graduate Institute, Carpinteria, CA, February, 2013.

Robbins, B. D., Higgins, M., Fisher, M., & Over, K. (2011). Conflicts of interest in research on antipsychotic treatment of pediatric bipolar disorder, temper dysregulation disorder, and attenuated psychotic symptoms syndrome: Exploring the unholy alliance between big pharma and psychiatry. *Journal of Psychological Issues in Organizational Culture, 1*(4), 32–49.

Romanyshyn, R. (1989). *Technology as symptom and dream*. New York, NY: Routledge.

Roysircar, G. (2011). The big picture of advocacy: Counselor, heal society and thyself. *Journal of Counseling & Development, 87*(3), 288–294.

Rudman, L. A., & Mescher, K. (2012). Of animals and objects: Men's implicit dehumanization of women and likelihood of sexual aggression. *Personality and Social Psychology Bulletin, 38*(6), 734–746.

Rummel-Kluge, C., Komossa, K., Schwarz, S., Hunger, H., Schmid, F., Lobos, C. A., . . . Leucht, S. (2010). Head-to-head comparisons of metabolic side effects of second generation antipsychotics in the treatment of schizophrenia: A systematic review and analysis. *Schizophrenia Research, 123*(2–3), 225–233.

Rummel-Kluge, C., Komossa, K., Schwarz, S., Hunger, H., Schmid, F., Kissling, W., . . . Leucht, S. (2012). Second-generation antipsychotic drugs and extrapyramidal side effects: A systematic review of meta-analysis of head-to-head comparisons. *Schizophrenia Bulletin, 38*(1), 167–177.

Santiago, C. D., Kaltman, S., & Miranda, J. (2012). Poverty and mental health: How do low-income adults and children fare in psychotherapy? *Journal of Clinical Psychology, 69*(2), 115–126.

Scheler, M. (1973). *Formalism and non-formal ethics of values: A new attempt toward the foundations of an ethical personalism*. (M. S. Frings & P. L. Funk, Trans.). Chicago, IL: Northwestern University Press.

Steinkraus, W. E. (1973). Martin Luther King's personalism and non-violence. *Journal of the History of Ideas, 34*(1), 97–111.

Stewart, A. (2009). Determinants of disparities. In P. Ruiz& A. Primm (Eds.), *Disparities in psychiatric care: Clinical and cross-cultural perspectives* (pp. 10–18). Hagerstown, MD: Lippincott Williams & Wilkins.

Stoppard, J. M. (2000). *Understanding depression: Feminist social constructionist approaches*. New York, NY: Routledge.

Trierweiler, S. J., Neighbors, H. W., Munday, C., Thompson, E. E., Binion, V. J., & Gomez, J. P. (2000). Clinical attributions associated with the diagnosis of schizophrenia in African American and non-African American patients. *Journal of Consulting & Clinical Psychology, 68*(1), 171–175.

Turney, K., Kissane, R., & Edin, K. (2013). After moving to opportunity: How moving to a low-poverty neighborhood improves mental health among African American women. *Society and Mental Health, 3*(1), 1–21.

Ussher, J. M. (2010). Are we medicalizing women's misery? A critical review of women's higher rates of reported depression. *Feminism & Psychology, 20*(1), 9–35.

Wahl, O. F. (2012). Stigma as a barrier to recovery from mental illness. *Trends in Cognitive Sciences, 16*(1), 9–10.

Wall, J., & Monahan, T. (2011). Surveillance and violence from afar: The politics of drones and liminal security-scapes. *Theoretical Criminology, 15*(3), 239–254.

Whaley, A. L. (2004). A two-stage method for the study of cultural bias in the diagnosis of schizophrenia in African Americans. *Journal of Black Psychology, 30*(2), 167–186.

Whitaker, R. (2002). *Mad in America: Bad science, bad medicine, and the enduring mistreatment of the mentally ill.* Philadelphia, PA: Basic Books.

Whitaker, R. (2010). *Anatomy of an epidemic: Magic bullets, psychiatric drugs, and the astonishing rise of mental illness in America.* New York, NY: Crown.

Whitaker, R. (2012). Weighing the evidence: What science has to say about prescribing atypical antipsychotics to children. In S. Olfman & B. D. Robbins (Eds.), *Drugging our children: How profiteers are pushing antipsychotics on our youngest and what we can do to stop it* (pp. 3–16). Santa Barbara, CA: Praeger.

Williams, D. (2005). *Who is my neighbor? Personalism and the foundations of human rights.* Washington, DC: Catholic University Press.

Williams, T. D., & Bengtsson, J. O. (2009). Personalism (n.p.). *Stanford encyclopedia of philosophy.* Retrieved from http://plato.stanford.edu/entries/personalism/

Wojtyla, K. (1995). *Love and responsibility.* (H. T. Willets, Trans.). New York, NY: Farrar, Straus, & Giroux.

Woznicki, A. N. (1980). *A Christian humanism: Karol Wojtyla's existential personalism.* New Britain, CT: Mariel Publications.

Wunderink, L., Nieboer, R. M., Wiersma, D., Systerra, S., & Nienhuis, M. A. (2013). Recovery in remitted first-episode psychosis at 7 years of follow-up of an early dose reduction/discontinuation or maintenance treatment strategy: Long-term follow-up of a 2-year randomized clinical trial. *JAMA Psychiatry.* Retrieved from http://archpsyc.jamanetwork.com

Yoshikawa, H., Abert, J. L., & Beardslee, W. R. (2012). The effects of poverty on the mental, emotional, and behavioral health of children and youth: Implications for prevention. *American Psychologist, 67*(4), 272–284.

Zito, J. M., Burcu, M., Ibe, A., Safer, D. J., & Madger, L. S. (2013). Antipsychotic use by Medicaid-insured youths: Impact of eligibility and psychiatric diagnosis across a decade. *Psychiatric Services, 64*(3), 223–229.

Chapter 5

The Psychology of Justice in the Workplace: Meaning, Perception, and Promotion

Poonam Oberoi and Gazi Islam

Nearly five decades ago, French (1964) coined the term *organizational justice* for fairness or justice-related issues in the workplace. Since then, organizational justice, which is concerned with social justice in workplace contexts, has become an important concept that is relevant to literature of many disciplines such as law (Lind, Kulik, Ambrose, & De Vera Park, 1993), politics (Tyler, Rasinski, & McGraw, 1985), organizations (Cropanzano & Greenberg, 1997), business (Kahneman, Knetsch, & Thaler, 1986), and society in general (Rawls, 1971). Across these disciplines, the topic of social justice has received considerable attention from various types of scholars, such as philosophers, legal scholars, political scientists, sociologists, economists, and psychologists, involving a diversity of theoretical and empirical approaches. Over the past three decades, studies on the social psychology of justice have emphasized the meaning of social justice (Colquitt, Conlon, Wesson, Porter, & Ng, 2001; Pillai, Schriesheim, & Williams, 1999), how justice judgments are formed (van den Bos, 2003), and the empirical consequences of perceived just and unjust actions (Greenberg, 1997; Ince & Gul, 2011; Lind, Greenberg, Scott, & Welchans, 2000).

Social justice in the workplace, as a concept, relates to the treatment of employees by the authorities in the workplace (Pillai et al., 1999). Research in organizational psychology considers justice to be under the influence of contextual factors (Fortin, 2008). Moreover, an act is considered just if different individuals perceive it to be so. Hence, what is fair or just relates to objective decision making and subjective perceptions of fairness or righteousness of the act (Fortin, 2008). More importantly, research has led to the development of four dimensions of social justice, which are distributive, procedural, interpersonal, and informational justice.

It is commonly acknowledged that employee satisfaction is essential for effective functioning of the organization (Bos, 2003). Hence, studies have been devoted to understanding how individuals react to fair or unfair treatment, with a focus on linking social justice with outcomes such as performance, employee's sense of citizenship, commitment and satisfaction with the firm, and with social authorities. For example, the perception of unjust treatment has been empirically linked to legal action (Lind et al., 2000) and antisocial behavior (Greenberg, 1997), whereas fair treatment by superiors has been linked to increased decision acceptance (Lind et al., 1993), as well as policy attitudes (Tyler et al., 1985), and conformity to regulation (Tyler, 1990).

Whereas some social psychologists focus on the effects of social justice, others emphasize how justice-related judgments are formed (Ambrose & Kulik, 2001; Van den Bos & Lind, 2002). Because justice-related judgments have important consequences, understanding how individuals (manager, police officer, or a court judge) form judgments is of crucial importance. Studies on the formation of justice-related judgments have shown that the social psychology of groups (e.g., Lind & Tyler, 1988; Tyler & Lind, 1992) and the affective state of mind of an individual (Bos, 2003) have significant impact on the judgment process.

In the following sections of this chapter, the focus will be on the various issues surrounding the topic of social justice. It is important to study these issues because they may foster insights into what precisely social justice is, how employees and managers act and feel regarding just and unjust actions, and how justice and its perceptions are influenced by contextual factors. The chapter first presents critical reflections on the concept of social justice, different dimensions of justice, and debates surrounding the construct discrimination and various theories related to social justice. The chapter then presents arguments explaining how justice perception differs based on the multilevel nature of the construct and varied contextual factors. The chapter ends with discussion on how to promote real organizational justice within firms.

CONCEPTUALIZATION OF JUSTICE

Academics from the domain of organizational psychology and other social sciences have offered varied conceptualizations of social justice. In the psychology literature, rationalist approaches state that moral judgments are formed primarily through the process of cognitive reasoning (Kohlberg, 1969; Piaget, 1975; Turiel, 1983). For example, the cognitive reasoning behind creating the law banning the display of religious symbols in public places is to emphasize secularism and to ensure clear identification of a person for security reasons. In contrast, intuitionist approaches argue that people's intuitive feelings about what is right or wrong cause moral judgments. The moral reasoning is usually a post hoc construction, generated after moral judgments have been reached (Haidt, 2001; Kagan, 1984). Such intuitionist approaches, for example, would help understand, and consider just, the moral reasoning of people suffering from religious discrimination at work.

Social scientists and organizational psychologists seem to agree on the definition of the concept of justice. They use the terms *justice* and *fairness* interchangeably, whereas when philosophers use these terms, they often pertain to distinct concepts (e.g., Rawls, 1971). For convenience, we choose to use these terms as they are employed within the broader organizational psychology and social science literature.

THE ROOTS AND DIMENSIONS OF ORGANIZATIONAL JUSTICE

In this section, we trace the emergence of organizational justice and elaborate on the continuing debate on social justice in organizations.

Distributive Justice

Early views of organizational justice were based in the *distributive* aspect of justice, and have their basis in Adams's equity theory (1965). Adams explained that people were not concerned with the absolute level of outcomes but whether the outcomes were fair with regard to two parameters: (1) the ratio of one's contributions or inputs (e.g., education, intelligence, and experience) to the outputs (e.g., salary, perks, recognition) received and (2) how this ratio stands in comparison to the input/output ratio of other employees.

Procedural Justice

As the social justice literature developed, Thibaut and Walker (1975) identified a second, *procedural* dimension of social justice. Whereas distributive justice involves judgments of relative distributions, procedural justice judgments concern the outcome allocation process or policy though which outcomes are decided. Thibaut and Walker (1975) studied such judgments in the arena of dispute resolution procedures, wherein disputants' reactions of the procedures could have important ramifications for disputes. Although, initially procedural justice discourse was concentrated in the domain of law, Leventhal, Karuza, and Fry (1980) extended the same to nonlegal organizational settings. In the process, Leventhal et al. stressed that justice procedures should be temporally consistent, bias-free, based on relevant information and error detection processes, consistent with prevalent ethical norms, and conscious of major stakeholders. Further studies (e.g., Cohen-Charash & Spector, 2001) emphasized the importance of fair processes as predictors of work attitudes and effective work behaviors.

Interpersonal or Interactional Justice

Bies and Moag (1986) observed a third dimension of social justice from an interpersonal interaction point of view. Earlier models had either neglected the interactional aspect altogether or had confounded interpersonal treatment with the issues of formal procedures. The idea of interactional justice is that interactions have an implicit idea of what being fairly treated consists of, at an interpersonal level, in terms of civility and quality of interaction. Even if policies and allocations are fair, when someone is treated with a lack of respect, is not accorded dignity or civility, or is not provided with clear information, he or she is liable to feel unfairly treated. Illustrations of interactional justice can be found in studies on recruitment (Bies, 1986) and police and courtroom interactions (Tyler, 1988). Outside of decision-making contexts, interactional justice takes place across a wide array of everyday encounters that can involve elements of deception, invasion of privacy, derogatory judgments, and disrespect (Bies, 2001). Building on past literature on the topic, Greenberg (1993) explained that the interpersonal dimension involved both quality of treatment and the explanation and information regarding the decision-making process. Based on these two elements, Colquitt et al. (2001) split the interpersonal dimension previously discussed into two component subdimensions, namely informational justice and interpersonal justice. They explain the newly proposed informational justice dimension as focusing on the information provided to people about why certain procedures were used in a certain way or why outcomes were distributed in a certain fashion.

Construct Discrimination

Elaborating on this point, an ongoing debate in the organizational justice literature is whether justice should be considered as a single construct or as multiple constructs (e.g. Fortin, 2008). Scholars engaged in the debate concerning social justice have different viewpoints regarding whether one should distinguish two, three, or four dimensions of justice. For example, the *interactional justice* component may be further broken down into interpersonal and informational elements (Sweeney & McFarlin 1993; Tyler & Bies 1990), with *interpersonal justice* referring to the quality of treatment and *informational justice* referring to whether individuals are adequately informed about organizational decisions and policies. Some, however, have argued that the interactional justice construct is superfluous, and can be subsumed under procedural justice (e.g., Lind & Tyler 1988). Conversely, other studies, noting that the two types are prima facie different and have different operationalizations, have concluded that the procedural and interpersonal elements of justice should be considered distinct (Bobocel & Holmvall, 2001). This conclusion has been supported by meta-analytic studies that show the two vary somewhat correlationally (Cohen-Charash & Spector, 2001; Colquitt et al., 2001).

There are also discussions regarding the question of whether the two elements of interactional justice, namely interpersonal treatment and the provision of adequate and timely information, should be treated as separate dimensions or not. The study by Colquitt et al. (2001) is the only meta-analysis of social justice differentiating between these elements. These scholars reviewed 183 studies and concluded that procedural, interpersonal, and informational justices have different correlates, and measuring the three separately explains incremental variance in fairness perceptions. They also deduced that a four-factor model fits the data better than one-, two- or three-factor models.

To generalize from the dimensionality debate, however, the three main questions that justice theorists have tried to answer are (1) why justice matters to people, (2) how fairness judgments are made, and (3) why and how people react to the outcomes. Different theories in relation to these questions can be grouped into process theories (Cropanzano, Byrne, Bobocel, & Rupp, 2001a; as cited by Fortin, 2008) and integrative theories (Blader & Tyler, 2005).

Process Theories

Process theories have brought forward several models to explain why people care about justice or fairness (for a detailed review, see Cropanzano, Rupp, Mohler, & Schminke, 2001). Some of the main models are the instrumental model, the relational model, and the moral virtues model. According to the instrumental model, individuals are concerned about fairness because it is a control mechanism to ensure the predictability and favorability of their outcomes (Tyler 1987). The relational model postulates that individuals care about fairness because receiving fair treatment indicates status and worth within a group. Folger (1998) argues that, in the moral virtue model, the presence of selfish motives does not preclude concerns for others at the same time.

Integrative Theories

Integrative theories of justice, as described by Fortin (2008), involve using the various dimensions of justice to answer broader questions of how people make and react to justice judgments (Blader & Tyler 2005). These integrative approaches tend to look at general psychological processes that are behind justice thinking in general, regardless of the specific type of judgment. For example, in Folger and Cropanzando's (2001) counterfactual approach to fairness judgments, individuals judge their own outcomes on the basis of how well-off others are, and how well-off they themselves could be. In contrast, the uncertainty management approach describes how fairness-related information can eliminate both uncertainty and related discomfort (Lind & Van den Bos, 2002; Van den Bos & Lind, 2002). The group engagement model explains why individuals cooperate in groups, organizations, and societies (Tyler & Blader, 2000, 2003). According to this model, identification within a group (the status or standing of the group, and one's status within the group) mediates the link between justice and cooperation (Blader & Tyler, 2005). These identification factors will shape the extent to which employees define themselves as members of the group, organization, or society.

To summarize, there is little clarity on what the ultimate goal of justice is, and whether there are altruistic goals of justice or only self-interested goals. However, people care about fairness for a number of reasons, and these include instrumental, relational, and moral concerns. Moreover, there is debate over why people react to justice judgments differently. The group engagement model, on the one hand, is suited to explaining positive attitudes and values, and cooperative behavior within social contexts. On the other hand, the uncertainty management and fairness approach do not explicitly link justice and cooperation (Blader & Tyler, 2005). One cannot conclude with certainty whether one of these theories explains overall justice dynamics better than the others.

Summary

The purpose of this section was to elaborate on the concept of organizational justice according to the business and organizational psychology literatures. We explained that organizational justice involves organizational relationships marked by distributive, procedural, informational, and interpersonal aspects, and that each of these aspects produces a specific version of justice concerns. We described how different dimensions of organizational justice emerged, and the ongoing debate regarding the distinguishability of these dimensions. We also discussed different theories that relate to organizational justice. In the following section, we explore why organizational justice is both a rich and complex construct.

MULTILEVEL FEATURES OF ORGANIZATIONAL JUSTICE

A review of extant literature reveals that organizational justice has been a topic of much intellectual exploration from a wide variety of angles. This has led to some extremely enriching debates about the meaning of social and organizational justice, varied stakeholder perceptions of this topic, and regarding the varied levels at which justice manifests itself. Even more interesting is the literature that covers a wide variety of contextual variables, again, at different levels, that influence the perception of justice. In this section, we summarize some of this literature to expose the readers to the richness as well as the complexity of the organizational justice construct.

Each social justice dimension represents a different type of justice. For example, distributive justice refers to the perceived fairness of outcome distribution, whereas procedural justice is regarding the fairness of the procedures used to determine the outcomes. Additionally, each dimension operates at a different level of analysis. For example, procedural justice refers to the fairness of justice procedures at the *organizational level* (Erdogan, 2002), whereas interactional justice is the fairness of treatment at the *interpersonal level*, for example, between hierarchical superior and employee (Masterson, Lewis, Goldman, & Taylor, 2000; Moorman, 1991). Therefore, in the existing literature, level (supervisor, organization) is equated to the type (procedural, interaction) of justice. Less studied, we may note, are the implications of organizational justice phenomena at the wider social level, in terms of how justice perceptions at work affect and are affected by wider patterns of social inequalities, ideologies, and power dynamics. Although research at this level has been sparse, and because interpersonal experiences at work may provide templates for wider views on social ties, and relationships more generally, examining the effects of organizational justice on social justice more generally is a fruitful area for exploration.

Although the link between social and organizational justice perceptions is yet to be fully explored, a wide literature linking macro phenomena with organizational justice perceptions exists. Within this literature, researchers have emphasized various individual-, interactional-, and cultural-level contextual factors that impact or moderate perceptions of justice and related reactions. Greenberg (1993) classified the contextual factors into two groups: structural and social determinants. *Structural determinants* are basically environmental factors, whereas *social determinants* focus on treatment of individuals. The consideration of different categories of antecedents emphasizes the importance of considering a broad range of factors influencing justice perceptions. Cropanzano et al. (2001) proposed that the type of processing and perception of justice may also depend on the availability of information, on time pressure, and on cognitive resources available. We review three particular contextual factors next, namely: team environment, cross-cultural consideration, and the role of power.

Team Environment

The team environment is an interactional contextual factor that was introduced by Mossholder, Bennett, and Martin (1998). The team environment factor points toward the importance of colleagues outside hierarchical relationships and the important role they play in justice dynamics. The level of agreement on justice judgments within a team, termed as justice climate strength, was found to be an important moderator in the relationship between procedural justice team perceptions and outcomes (Colquitt et al., 2002). Other studies (Liao & Rupp, 2005; Roberson, 2006) have demonstrated that team effects are powerful predictors of justice-related reactions.

Cross-Cultural Consideration

Greenberg (2001a; as cited by Fortin 2008) emphasized the significance of cultural contextual factors in justice perceptions. He argued that cross-cultural research helps one to better understand organizational justice. The concept of justice and justice-related norms differs between cultures[1] (Greenberg 2001b; Leung & Tong, 2004). Colquitt et al. (2005a; as cited by Fortin, 2008) explained that culture affects rules for judging, goals of fair treatment, choices made when applying principles, the process of forming judgments, and the effects of justice on outcomes. McFarlin and Sweeney (2001) found that the degree of collectivism versus individualism, as well as the degree of formality, strongly affects the judgment evaluation style in different cultures. Moreover, cultural differences explain not only the judgment process but also employees' reactions to justice outcomes (Blader, Chang, & Tyler, 2001). For example, Blader et al. (2001) explained in their cross-cultural study that Taiwanese were less likely to retaliate, as compared to Americans, to an unjust outcome.

Role of Power

Extant research also emphasizes the contextual role of power (emanating from position, organizational forms, and strategy) with regard to social justice. Leventhal et al. (1980) posited that the distribution of power impacts justice norms and reactions to justice-related decisions. Greenberg and Cohen (1982) proposed that powerful members determine which justice dimensions are more salient in an organization. Ambrose and Schminke (2003), in a similar fashion, explained that organizational forms could be an additional mechanism through which the powerful can influence justice judgments. They explain that, under different organization forms, different justice dimensions become important. In mechanistic organizations, for example, procedural justice and perceived organizational support are strongly linked, whereas in organic organizations, interactional justice and supervisory trust are more strongly linked. Studies have further described the impact of power strategies based on reward or punishment on justice-related outcomes to differ (Molm, Quist, & Wiseley, 1993).

Summary

In this section, we shed light on the richness and complexity of the organizational justice construct. First, we explained that, over and above the issue of multiple constructs and stakeholders, justice concepts might be considered at different levels of analysis, including both organizational and interpersonal levels. Furthermore, these multilevel justice dimensions are under the influence of multiple types of contextual factors (e.g., structural and social). To conclude, different justice dimensions have been related to different actions in the workplace within relevant literature. For example, in extant literature the action of performance appraisal is related to procedural and interactional justice (Erdogan, 2002), whereas resource allocation is related to distributive justice (Greenberg, 2004). Similarly, Sheppard (1985) related organizational dispute resolution (1984) with the traditional notion of procedural justice. These varied arguments contribute to the overall richness and complexity of the organizational justice construct. In order to draw out the implications for a broader understanding of justice, however, several important directions for development should be outlined.

FUTURE DIRECTIONS FOR JUSTICE RESEARCH IN ORGANIZATIONAL PSYCHOLOGY

Proactive versus Reactive Approaches

The key question that every scholar of organizational justice struggles with is: How can one promote organizational justice? The feeling of injustice in a job context takes several forms—such as stress, lack of productivity, and lack of corporate citizenship. Hence, promoting a sense of real justice is an important role of a manager.

Promoting organizational justice requires understanding the mechanisms by which injustice causes negative outcomes (Greenberg, 2004). Greenberg (2004) described how one kind of unjust behavior by a manager starts a series of negative reactions. For example, if an employee perceives an unfair distribution of a certain resource (distributive injustice), he or she might try to seek information about how fairly those outcomes were determined (procedural injustice). Concerns about procedural injustice compel the employee to seek information and support from his or her manager or hierarchical superiors, and the degree to which the hierarchical superior treats the employee in a respectful and caring manner will reflect the employee's perceptions of interactional justice. Therefore, Greenberg (2004) proposed the following three steps for managers to promote organizational justice. First, always explain the reasoning behind decisions in a dignified and respectful manner. Second, allow employees to give their opinion and try and provide due attention to their concerns. Lastly, use accurate, unbiased procedures and implement them transparently. Although some degree of injustice in the workplace is inevitable, following the aforementioned measures can mitigate most negative reactions. It is possible that, in certain situations, individuals may perceive these measures as ways to reduce negative employee perceptions, rather than remedies for actual injustices. Greenberg (2004) explains that both just action and employee perceptions may be improved through organizational justice measures. He insists that with these measures management will not only be "doing the right thing by people, but proactively cultivating one's image of fairness, ensuring that others know of your commitment to fairness" (Greenberg, 2004, p. 363). Moreover, we would suggest that along with the utilization of these measures management should enforce change, if and when required, so that these measures are not seen as just another suppression tactic. When management proposes the required change, then the measures of Greenberg (2004) do not appear to be just to mitigate the negative reactions, but actually to create a just working environment. There is a need for a shift in the attitude of managers, employees, and academics to further ensure the promotion of a just working environment, which will be discussed in the following section.

As mentioned earlier in this chapter, a large proportion of extant research on justice focuses on reactions to justice or injustices in the workplace (Greenberg, 1997; Ince & Gul, 2011; Lind et al., 2000;). This is termed as the *reactive approach* in justice literature. With this approach, researchers focus on people's attempts either to escape from or to avoid perceived unfair states. In contrast, the *proactive approach* focuses on behaviors designed to promote justice. With this approach in consideration, researchers examine managers' or hierarchical superiors' proactive behaviors attempting to create just work environments. If managers and organizational justice scholars actively engage in the proactive approach to justice, we believe that a radical shift from superficial impression management to creating a truly just and fair work environment can be achieved. Organizational justice scholars can then begin to address more profound issues, such as the creation and implementation of just policies and procedures.

Linking Organizational Justice to Wider Workplace Issues

The majority of organizational justice literature deals with the dyadic relationship between supervisors and employees (i.e., interactional justice) or the reactions of employees to specific workplace policies and procedures (i.e., procedural and distributive justice). For example, the organizational behavior, workplace deviance, and management literature have not only focused on negative reactions but also on the deviant outcomes of injustice in the workplace. Ambrose, Seabright, and Schminke (2002), for instance, explain that injustice is the most common cause of sabotage and retaliation. When employees feel a sense of powerlessness, frustration, and boredom at work, their sense of injustice increases and they try to damage, disrupt, or subvert the organization for personal purposes. Further, Greenberg (1990) linked injustice to dysfunctional workplace behavior such as theft. Early research on justice and deviance focused on distributive justice and suggested that the goal of sabotage or deviant actions was to restore equity (DeMore, Fisher, & Baron, 1988; Fisher & Baron, 1982; Sieh, 1987). However, recent research suggests that individuals may take revenge against someone who has mistreated them (Bies, Tripp, & Kramer, 1997). Hence, today the topic of deviant outcomes relates mostly to the interaction dimension of justice. Justice (Folger & Baron, 1996; Folger & Skarlicki, 1998; Giacalone & Greenberg, 1997; Greenberg, 1990; Neuman & Baron, 1997; Skarlicki & Folger, 1997) and powerlessness (Ambrose et al., 2002) are promising factors to understand workplace deviances and dysfunctional consequences. It could be useful for justice researchers to gain additional insight by considering other common characteristics such as importance of control for these two factors. Moreover, no empirical study has shown significant relationships between the source of injustice (organizational versus interpersonal) and who is harmed (organization or individual), nor has it been proven that there is a significant relationship between the source of injustice and the seriousness of the sabotage.

However, justice issues also loom in the vast changes marking the structure of workplaces and the labor market more generally (e.g., Kalleberg, 2009). For example, the increasing use of flexible and temporary job arrangements calls into question the solidarity of workers and their organizations, reframing work relationships in terms of "human capital" (e.g., Foss, 2008) rather than human dignity (c.f. Islam, 2012). Similarly, part-time employees are often not accorded the same job benefits and recognition as full-time employees, even when doing similar work, bringing up questions of equity and fairness. Although these wider labor market issues are clearly relevant to how one should think about justice in the workplace, they have remained largely absent from the organizational justice literature, which has tended to focus more on psychological (versus structural) features of benefits and relationships.

Moreover, whereas the psychological justice literature has focused to a large extent on employee voice as a (c.f. Fortin, 2008) correlate of justice perceptions, and an aspect of fair procedures, the issue of voice in this literature is usually treated as a managerial issue, neglecting the wider context of employee voice in the transformations of contemporary work (e.g., Kalleberg, 2009). For example, the decline of unions in the United States, as in most OECD countries, as a mechanism for employee participation provides the backdrop to organizational policies regarding voice and other procedural issues in managerial policies. Little work has been done as yet to explore how, for example, employee voice is linked to psychological justice perception when alternate means of worker expression, such as unions or work councils, are present versus when they are not. To engage in these kinds of studies would draw a link between the psychology and sociology of voice, and better allow researchers to make connections between these levels.

Viewing Workplaces as Templates for Wider Justice Concerns

Beyond the labor market in general, the experience of organizational justice and injustice may have implications for wider notions of social equity and justice. These aspects, often linking the individual psychology of justice perceptions with the sociology of work, involve the ways in which injustice at work can transfer over to nonwork life, through providing templates or schemas for social action more generally, or through creating inequitable outcomes that generate material and symbolic social inequities.

For example, regarding the increased precarity of work, some scholars claim that social drift and a sense of social alienation come about when work life is no longer seen in terms of solidarity and community (e.g., Deranty, 2008). Worker's experience of being denied dignity, autonomy, and individuality at work, key to the experience of injustice (van Prooijen & Willem, 2009), can erode the social recognition essential to the creation of social solidarity (Islam, 2012). Views of employees as substitutable, with skills decontextualized from their social contexts and packaged as individual "CVs" (Bernstein, 2006), create a kind of objectification of employees that denies human autonomy.

Beyond a sense of individual injustice and alienation, workplace injustice, particularly when distributional outcomes are unequal among class, racial, or ethnic lines, can exacerbate existing group-based social divisions (e.g., Gill & Pratt, 2008). For example, perceptions by group members that they are being treated unjustly by their organization on the basis of group categories are likely to view society as more unjust generally, such that the organization becomes the vehicle through which visions of society-at-large are created and reinforced. Further, as Christopherson (2008) claims, precarious work conditions can increase minority-group members' dependence on identity-based social ties and sources of support, leading to social fragmentation along identity lines and the loss of a sense of a just society in general.

In sum, the aforementioned avenues pose difficult questions about the relationships between individual justice perceptions, structures of work, and social justice more generally. Answering these questions will probably require increased collaboration between psychologists, organizational scholars, and sociologists. The multileveled nature of organizational justice requires a broad perspective, and as we have suggested, the payoffs for such an understanding of justice are significant.

CONCLUSION

In this chapter, we focused on the concept of organizational justice and elaborated existing theories regarding the meaning, perception, and promotion of the same. We started out by outlining the broad categories of research topics with regard to organizational justice that have been given due importance in business and industrial-organizational psychology literature. These research topics include understanding the meaning of organizational justice, understanding how individuals react to fair or unfair outcomes, and finally, understanding how justice-related decisions are made. We then discussed in depth the concept of organizational justice, its different dimensions, the debate surrounding the construct discrimination, and various theories related to social justice. Next, we also discussed the complexity of the organizational justice construct by evoking the multilevel nature of the construct, and the multilevel contextual factors that influence justice perceptions. We explained that the different dimensions of justice don't just mean different thing but they are also considered at different level of analysis. We then discussed further areas in which research can do justice to these different dimensions and levels, involving cross-level work in the promotion of just workplaces, the understanding of organizational justice against the backdrop of contemporary workplace changes, and the relevance of organizational justice for understanding social justice more generally.

NOTE

1. Almost all studies cited in this subsection rely on Hofstede's (1980) national culture model to differentiate cultures.

REFERENCES

Adams, J. S. (1965). Inequity in social exchange. In L. Berkowitz (Ed.), *Advances in experimental social psychology* (Vol. 2, pp. 267–299). New York, NY: Academic.

Ambrose, M. L., & Kulik, C. T. (2001). How do I know that's fair? A categorization approach to fairness judgments. In S. W. Gilliland, D. D. Steiner, & D. P. Skarlicki (Eds.), *Theoretical and cultural perspectives on organizational justice* (pp. 35–62). Greenwich, CT: Information Age.

Ambrose, M. L., & Schminke, M. (2003). Organization structure as a moderator of the relationship between procedural justice, interactional justice, perceived organizational support, and supervisory trust. *Journal of Applied Psychology, 88,* 295–305.

Ambrose, M. L., Seabright, M., & Schminke, M. (2002). Sabotage in the workplace: The role of organizational injustice. *Organizational Behavior and Human Decision Processes, 89,* 947–965.

Bernstein, J. (2006). All together now: Common sense for a new economy. San Francisco, CA: Berrett-Koehler.

Bies, R. J. (1986). Identifying principles of interactional justice: The case of corporate recruiting. Paper presented at the Moving beyond Equity Theory: New Directions in Research on Justice in Organizations, Symposium at the Annual Meeting of the Academy of Management, Chicago, IL.

Bies, R. J. (2001). Interactional (in)justice: The sacred and the profane. In J. Greenberg & R. Cropanzano (Eds.), *Advances in organizational justice* (pp. 89–118). Palo Alto, CA: Stanford University.

Bies, R. J., & Moag, J. F. (1986). Interactional justice: Communication criteria of fairness. In R. J. Lewicki, B. H. Sheppard, & M. H. Bazerman (Eds.), *Research on negotiations in organizations* (Vol. 1, pp. 43–55). Greenwich, CT: JAI.

Bies, R. J., Tripp, T. M., & Kramer, R. M. (1997). At the breaking point: Cognitive and social dynamics of revenge in organizations. In R. Giacalone & J. Greenberg (Eds.), *Antisocial behavior in organizations* (pp. 18–36). London: Sage.

Blader, S. L., Chang, C. C., & Tyler, T. R. (2001). Procedural justice and retaliation in organizations: Comparing cross-nationally the importance of fair group processes. *International Journal of Conflict Management, 12,* 295–311.

Blader, S., & Tyler, T. R. (2005). How can theories of organizational justice explain the effects of fairness? In J. Greenberg & J. A. Colquitt (Eds.), *Handbook of organizational justice* (pp. 329–354). Mahwah, NJ: Lawrence Erlbaum.

Bobocel, D. R., & Holmvall, C. M. (2001). Are interactional justice and procedural justice different? Framing the debate. In S. W. Gilliland, D. D. Steiner, & D. P. Skarlicki (Eds), *Theoretical and cultural perspectives on organizational justice* (pp. 85–108). Greenwich, CT: IAP.

Christopherson, S. (2008). Beyond the self-expressive creative worker: An industry perspective on entertainment media. *Theory, Culture & Society, 25*(7–8), 73–95.

Cohen-Charash, Y., & Spector, P. E. (2001). The role of justice in organizations: A meta-analysis. *Organizational Behavior and Human Decision Processes, 86,* 278–321.

Colquitt, J. A., Conlon, D. E., Wesson, M. J., Porter, C., & Ng, K. Y. (2001). Justice at the millennium: A meta-analytic review of 25 years of organizational justice research. *Journal of Applied Psychology, 86*(3), 425–445.

Cropanzano, R., Byrne, Z. S., Bobocel, R., & Rupp, D. (2001). Moral virtues, fairness heuristics, social entities and other denizens of organizational justice. *Journal of Vocational Behavior, 58,* 164–209.

Cropanzano, R., & Greenberg, J. (1997). Progress in organizational justice: Tunneling through the maze. In C. L. Cooper & I. T. Robertson (Eds.), *International review of industrial and organizational psychology* (pp. 317–372). New York, NY: Wiley.

Cropanzano, R., Rupp, D. E., Mohler, C. J., & Schminke, M. (2001). Three roads to organizational justice. In J. Martocchio (Ed.), *Research in personnel and human resource management* (Vol. 20, pp. 1–113). Bingley, UK: Emerald.

DeMore, S. W., Fisher, J. D., & Baron, R. M. (1988). The equity-control model as a predictor of vandalism among college students. *Journal of Applied Social Psychology, 18,* 80–91.

Deranty, J. P. (2008). Work and the precarisation of existence. *European Journal of Social Theory, 11(4),* 443-463.

Erdogan, B. (2002). Antecedents and consequences of justice perceptions in performance appraisals. *Human Resource Management Review, 12,* 555–578.

Fisher, J. D., & Baron, R. M. (1982). An equity based model of vandalism. *Population and Environment, 5,* 182–200.

French, W. 1964. *The personal management process: Human resource administration.* Boston, MA: Houghton Mifflin.

Folger, R. (1998). Fairness as a moral virtue. In M. Schminke (Ed.), *Managerial ethics: Moral management of people and processes* (pp. 13–34). Mahwah, NJ: Lawrence Erlbaum.

Folger, R., & Baron, R. A. (1996). Violence and hostility at work: A model of reactions to perceived injustice. In G. R. VanderBos & E. Q. Bulatao (Eds.), *Violence on the job: Identifying risks and developing solutions* (pp. 51–85). Washington, DC: American Psychological Association.

Folger, R., & Cropanzano, R. (2001). Fairness theory: Justice as accountability. In J. Greenberg & R. Cropanzano (Eds.), *Advances in organizational justice* (pp. 1–55). Palo Alto, CA: Stanford University.

Folger, R., & Skarlicki, D. P. (1998). A popcorn metaphor for employee aggression. In R. W. Griffin, A. O'Leary-Kelly, & J. M. Collins (Eds.), *Dysfunctional behavior in organizations, Part A: Violent and deviant behavior* (pp. 43–82). Stamford, CT: JAI Press.

Fortin, M. (2008). Perspectives on organizational justice: Concept clarification, social context integration, time and links with morality. *International Journal of Management Reviews, 10*(2), 93–126. doi: 10.1111/j.1468-2370.2008.00231.x

Foss, N. J. (2008). Human Capital and Transaction Cost Economics, SMG Working Paper No. 2, Copenhagen Business School Working Paper Series.

Giacalone, R. A., & Greenberg, J. (1997). *Antisocial behavior in organizations.* Thousand Oaks, CA: Sage.

Gill, R., & Pratt, A. (2008). In the social factory? Immaterial labour, precariousness and cultural work. *Theory, Culture & Society, 25*(7–8), 1–30.

Greenberg, J. (1993). The social side of fairness: Interpersonal and informational classes of organizational justice. In R. Cropanzano (Ed.), *Justice in the workplace: Approaching fairness in human resource management* (pp. 79–103). Hillsdale, NJ: Lawrence Erlbaum.

Greenberg, J. (1997). A social influence model of employee theft: Beyond the fraud triangle. In R. J. Lewicki, R. J. Bies, & B. H. Sheppard (Eds.), *Research on negotiation in organizations* (Vol. 6, pp. 29–52). Greenwich, CT: JAI.

Greenberg, J., (2001). The seven loose can(n)ons of organizational justice. In J. Greenberg & R. Cropanzano (Eds.), *Advances in organizational justice* (pp. 245–272). Palo Alto, CA: Stanford University.

Greenberg, J., & Cohen, R. L. (1982). Why justice? Normative and instrumental interpretations. In J. Greenberg & R. L. Cohen (Eds.), *Equity and justice in social behavior* (pp. 437–469). New York, NY: Academic.

Haidt, J. (2001). The emotional dog and its rational tail: A social intuitionist approach to moral judgment. *Psychological Review, 108,* 814–834.

Ince, M., & Gul, H. (2011). The effect of employees' perceptions of organizational justice on organizational citizenship behavior: An application in Turkish public institutions. *International Journal of Business and Management, 6*(6), 134–149.

Islam, G. (2012). Recognition, reification and practices of forgetting: Ethical implications of human resource management. *Journal of Business Ethics, 111*(1), 37–48.

Kagan, J. (1984). *The nature of the child.* New York, NY: Basic Books.

Kahneman, D., Knetsch, J. L., & Thaler, R. H. (1986). Fairness as a constraint on profit seeking: Entitlements in the market. *The American Economic Review, 76,* 728–741.

Kalleberg, A. L. (2009). Precarious work, insecure workers: Employment relations in transition. *American Sociological Review, 74,* 1–22.

Kohlberg, L. (1969). Stage and sequence: The cognitive–developmental approach to socialization. In D. A. Goslin (Ed.), *Handbook of socialization theory and research* (pp. 347–480). Chicago, IL: Rand McNally.

Leung, K., & Tong, K. K. (2004). Justice across cultures: A three-stage model for intercultural negotiation. In M. Gelfand & J. Brett (Eds.), *The handbook of negotiation and culture* (pp. 313–333). Palo Alto, CA: Stanford University Press.

Leventhal, G. S., Karuza, J., & Fry, W. R. (1980). Beyond fairness: A theory of allocation preferences. In G. Mikula (Ed.), *Justice and social interaction* (pp. 167–218). New York, NY: Springer-Verlag.

Liao, H., & Rupp, D. E. (2005). The impact of justice climate and justice orientation on work outcomes: A cross-level multifoci framework. *Journal of Applied Psychology, 90,* 242–256.

Lind, E. A., Kulik, C. T., Ambrose, M., & De Vera Park, M. V. (1993). Individual and corporate dispute resolution: Using procedural fairness as a decision heuristic. *Administrative Science Quarterly, 38,* 224–251.

Lind, E. A., Greenberg, J., Scott, K. S., & Welchans, T. D. (2000). The winding road from employee to complainant: Situational and psycho-logical determinants of wrongful termination claims. *Administrative Science Quarterly, 45,* 557–590.

Lind, E. A., & Tyler, T. R. (1988). *The social psychology of procedural justice.* New York, NY: Plenum Press.

Lind, E. A., & Van den Bos, K. (2002). When fairness works: Towards a general theory of uncertainty management. In B. M. Staw & R. M. Kramer (Eds.), *Research in organizational behavior* (Vol. 24, pp. 181–223). Boston, MA: Elsevier.

Masterson, S. S., Lewis, K., Goldman, B. M., & Taylor, M. S. (2000). Integrating justice and social exchange: The differing effects of fair procedures and treatment on work relationships. *Academy of Management Journal, 43,* 738–748.

McFarlin, D. B., & Sweeney, P. D. (2001). Cross-cultural applications of organizational justice. In R. Cropanzano (Ed.), *Justice in the workplace: From theory to practice* (Vol. 2, pp. 67–96). Mahwah, NJ: Lawrence Erlbaum.

Molm, L. D., Quist, T. M., & Wiseley, P. A. (1993). Reciprocal justice and strategies of exchange. *Social Forces, 72*(1), 19–44.

Moorman, R. H. (1991). Relationship between organizational justice and organizational citizenship behaviors: Do fairness perceptions influence employee citizenship? *Journal of Applied Psychology, 76,* 845–855.

Mossholder, K. W., Bennett, N., & Martin, C. L. (1998). A multilevel analysis of procedural justice context justice. *Organizational Behavior and Human Decision Processes, 89,* 925–946.

Neuman, J. H., & Baron, R. A. (1997). Aggression in the workplace. In R. Giacalone & J. Greenberg (Eds.), *Antisocial behavior in organizations* (pp. 37–67). London: Sage.

Piaget, J. (1975). *The moral judgment of the child.* London, UK: Routledge and Kegan Paul. (Original work published 1932).

Pillai, R., Schriesheim, C. A., & Williams, E. S. 1999. Fairness perceptions and trust as mediators for trans-formational and transactional leadership: A two-sample study. *Journal of Management, 25,* 897–933.

Rawls, J. (1971). *A theory of justice.* Oxford, UK: Oxford University Press.

Roberson, Q. M. (2006). Justice in teams: The activation and role of sensemaking in the emergence of justice climates. *Organizational Behavior and Human Decision Processes, 100,* 177–192.

Sheppard, B. H. (1985). Justice is no simple matter: Case for elaborating our model of procedural fairness. *Journal of Personality and Social Psychology, 49,* 953–962.

Sieh, E.W. (1987). Garment workers: Perceptions of inequity and employee theft. *British Journal of Criminology, 27,* 174–191.

Skarlicki, D. P., & Folger, R. (1997). Retaliation in the workplace: The roles of distributive, procedural, and interactional justice. *Journal of Applied Psychology, 60,* 635–637.

Sweeney, P. D., & McFarlin, D. B. (1993). Workers' evaluation of the "ends" and the "means": An examination of four models of distributive and procedural justice. *Organizational Behavior and Human Decision Processes, 55,* 23–40.

Thibaut, J., & Walker, L. (1975). *Procedural justice: A psychological analysis.* Hillsdale, NJ: Erlbaum.

Turiel, E. (1983). *The development of social knowledge: Morality and convention.* Cambridge, UK: Cambridge University Press.

Tyler, T. R. (1987). Conditions leading to value-expressive effects in judgments of procedural justice: A test of four models. *Journal of Personality and Social Psychology, 52,* 333–344.

Tyler, T. R. (1988). What is procedural justice? Criteria used by citizens to assess the fairness of legal procedures. *Law and Society Review, 22,* 301–335.

Tyler, T. R. (1990). *Why do people obey the law? Procedural justice, legitimacy, and compliance.* New Haven, CT: Yale University Press.

Tyler, T. R., & Bies, R. J. (1990). Beyond formal procedures: The interpersonal context of procedural justice. In J. S. Carroll (Ed.), *Applied social psychology and organizational settings* (pp. 77–98). Hillsdale, NJ: Erlbaum.

Tyler, T. R., & Blader, S. (2000). *Cooperation in groups: Procedural justice, social identity, and behavioral engagement.* Philadelphia, PA: Psychology.

Tyler, T. R., & Blader, S. (2003). The group engagement model: procedural justice, social identity, and cooperative behavior. *Personality and Social Psychology Review, 7,* 349–361.

Tyler, T. R., & Lind, E. A. (1992). A relational model of authority in groups. In M. P. Zanna (Ed.), *Advances in experimental social psychology* (Vol. 25, pp. 115–191). San Diego, CA: Academic Press.

Tyler, T. R., Rasinski, K. A., & McGraw, K. M. (1985). The influence of perceived injustice on the endorsement of political leaders. *Journal of Applied Social Psychology, 15,* 700–725.

van den Bos, K. (2003). On the subjective quality of social justice: The role of affect as information in the psychology of justice judgments. *Journal of Personality and Social Psychology, 85*(3), 482–498.

van den Bos, K., & Lind, E. A. (2002). Uncertainty management by means of fairness judgments. In M. P. Zanna (Ed.), *Advances in experimental social psychology* (Vol. 34, pp. 1–60). San Diego, CA: Academic Press.

van Prooijen, J., & Willem, V. (2009). Procedural justice as autonomy regulation. *Journal of Personality and Social Psychology, 96*(6), 1166–1180.

Chapter 6

Empowering Communities for Health Promotion

Carolyn M. Tucker, Tya M. Arthur, Julia Roncoroni, Whitney Wall, Jackeline Sanchez, Tasia M. Smith, and Dynora Pierre-Louis

Empowerment is described as the process by which people, organizations, and communities gain control or power over their lives and health (Labonte, 2010). Empowerment also has been described as the process by which groups with little power (e.g., racial and ethnic minorities, the poor) work together to increase control and power over events that influence their lives and health. This power and control is gained by groups and individuals through their own efforts rather than bestowed by others. However, those with more power, or who have access to it, must help create conditions that enable those with little power to gain control and power over their own lives and health (Laverack, 2011).

Empowering communities to control or have power over their own health (i.e., community health empowerment) involves enhancing the capacity of community-based organizations to identify community health needs, and to implement culturally and contextually appropriate health promotion and disease prevention interventions to address these needs (Freudenberg, 2004; Goodman, Speers, McLeroy, & Fawcett, 2009). This capacity enhancement involves organizational empowerment, which requires (1) viability, leadership, and trust among organization members to engage in community change actions; (2) collaborations and alliances with other organizations; and (3) disseminating information, marshaling resources, and developing new programs and projects to benefit the community (Peterson & Zimmerman, 2004).

Community health promotion is a growing national priority in the United States and in many other countries around the world (Agency for Healthcare Research and Quality [AHRQ], 2011). The major variables providing impetus for making community health promotion a high priority in the United States include (1) widening prevalence of health disparities, (2) skyrocketing general health care and health disparities-related costs, (3) increasing awareness of the high prevalence of limited health literacy, and (4) increasing recognition of health promotion as an integral part of social justice. These variables are discussed in the following sections.

HEALTH DISPARITIES

Health disparities are differences in health status, health care quality, health care access, health outcomes, disease prevalence, and death rates in association with demographic variables, including race and ethnicity, gender, age, education, income, sexual orientation, disability status, and geographical location (U.S. Department of Health and Human Services [HHS], 2011). Racial and ethnic minorities, the poor, and the medically underserved are disproportionately affected by health disparities. Specifically, these groups have the highest prevalence of chronic diseases and death rates from these diseases because of limited health literacy, lack of access to preventive care, the absence of affordable care options, provision of low-quality health care by providers, and treatment non-adherence related to unsatisfactory care in general and culturally insensitive health care in particular (AHRQ, 2011).

The United States is the wealthiest country in the world, has the greatest access to education, and is a world leader in health care services and medical technology, yet ranks near the bottom among developed countries on most health status measures (Schroeder, 2007). Disparities in health status are large in the United States and globally, and are an impediment to improving national health rankings. The underlying core contributors to health disparities in the United States, and in other countries, are (1) an economic and social structure that keeps most resources, including health and economic resources, in the control of individuals and groups with higher versus lower incomes and social status; and (2) an understandable resistance or reluctance by individuals and groups with higher incomes and social status to change this status quo.

SKYROCKETING GENERAL HEALTH CARE AND HEALTH DISPARITIES-RELATED COSTS

The cost of health care continues to rise due to a combination of factors, including greater use of expensive health care services (e.g., emergency care), increases in medical technology and pharmaceutical costs, and growing numbers of health care users (e.g., individuals with chronic health problems) (Department of Defense, 2007). Additionally, the total economic cost of health disparities in the United States is more than $300 billion annually (LaViest, Gaskin, & Richard, 2009). The ultimate outcome of these realities is higher costs for all. Given that racial and ethnic minorities and the poor are most negatively impacted by health disparities and are least likely to afford increasingly more costly health promotion and health care services—and thus have less personal control over their health as a result, it is clear that economic and health empowerment in minority and low-income communities is needed. It is not surprising, therefore, that economic empowerment and community participation are considered major strategies worldwide for reducing health disparities (Tsey, Harvey, Gibson, & Pearson, 2009).

HIGH PREVALENCE OF LIMITED HEALTH LITERACY

Health literacy is defined in the 2010 Patient Protection and Affordable Care Act (ACA) as the capacity to obtain, communicate, process, and understand basic health information and services to make appropriate health decisions. Limited health literacy impedes health promotion. Specifically, limited health literacy (1) lowers the ability to understand food labels, and thus the ability to make healthy dietary choices; and (2) lowers the ability to understand medication labels, and thus the ability to follow treatment recommendations. Limited health literacy also has been positively linked to a lower likelihood of receiving preventive care, greater use of costly emergency care, worse health status, and higher mortality rates among the elderly (Berkman, Sheridan, Donahue, Halpern, & Crotty, 2011).

The inclusion of a focus on health literacy in the ACA called attention to the prevalence of limited health literacy in the United States. A national population-level study of health literacy skills reported that only 12 percent of U.S. adults have the needed health literacy skills to understand and use health information effectively, and more than a third of adults in the United States have basic or below basic health literacy (DHHS, 2008).

Health policies such as the ACA, the Department of Health and Human Services' 2010 National Action Plan to Improve Health Literacy, and the Plain Writing Act of 2010 have been set forth to promote health literacy within the culturally diverse communities of the United States. This policy approach to promoting health literacy results from national recognition that (1) limited health literacy is a multifaceted problem involving individuals, their health care providers, and health and health care organizations within their communities; and (2) promoting health literacy, and therefore health, requires system-level changes for both health professionals and organizations within communities (Institute of Medicine [IOM], 2011). For example, providers must be trained to communicate with patients in a clear, understandable manner and to be culturally competent and sensitive, and health and health care organizations must be designed to enable patients to successfully navigate in them and obtain needed health services.

RECOGNITION OF HEALTH PROMOTION AS AN INTEGRAL PART OF SOCIAL JUSTICE

There is increasing recognition that health promotion is positively influenced not only by individual engagement in health-promoting behaviors, but also by the following conditions that impact health: (1) behavioral conditions such as healthy community norms with regard to healthy eating, exercise, and abstinence from tobacco products (NPA, 2011); (2) environmental conditions such as the absence of lead exposure, safe workplaces, and safe living conditions; and (3) social conditions such as middle to high socioeconomic status, employment, and educational attainment beyond high school, food security, available housing and transportation, absence of perceived racism, and access to affordable, quality health care (Andrulis, Siddiqui, Purtle, & Duchon, 2010; Centers for Disease Control and Prevention, 2011; Law et al., 2010). These conditions do not exist across all communities, and the power to change this reality is typically held by the members of communities who experience these conditions. This state of affairs has contributed to the increasing advocacy for social justice to address social conditions that negatively impact peoples' lives (e.g., health disparities). *Social justice* has been defined as a balance of benefits and burdens within communities, and society at large, so that everyone experiences equitable living and full participation in decisions and activities affecting each other (Buettner-Schmidt & Lobo, 2012).

When considered in a health care context, social justice has been termed health care justice. Specifically, *health care justice* encompasses fairness, equal distribution of health care resources and power, fair health care organizations and policies, and equal human rights and well-being for all involved in the provision and experience of health care within health care organizations (Buettner-Schmidt & Lobo, 2012). The occurrence of physicians and health care organizations having and exerting power over their patients (e.g., by formulating health care policies and procedures without patient input, making treatment decisions about patients with no or little input from patients) can be described as health care injustice. Documented racial bias in the treatment of racial and ethnic minority patients (Schulman et al., 1999) is also an example of health care injustice. Typically, individuals and patients with little economic or social power (e.g., racial/ethnic minorities, the poor, and the medically underserved) are easier to exclude from decision-making processes regarding their health and well-being and are more likely to report experiencing racial bias in the health care process.

CONTRIBUTIONS OF PSYCHOLOGY TO THE EMERGENCE OF COMMUNITY EMPOWERMENT FOR HEALTH PROMOTION

The field of psychology has contributed significantly to the increasing focus on community empowerment for health promotion. The initial psychology perspectives and theories and models that addressed health promotion viewed the health of individuals as influenced primarily by psychological variables (e.g., perceived control, motivation), skills, and knowledge that are modifiable with individual-focused interventions that may or may not include the support of significant others (e.g., family). Presently, however, there is much consensus that the health of individuals (i.e., community members) is influenced by external variables (e.g., air pollution, lack of access to potable water, food insecurity due to poverty) over which they have limited individual control, but over which they can have much control when working as part of a mobilized community with a health promotion goal. Examples of the psychology perspectives and theories and models that have informed community empowerment for health promotion are described in the following sections.

Critical Psychology

An impetus for the movement toward community empowerment for health promotion is critical psychology, which emphasizes the importance of exploring the connection between human behaviors and activities (e.g., health behaviors), and both social and material conditions (e.g., poverty, absence of parks for children) and power structures (e.g., health policy boards without representation from culturally- and economically diverse communities). Critical psychology includes an emphasis on research to understand the experience of social exclusion, marginalization and suffering that comes with social exclusion, and unequal social structures, processes, and access to power (Murray & Polland, 2006). Such research has provided an impetus for community empowerment (e.g., community mobilization to vote for political leaders that support health care in poor communities) that leads to social, economic, environmental, and other conditions conducive to the health and well-being of community members.

Community Psychology

A major contribution of community psychology to community empowerment for health promotion is its view of communities as important social forces in the process of change (e.g., the process of transforming social inequality to social justice; Nelson & Prilleltensky, 2004). The core aspects of community psychology are: (1) understanding community-level conditions and individual-level variables that together enable community members to engage in healthy lifestyles and (2) promoting changes at the community level that enable these healthy lifestyles. This community-level change typically involves changes in existing power structures and distribution of community resources through the efforts of community members to enable individual-level empowerment for engaging in healthy lifestyles (Campbell & Murray, 2004).

Health Psychology

This was the most popular area of psychology in the past decade, likely because of its focus on understanding and influencing health promotion and disease prevention. Health psychology utilizes a biopsychosocial model, considers direct and indirect linkages between psychology and health, views health as a continuum, and seeks to understand variability in health (Ogden, 2012). This area of psychology has provided leadership in viewing health not as an absence of disease but rather as a goal in itself that includes happiness, well-being, and an overall health-related quality of life (Schmidt, Raque-Bogdan, Piontkowski, & Schaefer, 2011). Core perspectives of health psychology are that promotion and maintenance of health is a key strategy for the prevention of disease and that health promotion plays a role in treating and minimizing the negative impact of illness. A key defining characteristic of health psychology is the use of theory and research to develop, test, and evaluate interventions to promote health and prevent disease.

Subspecialty areas within health psychology include the following: (1) clinical health psychology—an area that targets the health care system for the purposes of both health promotion and treatment of illness (Marks 2002); (b) public health psychology—an area concerned with health promotion rather than treatment of illness with major attention to the social, economic, political, and individual determinants of health, epidemiological studies, and implementation and evaluation of public health interventions (Carroll, Davey, Smith, & Bennett, 1996); (3) critical health psychology—an area focused on achieving health equity through changing the governmental, political, and commercial power structures that foster health inequity (Marks, 2002); and (4) community health psychology—an area concerned with social change that enables individuals in vulnerable communities to be empowered to take charge of their health individually and collectively through changes in social structures and to the control of economic resources that render them at risk for poor health (Campbell & Murray, 2004; Marks, 2002). Community health psychology has been most instrumental in bringing national and international attention to the need for and value of empowering communities for health promotion.

CONTEMPORARY THEORIES/MODELS USED TO INFORM INTERVENTIONS TO FOSTER HEALTH PROMOTING BEHAVIORS AMONG COMMUNITY MEMBERS

An important aspect of community health empowerment is empowering individuals and groups in communities to engage in health-promoting behaviors (e.g., eating foods lower in sodium, fat, and sugar, walking up stairs rather than taking an elevator). Promoting individual health empowerment is an important supplement to—not a replacement for—efforts to promote community empowerment needed to create conditions and actions in communities for community health promotion (e.g., enacting policies that ensure pure and safe drinking water).

The socio-ecological model (Bronfenbrenner, 1979) and social cognitive theory (Bandura, 1986) are two well-known theories for understanding health promoting behaviors and developing interventions to promote these behaviors. A relatively new theory, called health self-empowerment theory (Tucker, Butler, Loyuk,

Desmond, & Surrency, 2009; Tucker, Daly, & Herman, 2010), has been set forth as a culturally sensitive theory for use in understanding and facilitating health promoting behaviors of individuals who experience limited power in important aspects of their lives (e.g., racial and ethnic minorities, the poor). Additionally, a relatively new model—the patient-centered culturally sensitive health care model (Tucker, Rice, Marsiske, Nielson, & Herman, 2011)—has been developed to explain and increase health-promoting behaviors and treatment adherence among culturally diverse patients.

Socio-Ecological Model

This model asserts that multilevel and multidimensional factors influence health and offers a framework for understanding and facilitating health promotion based on that context. These factors may include individual variables, social interactions, organizational influences, community environment and policies, geographic location and associated resources and systems, and system- and government-level variables that impact public health. According to this model, successful health promotion interventions must consider and address those factors relevant to health promotion among the target individual, group, or community (Bronfenbrenner, 1979; Smedley & Syme, 2000).

Social Cognitive Theory

This theory asserts that cognitive/personal variables (e.g., self-efficacy, self-motivation) and social/environmental variables (e.g., poverty, limited access to health care) are important determinants of health behaviors (Bandura, 1998, 2004). According to Bandura (2004), social cognitive theory emphasizes self-regulation as the core influence of health behaviors. This self-regulation occurs through knowledge of the positive and negative impact of different health practices on health, perceived self-efficacy in relation to health habits, outcome expectations for different health habits, one's health goals and plans and strategies for achieving these goals, and the perceived facilitators and barriers to desired health-related changes (Bandura, 2004).

Health Self-Empowerment (HSE) Theory

HSE theory acknowledges the influence of social, environmental, and economic conditions on health behaviors, but asserts that, given the intractable nature of these variables in many communities—including racial and ethnic minority and low-income communities—self-empowerment-oriented self-variables are key target variables for understanding and modifying the health behaviors of community members. These self-variables are described as literature-based, modifiable, self-empowerment-oriented, and cognitive-behavioral (Tucker et al., 2009, 2010).

HSE theory asserts that engagement in health-promoting behaviors is influenced by the following self-empowerment variables: (1) health self-efficacy and perceived behavioral control, (2) health motivation, (3) self-praise of health-promoting behaviors, (4) health responsibility and knowledge, and (5) active coping strategies and skills for managing stress and depression—variables that have been linked to health status. Support for this assertion comes from research showing that these health self-empowerment variables are significant predictors of health-promoting behaviors in African American women (Tucker et al., 2009).

According to HSE theory, the following occurs: (1) health self-praise directly reinforces and shapes the occurrence of health promoting behaviors, and consequently serves to sustain these behaviors; (2) health self-praise also directly influences health motivation, which influences and is influenced by health knowledge and responsibility; (3) health motivation directly influences health-promoting behaviors; and (4) the influences of health knowledge and responsibility and coping style and skills on health-promoting behaviors are mediated by health self-efficacy, which directly influences health-promoting behaviors. This theory is culturally sensitive in that it recognizes the importance of self-empowerment for health promotion among individuals or groups—particularly those who typically have low perceived or actual power such as racial and ethnic minorities—under whatever intractable cultural, social, economic, and environmental conditions that exist (Tucker et al., 2009, 2010). Research is needed to evidence the usefulness of this theory.

Patient-Centered Culturally Sensitive Health Care Model

According to this model, patient-centered culturally sensitive health care has the following specific characteristics: (1) it emphasizes the demonstration of patient-desired, modifiable, provider and office staff behaviors and attitudes; (2) it adheres to health care center policies that culturally diverse patients identify as indicators of respect for their culture and that enable these patients to feel comfortable with, trusting of, and respected by their health care providers and office staff; (3) it conceptualizes the patient-provider relationship as a partnership that emerges from patient-centeredness; and (4) it is patient-empowerment-oriented (Tucker et al., 2007a, 2007b). Furthermore, this model posits that providers' cultural sensitivity impacts patients' sense of trust in their provider, satisfaction with their provider's care, and sense of interpersonal control (i.e., empowerment in the patient-provider relationship). The model also posits that (1) patients' satisfaction with their provider's care and sense of interpersonal control indirectly affect treatment regimen adherence indicators (e.g., engagement in health-promoting lifestyles, medication, and dietary adherence); and (2) patients' physical stress, satisfaction with their providers' care, and sense of interpersonal control also have direct effects on the treatment regimen adherence indicators (Tucker et al., 2011a).

A test of this model in a community-based primary care clinic with low-income African American and non-Hispanic White patients revealed support for the model. Particularly noteworthy were the following findings: (1) perceived provider cultural sensitivity had a significant positive direct effect on dietary adherence for the African American patients only; and (b) the effect of perceived interpersonal control on health-promoting lifestyles was significantly larger for the African American patients than for the non-Hispanic White patients (Tucker et al., 2011a). These findings suggest that different health care variables may influence health-promoting behaviors of each racial and ethnic or cultural patient group and that provider cultural sensitivity as defined by culturally diverse patients likely influences these behaviors.

NEED FOR COMMUNITY HEALTH EMPOWERMENT AROUND THE WORLD

Community health empowerment (i.e., empowering communities for health promotion) involves enhancing the capacity of community-based organizations to identify community health needs and to implement culturally and contextually appropriate health promotion and disease prevention interventions designed to address the unequal environmental conditions that adversely impact the health of community members (Freudenberg, 2004; Goodman et al., 2009). Community health empowerment is informed by theories and models, such as some of those mentioned earlier in this chapter, which assert that changes in social problems (e.g., health disparities) and the promotion of health require actions that reflect the values of social justice, equity, and community participation (Zimmerman, 2000).

There are three indications of the need for community health empowerment around the world. First, community empowerment has been strongly advocated as a key strategy for reducing health disparities—a problem that plagues the United States and other countries internationally (Andrulis et al., 2010; Griffith et al., 2010). This problem is exacerbated by the increased movement of individuals, many of whom live in poverty, to other countries for jobs or other reasons (e.g., refuge, education). These documented or undocumented visitors and immigrants (who often seek to become citizens of the county to which they migrate) become a part of existing communities or create their own, and become users of the health care system in their new home country. Because of barriers such as language and income, these visitors and immigrants often do not have access to health care or experience poor quality care. It is only through culturally sensitive community health empowerment that the health disparities that these visitors and immigrants face can be eliminated. Such community health empowerment requires assessment of culture-related health issues and respect for, as well as responsiveness to, these issues when formulating community plans and actions for health promotion among all community members.

Second, community health empowerment is needed around the world to address the problems of high health care costs and the shortage of health care providers internationally, including in the United States. Given that these problems are greatest in low-income and rural communities, these communities need to be involved in creating health policies, systems, and interventions that enable satisfactory health care and health promotion among members of their communities.

Third, there is a need for community health empowerment that conceptualizes nations as communities and involves these national communities working collaboratively to develop health policies and programs that address global health challenges. Global health challenges include, but are not limited to, unsafe water, air pollution, malnutrition, and physical injuries and mental disabilities due to violence. Achieving such collaborations is consistent with the calls of Lee (2006) for identifying ways that globalization can enable people to increase control of and improve their health.

Sample Assessment Tools That Enable Community Empowerment for Health Promotion

A key strategy for empowering communities to take charge of their own health promotion is to involve them in the development and use of practical assessment tools that can be used to obtain data to guide interventions to promote health and prevent and manage disease. Given that there is increasing cultural diversity among and within communities, it is important that such assessments are developed with input from culturally diverse individuals. These individuals are the true experts on the variables that influence their own health-promoting behaviors and their health care behaviors for disease prevention and management. Following are a few examples of practical assessment tools that can be used in community efforts to promote health and prevent or manage disease.

Motivators of and Barriers to Health-Smart Behaviors Inventory (MB-HSBI)—Adult Form (Tucker et al., 2011b) and Youth Form (Tucker et al., 2012)

Both the Adult Form and Youth Form of the MB-HSBI assess the extent to which certain variables are motivators of, or barriers to, engaging in four health-promoting (health-smart) behaviors using a 4-point scale from 1 (*strongly disagree*) to 4 (*strongly agree*). The four health-smart behavior domains of each form of the MB-HSBI are as follows: (1) eating a healthy breakfast, (2) eating healthy foods and snacks, (3) drinking water and other healthy drinks, and (4) engaging in physical activity. For each of these four health-smart behavior domains, the MB-HSBI includes a motivators scale and a barriers scale.

Development of each form of the MB-HSBI involved having race and ethnicity-, gender-, and age-concordant focus groups identify the motivators of and barriers to health-promoting (health-smart) behaviors. These focus groups included low-income African American, Hispanic/Latino, and non-Hispanic White children, adolescents, and adults (Bragg, Tucker, Kaye, & Desmond, 2009). The inventories were used in a national study involving 926 adults and 576 youth (9 to 17 years) to establish their reliability and validity. Factor analyses revealed that both inventory versions consist of scales that have adequate-to-high internal consistencies. Additionally, both inventory versions were found to have concurrent, convergent, and discriminant validity (Tucker et al., 2011b, 2012).

Tucker Culturally Sensitive Health Care Provider Inventory (T-CSHCPI; Tucker, Nghiem, Marsiske, & Robinson, 2012)

The T-CSHCPI assesses patients' perceived levels of patient-centered cultural sensitivity displayed by their providers. It consists of 27 behaviors, attitudes, and types of provider knowledge (i.e., cultural sensitivity indicators) that were identified through culturally diverse focus groups as enabling patients to feel comfortable with, trusting of, and respected by their providers (Tucker et al., 2003). The instructions on the T-CSHCPI are to rate level of agreement that the provider, seen most often at one's health care site, shows the listed cultural sensitivity indicators, using a Likert rating scale from 1 (*strongly disagree*) to 4 (*strongly agree*). Analyses of data from administration of the T-CSHCPI to a culturally diverse national sample of outpatients revealed that the inventory's overall reliability and the reliability of each of its three subscales was >.90. This inventory also was shown to be valid when used with this national sample (Tucker et al., 2012).

Tucker Culturally Sensitive Health Care Office Staff Inventory (T-CSHCOSI; Tucker, Wall, Marsiske, Nghiem, & Roncoroni, 2014)

The T-CSHCOSI assesses patients' perceived levels of patient-centered cultural sensitivity displayed by the front-desk office staff at their health care site. It consists of 18 cultural sensitivity indicators that were identified through culturally diverse focus groups as enabling patients to feel comfortable with, trusting of, and respected by the front desk office staff at their health care site. The instructions for this inventory are to rate level of agreement that the front desk office staff at one's health care site show the listed office staff cultural sensitivity indicators on a Likert scale from 1 (*strongly disagree*) to 4 (*strongly agree*). Data from a culturally diverse national sample of patients who receive care at hospitals, community centers and clinics, or private practice offices showed that the T-CSHCOSI and its two subscales were reliable and that the inventory was valid when used with this sample of patients.

Tucker Culturally Sensitive Health Care Environment Inventory (T-CSHCEI; Tucker, Roncoroni, Marsiske, Nghiem, & Wall, 2014)

This is a nine-item self-report measure designed to assess patients' perceived levels of patient-centered cultural sensitivity in the physical environment and policies of their health care site. These items were generated in culturally diverse adult focus groups in which patients were asked to identify characteristics of their health care site that enabled them to feel comfortable, trusting, and respected. The instructions on the T-CSHCEI are to rate level of agreement that the listed health care site characteristics and policies exist at their health care site using a Likert scale from 1 (*strongly disagree*) to 4 (*strongly agree*). The T-CSHCEI was shown to be valid and reliable ($\alpha = .93$) when administered to a culturally diverse national sample of patients.

Community Health Promotion Intervention Development, Testing, and Evaluation

There is growing consensus that successful interventions to promote community health involve a collaborative partnership with the community and are community empowerment-oriented, assessment-based, culturally sensitive, responsive to the needs, strengths, values, and context of the community, consistent with a social justice orientation, evaluated to determine their effectiveness, and sustained through strategies planned when developing the interventions. The Principles of Community Engagement (National Institutes of Health [NIH], 2011), the Community-Based Participatory Research approach (Minkler & Wallerstein, 2003), and the RE-AIM Framework (Glasgow, Vogt, & Boles, 1999) are useful in guiding the development, testing the effectiveness, and evaluating the public health impact of such interventions, respectively.

Intervention Development: Principles of Community Engagement

There is increasing agreement that interventions to promote health in communities must involve community leaders as highly respected research collaborators and must enable communities to play the leading roles in every aspect of the intervention, starting with determining the health issue that is of concern to the community and for which an intervention is desired. Furthermore, there is increasing agreement that such interventions, and the research to test their effectiveness, must engage the target community in ways that facilitate community empowerment. An example of the growing commitment to community-engaged research is the increased funding of community-engaged translational research and community-university collaborative research by the National Institutes of Health (NIH). Other examples of this commitment are the decision of AHRQ to advocate for engaging patients and families in the redesign of medical care (Scholle, Torda, Peikes, Han, & Genevro, 2010), and the emphasis in *Healthy People 2020* on collaboration among diverse groups as a strategy for health promotion.

To promote successful community engagement for the development of health promotion interventions, much attention has been given to defining and describing community engagement. For example, it has been described as follows:

> [T]he process of working collaboratively with and through groups of people affiliated by geographic proximity, special interest, or similar situations

> to address issues affecting the well-being of those people. It is a powerful vehicle for bringing about environmental and behavioral changes that will improve the health of the community and its members. It often involves partnerships and coalitions that help mobilize resources and influence systems, change relationships among partners, and serve as catalysts for changing policies, programs, and practices. (CDC, 1997, p. 9)

Furthermore, community engagement should be consistent with the ideals of community organization, which include social justice, empowerment, participation, and self-determination for community members (Chávez, Minkler, Wallerstein, & Spencer, 2007; Wallerstein & Duran, 2006).

The NIH (2011) has set forth nine principles of community engagement that can guide researchers and community members. Specifically, to prepare for community engagement one must (1) be clear about the intervention and research planned; and (2) learn about the culture, history, power structures, and experiences with and attitudes toward past health promotion efforts/researchers. In order for community engagement to actually occur one must (1) meet in the community with the goal of establishing trusting relationships involving researchers and interventionists and community leaders and forging commitments to collaborating for community engagement; and (2) respect that the community has the right to determine what it will and will not do and that interventions/research must occur in accordance with this right and existing community power structures. Finally, for community engagement to be successful one must (1) use a respectful community partnership approach; (2) be culturally sensitive; (3) identify and help develop community strengths and resources that will empower the community to act in self-determined ways to sustain health promotion gains; (4) be flexible and prepared to relinquish control of interventions and other activities to the community; and (5) be prepared for the needed long-term commitment to the forged partnership and collaboration.

Testing: Community-Based Participatory Research (CBPR) Approach

CBPR has become increasingly more common as a research approach to conducting health promotion research in communities. Its defining characteristics include forging a research collaboration to conduct research—a collaboration in which the collaborators (i.e., researchers and community leaders) are equal partners in all aspects of the research process and recognize and respect the important strengths that each brings to this process. Additionally, core aspects of CBPR include (1) having the community identify the health issue that is the focus of the research, and (2) participating in social change that enables community members to assume leadership in successfully addressing the identified health issue (Minkler & Wallerstein, 2003). A likely outcome of the CBPR approach is community ownership of the health promotion intervention, which will in turn increase the likelihood of the intervention being institutionalized within the community. Such institutionalization will enable long-term health promotion benefits of the intervention among community members.

Evaluation: RE-AIM Framework

The RE-AIM framework is often used to evaluate the public impact of an empirically demonstrated efficacious intervention (Glasgow et al., 1999). This framework allows the determination of whether such interventions will likely benefit the community-at-large, not just the individuals similar to the research participants.

The factors in this framework that are used to evaluate the public impact or usefulness of an intervention are as follows: (1) reach, (2) efficacy and effectiveness, (3) adoption, (4) implementation, and (5) maintenance. Reach refers to the level of individual participation (e.g., participation rate) and representativeness of the participating sample. Efficacy and effectiveness refers to negative and positive outcomes and impact on a variety of variables (e.g., quality of life), not just physiological variables. Adoption involves assessing the variety of settings that utilize an intervention or policy. Implementation refers to the level at which an intervention protocol is followed by individuals (e.g., treatment adherence) or staff at an intervention setting. Maintenance involves the degree to which behavior changes are sustained over time or an intervention or policy becomes routine (Glasgow et al., 1999).

Example Community Interventions for Promoting Community Health

Interventions to empower communities for health promotion often have occurred in churches and schools, as these organizations are stable, have major influence on the behaviors of children and adults, and have policies, structures, and networks of influential leaders (e.g., pastors, teachers) who can be effective collaborators in efforts to promote health in their communities. Other interventions to foster community health promotion typically have involved developing or changing state- or federal-level health policies; however, these policy-focused interventions usually have originated on a local level within a community or communities concerned with a health issue.

Church-Based Interventions for Health Promotion

These interventions can emerge from within churches (e.g., health ministries), outside churches (i.e., researcher implemented), or can be the product of collaborative partnerships between researchers and church leaders. The interventions that emerge from within churches often do not include research data to evaluate adequately their effectiveness; however, studies have reported all three types of church-based interventions to be effective. Based on a review of these studies, it was concluded that collaborative research studies to develop, evaluate, and test church-based interventions are recommended for community health promotion (DeHaven, Hunter, Wilder, Walton, & Berry, 2004).

Perhaps the most well-known church-based health-promotion intervention is *Body and Soul*, an evidenced-based intervention—mostly administered by church members—to increase food and vegetable consumption. Sixteen predominantly African American churches participated in the intervention, which included church-wide events, pastor support, policy change (e.g., serving fruit and vegetables at events), self-help print and video materials, and motivational interviewing conducted by trained volunteers. At six-month follow-up, church members in the intervention group showed a significant net increase in food and vegetable consumption relative to the control group as well as a significant decrease in fat intake, greater intrinsic motivation to eat fruit and vegetables, and greater social support and self-efficacy for eating fruits and vegetables (Resnicow et al., 2004). However, in a subsequent study using the RE-AIM framework to evaluate Body and Soul, implementation and maintenance problems were identified (Campbell, Resnicow, Carr, Wang, & Williams, 2007). It may be that the CBPR approach would have allowed greater attention to training and planning to prevent such problems during the intervention. Future health promotion research in churches that uses this empowerment-oriented research approach and includes cultural and spiritual sensitivity aspects (e.g., discussion of beliefs about the causes of disease) in the intervention is needed (Campbell et al., 2007).

School-Based Interventions for Health Promotion

Schools are ideal venues for empowering communities for health promotion because they are widespread throughout the community, and typically have the organizational structure, leaders (e.g., teacher, administrators), modifiable policies and curricula, and physical resources (Brown & Summerbell, 2009). Schools also have the commitment to social justice and respect from their larger community that enables such an empowerment role. Furthermore, schools have consistent access to students, who can be targets of health promotion activities and major catalysts for their parents' engagement in these activities. Thus, schools are often settings for promoting health and preventing many public health problems, including obesity, smoking, sexual health, injury prevention, and mental health (Pearson et al., 2012).

An example of a school-based health-promotion program is the five-semester school-based intervention program that was implemented by Siega-Riz et al. (2011) to improve dietary intake of middle school students. The study included both intervention and control schools. The intervention program consisted of integrating multiple dietary health promotion components (i.e., nutrition, physical education, behavior change, and social-marketing-based communications components) into the school curriculum. At the end of the study, the children at the intervention schools, as compared to the children at the control schools, reported consuming significantly more fruit and water.

Public Health Policy Interventions

Communities often have addressed problems (e.g., air pollution, smoking among adolescents) that impact their health by partnering with their local, state, and national representatives and/or with community organizations (e.g., schools, civic organizations) to advocate for policy changes to reduce or eliminate these problems. Keys to the success of such advocacy and partnerships include having research data evidencing the magnitude of the problem, economic impact data (e.g., medical costs), media coverage, and legal, practice, and research experts who can explain the data and the related proposed health policies in simple ways that lawmakers and the public can understand (Brownson, Chriqui, & Stamatakis, 2009). In other words, public health policy interventions are complex and require multilevel and multidimensional participation (Glanz, Rimer, & Viswanath, 2008). Additionally, they often are adopted state by state over time. However, public health policy interventions have the advantage of promoting health in communities across the nation and the world.

An example of a type of health policy that has promoted health in communities around the world is smoking policies that ban smoking in most or all public places. Specifically, it has been shown that following smoking bans in Pueblo, Italy, Scotland, and the United States, there have been rapid and substantial reductions in hospitalization for acute coronary events (Lloyd-Jones et al., 2010). Such research has magnified the importance of evidence-based public health policies for health promotion (Brownson et al., 2009). However, community empowerment aimed at advocating for public health policies is a critical component in making these policies become reality.

CONCLUSION

There are two overall approaches to empowering communities for health promotion—one that is individual- and family-level focused and one that is system-level focused. These approaches can and likely should be viewed as complementary rather than competing.

The individual- and family-level approach emphasizes providing community members and their families with knowledge, cognitive-behavioral strategies, and skills for taking control of their health under whatever social, economic, environmental, and educational barriers to health promotion exist. This approach recognizes that these barriers are intractable and the goal of health cannot wait for the social justice, policy changes, and other societal changes needed to alleviate these barriers. Psychologists have historically taken a leadership role in developing the psychological theories and testing the theory-based interventions that have been shown to be effective in empowering community members and their families for health promotion. This research is increasingly occurring with various levels of partnership and collaboration with community members.

The system-level approach to empowering communities for health promotion is responsive to the reality that health and health promotion are influenced tremendously by multiple factors over which individuals and families have little or no control, including poverty, poor access to fresh fruits and vegetables, racism, culturally insensitive health care providers, health illiteracy, and all other forms of social, economic, health, and health care injustice. This approach recognizes that multilevel and multidimensional partnerships that involve community members and organizations (e.g., churches, schools) and other health-focused groups (e.g., universities, health policy makers, health care providers and organizations, social justice advocates) are needed to empower communities for health promotion. Psychologists have played important roles in developing theories and testing theory-based interventions for system-level community empowerment for health promotion. However, psychologists and other researchers and interventionists need additional training and experiences to promote this community empowerment.

For psychologists to be better prepared for system-level community empowerment for health promotion it is clear that their training must be expanded to include a much increased focus on social justice and global health and the impact of these on community and individual health. Because cultural sensitivity and health care justice are important in individual- and family-level and system-level approaches to community empowerment for health promotion, it is important that psychologists receive additional training in multicultural health counseling and culturally sensitive health care (Tucker et al., 2010) and in the principles of community engagement (NIH, 2011).

Finally, it is important for psychologists to incorporate interdisciplinary research and interventions into their work, and to spend time doing activities that are community-based when they are not working, such as attending inner-city churches or community events in underserved rural communities. Such activities help to build relationships and the trust needed for community engagement—the first step to community empowerment for health promotion.

REFERENCES

Agency for Healthcare Research and Quality. (2011). *2010 National healthcare disparities report* (AHRQ Publication No. 11-0005). Retrieved from http://www.ahrq.gov/qual/nhdr10/nhdr10.pdf

Andrulis, D. P., Siddiqui, N. J., Purtle, J. P., & Duchon, L. (2010). *Patient Protection and Affordable Care Act of 2010: Advancing health equity for racially and ethnically diverse populations.* Retrieved from http://www.nashp.org/sites/default/files/files/webinars/joint.center.ppaca_.health.equity.report.pdf

Bandura, A. (1986). *Social foundations of thought and action: A social cognitive theory*. Englewood Cliffs, NJ: Prentice Hall.

Bandura, A. (1998). Health promotion from the perspective of social cognitive theory. *Psychology & Health, 13*, 623–649. doi: 10.1080/08870449808407422

Bandura, A. (2004). Health promotion by social cognitive means. *Health Education & Behavior, 31*, 143–164. doi: 10.1177/1090198104263660

Berkman, N. D., Sheridan, S. L., Donahue, K. E., Halpern, D. J., & Crotty, K. (2011). Low health literacy and health outcomes: An updated systematic review. *Annals of Internal Medicine. 155*, 97–107. Retrieved from http://www.annals.org

Bragg, M. A., Tucker, C. M., Kaye, L. B., & Desmond, F. F. (2009). Motivators of and barriers to engaging in physical activity: Perspectives of culturally diverse adolescents and adults. *American Journal of Health Education, 40*(3), 146–154. Retrieved from http://www.aahperd.org/aahe/publications/ajhe/

Bronfenbrenner, U. (1979). *The ecology of human development: Experiments by nature and design*. Cambridge, MA: Harvard University.

Brown, T., & Summerbell, C. (2009). Systematic review of school-based interventions that focus on changing dietary intake and physical activity levels to prevent childhood obesity: An update to the obesity guidance produced by the National Institute for Health and Clinical Excellence. *Obesity Reviews, 10*(1):110–141. doi: 10.1111/j.1467-789X.2008.00515.x

Brownson, R. C., Chriqui, J. F., & Stamatakis, K. A. (2009). Understanding evidence-based public health policy. *American Journal of Public Health, 99*, 1576–1583. doi: 10.2105/AJPH.2008.156224

Buettner-Schmidt, K., & Lobo, M. L. (2012). Social justice: A concept analysis. *Journal of Advanced Nursing, 68*(4), 948–958. doi: 10.1111/j.1365-2648.2011.05856.x

Campbell, C., & Murray, M. (2004). Community health psychology: Promoting analysis and action for social change. *Journal of Health Psychology, 9*(2), 187–95. doi: 10.1177/1359105304040886

Campbell, M. K., Hudson, M. A., Resnicow, K., Blakeney, N., Paxton, A., & Baskin, M. (2007). Church-based health promotion interventions: Evidence and lessons learned. *Annual Review of Public Health, 28*, 213–234. doi: 10.1146/annurev.publhealth.28.021406.144016

Campbell, M. K., Resnicow, K., Carr, C., Wang, T., & Williams, A. (2007). Process evaluation of an effective church-based diet intervention: Body & soul. *Health Education & Behavior, 34*(6), 864–880. doi: 10.1177/1090198106292020

Carrol, D., Davey Smith, G., & Bennett, P. (1996). Some observations on health and socioeconomic status. *Journal of Health Psychology, 1*, 23–39. doi: 10.1177/135910539600100103

Centers for Disease Control and Prevention. (1997). *Principles of community engagement* (1st ed.). Atlanta, GA: CDC/ATSDR Committee on Community Engagement.

Centers for Disease Control and Prevention. (2011). CDC health disparities and inequalities report—United States, 2011. *Morbidity and Mortality Weekly Report, 60*(Suppl). Retrieved from http://www.cdc.gov/mmwr/pdf/other/su6001.pdf

Chávez, V., Minkler, M., Wallerstein, N., & Spencer, M. S. (2007). Community organizing for health and social justice. In L. Cohen, V. Chávez, & S. Chehimi (Eds.), *Prevention is primary: Strategies for community well-being* (1st ed., pp. 95–120). San Francisco, CA: John Wiley and Sons.

DeHaven, M. J., Hunter, I. B., Wilder, L., Walton, J. W., & Berry, J. (2004). Health programs in faith-based organizations: Are they effective? *American Journal of Public Health, 94*(6), 1030–1036. doi: 10.2105/AJPH.94.6.1030

Department of Defense, Task Force on the Future of Military Health Care. (2007). *Task force on the future of military health care: Interim report.* Retrieved from http://health.mil/dhb/meetings/2007-05-23/Task_Force_Interim_Report_053107.pdf

Freudenberg, N. (2004). Community capacity for environmental health promotion: Determinants and implications for practice. *Health Education & Behavior, 31*(4), 472–490. doi: 10.1177/1090198104265599

Glanz, K., Rimer, B. K., & Viswanath, K. (Eds.). (2008). *Health behavior and health education: Theory, research, and practice* (4th ed.). San Francisco, CA: Jossey-Bass.

Glasgow, R. E., Vogt, T. M., & Boles, S. M. (1999). Evaluating the public health impact of health promotion interventions: The RE-AIM framework. *American Journal of Public Health, 89*(9), 1322–1327. Retrieved from http://ajph.aphapublications.org/doi/pdf/10.2105/AJPH.89.9.1322

Goodman, R. M., Speers, M. A., McLeroy, K., & Fawcett, S. (2009). Identifying and defining the dimensions of community capacity to provide a basis for measurement. *Health Education & Behavior, 25*(3), 258–278. doi: 10.1177/109019819802500303

Griffith, D. M., Allen, J. O., DeLoney, E. H., Robinson, K., Lewis, E. Y., Campbell, B., . . . Reischl, T. (2010). Community-based organizational capacity building as a strategy to reduce racial health disparities. *The Journal of Primary Prevention, 31*(1), 31–39. Retrieved from http://link.springer.com/journal/10935

Institute of Medicine. (2011). *Health literacy implications for health care reform: A workshop summary.* Washington, DC: National Academies Press.

Labonte, R. (2010). Health promotion and empowerment: Reflections on professional practice. In J. M. Black, S. R. Furney, H. M. Graf, & A. E. Nolte (Eds.), *Philosophical foundations of health education* (pp. 179–195). San Francisco, CA: Jossey-Bass.

LaViest, T. A., Gaskin, D. J., & Richard, P. (2009). *The economic burden of health inequalities in the United States.* Retrieved from http://www.jointcenter.org/research/the-economic-burden-of-health-inequalities-in-the-united-states

Laverack, G. (2011). Improving health outcomes through community empowerment: A review of the literature. *Journal of Health, Population, and Nutrition, 24,* 113–120. Retrieved from http://www.jhpn.net/index.php/jhpn/index

Law, G., Pope, J., Lalani, S., Silverman, E., Cooper, G., Fortin, P., . . . Peschken, C. (2010). Barriers to health care in a multiethnic cohort of systemic lupus erythematosus (SLE) patients: Patient and physician perceptions. *Revista Romana de Reumatologie, 19*(1), 12–20. Retrieved from http://journals.lww.com/md-journal/pages/default.aspx

Lee, K. (2006). Global health promotion: How can we strengthen governance and build effective strategies? *Health Promotion International, 21*(Suppl 1), 42–50. doi: 10.1093/heapro/dal050

Lloyd-Jones, D. M., Hong, Y., Labarthe, D., Mozaffarian, D., Appel, L. J., Van Horn, L., . . . Rosamond, W. D. (2010). Defining and setting national goals for cardiovascular health promotion and disease reduction: The American Heart Association's strategic impact goal through 2020 and beyond. *Circulation, 121*(4), 586–613. doi: 10.1161/CIRCULATIONAHA.109.192703

Marks, D. F. (2002). Freedom, responsibility and power: Contrasting approaches to health psychology. *Journal of Health Psychology, 7*(1), 5–19. doi: 10.1177/1359105302007001066

Minkler, M., & Wallerstein, N. (2003). *Community-based participatory research in health.* San Francisco, CA: Jossey-Bass.

Minority Health and Health Disparities Research and Education Act of 2000, S. 1880, 106th Cong., 2nd Sess. (2000). Retrieved from https://www.govtrack.us/congress/bills/106/s1880/text

Murray, M., & Poland, B. (2006). Health psychology and social action. *Journal of Health Psychology, 11*(3), 379–384. doi: 10.1177/1359105306063308

National Institutes of Health. (2011). *Principles of community engagement* (2nd ed.). NIH Publication No. 11-7782. Retrieved from http://www.atsdr.cdc.gov/community engagement

National Partnership for Action to End Health Disparities [NPA]. (2011). *National stakeholder strategy for achieving health equity.* Rockville, MD: U.S. Department of Health and Human Services, Office of Minority Health.

Nelson, G., & Prilleltensky, I. (2004). *Community psychology: In pursuit of liberation and well-being.* London, UK: Palgrave/Macmillan.

Ogden, J. (2012). *Health psychology: A textbook* (5th ed.). Maidenhead, UK: Open University.

Pearson, M., Chilton, R., Woods, H. B., Wyatt, K., Ford, T., Abraham, C., & Anderson, R. (2012). Implementing health promotion in schools: Protocol for a realist systematic review of research and experience in the United Kingdom (UK). *Systematic Reviews, 1*(1), 48–54. doi: 10.1186/2046-4053-1-48

Peterson N. A., & Zimmerman, M. A. (2004). Beyond the individual: Toward a nomological network of organizational empowerment. *American Journal of Community Psychology, 34*(1–2), 129–145. doi: 10.1023/B:AJCP.0000040151.77047.58

Resnicow, K., Kramish Campbell, M., Carr, C., McCarty, F., Wang, T., Periasamy, S., . . . Stables, G. (2004). Body and soul: A dietary intervention conducted through African-American churches. *American Journal of Preventive Medicine, 27*(2), 97–105. Retrieved from http://dx.doi.org/10.1016/j.amepre.2004.04.009

Schmidt, C. K., Raque-Bogdan, T. L., Piontkowski, S., & Schaefer, K. L. (2011). Putting the positive in health psychology: A content analysis of three journals. *Journal of Health Psychology, 16*(4), 607–620. doi: 10.1177/1359105310384296

Scholle, S. H., Torda, P., Peikes, D., Han, E., & Genevro, J. (2010). *Engaging patients and families in the medical home.* AHRQ Publication No. 10-0083-EF. Rockville, MD: Agency for Healthcare Research and Quality.

Schroeder, S. A. (2007). We can do better—Improving the health of the American people. *New England Journal of Medicine,* 357(12), 1221–1228. doi: 10.1056/NEJMsa073350

Schulman, K. A., Berlin, J. A., Harless, W., Kerner, J. F., Sistrunk, S., Gersh, B. J., . . . Escarce, J. J. (1999). The effect of race and sex on physicians' recommendations for cardiac catheterization. *New England Journal of Medicine, 340*(8), 618–626. doi: 10.1056/NEJM199902253400806

Siega-Riz, A. M., El Ghormli, L., Mobley, C., Gillis, B., Stadler, D., Hartstein, J., . . . Bridgman, J. (2011). The effects of the HEALTHY study intervention on middle school student dietary intakes. *International Journal of Behavioral Nutrition and Physical Act, 8*(7), 1–8. doi: 10.1186/1479-5868-8-7

Smedley, B. D., & Syme, S. L. (2000). *Promoting health: Intervention strategies from social and behavioral research.* Washington, DC: National Academies Press.

Tsey, K., Harvey, D., Gibson, T., & Pearson, L. (2009). The role of empowerment in setting a foundation for social and emotional wellbeing. *Advances in Mental Health, 8*(1), 6–15. doi: 10.5172/jamh.8.1.6

Tucker, C. M., Butler, A. M., Loyuk, I. S., Desmond, F. F., & Surrency, S. L. (2009). Predictors of a health promoting lifestyle and behaviors among low-income African American mothers and White mothers of chronically ill children. *Journal of the National Medical Association, 101*(2), 103–110. Retrieved from http://www.nmanet.org/index

Tucker, C. M., Daly, K., & Herman, K. (2010). Customized multicultural health counseling: Bridging the gap between mental and physical health for racial and ethnic minorities. In J. G. Ponterotto, J. M. Casas, L. A. Suzuki, & C. M. Alexander (Eds.), *Handbook of multicultural counseling* (3rd ed., pp. 505–516). Thousand Oaks, CA: Sage.

Tucker, C. M., Herman, K. C., Pedersen, T. R., Higley, B., Montrichard, M., & Ivery, P. (2003). Cultural sensitivity in physician-patient relationships perspectives of an ethnically diverse sample of low-income primary care patients. *Medical Care, 41*(7), 859–870. Retrieved from http://journals.lww.com/lww-medicalcare/pages/default.aspx

Tucker, C. M., Herman, K. C., Ferdinand, L. A., Bailey, T. R., Lopez, M. T., Beato, C., . . . Cooper, L. L. (2007a). Providing patient-centered culturally sensitive health care: A formative model. *The Counseling Psychologist, 35*(5), 679–705. doi: 10.1177/0011000007301689

Tucker, C. M., Mirsu-Paun, A., Van den Berg, J. J., Ferdinand, L., Jones, J. D., Curry, R. W., . . . Beato, C. (2007b). Assessments for measuring patient-centered cultural sensitivity in community-based primary care clinics. *Journal of the National Medical Association, 99*(6), 609–619. Retrieved from http://www.ncbi.nlm.nih.gov.lp.hscl.ufl.edu/pmc/articles/PMC2574382/pdf/jnma00205-0011.pdf

Tucker, C. M., Rice, K. G., Marsiske, M., Jones Nielson, J., & Herman, K. C. (2011a). Patient-centered culturally sensitive health care: Model testing and refinement. *Health Psychology, 30,* 342–350. doi: 10.1037/a0022967

Tucker, C. M., Rice, K. G., Hou, W., Kaye, L. B., Nolan, S. E., Grandoit, D. J., . . . Desmond, F. F. (2011b). Development of the motivators of and barriers to health-smart behaviors inventory. *Psychological Assessment, 23*(2), 487–503. doi: 10.1037/a0022299

Tucker, C. M., Rice, K. G., Desmond, F. F., Hou, W., Kaye, L. B., & Smith, T. M. (2012). The youth form of the motivators of and barriers to health-smart behaviors inventory. *Psychological Assessment, 24*(2), 490–502. doi: 10.1037/a0026262

Tucker, C. M., Nghiem, K. N., Marsiske, M., & Robinson, A. C. (2012). Validation of a patient-centered culturally sensitive health care provider inventory using a national sample of adult patients. *Patient Education Counseling, 9,* 344–349.

Tucker, C. M., Roncoroni, J., Marsiske, M., Nghiem, K. N., & Wall, W. (2014). Validation of a patient-centered culturally sensitive clinic environment inventory using a national sample of adult patients. *Journal of Transcultural Nursing, 25,* 80–86.

Tucker, C. M. Wall, W. Marsiske, M., Nghiem, K., & Roncoroni, J. (in press). Validation of a patient-centered culturally sensitive health care office staff inventory. *Primary Healthcare Research & Development.*

U.S. Department of Health and Human Services. (2008). *America's health literacy: Why we need accessible health information.* (Issue Brief). Retrieved from http://www.health.gov/ communication/literacy/issuebrief/

U.S. Department of Health and Human Services, Office of Disease Prevention and Health Promotion. (2011). *Healthy people 2020: Disparities.* Retrieved from http://healthypeople.gov/2020/about/disparitiesAbout.aspx

Wallerstein, N. B., & Duran, B. (2006). Using community-based participatory research to address health disparities. *Health Promotion Practice, 27*(3), 312–323. doi: 10.1177/1524839906289376

Zimmerman, M. A. (2000). Empowerment theory: Psychological, organizational, and community levels of analysis. In J. Rappaport & E. Seidman (Eds.), *Handbook of community psychology* (pp. 43–63). New York, NY: Kluwer Academic/Plenum.

Chapter 7

Surviving the Peace: Redefining Community-Based Veteran Services through the DryHootch Partnership

Zeno Franco, Mark Flower, Robert Curry, Karen J. Berte, and Jeff Whittle

INTRODUCTION

The social justice considerations surrounding military service and the aftermath of military duty are deep and complex, ranging from how service members are selected, who among these are eligible for combat, how medical and mental health services are provided upon return from duty, and how society as a whole addresses the reintegration of veterans. At least three of the main domains of social justice—distributive, procedural, and restorative justice—have clear relevance when considering the life outcomes of military service members and veterans.

For example, in terms of distributive justice, conscripted military service in the United States was used to fill the military ranks for World War I, World War II, the Vietnam War, as well as many of the interwar years. While the draft was never entirely equitable in its distribution of chance of service in combat, these concerns were magnified with the transition to an all-volunteer force given the evidence that those from lower socioeconomic status (SES) backgrounds are more likely to bear the burden of military duty (Bachman, Segal, Freedman-Doan, & O'Malley,

2000). Furthermore, recruitment from lower SES groups may be linked to higher premilitary trauma exposure, increasing the likelihood that accumulated trauma results in posttraumatic stress disorder (PTSD) (Roberts, Gilman, Breslau, Breslau, & Koenen, 2011). Procedural justice considerations in the military include how women and gays have until recently been systematically excluded from military service or from combat duty through laws and regulations (McIntyre, Bartle, Landis, & Dansby, 2002; Miner-Rubino & Cortina, 2007; Wexler, 1996).

This chapter focuses broadly on restorative justice for military veterans reintegrating into civilian life. Since 1636 some form of social support for military veterans has been legally prescribed in the territories that would become United States.[1] The Veterans Administration was established in 1930 and has grown from 54 hospitals to 152 hospitals, 800 community-based outpatient clinics, 126 nursing home care units, and 35 domiciliaries according to the Veteran Health Administration (VHA; U.S. Department of Veteran Affairs, 2013b). The Department of Veterans Affairs in its current form was established in 1989, a year after the legislation was passed ("The Department of Veterans Affairs Act," 1988). Although the VHA focuses on professionally led mental health care, dissatisfaction with this model after the Vietnam war led to the creation of community-based Vet Centers, and more recent focus on the effectiveness of veteran peer-led mental health services (Resnick, Armstrong, & Sperrazza, 2004; Resnick & Rosenheck, 2008) as an integral part of the service continuum, gradually paving the way for para-professional roles in VHA mental health services.

This transition toward integration of professional and veteran-led services supports the overall goal of restorative justice in that it increasingly puts veterans in the driver's seat in defining care priorities and approaches; however, true integration is not a simple process. This chapter attempts to accomplish four tasks revolving around this discussion of restoration of physical, social, and mental health to those who have sacrificed for their nation: First, we outline a number of the health disparities faced by veterans—highlighting the unjust distribution of burden veterans face; second, we present veteran peer mentorship as a restorative, consumer-driven approach to veteran care; third, we summarize the history of a community-academic partnership for veteran health undertaken by a community-based veterans organization, a major VA hospital, and a civilian medical school as part of a journey toward community-based veteran peer services; fourth, we offer some lessons learned through this partnership to help inform a broader discussion about socially just approaches to veteran care, seeking to better integrate veteran services across a wide range of stakeholders.

PHYSICAL, SOCIAL, AND MENTAL HEALTH DISPARITIES IN U.S. MILITARY SERVICE PERSONNEL AND VETERANS

Mental health and reintegration problems faced by combat veterans returning to civilian life have profound consequences for personal and community health (Beckham, Moore, & Reynolds, 2000; CDC, 2005; Ferrada-Noli, Ormstad,

Lundin, & Sundbom, 1998; Kotler, Iancu, Efroni, & Amir, 2001; Rosenheck, Frisman, & Kasprow, 1999). Veterans returning to civilian life after service in the current conflicts in Afghanistan and Iraq (Operations Enduring Freedom and Iraqi Freedom or OEF/OIF) are at disproportionate risk of developing mental health disorders with life-long consequences for individuals, families, and communities. First, because veterans are exposed to extraordinary trauma, they are more likely than the general population to suffer from PTSD (Kessler, 2000; Magruder et al., 2005). Department of Defense (DoD) mental health screenings conducted immediately and six months post-deployment found 20.3% of deployed active duty military personnel and 42.4% of deployed reservists warranted referral; however, most do not receive the care they need—often because they do not get or fail to show up for follow-ups (Milliken, Auchterlonie, Hoge, McGurk, & Thomas, 2007).

After controlling for other factors, PTSD predicts substance abuse, cigarette smoking, hypertension, and obesity (Coughlin, 2012). Combat-related traumatic brain injury (TBI), the "signature wound" of the current wars, can cause difficulty with attention, processing speed and emotional liability, hampering social, vocational, and scholastic performance (Hoge, et al., 2008). These difficulties are compounded by prolonged separation from family member and jobs, creating increased risk for familial discord, unemployment, and social isolation (Sayers, Farrow, Ross, & Oslin, 2009; Sherman, Sautter, Jackson, Lyons, & Han, 2006). Moreover, higher levels of substance abuse, homelessness, impulsivity, and anger control put veterans at increased risk for interpersonal violence, suicide, and unintentional injury as compared to their civilian counterparts. For example, data show that 46% of veterans in college report experiencing suicidal thoughts and 7.7% make an attempt, as compared to 6% reporting thoughts and 1.3% attempting among nonveteran students (Rudd, Goulding, & Bryan, 2011). A recent, large-scale epidemiological study using the National Violent Death Reporting System found the suicide completion rate for veterans was twice that of nonveterans [OR 2.04, 95%CI 1.10–3.80] (Kaplan, Huguet, McFarland, & Newsom, 2007). Younger veterans with comorbid PTSD and depression are at greater risk for suicide completion than older veterans with the same diagnoses (Zivin et al., 2007). The severity of this issue cannot be overstated as about one U.S. active duty service member—and as many as 18 veterans—commits suicide daily (Thompson & Gibbs, 2012).

Veterans face barriers to accessing mental health care, both in the Veterans Health Administration and in civilian care settings. For example, fewer than 30% of OEF/OIF veterans in VHA care complete recommended, evidence-based treatment for new PTSD diagnoses within one year (Seal et al., 2010). In civilian care settings, most primary care and community providers do not screen for veteran status, are not familiar with the jargon and culture of the military, and often misdiagnose veterans because of unfamiliarity with the clinical presentations of combat PTSD and other sequelae of military service (Hinojosa, Hinojosa, Nelson, & Nelson, 2010).

VETERAN PEER MENTORING AS A RESTORATIVE, INCLUSIVE INTERVENTION

A growing evidence base shows that peer mentorship is an effective treatment modality for mental health problems. Moreover, some veterans may be more likely to use peer services since this approach does not have the stigma associated with seeking professional mental health care (Resnick et al., 2004; Resnick & Rosenheck, 2008). Recognizing the importance of this model, especially as many veterans report feeling more comfortable discussing their military experience with others who share this background, VHA is increasingly hiring veterans into these paraprofessional roles. Standards for how these peers should be trained and ideas regarding how they best fit into the continuum of care are rapidly evolving (Barber, Rosenheck, Armstrong, & Resnick, 2008). However, there are several limitations to this model, including hospital centric delivery of services, desire on the part of some veterans to access services that are entirely anonymous or at least delivered in less formal settings (Burnam, Meredith, Tanielian, & Jaycox, 2009), and the sense among some younger veterans that they feel out of place among the older veterans who make up the bulk of VHA users (Bowman, 2010).

These considerations underscore the importance of refining peer mentor interventions for younger veterans. Thus, such programs should be sensitive to younger veterans' unique needs (e.g., available after-hours on college campuses where many are currently enrolled), use communication strategies that meet their expectations (e.g., using up-to-date technologies), and address critical gaps in the care of service-related mental health problems (e.g., using peer interactions to facilitate referral to veteran-friendly civilian providers and to improve care hand-offs from community to VHA care when needed) (Kaplan et al., 2007). Although VHA-delivered peer mentor services are an important component of care, community-based veterans' organizations advocate for alternative peer models that are more flexible.

THE DRYHOOTCH/MILWAUKEE VA/MEDICAL COLLEGE OF WISCONSIN COMMUNITY-ACADEMIC PARTNERSHIP FOR VETERAN HEALTH

DryHootch is a veteran-led community outreach effort based on Brady Street in the city of Milwaukee's bustling East Side business district. *Hootch* was the term for a hut or other safe place to sleep, commonly used in the Vietnam combat theater, and is also a play on the word's association with alcohol—one of the major problems for veterans of all eras. The term *dry* denotes the organization's mission to provide a social gathering place that is free of alcohol. Thus the concept behind DryHootch is a desire to establish a coffee house or café-like environment that is dedicated to "helping veterans who survived the war, survive the peace." Although DryHootch is a small organization, it has grown from being a dream held by a number of veterans who were in conversation with the Milwaukee VA about creating an alternative social space around 2007, to owning a building near Downtown Milwaukee and opening services there in 2010, to expanding to several satellite locations throughout the state in 2012. DryHootch views its primary mission as developing and providing an innovative, veteran-led peer mentorship program that provides services to a wide range of veterans, some of whom may not even be eligible for VHA services (e.g., because of dishonorable discharge status).

DryHootch's primary location is near the University of Wisconsin-Milwaukee (UWM) campus, which has the largest number of veteran students of any college campus in the state. The location also places the storefront squarely in a high traffic retail hub. DryHootch volunteers, local firefighters, union plumbers, and other skilled laborers who donated their time substantially remodeled the building. The first floor and patio are dedicated to retail coffee sales—many of the customers are veterans, but the public is also welcome to drink coffee and enjoy a wide variety of activities that occur in this space.

The second floor provides a private area for veterans where a number of different groups meet focusing on the problems associated with demobilization and reintegration into civilian life. Using this space, DryHootch offers peer-to-peer support to veterans of all eras, including those who are now returning from Iraq and Afghanistan.

A BRIEF HISTORY OF THE DRYHOOTCH/ZVAMC/ MEDICAL COLLEGE OF WISCONSIN

Community-Academic Partnership

The Community-Academic Partnership for Veteran Health partnership began in 2007, when the veteran leaders of the nascent DryHootch organization approached the leadership of the Clement J. Zablocki VA Medical Center (ZVAMC; also called simply the Milwaukee VA) with the idea of creating a venue on the ZVAMC campus for veteran engagement focused on informal social interaction rather than formal treatment. The leadership at ZVAMC was interested in this idea since it aligned well with the VHA's objectives to provide comprehensive services to veterans, although it fell slightly outside the primary clinical activities of a VA hospital. The ZVAMC was among the first three facilities created in response to President Lincoln's second inaugural address, in which he urged the nation "to care for him who shall have borne the battle and his widow and his orphan" in the last days of the Civil War (U.S. Department of Veteran Affairs, 2013a, para. 1). It is a tertiary care VA Medical Center located on 125 acres within the city of Milwaukee. Initial discussions were sparked by the recognition that much of the prime real estate belonging to ZVAMC was underused, placing it at risk for being repurposed away from veteran service.

DryHootch, the Milwaukee VA Medical Center, and the Medical College of Wisconsin formally created a community academic partnership for veteran health in 2008[2] in an attempt to use DryHootch's unique position in the community in concert with the expertise in veterans' mental health treatment available through the VA and the MCW's expertise in public health-related interventions and research.

Partnership Challenges

Difficulties within community-academic partnerships are quite common given the complexity of articulating and negotiating between the cultures, objectives, and styles represented in the collaborating organizations (Minkler & Wallerstein, 2010). The DryHootch/VA/MCW partnership is no exception. We briefly summarize some of the challenges and successes encountered by this partnership as they closely mirror the types of issues found in all Community-Based Participatory Research efforts (CBPR; Ahmed, Beck, Maurana, & Newton, 2004; Minkler & Wallerstein, 2010). These experiences are nuanced by the specific worries, aspirations, and tensions involved in bringing together a veteran serving nonprofit organization and a major VA hospital to work on improving continuity of services and social support between community outreach programs and hospital-based care.

A History of Miscommunication and Mistrust

Trust issues between DryHootch and the VA—which may reflect, in part, historical problems left over from the Vietnam era—created tension at the beginning of the partnership. This was perhaps best reflected in the selection of a physical site for DryHootch operations. DryHootch members recall that ZVAMC leadership proposed that DryHootch use an unused building on the ZVAMC campus to house peer support groups and other programming for $1. From the perspective of the DryHootch, this building was to be theirs to renovate and transform into their vision of a social space for veterans, distinct from the VA, yet on the VA campus.

However, what had not been clarified was that the proposed space was a designated historical building, part of the National Soldiers Home Historic District, dating to the post–Civil War period. Local VA leadership was concerned that renovations undertaken by the DryHootch veterans could violate the rules associated with modifications to historic buildings and that offering alternative, non-VA programming on a VA campus could cause problems with JCAHO accreditation. DryHootch describes the offer to use this facility as being revoked after more than 100 hours of labor were spent on renovations, and after *pro bono* architectural planning support was already secured. For the community partner, this underscored a sense that the VA was not supportive of the DryHootch idea. Leadership at the ZVAMC similarly felt that DryHootch did not understand the legal and regulatory constraints faced by a large hospital. This conflict ultimately resulted in DryHootch renting and later purchasing a building in a retail district near downtown Milwaukee, which the community partner has come to regard as a "blessing in disguise"—offering greater freedom, and placing them closer to many veterans who might not be using VA services.

Notably, each member of the partnership recalls the facts of what occurred and the meaning associated with these events very differently.[3] At the time of this writing we have simply agreed that the preceding text represents a relatively unbiased summary, while residual tensions over the specific events and their implications remain. Yet, we have learned to negotiate through those differences and the ongoing disagreement itself may have served a purpose in binding us together through our occasionally contentious history.

Mission and Risk Management

At its inception, the partnership stated that a major part of its mission was to provide peer-led veteran support for practical and mental health problems, based largely on the Vet-to-Vet model (Resnick et al., 2004; Resnick & Rosenheck, 2008). However, DryHootch brought in a clinician on a volunteer basis who, early on in the partnership, was interested in providing one-on-one counseling, therapeutic retreats, and practicums for student clinicians from the local university (as director of peer programming). The medical and mental health providers from the VA and MCW were uncomfortable with this direction because DryHootch did not have the basic infrastructure they believed was needed to safely run a mental health clinic (i.e., a system for keeping progress notes, procedures for handling protected health information, or a process for handling crisis situations, and so on). Over several months, MCW and VA partners repeatedly approached senior DryHootch leaders with their concerns, including the possible legal and financial risks to DryHootch, the potential for negative press that might harm the VA, and potential risk to veterans if they received inappropriate care.

DryHootch partnership members responded that they felt this was an example of the partnership being used to influence the day-to-day operations of their organization so that it would conform to the wishes of the VA. This problem arose while a large grant was being prepared for submission; some academic members of the partnership felt DryHootch's change in mission away from peer-to-peer services represented a serious enough risk to abandon the grant writing effort. When this sentiment was expressed to DryHootch, it was viewed as a pressure tactic that had the potential to disassemble the partnership, rather than a genuine expression of concern. Ultimately, the community-based clinician working for DryHootch departed, the leadership at DryHootch resumed course toward peer-to-peer services, and the partnership resumed its normal activities.

Research Difficulties

One of the principles of CBPR is the timely production of research materials that can be disseminated to various stakeholders that is collaboratively developed as part of the partnership. Although the partnership fielded an initial survey of veterans quite rapidly, some of the VA partners were unhappy with the wording of a draft report summarizing descriptive statistics from the instrument. The objections were focused on items that were designed to identify nonusers of the VA and reasons these participants did not want to seek care through the VA Healthcare System. Individuals at the ZVAMC were concerned that this information might paint an unduly negative picture of the VA, and it noted that the survey instrument did not contain any items probing for positive experiences with VA care. In contrast, DryHootch viewed these questions as central to better understanding how it might fill gaps and that these data might also provide important information for the VA. Other academic partners from MCW struggled to obtain input and edits from DryHootch—in part because the relative value of this research activity was not fully understood by the community partner.

Ultimately, as wording compromises were agreed upon and a final report for the partnership was printed, ZVAMC fears about misuse of the data were reduced and the value of the product as a way of communicating with stakeholders became obvious to DryHootch leadership. We also note that many of the positive aspects of VA care generally, and ZVAMC in particular, emerged through the qualitative data analysis of open-ended items from the survey. These steps ultimately resulted in greater mutuality around research design and execution within the partnership.

Partnership Successes

Weathering Storms

The difficulties noted within the partnership around mutual agreement of the mission and risk management resulted in the academic members of the partnership—particularly the mental health professionals—reducing formal contact with DryHootch and shifting to a wait-and-see stance in large part to reduce risk exposure for the institutions involved. At the same time, we dramatically increased the informal contact between the partners, with one member of the academic team shuttling between the individuals who make up the actual fabric of the partnership. An informal dinner and retreat was also held in the home of one of the senior academic partners. Although the CBPR literature stresses the importance of these types of contacts as a way to improve mutual understanding and identification with the partnership (not just one's home institution), most members of the partnership were new to the CBPR process; all were more concerned with pursuing grant funding and program development than with these more foundational partnership activities.

Once grievances were aired—and perhaps more importantly, once all members understood that areas of contention had personal impact for individual partners rather than just being organizational or institutional constraints, many of the strains on the partnership were reduced. For example, mental health professionals' concerns about risk were related to issues such as licensing, and some of the partners' unavailability to respond to some invitations to participate in community events by DryHootch was not due to lack of interest, but rather time constrains associated with their respective positions. Conversely, the feedback from DryHootch through these personal contacts helped the academic partners to understand that some of the invitations to participate in community outreach events were not intended to create more work—they were not necessarily invitations to formally present or to be experts, but to provide silent support and credibility to the organization simply by being at the table with them.

Shared Workflow

As these trust considerations gradually resolved over the following months, greater agreement about goals for the partnership emerged. During the next round of collaborative grant writing, we were able to address difficult issues more directly—but perhaps more importantly, the brainstorming process began to feel more mutual, and instead of meeting at a neutral place located physically in between the partnering organizations, smaller breakout meetings began occurring on an *ad hoc* basis at DryHootch and MCW—bringing the actual flow of work associated with grant writing closer to the operation level of each of the organizations. This gradual process of transitioning toward seeing the work of the partnership as a part of everyday operations continued through the analysis of the survey data. At this point, when coding issues were discussed over email, several members of DryHootch staff would respond, not just the academic members with an interest in the publishing the results. In fact, attempts to formalize the process of research (e.g., to address issues such as cross-organization inter-rater reliability) were often met with silence, whereas more spontaneous requests for assistance with data analysis seemed fun and engaging. In this way, the research process also took on some of the ethos and improvisational style of the community organization.

Creating a Shared Language and Culture

Community-academic partnerships are clear examples of *ad hoc* organizations or "adhocracies" (Bailey & Koney, 1996). These partnerships are formed between members of existing organizations, each with their own cultures, expectations, and reward systems. Existing in the liminal space between these institutions can create discontinuities that make sustaining a partnership difficult or impossible, yet truly innovative approaches to addressing public health problems are perhaps best formed within this marginal, trans-organizational space (Sandy, 2005). In part through deliberate actions, and also through time and chance, the DryHootch/VA/MCW partnership began developing a shared experience. For several months during formal meetings, we spent more time directly talking about the principles of CBPR—in part, recognizing that because this was new ground for almost all of us, the partnership had to educate itself about the very idea of what a partnership is supposed to be. We also began using the term *partnership* and going over the history of the group very deliberately during meetings to reinforce the notion that when we were gathered in this way, we represented a distinct entity—not just our home organizations.

Other areas of increasing mutuality occurred by happenstance. For example, during the retreat and dinner described previously, one of the DryHootch members left a pack of cigarettes at the home of one of the senior researchers who is deeply involved in cardiovascular health. Efforts to return this pack of cigarettes were repeatedly foiled, resulting in a number of humorous exchanges. Other inside jokes gradually evolved. These have served as touchstones within the partnership, allowing tensions to be defused when necessary both through the humor itself and through the recognition of a shared history that equalizes interpersonal relationships (Sandy, 2011).

More serious issues around creating a shared language came up during a later, more formal, half-day planning retreat. In response to a discussion of some of the difficult moments in the partnership and the academic partners' efforts to provide early warning about these potential issues, DryHootch senior staff noted that these warnings were too subtle and did not fully register with DryHootch until after the problem had reached the boiling point. DryHootch reminded the academic partners that they are military veterans, many of whom have attendant concentration problems associated with PTSD or long-term substance abuse, trying to run a small organization and often working at the limits of their capacity. DryHootch requested that important messages should be flagged as such in order to differentiate them from the wash of information they experience as a start-up nonprofit. DryHootch staff suggested that the partners use the term *red flag* (or other colors as appropriate) to denote important communications intended to head off potential crises. So far, we have not had to do so, but this is an important example of deliberately defining partnership language as a distinct set of communication strategies that are specific to the group—rather than relying on more subtle strategies that might be more effective or acceptable in a large, institutional setting.

LESSONS LEARNED

At their best, community-academic partnerships have the ability to create transformative change in how health care is delivered and consumed. We often think about this transformative change as having an external impact, but the internal changes and learning occurring within and among the partners remain important to capture. The *pain points* within partnerships often distill the tensions involved in improving health service delivery for marginalized groups, as well as illuminate actionable solutions. For us, this has been a five-year process, which the DryHootch partners view as part of their overall journey toward consumer-driven mental health care and improving access for veterans from all walks of life, but particularly those who are most vulnerable to falling through the cracks.

We do our best here to summarize some of the key lessons we have learned in the hopes that they provide groundwork for a continuing discussion about how the Veterans Health Administration and small, nonprofit veteran-serving organizations in community settings can work together to improve the continuum of care for military service personnel transitioning to civilian life.

One of the touchstones for the partnership was a trip that two of us took to co-present about the partnership during a Wisconsin snowstorm. Throughout a three-hour drive in treacherous conditions, questions about the differences between professional clinical psychology and DryHootch's peer mentorship approach were discussed in occasionally pointed detail. Issues around boundary setting and the potential for harmful dual relationships between peer mentors and their mentees were pointed out to the DryHootch partner. The community partner noted that one of the ways that professional clinical psychology fails to serve is that many of the people who most need the help cannot be reached without creating dual relationships, and that this approach often allows veterans who are at greatest risk to not be turned off by a relationship that is purely designed to deliver an intervention. The community partner suggested that many of the rules of professional clinical psychology (except for those dealing with imminent harm to self or others) serve as a fundamental barrier to obtaining needed services that can start a veteran on the road to recovery and lay the groundwork for entering a formal therapeutic relationship with a counselor or psychologist at a later time. Although some concerns about this perspective remain among the professional providers in our group, this line of thought has certainly influenced our thinking about how best to manage veterans in the early stages of recovery and it points out the potential importance of pairing professional and paraprofessional services more deliberately to optimize outreach to those least likely to seek professional care.

Simultaneously with this discussion about our (the academics) concerns regarding the boundary setting of DryHootch's peer mentors, we realized that one of the mistakes that we made early on was viewing our interactions with DryHootch solely through the lens of clinical psychology—worrying primarily about individual situations that we thought DryHootch might not be prepared to handle in ways consistent with academic and clinical psychology norms. Other psychologists with more experience doing community psychology pointed out that we needed to begin viewing our interactions with DryHootch through the lens of organizational psychology. From this perspective, we reconceptualized our role as primarily as an organizational consulting role, working to strengthen DryHootch's ability to provide appropriate services and deal effectively with veteran crises, rather than trying to intervene at an individual level on a case-by-case basis.

We also gradually stopped viewing ourselves as the experts, coming to see ourselves as just one voice among many within the partnership, all with different types of expertise, and all bound by the common value of improving veteran care. This release of the mantle of expert was something that DryHootch had asked for (e.g., with comments such as, "can you please just show up to this meeting, you don't have to say anything, but we need you at the table"); however, it took time just to see how pervasive this internalized role was. We often did not see the point of showing up if we were not leading a conversation or presenting a talk, and so on. Relatedly, the fundamental value of friendship and the implicit and expressed view that the partnership would remain intact regardless of short-term disagreements, lack of funding, or other issues fundamentally changed the dynamics of the group. These changes in academic and professional provider attitudes toward the partnership are not to say that we no longer offer critical feedback to DryHootch. Rather, it is given in a more constructive way, with a deeper awareness of the operational constraints of a small nonprofit as well as how the personal relationships assist in making clear that the intention is to build capacity rather than create roadblocks.

From the perspective of DryHootch's leadership, the primary partners in this group, some of the main lessons learned include developing a deeper understanding of the rules and regulations the academic partners face—but not in the abstract. Through the interpersonal relationships, it is possible for DryHootch to better understand that these rules often create personal constraints or risk for individual academic partners. In this sense, one of the charges that DryHootch gave to the academic partners about acceptance of their views has also been mirrored (Franco, Flower, Sandy, & Whittle, in press), with DryHootch challenging itself to practice a more radical acceptance of the VA health care system for what it is and what it does best.

DryHootch partners also have noted that they have personally changed through this process, feeling less need to forcefully point out the "rules that hurt" in the health care systems with which they interact. They also find that opportunities to negotiate about these rules, barriers, and other issues that diminish care for veterans seem to come up naturally in conversations and that there is a right time to express views about these problems. Waiting for these natural opportunities to talk about these issues is perceived by DryHootch as a way to better catalyze action than the somewhat confrontational approach they used in the beginning years of the partnership.

Although identified throughout the literature on best practices in community academic partnerships, in discussing these lessons learned DryHootch noted the importance of reemphasizing that the most effective conversations within the partnership are deeply honest, revealing the personal rather than just institutional constraints faced by each individual at the table. This process allows for the identification of action steps and mutually agreeable work-arounds. The work-arounds that accommodate all of the needs within the partnership are the foundation of our work together and they represent in tangible ways equitable, just, and restorative interpersonal practice and governance that sets an example for how large and small entities can work together toward a commonly held goal: in this case, improving veteran health care across an entire community.

NOTES

1. http://www.va.gov/about_va/vahistory.asp

2. The partnership later expanded to include faculty of the University of Wisconsin—Milwaukee, Marquette University, Mental Health America. At present, additional partners are currently being recruited to serve on a broader "Veteran Health Coalition" intended to address broader systemic barriers to veteran care.

3. The views expressed here do not necessarily represent those of the Zablocki (Milwaukee) VA Medical Center or DryHootch of America, Inc. They are instead the product of an ongoing conversation between individuals from all agencies in the partnership about their recollection of events.

REFERENCES

Ahmed, S., Beck, B., Maurana, C., & Newton, G. (2004). Overcoming barriers to effective community-based participatory research in US medical schools. *Education for Health, 17*(2), 141–151.

Bachman, J. G., Segal, D. R., Freedman-Doan, P., & O'Malley, P. M. (2000). Who chooses military service? Correlates of propensity and enlistment in the US Armed Forces. *Military Psychology, 12*(1), 1–30.

Bailey, D., & Koney, K. M. (1996). Interorganizational community-based collaboratives: A strategic response to shape the social work agenda. *Social Work, 41*(6), 602–611.

Barber, J., Rosenheck, R., Armstrong, M., & Resnick, S. (2008). Monitoring the dissemination of peer support in the VA Healthcare System. *Community Mental Health Journal, 44*(6), 433–441. doi: 10.1007/s10597-008-9146-7

Beckham, J. C., Moore, S. D., & Reynolds, V. (2000). Interpersonal hostility and violence in Vietnam combat veterans with chronic posttraumatic stress disorder: A review of theoretical models and empirical evidence. *Aggression and Violent Behavior, 5*(5), 451–466.

Bowman, T. (Producer). (2010). *The changing veteran poses challenges for the VA*. Retrieved from http://www.npr.org/templates/story/story.php?storyId=126672675

Burnam, M. A., Meredith, L. S., Tanielian, T., & Jaycox, L. H. (2009). Mental health care for Iraq and Afghanistan war veterans. *Health Affairs, 28*(3), 771–782.

CDC. (2005). Deaths from violence: A look at 17 states—Data from the National Violent Death Reporting System: Centers for Disease Control.

Coughlin, S. S. (2012). *Post-traumatic stress disorder and chronic health conditions*. Washington, DC: American Public Health Association.

The Department of Veterans Affairs Act of 1988, Pub L. No. 100-527 (1989).

Ferrada-Noli, A., Ormstad, L., & Sundbom, E.. (1998). Suicidal behavior after severe trauma. Part 1: PTSD diagnoses, psychiatric comorbidity, and assessments of suicidal behavior. *Journal of Traumatic Stress, 11*, 103–112.

Franco, Z., Flower, M., Sandy, M., & Whittle, J. (in press). Professional ethics and virtue ethics in community engaged healthcare training. In D. Mitchell & R. Ream (Eds.), *Professional responsibility: The fundamental issue in education and healthcare reform*. New York, NY: Springer.

Hinojosa, R., Hinojosa, M. S., Nelson, K., & Nelson, D. (2010). Veteran family reintegration, primary care needs, and the benefit of the patient-centered medical home model.

The Journal of the American Board of Family Medicine, 23(6), 770–774. doi: 10.3122/jabfm.2010.06.100094

Hoge, C. W., McGurk, D., Thomas, J. L., Cox, A., Engel, C., & Castro, C. (2008). Mild traumatic brain injury in U.S. soldiers returning from Iraq. *New England Journal of Medicine, 358,* 453–463.

Kaplan, M. S., Huguet, N., McFarland, B. H., & Newsom, J. T. (2007). Suicide among male veterans: A prospective population-based study. *Journal of Epidemiology and Community Health, 61*(7), 619–624. doi: 10.1136/jech.2006.054346

Kessler, R. (2000). Posttraumatic stress disorder: The burden to the individual and to society. *Journal of Clinical Psychiatry, 61,* 4–12.

Kotler, M., Iancu, I., Efroni, R., & Amir, M. (2001). Anger, impulsivity, social support, and suicide risk in patients with posttraumatic stress disorder. *Journal of Nervous & Mental Disease. 189*(3), 162–167.

Magruder, K., Frueh, B., Knapp, R., Johnson, M., Vaughan III, J., Carson, T., . . . Hebert, R. (2005). PTSD symptoms, demographic characteristics, and functional status among veterans treated in VA primary care clinics. *Journal of Traumatic Stress, 17*(4), 293–301.

McIntyre, R. M., Bartle, S. A., Landis, D., & Dansby, M. R. (2002). The effects of equal opportunity fairness attitudes on job satisfaction, organizational commitment, and perceived work group efficacy. *Military Psychology, 14*(4), 299–319.

Milliken, C. S., Auchterlonie, J. L., Hoge, C. W., McGurk, D., & Thomas, J. L. (2007). Longitudinal assessment of mental health problems among active and reserve component soldiers returning from the Iraq War. *JAMA, 298*(18), 2141–2148.

Miner-Rubino, K., & Cortina, L. M. (2007). Beyond targets: Consequences of vicarious exposure to misogyny at work. *Journal of Applied psychology, 92*(5), 1254.

Minkler, M., & Wallerstein, N. (2010). *Community-based participatory research for health: From process to outcomes.* San Francisco, CA: Jossey-Bass.

Resnick, S. G., Armstrong, M., Sperrazza, M., Harkness, L., & Rosenheck, R. A. (2004). A model of consumer-provider partnership: Vet-to-vet. *Psychiatric Rehabilitation Journal, 28*(2), 185–188.

Resnick, S. G., & Rosenheck, R. A. (2008). *Integrating peer-provided services : A quasi-experimental study of recovery orientation, confidence, and empowerment* (Vol. 59). Arlington, VA: American Psychiatric Association.

Roberts, A. L., Gilman, S. E., Breslau, J., Breslau, N., & Koenen, K. C. (2011). Race/ethnic differences in exposure to traumatic events, development of post-traumatic stress disorder, and treatment-seeking for post-traumatic stress disorder in the United States. *Psychological Medicine, 41*(01), 71–83.

Rosenheck, R. A., Frisman, L. K., & Kasprow, W. (1999). Improving access to disability benefits among homeless persons with mental illness: An agency-specific approach to services integration. *American Journal of Public Health, 89*(4), 524–528.

Rudd, M. D., Goulding, J., & Bryan, C. J. (2011). Student veterans: A national survey exploring psychological symptoms and suicide risk. *Professional Psychology: Research and Practice, 42*(5), 354–360.

Sandy, M. (2011). Practical beauty and the legacy of pragmatism: Generating theory for community-engaged scholarship. *Interchange, 42*(3), 261–285. doi: 10.1007/s10780-012-9159-6

Sandy, M. (2005). *Hermeneutic passages in academia and community* (Doctoral dissertation, Claremont Graduate University).

Sayers, S. L., Farrow, V. A., Ross, J., & Oslin, D. W. (2009). Family problems among recently returned military veterans referred for a mental health evaluation. *J. Clin Psych, 70,* 163–170.

Seal, K. H., Maguen, S., Cohen, B., Gima, K. S., Metzler, T. J., Ren, L., . . . Marmar, C. R. (2010). VA mental health services utilization in Iraq and Afghanistan veterans in the first year of receiving new mental health diagnoses. *Journal of Traumatic Stress, 23*(1), 5–16. doi: 10.1002/jts.20493

Sherman, M. D., Sautter, F., Jackson, M. H., Lyons, J. A., & Han, X. (2006). Domestic violence in veterans with Post Traumatic Stress Disorder who seek couples therapy. *Journal of Marital and Family Therapy, 32*(4), 479–490.

Thompson, M., & Gibbs, N. (2012). One a day: Why can't the Army win the war on suicide. *Time, 180*(4), 22–31.

U.S. Department of Veteran Affairs. (2013a). *About VA*. Retrieved from http://www.va.gov/about_va/

U.S. Department of Veteran Affairs. (2013b). *History-VA history*. Retrieved from http://www.va.gov/about_va/vahistory.asp

Wexler, D. B. (1996). Applying the law therapeutically. *Applied and Preventive Psychology, 5*(3), 179–186.

Zivin, K., Kim, H. M., McCarthy, J. F., Austin, K. L., Hoggatt, K. J., Walters, H., & Valenstein, M. (2007). Suicide mortality among individuals receiving treatment for depression in the Veterans Affairs Health System: Associations with patient and treatment setting characteristics. Washington, DC: American Public Health Association.

Chapter 8

Disasters, Psychology, and Social Justice

Diane Bretherton and Anouk Ride

Natural disasters affect communities around the world and have become a daily event in global news. However, despite the frequency of natural disasters, disaster management, development, social welfare, and psychology fields continue to conceptualize these events as outside of the broader concerns of social justice. This chapter briefly describes our research into community resilience as a context for reflecting on social justice issues embedded in the experience of, and response to, disasters. It considers how outsiders try to help communities, how psychologists might be involved, what actually helps communities, and concludes with a suggestion that psychology could focus less on a treatment role and more on working in partnership with communities to better adapt to changing environments.

For psychologists, their role in disasters is largely seen as that of practitioners who can design psychosocial programs and provide psychological assistance for the victims of trauma. For example, Saraceno (2006) explains, "Disaster psychology deals with psychological trauma . . . as a risk factor for mood and anxiety disorders and for nonpathological physical and emotional distress" (p. xii). In our research into community resilience in natural disasters (Ride & Bretherton, 2011) we found psychologists working not only in this specialized role, but also as survivors, rescue workers, leaders of organizations, academics, researchers, and engaged members of the community.

The general public responds to news of disasters with a rush of concern for survivors and a sense that one should do something to help. Indeed, funding for assistance relies on this altruistic response with organizations and aid agencies expecting the public to respond generously with donations. The impulse to urgency also affects the organizations involved in the rescue operations, with a feeling that every second counts and each minute will add to the death toll. In this emotional atmosphere there is a call to *do something*, and a more analytic view of what form that something should take may seem cold, even callous. In the heat of the moment, reflection on what sort of response is most appropriate and awareness of the social justice issues involved suffers. However, it could be that just doing an unspecified something appeases the emotion of the helper, but violates the principles of "do no harm" (Anderson, 1999; Anderson & Woodrow, 1998). In this chapter we explore some of the social justice issues that lie just below the surface of immediate responses to disasters and find that greater attention to these aspects could lead to a more proactive, culturally sensitive, role for psychology and psychologists in helping communities adapt to natural disasters.

Community Resilience in Natural Disasters

Rather than looking at disasters primarily from the point of view of the emergency services and aid agencies, as is common in the field (see, e.g., Lomitz, 1998), we examined the experience of the communities that have lived through them (Ride & Bretherton, 2011). We use the term *natural disasters* to refer to large natural events that impact human communities, and are measured not so much by the scale of the event but by the scale of the damage to people and property. This differs from an *emergency*, which, in the development field, is seen as a state demanding immediate action for humanitarian reasons (e.g., civilian deaths in war or starvation). For government, emergency is a situation that is officially declared as a "state of emergency" to facilitate a quick response by relevant agencies. Although many disasters are also declared as emergencies, we would argue that this terminology should not belie the need to look at what communities are doing on their own to respond to the disaster and the need to build local strengths. Indeed, often the state of emergency is declared long after the first two to three days when deaths, injuries, and other harm are most likely to occur and the community is largely responding without outside assistance from aid agencies or government.

Although we use the term natural disaster, we understand that few are entirely natural in their causes—for example, building on a flood plain will cause a flood to be highly damaging to those settlements, so the cause of the damage stems from the weather as well as social, economic, and historical reasons as to why people settled on the flood plain. This leads to understanding that natural disasters are an interaction between people and the environment, what one might call a *socio-ecological event* (Resilience Alliance, 2012). Understanding natural disasters as having a man-made component, and as being a question of governance, then leads on to questions about the site of the affected settlement, the building materials used, access to communication, ability to move out of the settlement if there is a threat, and whether the government is transparent about the dangers. The social justice issues start to emerge: Who decided where the people should live? How was the decision made? How well adapted are the buildings to the environment? How safe are the living conditions? Having looked at natural disasters within this framework, it comes as no surprise to find that the statistics (see, e.g., Fothergill & Peek, 2004) show that the people who are most at risk of experiencing natural disasters are often those who are least equipped in terms of material resources to respond and recover.

We looked at a range of types of disasters in a number of countries. Here we provide a brief overview of our findings, as a basis for discussion of the social justice issues. For a more comprehensive report of the research see Ride and Bretherton (2011). We used enhanced case studies, which consisted of a review of the information available about the country and the disaster and then interviews with local community leaders. The disasters that formed the basis of our case studies were the 2004 tsunami in Aceh, Indonesia, the 2005 earthquake in Pakistan, the 2007 tsunami in the Solomon Islands, the 2008 cyclone in Myanmar. In addition we had personal experience of the 1985 earthquake in Mexico and the 2009 fires in Australia. The interviews were conducted in the local language (e.g., Bahasa Indonesian, Urdu, Solomon Islands Pijin, and Swahili) and English, or a mixture, depending on the comfort of the person being interviewed, and then transcribed into English. The interviewer used a structured interview schedule, but the questions encouraged a narrative approach, starting with personal experience of the disaster, moving on to community response, and then the aftermath and recovery stages. Finally, the interview allowed space for reflection about what helped and did not help and the impact of the disaster on relationships, both within the community and between the community and the organizations and people who had provided aid. Our local researchers were people who could bridge the gap between the local and the international communities in terms of language, knowledge of local culture, and ability to conduct and report on research. The participants were civil society representatives from women's groups, cultural and arts networks, local relief and rescue workers, educators, youth workers and youth representatives, and religious and local government representatives.

It quickly became clear that there is quite a contrast between the distant view of disaster, shaped by the media, and the experience of those who live through the event. The media tends to portray community members as victims, stressing their helplessness, passivity, and need of rescue. The picture presented by the media can be even more negative, with accounts of looting and chaos suggesting that a natural disaster is a breakdown of civic order, a desperate game of every man for himself. The message is that powerful outsiders are needed to rescue the helpless, contain the lawlessness, and bring order to chaos. We, ourselves, were not immune to this victim stereotype, and began our research with a question as to what made some communities resilient rather than passive, as if resilience were the exception rather than the norm. We found instead that all the communities we studied were resilient, but that this resilience is rarely the subject of media attention. Furthermore, we found that the sense of urgency that permeates responses to emergencies is somewhat misleading. There is a time lapse between the sudden onset of disaster and the arrival of rescuers, wherein the local community is self-organizing.

Consider, for example, the earthquake in Mexico (Cessaro & Romero, 1987; Poniatowska, 1988). Seeing Mexico City as a dangerous, poor, insecure, and chaotic place, the Western media spread a dramatic montage of images—the discovery of bodies crushed by debris, faces of the traumatized victims, and damaged buildings dotted like crumpled pieces of paper through the cityscape. There was, however, undetected by the media, another force at work. Survivors called out and identified family members, friends, and colleagues, trapped under the rubble, quickly forming groups of people to lift, piece-by-piece, chunks of cement and bricks to try and reach them. Volunteer rescuers, who came to be known as "moles," formed teams of people who followed the direction of locals to go into the smallest spaces to try and rescue survivors. When word went out that rescuers needed picks, shovels, and torches, donations of equipment began to arrive from stores and peoples' garages. Road workers, mechanics, boot makers, and many others helped deliver equipment. This locally organised help, which draws upon networks of existing relationships and utilizes local knowledge, cannot be replaced by outside assistance. Outside assistance, for example, in the form of mechanised digging equipment, is helpful only insofar as it works with and builds upon the local efforts. The international experts who are flown in tend to be experts only in particular types of disasters, rather than experts in the language, the local culture, or in community development. If the international experts see themselves as superior to the locals, then problems arise.

This is not to deny that outside help is needed, but to caution that the integrity of the local response should be respected and that if there is an intervention from outside then some thought and discussion is needed as to what will be helpful, both in the short and in the long run. Further, as an emergency response is necessarily colored by emotion and a sense of urgency, attention needs to be paid to adaptation, before, during, and after the emergency.

Help from Outside the Community

In the interviews from our research are many examples of aid from outside that was well intended but culturally inappropriate, or even politically provocative. One simple but obvious example comes from Aceh, where people are predominately Islamic and therefore reject Christian symbols and idolisation. The coordinator of a local Aceh NGO, receiving assistance after the 2004 tsunami, recounts an experience of this:

> I was once given 1500 dolls, and after sorting them, we could only use about 800. The ones that may not be used are dogs, pigs, and Santa Claus. They're really sensitive, so we got rid of them. Someone who brought the dolls to me asked: "Then where should I take these, ma'am?" "Don't return things and don't throw them away, because its people's gift, we have to accept it, thanks be to Allah. Just go to the Chinese barrack (camp), just give it all to them." "Really?" "Yes." They must be happy there in Chinese barrack. . . . We had an activity at Tungkup mosque, at the front of the mosque. We were playing story telling with the kids, using dolls. Then a Tengku (royal) came with anger, ". . . it's a statue, blah blah blah." He was saying it's an idolization. We started to get scared and back down: "It's okay, relax. We keep the dolls here, but we can use it in other places." "Just don't play with dolls at the mosque." (Pelupessy, Bretherton, & Ride, 2011, p. 43)

Such examples of inappropriate aid show not only a waste of money, as the funding and transport of the dolls could have been spent on a useful product, but also a degree of ignorance of the local culture that is so marked as to be insulting. The coordinator of the agency was handed a problem, not a solution. Accepting the outside aid would incur the wrath of local authorities and place local operations at risk, whereas failure to accept the aid would threaten the relationship with the international aid agencies. Although any doll might be seen as an offensive form of idol, the suspicion that outsiders have a secret agenda and are exploiting the situation to spread propaganda would be reinforced by the implication that local children should celebrate and enjoy playing with Father Christmas dolls.

We found many such examples across all the locations we studied for example, people resisting projects to build close to the sea in Solomon Islands after the tsunami, Pakistani village people staying in their ruined homes rather than following directions to refugee camps, which they considered insecure, and Mexican volunteers protested against the cordoning off disaster zones by the armed forces. In Aceh, too, people did not accept the role of local and foreign military sent to help, as one anonymous interviewee described: "The military were still around. There was this American soldier who hit a kid. We said: 'You can't do that,' and so we didn't accept that soldier. The people didn't really fit with the army" (Pelupessy et al., 2011, p. 35).

An important omission from our research was a case study on Hurricane Katrina. We did commission a researcher to undertake interviews in New Orleans and when the researcher failed to do the interviews we commissioned a further researcher. When in turn the second researcher was unable to complete the case study, we were running close to our publication deadline and had to go ahead without including this case study. Although the approach of Gheytanchi et al. (2007) is somewhat different to ours, in that theirs' is less about listening to community experience and more a comprehensive analysis of the failure of the various levels of government to relate to the communities in New Orleans, it identifies themes that parallel our case studies. They note:

> Despite billions of dollars spent following 9/11 to improve emergency coordination, the response to Hurricane Katrina utterly failed. An understanding of the behavioral aspects of both disaster management personnel and the civilians impacted by catastrophes is essential to improving response performance. Psychologists must begin to conceptualize their contribution to disaster response beyond just treating acute stress reactions in victims, instead expanding their view to include the treatment of an entire policy, planning, and response system that appears to be badly broken. (p. 119)

PSYCHOLOGY, SOCIAL JUSTICE, AND DISASTERS

One difficulty in discussing the role of psychology and psychologists in coming to the aid of people in disasters is that there are many subdisciplines and various kinds of practitioners of psychology. A common role for disaster psychologists is that of clinical or counseling psychologists who come in after the disaster and help people deal with trauma. Although there is doubtless a role for clinical work in the aftermath of a disaster, the setting may not lend itself to work with individual clients. This may be a physical matter, with people crowded into shelters or tents and no facilities for a private face-to-face consultation. Or it might be a cultural issue, with people preferring a group setting and a more collectivist approach. Furthermore, there may be whole populations, rather than individuals, or groups of individuals, who are traumatized and logistically the therapist could barely scratch the surface of the problem on a one-on-one basis. Also a clinical approach may see the trauma as a form of pathology, and in a number of cultures any suggestion of mental illness may carry such stigma that singling out people for treatment could create flow-on problems for them.

A further problem with a more clinical and therapy oriented approach is that it tends to focus on individuals putting aside intrusive memories and forgetting the traumatic event, whereas it may be, from the point of view of adaptation, just as important to remember as to forget. In fact, one salient point about survivor perception of disaster that came out of our research in the various locations is that people do not talk about recovery or forgetting as being goals, instead they talk about remembering the disaster in a way that makes sense to them and infuses their experience with meaning. Each community we studied had a culturally relevant way of marking the event—from naming it to tattoos and community art to memorials in public parks. In Aceh, one NGO manager said far from the tsunami being something to forget, local people wanted to pass the stories on and retell them: "There was a woman that was pregnant when the tsunami happened. She gave birth afterwards. Or another woman even gave birth in the water. It became like, my children will inherit this story, and they have to know, so this story will be told, and will run in the family as a history" (Pelupessy et al., 2011, p. 45).

Treatment techniques, whether for individuals or groups, developed in one culture may not be fitting in another. One NGO coordinator in Islamic Aceh said:

> People needed to do some coping—they needed to tell their stories and share the problems they had. That assistance suited the culture here. But there was also a thing that didn't suit the culture. One time I saw, mothers were asked to dance and sing. It made them uncomfortable. . . . I think that those people just don't know that things like that are taboo in Aceh. (Pelupessy et al., 2011, p. 43)

Goodman et al. (2004) bring together literature from feminist and multicultural psychology to come up with some suggestions as to how counseling psychologists might work for social justice. Drawing on Bronfenbrenner's (1977) ecological model of social analysis, they suggest that social justice occurs on the micro-, meso-, and macro-levels. In the past, much of psychology focused on working with individuals but a social justice approach needs to also consider communities and organizations (meso-systems) and the overarching social structures, policies, and ideologies (macro-systems). The idea that psychologists interested in social justice must, Goodman et al. (2004) suggest, work to change social structures, not just individuals, is implicit in this conceptualization; the target of intervention in social justice work is not just the individual but the social context. They suggest six principles for putting social justice into practice in psychology. These are (1) ongoing self-examination, (2) sharing power, (3) giving voice, (4) facilitating consciousness raising, (5) building on strengths, and (6) leaving clients with the tools for social change. They suggest these tenets are useful across a range of social justice practices, including research, program design, policy development, and community intervention.

In practice, these distinctions should become artificial. Research is done to determine community needs; programs are developed to meet those needs, and then are evaluated to determine their effectiveness in ameliorating problems; and this research then informs policy. These principles apply not only to working with multicultural communities within one's own society but also to working with communities overseas. Rather than coming in as an expert with set ideas, the psychologist will need to listen and become a co-learner, with skills, knowledge, and experience to contribute, but with some humility about applying them in this new situation.

In terms of research, a social justice approach requires that psychology students learn to listen to others and learn interviewing skills, and that qualitative as well as quantitative methods of research are taught. This will mean that students have the skills to give voice to those who are not heard and critically question the structures of society (Kidder & Fine, 1997). Psychologists could also support research that links with contexts and sends students out to work with and learn about communities (Montero, 2009). It is important to inform interventions and adapt them to be locally appropriate rather than adopt a one-size-fits-all approach. We term these *intelligent methods*, ones that can be changed as we learn and provide feedback into the process. In our research, we found that the aid evaluations predominantly are focused on the question "did the agency achieve its goals?" rather than how local people saw, evaluated, and responded to the aid they were given, or how the interventions had altered the political landscape.

We find the basic thesis that Goodman et al. (2004) put forward to be sound, and in line with understandings drawn from critical, liberation, and community psychology, and their tips to be very useful. We take issue with the idea that psychology students must learn to become agents of social change, as if social change is an addendum, something extra to the basic role of the psychologist. Rather we stress that *all* interventions by psychologists occur in a social context and that psychologists are social agents. They may be unaware of the effects of their presence and their work on their social context, but structuration theory decries that their actions either produce or reproduce the social structures in the environment (Jabri, 1996). Even if their work is highly theoretical and scientific, history provides many examples of how scientific ideas influence and can be used to justify social policies and political ideologies. With the idea in mind that silence and lack of awareness by academics may be just as political as action, we emphasize the ability to listen and observe as the first step toward social justice as well as the principle of self-examination, but add to that the importance of monitoring changes in the context, be it micro, meso or macro. Peace theorists such as Lederach (2005) would place listening as the first priority. We might recall the influence of Carl Rogers and his fundamental contribution to counseling psychology through emphasizing the importance of listening to the client and responding empathically. Although Lederach works with different cultural groups and likes to formulate his response as a metaphor, the process is similar, and other cultures have also discovered for themselves the value of active listening. (See, e.g., Bretherton & Zhaoying, 2009).

Reflecting on Goodman et al.'s (2004) six principles, the negative impact of stereotyping victims of disaster becomes clear. The image of the survivor as a helpless individual existing in a social vacuum, needing rescue from more powerful and well-resourced outsiders, undermines the option to work cooperatively with local agencies. The urgency of the situation can be used as justification for neglecting reflection about self or the social context. The idea of power sharing is undermined by the image of helpless victims needing rescue. The "victims" are painted as being shattered and not able to speak for themselves, mentally shocked, without strengths to build on and not capable of wielding new tools.

Social psychology—with its study of topics like stereotyping, prejudice, and discrimination and its focus on group behavior—has much to offer in terms of understanding the dynamics of a community. However, sometimes the findings and understandings remain in academic journals and the laboratory, without the seamless application to community needs that Goodman and others (2004) envisage. It can be difficult to equate the relatively safe and slight laboratory manipulations of, for example, prejudice, with the degree of enmity that may prevail in real-life situations. Nonetheless, the theoretical understandings can help the practitioner in the field not only to understand the dynamics of the community but also to reflect on his or her own biases and blind spots, if the findings are used in context.

The founding fathers of social psychology were less laboratory-bound and their practices would be as sound today as they were in the past in preparing psychology students to work in demanding contexts. For example, Deutsch, following pioneers like Lewin (1936) and Sherif (see, e.g., Macleod, 2008, who describes Sherif's Robbers Cave Experiment), established a social psychology laboratory, but also maintained an ongoing practice as a psychologist and spent time with his students discussing current issues, consulting with them, and reflecting on the meaning of experiments, thinking about applications to therapy, issues of social justice, and how life should be lived (Frydenberg, 2005). He provided his students with a model for research, practice, creating cooperative learning environments, and working toward creating a more just world. And although this description may seem very male-dominated to feminist psychologists, this is a feature of the history of psychology, and he marks among his students and mentees some outstanding feminist psychologists, such as Michelle Fine (1992).

An approach that is open to learning together allows for evolution and transformation. In this stream of psychology, social justice, and linking theory to practice, was always integral, not only to peace psychologists but psychology as a whole discipline. Frydenberg quotes Deustch as attributing to his teacher Lewin the following approach:

> Practitioners identify significant problems to be solved, theorists develop a valid view of reality that contains the keys for solving the problems and practitioners apply the theory. Practitioners keep theorists in contact with social reality, and theorists provide practitioners with a deeper understanding of the social problems that confront them. (2005, p. 161)

Our point here is that social justice is not something new to the discipline of psychology but is tied up in its early development. Nor is social justice in contradiction to the scientific foundations of the discipline. A theory of human behavior that applies in the laboratory but not in the field, or is based on data from, and only applies to, first-year psychology students in an industrial nation does not provide a "valid view of reality" and is not a comprehensive scientific theory.

To see social justice as something applied, as an add-on course in advocacy, is, we believe, selling the discipline short. The basic academic value of seeking for truth should lead us to an appreciation of considering how our theories and findings hold up when put to the test of varying sociohistorical contexts. Rather than imposing our preconceived ideas of what will help, psychologists need to be open to finding out if existing practices do actually help in a new situation and be open to rethinking theories and practices when expectations are not met. This is not to devalue the work of psychologists who do act as advocates or the work of organizations like Psychologists for Social Responsibility. It is rather to say that the fact that some organizations undertake advocacy work does not absolve the rest of the profession from its obligation to try and understand the social justice implications of our work.

Peace psychologists such as Christie, Wagner, and Winter (2001) and McNair (2003) have given much thought to social justice issues. Christie (2006) distinguishes physical violence from structural violence. Although physical violence is episodic, overt and observable, structural violence is covert and built into the structures of society. The situation of the Australian Aborigines provides one example. When the British arrived in Australia 200 hundred years ago, they deemed the Aborigines to be part of the flora and fauna. The land was deemed to be empty of human occupation. This doctrine of "terra nullius" has caused Aboriginal people great suffering (see e.g., Bretherton & Mellor, 2006). Even today Aboriginal people can be shown to be disadvantaged in terms of longevity, overrepresentation in the legal system, housing, education, and other such indicators of well-being. Social psychology experiments suggest that Australians more easily associate a White face with a symbol of Australia than they can the picture of an Aboriginal face (Louis, Barlow, & Greenaway, 2012). This type of violence is harder to recognize but can be just as destructive in its effects as outbreaks of physical violence. The onus is on the peace psychologist to become aware of the inequalities and imbalances of power and to work with communities to address these. In this view healing is not only needed at the individual and communal levels but also at the macro-system level. An analysis of the structural violence in a disaster would pay attention to the inequalities in resources and political power that leads to poorer people living in more crowded and dangerous places, in lower-quality buildings with fewer chances to escape the disaster and fewer material resources to rebuild afterward. This analysis would also be aware of the inequalities in the recovery process, for example, the vastly different rates of pay between international experts and local aid workers. So, if the former goes home to a luxury hotel and the latter to a hovel, then an exemplary model of practice such as that described by Goodman et al. (2004), which stresses sharing and cooperative work, might seem rhetorical rather than authentic. Aid that does not take into account of the structural issues can feed into existing divisions and serve to increase rather than decrease the inequalities in a society. This is well recognized by international aid agencies in respect of age and gender, and many have a specific policy to make sure women and young people benefit from funds given.

In our research we found that psychologists were to be found among the survivors of disaster, the local rescuers and aid workers, and the outside parties coming in to help as well as contributing their theories to the design of intervention programs. However, we suggest that with a greater insight into the importance of the socioecological context, psychologists, along with others who work in aid, might in future play a stronger role in using their theory and practice to enhance adaptation before and after, as well as during, disasters.

WHAT HELPED COMMUNITIES RESPOND TO DISASTERS

We had expected that different types of disaster would give rise to very different experiences but found instead themes that recurred irrespective of the type of disaster or location of a community. A key factor was communication. People responded collectively to the disaster, working together to try and find out what was happening, to gather information about what was going on. Often, in a disaster, communications are disrupted but people used resources that were available to find out more, telephoning people elsewhere, passing on news from the media, where this was possible. After the emergency period, there is a need in the community for listening to each other and exchanging stories. A number of the helpers we interviewed had done a lot of listening but had not had an opportunity to tell their own stories.

Far from fleeing individually in an every-man-for-himself style, people gathered up elderly relatives and children who needed help and responded as a social unit. These stories of togetherness and cooperation were often celebrated as part of the memorialization and remembering of disaster, with community-led efforts to remember such as memorials, graffiti, tattoos, and other locally culturally relevant actions forming a basis for personal and collective memory of the disaster. In the case of the Aceh tsunami, the disaster was incorporated into a local identity of being strong and independent as a street children worker commented: "I think you already know about Acehnese. They used to face conflicts. They have a strong mentality to handle challenging situations. We have those capacities. We used to find ways to survive. Anything. We do everything to survive" (Pelupessy et al., 2011, p. 45).

People used their strengths, sometimes in surprising ways; for example, after the 2005 earthquake, on their own initiative, some Pakistani boys scouts used their first aid training to set up stations to bandage people with wounds, especially for children with wounds. As the risk of death through infection is very high, they provided a valuable service and probably saved many children from additional health problems. Existing social networks were very important and could be mobilized to respond to the disaster. In a number of the cases we studied the local psychology services responded very effectively. Rashida and Ali, psychologists in Pakistan, responding to the 2005 earthquake, describe how they would do relief work with groups of people in Pakistan:

> Rashida: You know, as we did all the relief work and what we did was, which was not really planned as a psychosocial support or anything, but we decided to all stay in the office. So we used to live there, that was where the warehouse was and since it was Ramadan we decided to give meals to the

> staff because they were all going, you know, 9 or 10 hours. When they would come back there would be very forced laughter. We had all heard, terrible, terrible stories of absolutely devastating things that had happened to people. And then we started realized and sort of, noticing differences in behavior and the way they were relating and those shared meals I think was a form of providing support.

For Rashida and Ali the focus of the media on what the government and army were doing, rather than civil society and many volunteers, did not tell the true story of the disaster.

> **Rashida:** What was absolutely fabulous is how ordinary Pakistanis came forward, the rich, the poor, middle class, and a lot is said about that, which is very well-deserved and I found it extremely humbling the way people responded. But, I think, still the stories that are still not well-known are of the survivors themselves and how they too played such an incredible role in helping each other, whether it was sharing goods or sharing food or just the solidarity of grief, so you know together dig graves and stuff like that.
>
> **Ali:** You know there were heroes at every point . . .
>
> **Rashida:** Every point (Bedar, Bretherton, & Ride, 2012, p. 52).

Local people did not keep to their professional or social roles but took an attitude of "we are all in this together" and "we will all do what we can." Local services were able to respond in a culturally appropriate way, bring together local networks, and often form new bonds across religious or ethnic backgrounds. This was a feature of the disaster response after Cyclone Nargis in Myanmar where NGOs previously worked with a particular sector of society (often a religious or ethnic group) rather than broadly with communities.

Distant parties could help support these local networks; interviewees described their appreciation for relationships preexisting to the disaster that then enabled funding to flow to local organizations quickly and without too much bureaucracy. Demands to local practitioners from international practitioners flown in to assist with disaster response and recovery were often a cause of stress rather than help in difficult times. As one local journalist in New Orleans commented in relation to flown-in media after Hurricane Katrina: "A crisis is not time to be making new friends" (Deutsche Welle Global Media Conference, 2010).

BEFORE, DURING AND AFTER THE DISASTER: WHAT CAN PSYCHOLOGISTS DO?

Throughout its history, psychology has tended to work at an individual level. There are exceptions; for example, we mentioned the work of Sherif who was interested in investigating the environmental conditions that would make groups more or less cooperative. Meyers (2002) writes about incorporating social justice into the teaching of psychology and noted that "our field often emphasizes individual-level functioning instead of broader social, cultural, and political forces" (para. 7). He suggests that a focus on social justice asks professors to seek out new connections that relate course topics to issues of social importance and inequalities: "This coverage draws attention to potential applications of psychological knowledge and the ways in which it can create change" (para 7). A more radical approach would suggest that a study of human behavior might contribute to an understanding of social, cultural, and political forces. For example, psychoanalysts felt that broad social, cultural, and political events were the business of psychologists and wrote extensively, for example, about war and fascism. It also follows from finding that natural disasters are in part human disasters, then the study of human behavior might contribute in a more fundamental way to understanding why disasters happen, how people respond, what can be done to mitigate and prevent disasters, and how people better adapt to the physical environment.

In more immediate practical terms, psychologists cannot suddenly acquire the cultural competence and links with local people in response to the emergency situation. Rather, the ability to respond appropriately will depend on a prior context of intercultural understanding and strong networks. As professionals psychologists are in a good position to learn about the work of colleagues in other cultures and nations and to help strengthen each other's work, a number of psychological associations in developed nations, like the American Psychological Society, are making an effort to reach out to international psychologists but this can be further enhanced if the utility of a more global approach is appreciated. Measures to help develop the skills and resources of local people will then see them well equipped to deal with an emergency in their homeland. Those of our researchers who were local people, practicing in the local community, but who had studied overseas for higher degrees provide an example. Psychologists at major universities and in well-resourced practices can strengthen networks by visiting overseas universities and clinics, finding opportunities for overseas psychologists to visit to study or attend conferences, send psychology books, and so on. A positive example is the Committee for the Psychological Study of Peace (CPSP), which builds stronger global links either by meeting in conjunction with major international congresses or holding a smaller symposium that occurs every second year in a conflict zone. The meeting allows local psychologists to meet with internationals. The registration fees are high, but the costs are kept low so the attendance of some psychologists from poorer nations can be sponsored. A CPSP site visit to an earthquake recovery zone in Indonesia, where highly cooperative community work had rebuilt in a very short time, provided some of the inspiration for our work on community response to disasters.

The value of such exchanges between psychologists from different nations is undermined if visitors are not treated as equals, as co-learners with something important to offer as well as something to learn. If international students are obliged to follow a supervisor's interest in a highly abstract area that is irrelevant to development in their home context, or treated as remedial students who have not fully mastered English, then the potential of the visit, for both visitor and host, will not be realized. More generally if the real-world experience of our students is appreciated, as well as their skill in carrying out laboratory projects or writing essays, then the multicultural experience in psychology classrooms can be appreciated. The use of more interactive learning and collaborative learning methods will further draw out the strengths of the students. International practitioners need to allow local people to contribute (rather than feel we need to empower them).

Educating outsiders about the cultural appropriateness of their actions and local culture is a task best done before entering the disaster zone. In a presentation at APA 2011, U.S. students returning from a trip to disaster-ravaged Haiti expressed surprise that Haitian children would share gifts and supplies—failing to understand the communal nature of such communities as opposed to the Western, more individualistic approach. This "surprise" really evidences a lack of cultural understanding of the students and preparation by their professors and sponsor organizations before undertaking the trip. Instead, taking students to cultures both within your own nation (where multicultural groups may have less power and you can argue that they should learn to adjust to the dominant culture) and outside (where other cultures have more power than you) can elicit two-way learning and exchange provided psychologists need to be aware that they may put people at risk (e.g., male counselors in Pakistan talking to women in villages may create tension for the villagers and the counselor concerned because of local norms around gender relations).

CONCLUSION

Adaptation refers to learning the lessons from the disaster and changing behaviour on the basis of the insights gained. Adaptation could mean better preparation for disasters, and improving disaster response, or it could necessitate more extensive shifts, such as deciding not to rebuild settlements in the same place or in the same way. It could also mean forming different relationships within the community, or between the community and the nation and the international arena. Like Goodman et al. (2004) we used Bronfenbrenner's map of human ecology but we took a wider focus to include different nations and macro-systems with the international community as our overarching system, for disasters have worldwide effects and call for a worldwide response.

From the accounts of our informants we identified a number of features that a psychologist would need to have to be able to most effectively assist in a disaster situation. These were to understand the strengths of community members as well as their vulnerabilities, to go beyond working with individuals and extend our work to communities and the wider sociopolitical sphere, and to go beyond working with immediate stresses and extend our efforts to helping better adaptation before, during, and after a disaster. It is possible to find psychologists from different divisions who do some of these things. Positive psychologists look for individual strengths and are beginning to identify posttraumatic growth as a possibility (see, e.g., Clay & Joseph, 2009). Community psychologists work with communities to improve health and are increasingly aware of the political implications of their work (see, e.g., Montero, 2009). Social psychologists are alert to the destructive role that may be played by prejudice and stereotypes (see, e.g., Louis et al., 2012). A number of practitioners working in the area of disaster management are increasingly critical of government policy (see, e.g., Gheytanchi et al., 2009). It is as if a new approach is emerging from different divisions of psychology, but that a conversation between the different types of psychologists would be constructive in developing a more integrated approach that is more firmly grounded in the discipline of psychology.

In conducting this research we learned a great deal about the strengths of individuals and communities. We tried to follow the principles of social justice in our conduct of the research, emphasising listening, working in partnership with local organisations, learning from our informants and local researchers, and sharing our findings together. We found there is a need to see disaster, environment, and community together as interlinked sets of systems such that it does not make sense to consider one part without the others. So then, an approach incorporating social justice, psychology, and natural disaster might be very different to the "expert helper-uninformed helpless" dichotomy that informs many interventions in disaster zones. It might emphasize listening and response to disaster, nature, community, and culture with the psychologist playing a role to help us realise the significance of the disaster and the new realisation the disaster may bring about community life at a time of both danger and opportunity. In this way, the psychologist can have a role in befriending a community as it pursues social justice.

REFERENCES

Anderson, M. B. (1999). *Do no harm: How aid can support peace—or war.* Boulder, CO: Lynne Reinner.

Anderson, M. B., & Woodrow, J. P. (1998). *Rising from the ashes: Development strategies in times of disaster.* Boulder, CO: Lynne Rienner.

Beda, A., Bretherton, D., & Ride, A. (2011). Pakistan. In A. Ride & D. Bretherton. (Eds.), *Community resilience in natural disasters* (pp. 51–90). New York: Palgrave Macmillan.

Bretherton, D., & Mellor, D. (2006). Reconciliation between Aboriginal and other Australians: The "Stolen Generations." *Journal of Social Issues, 62*(1) 81–98.

Bretherton, D., & Zhaoying, H. (2009). Listening with the ear, eye and heart: Conflict transformation in China. In D. Bagshaw & E. Porter (Eds.), *Mediation in the Asia Pacific Region* (pp. 182–197). London, UK; New York, NY: Routledge.

Bronfenbrenner, U. (1979). The ecology of human development: Experiments by nature and design. Cambridge, MA: Harvard University.

Cessaro, M. A & Romero, E. M. (Eds.). (1987). *The Mexico Earthquakes 1985: Factors involved and lessons learned.* New York, NY: American Society of Civil Engineers.

Christie, D. J. (2006). What is peace psychology the psychology of? *Journal of Social Issues, 62,* 1–17.

Christie, D. J., Wagner, R., & Winter, D. (2001). *Peace, conflict, and violence: Peace psychology for the 21st century.* Upper Saddle River, NJ: Prentice-Hall.

Clay, R., Knibbs, J., & Joseph, S. (2009). Measurement of posttraumatic growth in young people: A review. *Clinical Child Psychology and Psychiatry, 14*(3), 411–422.

Deutsche Welle Global Media Conference, Bonn, June 21–23 2010, Dart Centre moderated panel transcript as retrieved from http://dartcenter.org/content/transcript-witnessing-human-cost-climate-change.

Fine, M. (1992). *Disruptive voices: The possibilities of feminist research.* Ann Arbor: University of Michigan.

Fothergill, A. & Peek, L. (2004). Poverty and disasters in the United States: A review of recent sociological findings. *Natural Hazards, 32,* 89–112.

Frydenberg, E. (2005). *Tough minded and tender hearted: The life and work of Morton Deutsch.* Toowong, QLD: Australian Academic Press.

Gheytanchi, A., Joseph, L., Gierlach, E., Kimpara, S., Housley, J., Franco, Z. E. & Beutler, L. E. (2007). The dirty dozen: Twelve key failures of the Hurricane Katrina response & how psychology can help. *American Psychologist, 62,* 118–130.

Goodman, L. A., Liang, B., Helms, J. E., Latta, R. E., Sparks, E., & Wentraub, S. R. (2004). Training counseling psychologists as social justice agents: Feminist and multicultural principles in action. *The Counseling Psychologist, 32,* 763–837.

Jabri, V. (1996). *Discourses on violence: Conflict analysis reconsidered.* Manchester, UK: Manchester University Press.

Kidder, L. H., & Fine, M. (1997). Qualitative inquiry in psychology: A radical tradition. In D. Fox & I. Prilleltensky (Eds.), *Critical psychology: An introduction* (pp. 34–50). Thousand Oaks, CA: Sage.

Lederach, J. P. (2005). *The moral imagination: The art and soul of building peace.* Oxford, MA: Oxford University Press, 2005.

Lewin, K. (1936). *Principles of topological psychology.* New York, NY: McGraw Hill.

Lomitz, C. (1998). Book review of E. L. Quantantelli (Ed.).What is a disaster? In *Natural Hazards, 18,* 87–88.

Louis, W., Barlow, F., & Greenaway, K. (2012). National identity, Australian values and outsiders. In D. Bretherton & N. Balvin (Eds.), *Peace psychology in Australia* (pp 87–104). New York, NY: Springer.

MacNair, R. M. (2003). *The psychology of peace: An introduction.* Westport, CT: Praeger.

McLeod, S. A. (2008). Robbers Cave Experiment/Realistic conflict theory. Retrieved from http://www.simplypsychology.org/robbers-cave.html/

Meyers, S. A. (2002). *Putting social justice into practice in psychology courses. Observer.* Retrieved from www.psychologicalscience.org/observer/getArticle.cfm?id=2241

Montero, M. (2009). Community action and research as citizen construction. *American Journal of Community Psychology, 43,* 149–161.

Pelupessy, D., Bretherton, D., & Ride, A. (2011). Indonesia. In A. Ride & D. Bretherton (Eds.), *Community resilience in natural disasters* (pp. 19–49). New York, NY: Palgrave Macmillan.

Poniatowska, E. (1988). *Nothing, nobody: The voices of the Mexico City earthquake.* Philadelphia, PA: Temple University Press.

Resilience Alliance. (2012). Retrieved from www.resalliance.org

Ride, A., & Bretherton, D. (Eds.) (2011). *Community resilience in natural disasters.* New York, NY: Palgrave Macmillan.

Saraceno, B. (2006). Foreword. In G. Reyes & G. Jacobs (Eds.), *Handbook of international disaster psychology: Fundamentals and overview* (pp. xii–xiv). Santa Barbara, CA: Praeger.

Chapter 9

Compassion, Suffering, and Human Flourishing: Toward a Moral and Jurisprudential Psychology of Social Justice[1]

Christopher R. Williams and Bruce A. Arrigo

In two recent volumes, Arrigo and Milovanovic (2009) and Arrigo, Bersot, and Sellers (2011) articulate a provocative and globally relevant thesis about the existential, corporeal, material, and cosmopolitan forces of self/other captivity and of self/other risk management. Captivity refers to the forces that bind or check individual and collective consciousness. Risk management refers to the forces of human social capital as difference (i.e., as latent potential and as unharnessed possibility) that are reduced (i.e., difference as *otherized*; thus, limits to one's being) or repressed (i.e., difference as territorialized; thus, denials of one's becoming). The authors contend that the maintenance of these captivity and risk management forces is harmful. Indeed, this maintenance functions as a kind of social dis-ease or societal madness.

The forces of captivity and risk management destructively nurture a society of captives that encompasses many imprisoned individuals, groups, or collectives (Arrigo & Milovanovic, 2009). They include the kept (i.e., to those held existentially, corporeally, and materially captive) as well as to their keepers (i.e., to those whose risk management includes the policing and domestication of human social capital), regulators (i.e., to those who administrate over, legislate for, or educate about risk management's safeguarding or normalization), and watchers (i.e., to those who fearfully and desperately submit to captivity-through-risk-management as the healthy and natural path to human social progress). Arrigo et al. (2011) argued that sustaining these interdependent and co-productive conditions is pathological because the dynamics of captivity and risk management dangerously grow society's own systemic imprisonment. This condition is termed *totalizing confinement*. Under this condition, notions of self and other, citizenship and social justice, freedom and responsibility, community and society are no more than shadows of what they could be or could become for, by, and about one and all.

The thesis outlined earlier is linked to key insights derived from *psychological jurisprudence* (PJ) (e.g., Arrigo, 2010, 2011a, 2011b, 2012, in press). PJ is a novel and experimental theory, method, and type of praxis. It is a radical philosophical perspective and it is an emergent form of cultural criticism (Arrigo, 2004). To better specify how PJ advances the aims of human flourishing (i.e., unleashed potential, marshaled possibility), while serving as an ethical and jurisprudential framework for a psychology of social justice, this chapter briefly enumerates PJ's key philosophical constituents. However, to better specify PJ's moral and jurisprudential commitments, the dynamics of compassion and suffering are first reviewed. These dynamics suggest a great deal about the intrapersonal landscapes and interpersonal contexts that adjudicate the character (i.e., the flourishing or excellence) of social justice. As the chapter posits, PJ's Aristotelian-derived (1976; see also, Hughes, 2001)) virtue philosophy holds considerable promise for overcoming and transforming the conditions (i.e., the landscapes and contexts) of captivity that presently render the status of human social flourishing (as compassion) and human social injustice (as suffering) artifacts of increasingly destructive and pathological risk management dispositions.

THE DYNAMICS OF COMPASSION AND SUFFERING

Although social justice has been and continues to be variously defined and conceptualized, most if not all characterizations are rooted in ideals of human flourishing. At its core, the very notion of social justice seems wedded to the development of, or conditions that provide for the development of, human possibilities and potentialities. More specifically, concerns of social justice seem each to emanate from one crucial and overriding humanistic concern: the development and sustenance of social conditions within which all persons have the greatest opportunity to realize their possibilities and potentialities, as unique individuals and as members of greater communities and societies. In this light, issues of social justice might be most properly rooted in the Aristotelian (1976) *eudaimonic* tradition—one that takes human well-being, fulfillment, or flourishing as the highest good.

As a philosophical orientation, this tradition directly confronts the various personal, communal, institutional, and societal impediments that reduce and repress the realization of this good, this virtue of living excellently.

Critiques of social and organizational structure notwithstanding, the development and sustenance of conditions conducive to human fulfillment and flourishing has much to do with the ways in which people are mindful of and treat themselves as well as one another. That is to say, although concerns of social injustice are often linked with broader macrological forces, one should also recognize that, to a large extent, justice and injustice are intrapersonal and interpersonal realities. Put another way, they are concerns not only of institutional policy and practice (society) but also equally of moral psychology (self). In this respect, then, the possibility of social justice is completely proportional to the degree to which public and personal character is directed toward and facilitative of human excellence and flourishing. Ultimately, social justice must be grounded in a collective ethic that is "rooted in a sensitivity to the interests and needs of others, a rational awareness that my good is tied up with the good of others" (Kurtz, 1969, p. 10).

Rational awareness of the interdependency of individual goods is the foundation of a moral psychology that makes possible the types of human relationships and human communities necessary for the evolution of social justice and the conditions of human flourishing. At the same time, the absence of such awareness makes possible the types of thinking, feeling, and relating toward others that generate injustice—that create and sustain indifference, harm and suffering. As Richard Taylor (2000) suggests, "[t]he distinction between justice and injustice presupposes the existence of a multiplicity of beings . . . it is a distinction that applies, not to the things we find in the world, but to our behavior with respect to each other" (p. 238). Injustice feeds off of this multiplicity and the distinctions inherent in it; justice, in turn, "calls upon us to refuse to invest in a social ethic that separates us from one another and instead to visualize all people . . . as being connected" (Wozniak, 2000, p. 283).

Given the earlier observations, the virtue of compassion may very well be the most foundational of humanistic goods regarding communal and other forms of social health. Compassion is that disposition or way of being that is most fundamentally other-regarding—always interpersonal, always involving a concern for the good of the other (Blum, 1980). It expands the boundaries of the self rather than tightening or strengthening them (cf. Nussbaum, 2001, p. 300). In this respect, one might think of compassion as the vital generative force underlying the struggle for social justice—for the types of communities and relationships that make possible the realization of humanistic ideals of collective flourishing. Compassion informs and, in fact, makes possible an awareness of suffering as an impediment to sentient well-being, flourishing, and excellence. Thus, it is crucial to a moral psychology of nonharm and benevolence—one by which people refuse to add suffering to the world and, positively, are inclined to remedy existing suffering wherever and whenever it emerges.

Compassion might thus be understood as the *moral foundation of social justice*. Characterized by social and cultural conditions that provide the greatest opportunity for collective human flourishing, social justice is promoted by and perpetuated through the widespread embodiment of a fundamentally other-regarding moral psychology—of a collective value framework informed by a rational awareness of interconnectedness, sensitivity to the needs and interests of others, and rooted in the principle that "the highest moral prescription is for *humanity* as a whole" (Kurtz, 1969, p. 9).

In an important respect, then, the pursuit of social justice is the pursuit of human relationships and conditions of community that would allow for and promote the realization of human flourishing. Antithetical to such conditions and inimical to this pursuit are the realities of suffering that characterize contemporary social existence. Of special concern are the avertable, preventable, and remediable harms and pains that are created and perpetuated through our decisions and indecisions, actions and failures to act. More directly, it is not merely the presence of suffering that is of concern, but the ways in which individuals and institutions—both actively and passively—create communities and produce relationships and conditions within which suffering is likely to thrive (e.g., Quinney, 1991).

The harm and indifference that characterizes these relationships reflects the growing dormancy of people's innate capacity to be mindful of and treat themselves and others with dignity, care, and concern. In other words, the untapped potential and unleashed possibility of compassion in personal and social character and in subsequent individual and institutional behaviors informed by such character is held captive by such silence. Compassion as more fully affirming of human social flourishing and as an artifact of evolving self and society excellence is therefore rendered unimaginable, inexpressible, and uninhabitable. In sharp contrast to harm and indifference, compassion entails a sort of "suffering with"—experiencing the suffering of others in such a way that one is compelled to act toward its alleviation. It involves a rational awareness of and sensitivity to the suffering of others, relatedness to that suffering and those others, and a consequent experience of suffering within oneself. Thus, it is compassion that is both benefactor and adversary of suffering—its presence in the instance of the latter; its absence in that of the former.

If, as Thoreau (2012) once hinted, the personal always precedes the social, the pursuit of justice and the conditions of human flourishing are first and foremost an intrapersonal pursuit. In this view, the root of suffering and injustice and the root of compassion and flourishing are one and the same; namely, they are each grounded in cognitive and affective structures—informed as those may be by culture—by which individuals, as institutional representatives, make sense of and think, feel, and act about the realities of suffering with which they are presented. Crucially, the struggle for social justice thus entails a collective overcoming of obstacles that serve to inhibit the natural human disposition toward compassionate awareness—obstacles that are embedded in the very ways in which we think and feel about others and ourselves.

Compassionate awareness follows from and largely reflects shared appraisals of ourselves, of others, and of human suffering. Aristotle (2004) suggested as much in his *Rhetoric*, noting that in any given instance, compassion involves three key judgments: that the suffering of another is serious; that the suffering of another is undeserved; and that one's own possibilities are similar to those who are suffering. As such, compassion emerges from the evaluations of the relative seriousness of different forms of suffering as well as from a twofold judgment of the person or persons who are subjects of circumstances that lead them to suffer. These evaluations and judgments are themselves products of a more generalized (and, no doubt, culturally and institutionally shaped) cognitive and affective (i.e., psychological) framework through which people make sense of themselves, others, and the harms and hardships of human existence.

If compassion requires certain types of conclusions to be reached with regard to each of these evaluative engagements, it follows that each judgment represents a location from which the misguiding of our beliefs and self-other projections can erect barriers to compassionate awareness and serve as impediments to nonharmful and remedial (i.e., benevolent) action. Consequently, the more general framework that guides these beliefs and representations about the nature and scope of suffering gives rise to countervailing forces working against compassionate awareness and subsequent decisions and behaviors motivated by it. Between justice and its pursuit lie several crucial barriers. Recognizing these impediments—and the captivity that they engender—requires a landscape and a context for adjudicating self, other, and society differently: for transforming, indeed, revolutionizing human social flourishing as compassion and human social injustice as suffering.

THE INTRAPERSONAL LANDSCAPES AND INTERPERSONAL CONTEXTS OF SUFFERING

Virtues are dispositions; and dispositions, as Aristotle (1976) noted, require cultivation. To be sure, the disposition toward compassion surely seems a property of human nature—a possibility or potentiality that each individual has by virtue of being human (e.g., Ridley, 1996). Yet as Seneca (2009) suggested of virtue more generally, while people may be born *for* it, they are not born *with* it—"until you cultivate it there is only the material for virtue, not virtue itself." The cultivation of virtue of which both Aristotle and Seneca were concerned is not purely an individual struggle. At the same time, it is not purely a social or cultural struggle. In many ways, the cultivation of virtue—of compassion, tolerance, and all of those traits that seem central to the types of human relationships that engender comprise, community, and social justice—is bilateral and dynamic (Williams & Arrigo, 2004).

To borrow from Anderson (2002), we might say that part of the struggle for community and social justice is an "internal, existential struggle within all of us" (p. 238). The significance of its externalized manifestations notwithstanding, injustice is something that "lives within each of us, and until we overcome that internal form of violence . . . we will not be able to overcome its more external, social forms" (p. 238). Those barriers that impede the development and practice of compassion remain socially and culturally active only so long as they remain active psychological tendencies. They live in social character and are incorporated in cultural and institutional realities only so long as we fail in that "internal struggle" of which Anderson wrote.

We maintain that this is what Nussbaum (2001) had in mind as well when she observed that "compassionate individuals construct institutions that embody what they imagine" (p. 405). Similarly, we suppose that the degree to which unjust, harmful, and indifferent dispositions are active in individuals, they will remain active in the structures and institutions that society, as a collective of individuals, creates. Embedded in structures, institutions, and social character, in turn, they (these captivity-generating dispositions) become that much more formidable as "internal, existential" adversaries. These dispositions are the harm-generating limits and denials of human social capital that reductively and repressively manage the risk of social justice and the character that it therefore (dis)embodies.

At the same time that one's cultural, structural, and institutional realities are products of one's imagination, one cannot neglect to consider the ways in which collective consciousness is simultaneously shaped by existing macrological realities. Whereas structures and institutions tend to embody what one imagines, "institutions, in turn, influence the development of compassion in individuals" (Nussbaum, 2001, p. 405). To be sure, we do not expect the capacity and potentiality of virtue to materialize absent conditions conducive to their development and practice. Its scarcity in all spheres of human relating implicates not simply deficits of individual disposition, but perhaps more importantly the role of social character, socialization, social structure, and institutional arrangements and practices. As Fesmire (1997) noted, "There is no such thing as someone who is 'born' a saint or savage" (p. 285). Rather, one should understand tendencies toward virtue and vice as prominently shaped by and informed through one's interactions with the cultural, structural, and institutional elements of existence.

As Fesmire (1997) further explained, virtues "are not radically private possessions . . . and 'vices' do not merely result from 'weak wills' or 'sinful natures'" (p. 285). Characterlogical tendencies are best regarded as "products of interaction between the make-up of an individual on the one hand and objective elements of the social world on the other" (p. 285). There is thus an important sense in which separation between people in interpersonal spheres is "self-similar" (Williams & Arrigo, 2004, pp. 43–64) to the separations embedded within and promulgated by social structure and the policies and practices of social institutions.

In the interest of promoting social justice, it therefore becomes critical to consider the ways in which social institutions shape both social and individual character, as well as the ways in which intrapersonal and interpersonal disposition creates and sustains structures, institutions, and the regularized dynamics and practices that issue from them. Recognizing these dynamics is perhaps the first step toward "act[ing ethically and] intelligently for social progress" (Fesmire, 1997, p. 285).

PSYCHOLOGICAL JURISPRUDENCE AND RECOGNIZING THE MORAL DYNAMICS OF HUMAN SOCIAL PROGRESS

Psychological jurisprudence is a philosophy about the self in society; it diagnoses the social person. PJ emphasizes the cultivation of human social capital (i.e., dynamic potential in being, transformative possibility in becoming) for, by, and about one and all. As cultural criticism, PJ argues that these potentialities and possibilities await and long for recognition in human consciousness and in all facets of social relating. As such, PJ is a critical philosophy of ontology (a radical reading of who people could be/become as social beings) and ethics (a radical morality regarding the process of more fully realizing individual human flourishing and of actualizing latent, mutually generative, excellence). Thus, the ontology of PJ answers the question of will; its ethics responds to the question of way.

Moreover, PJ's epistemology represents a critique of discourse (i.e., an interrogation of the constructed narratives that define the social person) and the discursive, performative, and therefore situated properties that govern the texts of being in and of society. Stated differently, PJ's epistemology draws attention to the politics of discourse and the contested meaning-making terrain through which intention, choice, and action reside. This landscape, always and already politicized, tells the story of ontology (i.e., what it means to be a social being). Currently, this landscape is populated by stories of the self in society that are increasingly and alarmingly partialized and fragmented, fictionalized and false, virtualized and sensationalized. Among others, these include the de-realizing narratives of violence and victimization, crime and punishment, treatment and recovery, health and wellness, compassion and suffering, human agency and social reality.

The fact that PJ seeks to unleash human potential and possibility that await recognition or awareness in consciousness indicates that a constrained aesthetic (harm-generating images) about the social person presently (and far too routinely) maintains dominion over the topography of the (collective) psyche. This *jurisprudence of the mind* (e.g., Arrigo, 2004; Arrigo, Bersot, & Selllers, 2011; Arrigo & Milovanovic, 2009) both binds and checks human social capital. These constraints include the reductive and repressive conditions of bad faith (Sartre, 1956) and false consciousness (Marx, 1964) that repetitively caricaturize, trivialize, or sanitize the more dynamic and transformative properties of ontology. Overcoming both of these conditions (i.e., the self-deception and "escape" from freedom that bad faith nurtures; the hegemony of otherizing and territorializing and the fetishism of abstraction that false consciousness reproduces) requires a departure in how risk is presently managed within its various captivity-maintaining communal contexts and institutional settings. Risk refers to the regulation of difference, to self in society capital that could be otherwise, if each of person lived more dynamically (as beings moving toward unleashed potential), and that could become otherwise than being if each of person lived more transformatively (as beings dwelling within harnessed possibility). Thus, PJ's epistemology explains how the social reality of difference (e.g., the being and becoming of compassion and suffering) is currently reasoned and problematically scripted; PJ's aesthetics makes evident how these present-day renderings, when embraced and deployed as normal and healthy, often discipline and domesticate dynamic and transformative human social capital.

Embracing the critical philosophy of PJ—inhabiting the type of radical mindfulness that it promotes—requires a revolutionary attitude concerning the madness, citizenship, and social justice relationship. Appropriating this attitude is necessary because the madness of captivity (i.e., the society of captives) is sourced in its all-encompassing and mind-numbing ubiquity. Indeed, this madness extends not only to the kept (those who are confined and constrained) but also to those who keep them (those who monitor, treat, and correct the kept), regulate them (those who administrate to, educate about, or legislate over the kept), and watch them (those who passively and complacently accept captivity's normalizing strictures). The harm of this captivity is existential, corporeal, and material in its cultural composition and effects, and it includes harms of reduction (limits on being, forestalling one's humanity, otherizing) and harms of repression (denials of becoming, foreclosing one's possibilities, territorializing). These harms thwart human social capital. When the madness that the society of captives represents is reified, then a social pathology, a systemic dis-ease, and the condition of totalizing confinement are fetishized. Stated differently, when harms of reduction and repression are normalized, then the society-of-captives phenomenon gives way to society's total captivity. This is the point at which dynamic and transformative human social capital as progress is vanquished for, by, and about one and all. This is the point at which citizenship and social justice, compassion and suffering, human agency and social structure, and so on, appear within consciousness (i.e., the jurisprudence of the mind) as mere shadows of what they could become, humanistically, productively, and interdependently.

The principal cultural undertaking of PJ and its philosophy of aesthetics is to conceive of and generate human social capital as freedom, as a more completely liberated jurisprudence of the mind. Retrieving, replicating, and circulating these images holds the nearest promise of overcoming captivity's madness, and of revolutionizing individual and collective consciousness. These portraits of the social person are much more dynamic in their composition of being, and they include representations of the subject as "in-process," as moving toward unleashed potential. In addition, these images of the self in society are much more transformative in their composition of becoming, and they consist of visions of the subject as situated, as dwelling within harnessed possibility.

Reclamation of the sort described earlier summons latent potential in being (as in personal growth and human flourishing) and unleashes untapped possibility in becoming (as in collective change and social justice). This is the human social project as movement toward innovation, experimentation, and creativity; and as a body (intrapersonal and interpersonal, institutional and communal) without stasis, categories, or other captivity-generating limits or denials. This is the social person, always and already, as revolutionary (Deleuze, 1983), as being human and doing humanness differently (i.e., another way). When difference is envisioned as such, then the social person (i.e., as being and becoming revolutionary) requires a replacement method of risk management.

As method, PJ considers the question of managing risk by relying on the notion of citizenship. Stated otherwise, the possibility of restoring and the potential of revolutionizing difference occur when PJ's Aristotelian-derived (1976) normative theory guides the assessment (See also, Hughes, 2001). This theory holds that the embodied practice of excellence (or of living virtuously) is dynamic; it evolves. Cultivating human potential and dwelling within harnessed possibility, then, is about journeying toward and taking up residence within changing habits of character (e.g., living ever more compassionately, justly). These evolving habits of character, when exercised (i.e., conjured and consumed, spoken and inscribed, personified and deployed), hold the nearest power to ignite human social capital, to release people from captivity, and to re-diagnose the madness that presently renders one and all no more than shadows of being and becoming. To be clear, advancing this version of citizenship is a life-long quest. It is an ongoing pursuit in the service of living ever more humanely, productively, and interdependently as a mutating self in society for and about being and becoming increasingly excellent in each moment of life. This pursuit entails a careful reading (a genealogical deconstruction and de-territorialization; Deleuze & Guattari, 1987; Foucault, 1998) of the concealed values, obscured interests, and hidden assumptions lodged within the texts that define and regulate the social person's ontology. For example, legal documents, psychiatric records, release and discharge plans, treatment manuals, and professional codes of conduct are all texts (i.e., systems of thought). The content of these narratives mostly endorses a circumscribed and finite picture about what it means to be in and of society as an ex-offender, a recovering addict, a consumer of psychiatric services, or even as a provider of treatment and corrective services. These portraits often finalize being (Bahktin, 1982) and foreclose becoming (Deleuze, 1983). This is how the social person is captured (bound and checked) as shadow in consciousness.

There are many questions to ponder in this genealogy of human consciousness (Lacan, 1977, 1981) and its landscape, its jurisprudence, of the mind. To be in process and to be situated is to acknowledge how history and culture are constitutive of and interconnected to human social capital. In addition, PJ examines how and for whom notions of citizenship—of moving toward and dwelling within excellence or inhabitable virtues—are communicated through the narratives that classify, code, and correct the social person. This is a reference to PJ's radical morality and the process by which its philosophy of ethics first unpacks and then diagnosis the quality and extent of captivity that presently limits potential and presently denies possibility in the texts that discipline and domesticate the social person. The purpose of this excursion is to make more explicit how intention, choice, and action could be rendered more fully affirming of mutually generative potential and possibility. Thus, PJ's philosophy of ethics seeks to reveal how the presence of bad faith and false consciousness are located within the systems of thought that codify and regulate humanness (i.e., difference).

As praxis, PJ's therapeutic corrective about and treatment prescription for being and becoming excellent both dynamically and transformatively—of living ever more differently, productively, and interdependently—extends to and from the kept as well as their keepers, regulators, and watchers. Growing human social capital is an inexorably shared, although unfamiliar, undertaking. It is an uncharted venture into the latent potentialities and untapped possibilities of being and becoming. This strange departure affirms the interactive link between *thinking about* (imagining the in-and-of society self as more or other) and *doing* (making a difference because of one's difference) humanness. This is the crucible in which social justice awaits emergence as transpraxis (Nietzsche, 1968), as the overcoming that could more completely re-constitute and revolutionize the character of compassion and suffering for a people yet to come, for a people yet to be (Deleuze & Guattari, 1987). The possibility of instantiating this change (e.g., of growing individual well-being, communal good, and collective accord both dynamically and transformatively) begins as an exercise in critique (i.e., PJ's methodological solution).

On the question of captivity, risk management, and harm, the critique considers how the in-process and situated social person intends, chooses, and acts justly. This is thinking about and doing humanness as otherwise than what is—as continually moving toward and settling within signification that dignifies and affirms difference virtuously, treats and heals the harms of captivity dynamically, and restores and transforms one and all innovatively. This praxis strategy is about overcoming the conditions of captivity (i.e., the landscapes of bad faith and the contexts of false consciousness) that engender harm (reductive limits on being, repressive denials of becoming). For PJ, transcending these conditions entails an evaluation of how and for whom justice is symbolized (what are the images that dominate consciousness on matters of compassion and suffering intra-personally and interpersonally?), narrated (which texts inform the story of difference, of risk, within institutional settings and community-based contexts?), practiced (whose version of virtue, human flourishing, and social justice prevails collectively in consciousness?), and reproduced (how does the dissemination of these symbolizations, narrations, and practices emancipate ontology for one and all?). This is the journey of thinking about and doing social justice as transpraxis (Nietizsche, 1968; see also, Deleuze, 1983); as an unfinished and ever-freeing expedition; and as human social capital unleashed and harnessed ever more humanely, productively, and interdependently.

Commencing this journey anticipates all those within the society of captives who make meaning, discern choice, reach judgment, and undertake action as imprisoned social beings. The promise of release that follows from pursuing this journey represents a revolutionary ethic: a moral and jurisprudential psychology that seeks to recognize and transform the conditions of self-other captivity and self-other risk management. These conditions presently render the status of human social flourishing (as compassion) and human social injustice (as suffering) totalizing in their confinement. This is excellence as shadow: mere fragments and traces of the self, others, and society.

CONCLUSION

Compassion and suffering are two cornerstones of human social existence. How they are envisioned in consciousness, spoken of in interpersonal or communal exchanges, practiced in institutional or organizational environs, and reproduced in cultural situations and public settings, tells one a great deal about the nature of citizenship and the quality of social justice dignified by a particular society. The dynamics of compassion and suffering suggest that human flourishing for, by, and about one and all is limited (reduced) and that the common good as unleashed potential and harnessed possibility is denied (repressed). These conditions of self-society captivity are sustained often unwittingly through self-other risk management dispositions. Maintaining this state of affairs engenders a society of captives, and it assures totalizing confinement for the kept as well as their keepers, regulators, and watchers. Indeed, under these destructive and pathological circumstances, individual and collective consciousness is bound and checked; latent potential and untapped possibility are rendered unimaginable, inexpressible, and uninhabitable.

As a radical philosophical perspective and as an emergent form of cultural criticism, psychological jurisprudence diagnosis the forces that nurture social disease and that thwart human social capital. These forces are existential, corporeal, material, and cosmopolitan in essential composition. This chapter outlines PJ's Aristotelian-based theory, method, and praxis, and fits these insights to the dynamics of compassion and suffering. At issue are the intrapersonal landscapes and interpersonal contexts that adjudicate the character (i.e., the flourishing or excellence) of social justice, and the forces that await recognition in order overcome and transform the harms of this governance, the injustice of this domestication. As the chapter posits, these prophetic matters constitute an ethical and jurisprudential framework for developing a psychology of social justice.

NOTE

1. As with several of our collaborations, this chapter represents an integration of ideas based on insights that the two of us developed independent of one another. For additional commentary on the relationship between compassion and suffering, see, Williams, C. R. (2008). Compassion, suffering, and the self: A moral psychology of social justice.

Current Sociology, 56(1), 5–24. For additional commentary on psychological jurisprudence, see, Arrigo, B. A. (2013). Recognizing and transforming madness, citizenship, and social justice: Toward the revolution in risk management and the overcoming of captivity. *International Journal of Offender Therapy and Comparative Criminology, 57(6):* 712–719.

REFERENCES

Anderson, K. (2002). Richard Quinney's journey: The Marxist dimension. *Crime and Delinquency, 48* (2), 232–242.

Aristotle. (1976). *Ethics* (J. A. K. Thomson, Trans.). New York, NY: Penguin.

Aristotle. (2004). *Rhetoric* (W. Rhys Roberts, Trans.). New York, NY: Dove.

Arrigo, B. A. (Ed). (2004). *Psychological jurisprudence: Critical explorations in law, crime, and society.* Albany, NY: SUNY Press.

Arrigo, B. A. (2010). De/reconstructing critical psychological jurisprudence: Strategies of resistance and struggles for justice. *International Journal of Law in Context, 6*(4), 363–396.

Arrigo, B. A. (2011a). Madness, citizenship, and social justice: On the ethics of the shadow and the ultramodern. *Law and Literature, 23*(3), 404–441.

Arrigo, B. A. (2011b). Guest editorial: Forensic psychiatry and clinical criminology: On risk, captivity, and harm. *International Journal of Offender Therapy and Comparative Criminology, 55*(3), 347–349.

Arrigo, B. A. (2012). The ultramodern condition: On the phenomenology of the shadow as transgression. *Human Studies: A Journal for Philosophy and the Social Sciences, 35*(3), 429–445.

Arrigo, B. A. (in press). Managing risk and marginalizing identities: On the society of captives thesis and the harm of social dis-ease. *International Journal of Offender Therapy and Comparative Criminology.*

Arrigo, B. A., Bersot, H. Y., & Sellers, B. G. (2011). *The ethics of total confinement: A critique of madness, citizenship, and social justice.* New York, NY: Oxford University Press.

Arrigo, B. A., & Milovanovic, D. (2009). *Revolution in penology: Rethinking the society of captives.* New York, NY: Rowman and Littlefield.

Bakhtin, M. (1982). *The dialogic imagination: Four essays.* Austin: University of Texas Press.

Blum, L. (1980). Compassion. In A. O. Rorty (Ed.), *Explaining emotions* (pp. 507–518). Berkeley: University of California Press.

Deleuze, G. (1983). *Nietzsche and philosophy.* New York, NY: Columbia University Press.

Deleuze, G., & Guattari. F. (1987). *A thousand plateaus.* Minneapolis: University of Minnesota Press.

Fesmire, S. (1997). The social basis of character: An ecological humanist approach. In H. Lafollette (Ed.), *Ethics in practice: An anthology* (pp. 282–292). New York, NY: Blackwell Press.

Foucault, M. (1998). *The essential works of Foucault: Aesthetics, method, and epistemology* (Vol. 2). J. D. Faubion (Ed.). New York, NY: The New York Press.

Hughes, G. (2001). *Aristotle on ethics.* New York, NY: Routledge.

Kurtz, P. (1969). What is humanism. In P. Kurtz (Ed.), *Moral problems in contemporary society: Essays in humanistic ethics.* Englewood Cliffs, NJ: Prentice Hall.

Lacan, J. (1977). *Ecrits: A selection*. New York, NY: W. W. Norton.

Lacan, J. (1981). *The four fundamental concepts of psychoanalysis*. New York, NY: W. W. Norton.

Marx, K. 1964. *The economic and philosophical manuscripts of 1844*. New York, NY: International.

Nietzsche, F. (1968). *The will to power* (W. Kaufmann, Ed.). New York, NY: Vintage Books.

Nussbaum, M. (2001). *Upheavals of thought: The intelligence of emotions*. New York, NY: Cambridge University Press.

Quinney, R. (1991). The way of peace: On crime, suffering, and service. In R. Quinney & H. Pepinsky (Eds.) *Criminology as peacemaking*. Bloomington: Indiana University Press.

Ridley, M. (1996). *The origins of virtue: Human instincts and the evolution of cooperation*. New York, NY: Penguin.

Sartre, J. P. (1956). *Being and nothingness: An essay on phenomenological ontology*. New York, NY: Philosophical Library Press.

Seneca. (2009). *Dialogues and essays* (J. Davie, Trans.). New York, NY: Oxford University Press.

Taylor. R. (2000). *Good and evil*. Amherst, NY: Prometheus.

Thoreau, H. D. (2012). *Walden*. New York, NY: Empire Books.

Williams, C. & Arrigo, B. (2004). *Theory, justice, and social change: Theoretical integrations and critical applications*. New York, NY: Kluwer/Plenum.

Wozniak, J. (2000). The voices of peacemaking criminology: Insights into a perspective with an eye toward teaching. *Contemporary Justice Review, 3*(3), 267–289.

Chapter 10

Neuroscience and Psychology: Central Issues for Social Justice Leaders

Carlos P. Zalaquett and Allen E. Ivey

> Our interaction with clients changes their brain (and ours). In a not too distant future, counseling will be regarded as ideal for nurturing nature.
>
> —Óscar Gonçalves

Current neuroscience research on the brain has reached a state of precision wherein it now has immediate process and outcome implications for social justice action, whether individual, group, or community. The purpose of this chapter is to discuss key neuroscience and psychotherapy findings regarding mind, body, and environmental interactions and their relevancy for social justice leaders. The final section of this chapter offers suggestions as to how graduate students, practitioners, faculty, and policymakers can use neuroscience findings to advance a more just society.

WHY ARE NEUROSCIENCE AND COGNITIVE SCIENCE RELEVANT TO PSYCHOLOGY AND COUNSELING?

Neuroscience discoveries provide critical support for a new integration of research, prevention, and treatment. Continuing innovations and advances in positron emission tomography (PET) scans, functional magnetic resonance imaging (fMRI), and other methods such as a modern use of EEG equipment have opened up a new world and a paradigm shift for counseling and psychology. Neuroscientists can now measure changes in areas of the brain that light up or fire during normal conversation or individual counseling. Especially important for social justice advocates, developmental research reveals that social conditions such as trauma, poverty, abuse, and harassment measurably harm the formation of the brain. Using neuroimaging, it is now possible to track measurable functional and structural changes in people's brains resulting from developmental, environmental conditions and social interactions.

This progress in imaging techniques demonstrates that traditional dualism and separation between physical and mental health no longer exists. The body cannot be separated from the mind (Ivey & Zalaquett, 2011). This research also demonstrates the influential effect of environment and culture on individuals and groups (Likhtik, Popa, Apergis-Schoute, Fidacaro, & Paré, 2008; Lipina & Colombo, 2009). In addition, it reveals the critical effect of behavioral, cognitive, and interpersonal therapy on the brain (Grawe, 2007) and strongly supports the emphasis on listening, empathic understanding, and strength building. Conceptualizing the interview through microskill theory and practice reveals the central importance of the attention and attending behavior in the brain and how skills such as reflection of feeling become even more significant in emotional regulation (Ivey, Ivey, & Zalaquett, 2010).

Physicians have become increasingly aware that what happens in the body is deeply influenced by the mind. They report that 80% of medical issues involve the brain and stress, as stressful events leave a marked imprint on the brain (Ratey, 2008, 2011). Although some degree of stress is needed for learning and for physical growth, excessive stress can impair performance and produce neuronal damage. At the same time, the "stress cascade" can overwhelm clients and lead to serious psychiatric disorders such as depression and schizophrenia, including measureable DNA and brain changes (Corcoran et al., 2003; Drevets, Savitz, & Trimble, 2008).

The vast majority of work in counseling and psychotherapy includes stress as an underlying issue, and resolving stressors is critical in many styles of treatment. Neuroscience evidence demonstrates that stress management and lifestyle changes are necessary and effective routes toward both mental and physical health. Furthermore, stress management becomes central regardless of the psychological or medical model or chosen theoretical approach.

Neuroscience's findings on the brain also bring a more complete awareness of how environment and culture shape the individual. The neuroscientific evidence demonstrates that human beings are a unique social species with highly developed cultures and social institutions (Gazzaniga, 2008). Cacioppo, Bernstern, and Decety (2010) remarked that "our biology has helped shape the social environments we have created, and our social environment has helped shape our genes, brains, and bodies" (p. 676). Consider the impact of lifelong stressors on the developing child, which could range from inadequate nutrition to abuse to continuing urban environmental trauma.

HOW ARE NEUROSCIENCE AND COGNITIVE SCIENCE BRIDGING BIOLOGY AND MEDICINE WITH PSYCHOLOGY AND COUNSELING?

Neuroscience and cognitive science bridge biological and psychological approaches in several ways (see Grawe, 2007; Ratey, 2001, 2008). First, *neurogenesis*, the capacity of the brain to produce new neurons, advanced knowledge of brain development and complemented known information regarding its functional changes (e.g., establishing new neuronal connections or strengthening existing connections). Second, interaction with others changes the brain through the development of new neural networks. This is an example of *brain plasticity*. Throughout people's lives, millions of neurons, synapses, and neural connections are added and lost. Effective counseling and therapy helps develop new, useful neural pathways in the brain. Both psychotherapist and client's brain functioning can be measured through a variety of brain-imaging techniques, especially fMRI (Arehart-Treichel, 2001). Third, neuroscience research suggests most of psychology and counseling's theory and practice is on target. It also provides a clearer understanding of why what psychologists do works. Moreover, it provides ideas for improving work with clients, groups, and societies. And, surprisingly, it demonstrates that wellness, social justice, and context and environmentally based orientations are essential. Fourth, without a meaningful and effective environment, human beings cannot grow and change. In counseling and psychotherapy, this means that healing relationships are all the more important. Counseling and psychotherapy builds new brain networks that can assist in improving clients' mental health and well-being. Social justice complements the clinical relationship by attenuating conditions and actions that prevent or destroy the building of new brain networks that, in contrast, can be deleterious to clients' mental health and well-being. Fifth, poverty and stress are two key areas impacting brain development and functioning. Both are reviewed later in this chapter, followed by implications for social justice leaders.

Cacioppo and Decety (2009) stated that "psychological science in the 21st century can and should become not only the science of overt behavior, not only the science of the mind, but the science of brain function" (p. 12). They pointed out that major changes in psychology curriculum and practice will be necessary in this new world; furthermore, they suggested an integrated framework of research (Cacioppo & Decety, 2011). Not only has neuroscience demonstrated the need for updating psychology if it is to remain relevant, but it also suggests the need to update the field of social justice.

BASIC NEUROSCIENCE'S CONCEPTS RELEVANT FOR COUNSELING, PSYCHOLOGY, AND SOCIAL JUSTICE

The following neuroscience concepts represent central aspects of brain development and functioning. Each one of these can be harmed by stress and trauma, including the many aspects of oppression as defined by social justice advocates.

Neuroplasticity

The brain can change—it is not fixed and it responds to external environmental events and to actions initiated by the individual. The traditional assumption that brain anatomy and neurophysiology does not change is wrong. Throughout the lifespan new connections and new neural networks are developed. Regardless of age, genetic background, or life experience, change happens. As Schwartz and Begley (2003) noted, "Neuroplasticity can result in the wholesale remodeling of neural networks . . . a brain can rewire itself" (p. 13). Effective counseling not only changes minds, it changes brains as well—including those of helping practitioners. This area of study, known as *psychodynamic neurobiology*, focuses on the neural changes in both clinician and client and has become a recent focus in both clinical psychology pedagogy and clinical practice (Divine & Moore, 2010). New knowledge regarding the activation of neural networks as well as potential changes in neural structure within the clinical context further underscores what is known about processes of attachment, transference, and countertransference in the clinical relationship (see, e.g., Emotional Contagion; Hatfield, Cacioppo, & Rapson, 1994). Divino and Moore (2010) reflected on recent findings with regard to subtle neural and affective changes in the therapeutic context as follows:

> A combined focus on the content of a session, the patient's affect, the therapist's own affect, and any memories that may be kindled by the evoked affect is likely to reveal nonconscious aspects of the patient's communication. The neural circuits that are activated in the brain of the therapist may be linked to the therapist's own experiences that resonate with the experience the patient is trying to relay. (p. 342)

Neurogenesis

Counseling and psychotherapy can also support the building of new neurons (Ratey, 2001). One of the most startling findings is that completely new neurons can be generated in the learning process, even in older adults. The idea that the brain only deteriorates in later life has been proven wrong and there are many areas of the brain where neurogenesis occurs. Humans develop new neural networks throughout the lifespan in response to new situations and experiences in the environment. Exercise is particularly important as a lifetime process to ensure brain and physical health. Exercise increases blood flow and the release of positive neurotransmitters such as serotonin, and needs to be part of a psychotherapy treatment regime. Serotonin release is particularly helpful in mitigating depression and is released during exercise. If clients are sad—they should walk or run. If they cannot run, they should meditate and use relaxation training. Not only do clients feel better, their brains expand.

The Importance of Attention and Focus

Basic concepts of attention and attending behaviors are measurable through brain imaging and, of course, are required for the learning process that is counseling. When client and counselor attend to the story, the brains of both participants become involved (Siegel, 2012b). Factors in attention include *arousal* and *focus*. Arousal involves the reticular activating system, at the brain's core, which transmits stimuli to the cortex and activates neurons firing throughout many areas. The executive frontal cortex can determine the direction of attention. Central to this process is the microskill of attending behavior. If the practitioner attends with energy and interest, and this is communicated effectively, one can expect clients to see their counselors as a positive resource. An excellent treatment to facilitate client focus and attention is meditation. Benson and Proctor (2010) suggest that relaxation and meditation help clients switch off or switch on gene activity associated with health and disease (p. xii).

Clarifying the Understanding of Emotions

Brain imaging reveals that specific emotions fire neural activity in different parts of the brain (Davidson, 2000). The prefrontal cortex is a regulator of emotions, but can be overwhelmed by the limbic system in times of severe stress. The limbic systems' amygdala is the major seat of negative emotions such as sadness, anger, and fear, but it also energizes the process of learning and absorbing new input and memories in the hippocampus. Coupled with the hypothalamus, the pituitary and adrenal glands (the HPA axis), the amygdala activates behaviors to cope with external stress and danger (Ratey, 2008; Siegel, 2012a).

Many areas of the brain are activated by positive emotions. For example, positive emotions have been shown to influence executive functioning within the prefrontal cortex—a process that can facilitate an individual's cognitive performance on creative fluency tasks as well as his or her ability to switch from one task to something more novel; however, positive emotion has also been found to impair certain types of executive functioning such as planning and switching from one task to another task that includes previously encountered stimuli (Mitchell & Phillips, 2007). It is important to note the complexity of this process and that sufficient external sensory stimuli are needed both to stimulate positive and negative emotion and to observe the interplay between emotion and executive functioning occurring within the prefrontal cortex. Centrally, however, the TAP (i.e., thalamus, anterior cingulate cortex, and prefrontal cortex) stimulates the production of positive emotion from within. In this process, the nucleus accumbens sends out making it possible to focus on the positive.

Emotional expression is also important as it can affect others even without their awareness (Carter, 1999). It is possible to pick up the depressed mood and style of others and recommunicate this sadness back to others, thus reinforcing a cycle of negativity. Listening with energy and interest, and communicating this effectively, may help others receive that affect as a positive resource in itself. Active listening is a key aspect in developing positive relationships. As Carter (1999) explained:

> Expressions can . . . transmit emotions to others—the sight of a person showing intense disgust turns on in the observer's brain areas that are associated with the feeling of disgust. Similarly, if you smile, the world does indeed smile with you (up to a point). Experiments in which tiny sensors were attached to the "smile" muscles of people looking at faces show the sight of another person smiling triggers automatic mimicry—albeit so slight that it may not be visible. . . . [T]he brain concludes that something good is happening out there and creates a feeling of pleasure. (p. 87)

Focusing on Wellness and the Positives

Talking about strengths and resources impacts the brain in useful ways. For example, the neurotransmitter, dopamine, is released when situations are pleasant and positive, preparing the brain for new learning and the development of new neural networks. New learning will not occur unless the amygdala has enough stimuli so that it energizes the brain for opening to new information and ideas. At the same time, the amygdala is a basic seat of negative emotion—and certain types of stimuli will work against learning and change. Extreme external stimulation (war, rape, home break-in) can prompt too much stimulation, literally blowing the "fuse," and resulting in loss of neural connections.

Counselors and psychotherapists who focus primarily on negative issues and problems build a self-reinforcing circularity between the demons of the amygdala and the frontal cortex. The result is negative thinking, accompanied by negative feeling, and characteristics of depression. Pessimism feeds on itself. However, there is clear research evidence that an effective executive frontal cortex focusing on positives and strengths can overcome the negative (see Ratey, 2008; Siegel, 2012a). Appropriate medication (e.g., Lexapro, Wellbutrin) can enhance positive thinking through increasing the supply of serotonin. Ellis and Beck's cognitive behavioral therapy can do the same thing. Thus, counselors should accentuate the positive, and keep in mind that wellness activities such as exercise, positive reframing of old stories, interpersonal relationships, meditation, and leisure all facilitate the client's ability to control and modify negative thinking and feeling.

Empathy and Mirror Neurons

Empathy is not just an abstract idea; empathy is identifiable and measurable in the physical brain. Research on brain activity validates what the helping field has been saying for years (see Iacoboni, 2008). Decety and Jackson (2004) commented that "the basic building blocks [of empathy] are hardwired into the brain and await development through interaction with others. . . . empathy [is] an intentional capacity" (pp. 71, 93). Mirror neurons are neurons that fire when people behave, think, or feel and they also fire when they see others behave, think, or feel. Mirror neurons enable people to sense and understand what the client is saying and feeling. These neurons fire and even affect internal bodily responses when counselors truly empathically experience the world of the client. This is a natural talent that psychologists can encourage and develop by increasing their awareness of the client and noting what happens inside their own bodies (Siegel, 2012b).

In addition, psychotherapists awaken the mirror neurons in the client and facilitate their development of new connections in thoughts, feelings, and action. This awakening shows in verbal behavior of clients and the action that they take as a result of the interview. And, as the clients process their issues, new neural connections are born. Empathic behavior and the relationship are central to change. The empathic person's brain responds to another person's experience, even though he or she does not actually experience that person's world. Many studies over the years back up this central point (see Iacoboni, 2008). For example, children around their second year indicate concern for others cognitively, emotionally, and behaviorally by comprehending others' difficulties and trying to help. Consider two young children playing together. One falls and starts crying. Even though the second child has not been hurt, he or she also cries. This ability to observe the feelings of others could be considered the developmental roots of empathic understanding.

Decety and Jackson (2006) point out that the antisocial, criminal personality has reduced the ability to appreciate the emotions of others. There is less firing of mirror neurons in the prefrontal cortex, and this deficit also appears to be a dysfunction of the energizing amygdala and hippocampus (long-term memory). This breakthrough work with children diagnosed with conduct disorder again reveals less activity in mirror neuron areas of the brain. Susan Fiske (2007) presented another important finding. She investigated automatic prejudicial responses to the poor using MRI technology. She discovered that these responses go beyond prejudice as many individuals do not see the poor as humans. Research participants shown the photograph of a homeless man demonstrated brain activation patterns in areas that are "reliably implicated in disgust toward nonhuman objects such as garbage, mutilation, and human waste" (p. 157). Areas consistently associated with the perception of human beings failed to light up, "as if people had stumbled on a pile of garbage" (p. 157). It is possible that training in empathy and in microskills may increase the effectiveness of our mirror neurons and diminish responses.

HOW AND WHY ARE NEUROSCIENCE, COUNSELING, AND PSYCHOLOGY RELEVANT TO MULTICULTURAL AND SOCIAL JUSTICE LEADERS?

Key social justice issues such as poverty, abuse, bullying, racism, sexism, heterosexism, and discrimination against persons with disabilities, and other forms of oppression are all stressful. Stressful events can curtail normal brain development in newborns and youngsters and negatively affect brain neurogenesis and plasticity in adults and older adults; chronic stress leads to elevated levels of cortisol in the body, which can negatively impact neuronal networks "and even change the architecture of regions in the brain that are essential for learning and memory" (National Science Council on the Developing Child, 2011, p. 3). Thus, these social justice issues are detrimental to the psychological, physical, and social well-being of individuals. Two of these critical social justice issues, stress and poverty, are discussed next to illustrate the importance of advances in neuroscience and psychology for social justice leadership and the pursuit of a more just society.

Modern life is a stressful life as demonstrated by the high incidence of stress symptomatology observed across medical consultations. Stressful life conditions and events are observed in many societies worldwide. A moderate amount of stress, if not prolonged or too intense, is required for development and for physical health. Intense and long-term stress is damaging. Stressful experiences lead to dysfunctions of the prefrontal cortex, including critical areas regulating judgment, planning, decision making, moral reasoning, and sense of self. The subcortical arousal system bypasses the frontal lobe's executive functioning to prompt one's stress response. Out of this results a wide variety of so-called disorders, which are really a result of an often insane, oppressive environment. Discrimination shows in both the mind and body. Stressful experiences disengage the frontal lobes, which, over time, can lead to impulsivity, short-sightedness, aggressive behavior, increased anxiety, depression, alcohol and drug abuse, learning disorders, and stress-related diseases (National Science Council on the Developing Child, 2011). As Arán-Filippetti and De Minzi (2012) noted:

> it is feasible to hypothesize that these regions [the PFC] might be sensitive to childhood experience and SES. Supporting this hypothesis, Kishiyama et al. (2009) found that disparities affects PFC function in low SES children and this relationship could be explained by the influence of multiple factors associated with low-SES nurturing conditions, such as reduced access to cognitively stimulating materials and experiences and higher levels of stress. (pp. 406–407)

At the same time, stress is necessary for learning. People need mental and physical challenges to grow. Thus, psychotherapists should not necessarily aim for a totally neutral, peaceful environment, except as a rest period (for therapists and clients). During stress, glucocorticoids are released, which provide short-term pleasure; but long-term continued stress can result in damage to the brain and loss of brain plasticity (National Science Council on the Developing Child, 2011). During stressful times, excessive cortisol is released into the brain, which impacts one's attention and, if a sufficient amount is released in trauma or extended stress, long-term toxicity results with the loss of neural connections such as with post-traumatic stress.

Ratey (2008) noted that "cortisol is the long-acting stress hormone that helps to mobilize fuel, cue attention and memory, and prepare the body and brain to battle challenges to equilibrium. Cortisol oversees the stockpiling of fuel, in the form of fat, for future stresses. Its action is critical for our survival. At high or unrelenting concentrations such as those observed in post-traumatic stress cortisol has a toxic effect on neurons, eroding the connections between them and breaking down muscles and nerve cells to provide an immediate fuel source" (p. 277).

The report titled "Excessive Stress Disrupts the Architecture of the Developing Brain" (National Scientific Council on the Developing Child, 2005) provides a critical account of the effect of stress in children:

1. In the uterus, the unborn child responds to stress in the mother, while alcohol, drugs, and other stimulants can be extremely damaging.
2. For the developing child neural circuits are especially plastic and amenable to growth and change, but again excessive stress results in lesser brain development and in adulthood that child is more likely to have depression, an anxiety disorder, alcoholism, cardiovascular problems, and diabetes.
3. Positive experiences in pregnancy seem to facilitate child development.
4. Caregivers are critical to the development of the healthy child.
5. Children of poverty or who have been neglected tend to have elevated cortisol levels.

The release of cortisol (the main stress hormone) affects the hippocampus and the prefrontal cortex regions of the brain, leading to impaired memory and learning, and impaired executive functioning (e.g., attending and planning; Schibli & D'angiulli, 2011).

Social justice leaders should consider the varying positive and negative environments in which individuals and groups live. Poverty provides a clear illustration of the detrimental effects of unjust conditions. The World Health Organization (2000), the World Bank (2001), and the American Psychological Association (2000) have all documented the impact of environmental and social conditions on those who are poor. Their conclusion is that poverty is detrimental to the well-being of societies and individuals. Furthermore, the greater the income gap between the poorest and the wealthiest in a society, the higher the death rates for infants and adults and the lower the life expectancy for all members of that society, regardless of socioeconomic status.

Poverty and challenges such as racism and oppression negatively affect the brain. Incidents of racism result in the brain being hypervigilant, thus producing significant stress, with accompanying hyperfunctioning of the amygdala and interference with memory and other areas of the brain. Psychologists need to be aware that many environmental issues ranging from poverty to toxic environments to a dangerous community all work against neurogenesis and the development of full potential. Paul Krugman (2008) noted the following:

> Poverty in early childhood poisons the brain. . . . [N]euroscientists have found that many children growing up in very poor families with low social status experience unhealthy levels of stress hormones, which impair their neural development. The effect is to impair language development and memory—and hence the ability to escape poverty—for the rest of the child's life. (paras. 1 & 2)

Poverty is a global issue and extreme poverty is a worldwide health problem (Dashiff, DiMicco, Myers, & Sheppard, 2009) affecting 1.29 billion people (World Bank Group, 2012). It is observed around the world with wide country variations in ratio. Six percent of children live in poverty in Denmark, Finland, Norway, and Sweden; 7–9% in Austria, the Netherlands, and Switzerland; 10–15% in the Czech Republic, Germany, Australia, Luxembourg, and the United Kingdom; 16–20% in Estonia, Ireland, Canada, and Poland; 21% in the United States, and 30–32% in Guatemala and Brazil (after post-tax-and-transfer income; Gornick & Jäntti, 2012).

Poverty rates have increased in the new millennium due to economic downturns and show few signs of improvement in the near future. Hardship touches the lives of millions of American children, placing them at an elevated risk for school failure, physical, and mental health problems, delinquency, and reduced earnings and productivity (Mistry & Wadsworth, 2011). Beyond those living in poverty, many more children live in low-income families that earn between 100% and 200% of the federal poverty threshold (2013threshold is $23,550 for a family of four). Low-income parents also face significant challenges for making ends meet and their children exhibit greater academic, behavioral, and social competence problems as compared with children from middle-income and affluent families (Huston & Bentley, 2010; Wight, Chau, & Aratani, 2011; Wight, Chau, Thampi, & Aratani, 2010).

Using UNICEF Innocenti Research Centre's relative measure of poverty, which is defined as less than 50% of the median income, the United States has the second highest rate of child poverty at 21.9% (Anthony, King, & Austin, 2011). According to Anthony et al., the statistic that one in five children live in poverty in the United States has significant implications for the well-being of future generations, especially given the estimated social and economic losses associated with children growing up in poverty. Furthermore, with more families struggling in poverty (or just above the poverty level) and public assistance rates rising, the impact of poverty on many minority children is even more profound. The environment of poverty creates numerous stressful conditions that contribute to mental health problems for children and adults, including economic strain, family conflict, exposure to violence, and frequent moves or transitions. Poor families experience these poverty-related stressors more often, simultaneously, and for longer times than families in higher socioeconomic classes (Santiago, Etter, Wadsworth, & Raviv, 2012).

Poverty is associated with substandard housing, homelessness, inadequate childcare, unsafe neighborhoods, and underresourced schools. In addition, negative environmental factors such as pollutants and contaminants, and lack of portable water have detrimental effects on mental and physical development that both perpetuate and contribute to poverty. Men and women living in poverty have higher mortality rates and present higher incidence of osteoarthritis, hypertension, cervical cancer, coronary heart disease, AIDS/HIV infection, and other chronic health conditions. As a consequence, those who are poor are sicker and are more likely to have more disabilities than their higher SES counterparts, limiting their employment options, straining their financial resources, and increasing their stress levels. Furthermore, those living in poverty are over three times as likely to be uninsured. Lack of affordable health insurance, including mental health and substance abuse coverage, impedes health and well-being.

The impact of poverty on young children and adolescents is also significant and long lasting. Exposure to biological and psychosocial stressors affects the developing brain and compromises the development of children around the world (Ramiro, Madrid, & Brown, 2010). Inequalities in child development begin prenatally and, with cumulative exposure to developmental stressors, disparities widen (Sawyer et al., 2012; Walker et al., 2011). Children who are poor are at a greater risk than higher-income children for a range of problems, including poor academic achievement, poor socioemotional functioning, developmental delays, behavioral problems, poor nutrition, and low birth weight (Walker et al., 2011). Finally, low-income groups are the targets of discrimination based on their socioeconomic status as well as other social indicators such as gender. Those from middle and upper socioeconomic levels display attitudes and stereotypes that attribute poverty to personal failings rather than to socioeconomic structures and systems; and tend to ignore the strengths and competencies of those from low socioeconomic levels. Public policy and antipoverty programs also reflect these stereotypes. Counselors, psychologists, and other professionals also present such biases (Ivey & Zalaquett, 2011).

Low-income individuals are two to five times more likely to suffer from a diagnosable mental disorder than those of the highest socioeconomic levels, and poverty poses a significant obstacle to getting help for these mental health problems. Malnutrition is linked to poor brain development resulting in cognitive deficits and lower IQ; iron deficiency specifically is associated with a number of negative cognitive and motor development problems that can have long-lasting effects. In school-aged children, studies have shown that insufficient food can cause difficulties in the ability to concentrate and focus on academic tasks (Anthony et al., 2011; Fiese & Jones, 2012).

Not all children living in poverty will suffer negative outcomes. Poverty is not a neurological condition that can be directly mapped onto genetic makeup. Nonetheless, it is clear that the effects of poverty on children's brains are brought about by the environmental living situations (Schibli & D'angiulli, 2011). Research has documented both the negative influence of poverty on cognitive ability as measured by IQ tests and school achievement and the potential environmental and psychological factors explaining such differences; however, researchers are now reaching an understanding of the specific neurocognitive effects of poverty. Poverty and stress effects are disproportionate for certain neurocognitive systems, including language and executive functions (Hackman & Farah, 2009; Hackman, Farah, & Meaney, 2010; Rhoades, Greenberg, Lanza, & Blair, 2011), and brain lateralization (Boles, 2012) and flexibility (Clearfield & Niman, 2012) among children.

Worldwide poverty has detrimental effects on brain development, cognitive abilities, self-regulation, socioemotional functioning, and prosocial behaviors (Bandy & Ottoni-Wilhelm, 2012; Clearfield & Niman, 2012; Evans & Rosenbaum, 2008). Working and spatial memory, executive functioning, sensory memory, visuospatial skills, and phonological skills are among those negatively affected. Socially advantaged children exhibit superior executive attention processing and cognitive control via language compared with their low SES peers (Arán-Filippeti & De Minzi, 2012). Also, traumatic stress resulting from child mistreatment experienced in impoverished households is related to hippocampal alterations.

On the other hand, neuroscience and psychosocial research shows that by reducing the threats of biological and psychosocial stressors and risks and providing a caregiving environment that supports physical, cognitive, and socioemotional development, children can experience healthy brain development that enables them to achieve their developmental potential (Walker et al., 2011). With this strong foundation, they build lifespan developmental trajectories that enable them to benefit from, and contribute to family, community, education, and society and world.

Hackman and colleagues provided varied examples of studies demonstrating effective practices leading to improved cognitive and verbal abilities in poor children. One study reported improved language function in poor children whose families received additional income and education. Other studies identified interventions that promoted the development of specific neurocognitive systems using computerized games that train executive abilities. Diamond, Barnett, Thomas, and Munro (2007) reported that Tools of the Mind, a program that assists poor children practice in thinking aloud, planning pretend games, and other activities involving executive function, developed dramatically improved executive functions performance.

In sum, stress and poverty are detrimental to the physical, psychological, and social health of individuals; they represent but just a sample of the issues social justice leaders need to be aware of, knowledgeable about it, skilled in solving, and capable of taking action. On the other hand, effective interventions to promote early child development in low-income and middle-income countries exist either at scale or are potentially scalable. Interventions to reduce risks and support early child development will yield lifetime gains that contribute to the achievement and sustainability of improved development of next generations. By investing in early child development programs, communities have an opportunity to break the cycle of inequalities that has dominated the lives of millions of children and families in low-income and middle-income communities and countries.

By combining the framework of neuroscience, psychology, and social justice, psychologists have the potential to broaden our understanding of current societal problems more effectively. The more we reach such understanding, the more rationally psychologists can design programs for prevention and remediation. This is more important today because current data indicate that the normal human brain is considerably more flexible in its organization and function than is reflected in the neuroscience literature. For the social justice leaders the understanding of neuroscience advances, brain development and plasticity, and the mind/body and individual/context/culture interactions and interdependence is central for effective planning and action. This further advances the centrality of neuroscience for psychology and social justice leaders.

SOCIAL JUSTICE ACTIONS BASED ON OUR KNOWLEDGE AND NEW INFORMATION FROM NEUROSCIENCE

The following are suggested actions based on the succinct information presented in this chapter and framed within the ecological model proposed by Bronfenbrenner (1979). We suggest social justice leaders apply the bio-ecological model to guide interventions at the micro-, meso-, exo-, macro-, and chrono-systems level.

Learn about Neuroscience Findings and Research

Neuroscience research provides a biological foundation for understanding the impact of psychological and social justice work. The very act of counseling and therapy produces changes in client memory (as well as the therapists'). Therapists should note how new ideas and learning are being constructed in their interactions with clients, groups, and organizations. They should consider continued study and learn about brain structures and functions, as new findings may provide further support for their work and suggest specific guidelines for practice and social justice interventions.

Brain research is not in opposition to the cognitive, emotional, behavioral, and meaning emphasis of counseling and therapy. Rather, it will help psychology pinpoint types of interventions that are most helpful for clients. In fact, one of the clearest findings is that the brain needs environmental stimulation to grow and develop. Therapists need to offer a healthy atmosphere for client growth and development. Thus, we advocate for the integration of counseling, psychotherapy, neuroscience, molecular biology, and neuroimaging, and the infusion of knowledge from such integrated fields of study to practice, training, and research. We believe that each psychologist committed to social justice has the responsibility to start studying neuroscience and related fields. This will be time-consuming, but it is necessary to be ready for the next decade.

Educating Colleagues and Students

Not only do psychologists have a responsibility to learn neuroscientific findings, they also need to teach this information to others. Psychology and counseling programs have integrated social justice into their curriculums to varying degrees (Lewis, 2011; Toporek & Vaughn, 2010). Now is the time to integrate neuroscientific concepts into academic settings and course contents and publications related to social justice. Training effective change agents entails fostering their skills and knowledge in this area. Infusing neuroscience into mission statements and academic and professional foci, providing students with current neuroscientific findings, and helping them develop a firm grip of such information is critical. Psychologists should create curricula to teach students how this knowledge informs theories and practices and train them to apply neuroscience at multiple levels, teaching individual skills and more advanced competencies emphasizing social and institutional change as well as policymaking.

As Lipina and Colombo (2009) remind psychologists, there is also an ethical obligation to disseminate neuroscientific research findings and to dispel myths regarding brain development. Myths suggesting that rapid synapse formation only occurs during the first three years of life and that neurons cannot be produced after childhood have had a detrimental effect on the sciences, education programs, and public policies. As importantly, an effort should be made to educate others about healthy brain development.

Psychologists' Responsibility Does Not End with Individual Therapy

Oppression brings psychologists many clients—war, rape, abuse, poverty, racism, sexism—all forms of discrimination affect mental health. The family, groups, community, nation, and world can benefit from neuroscientific and psychological knowledge. Social justice leaders and psychologists have a responsibility to both inform clients about how oppression impacts their problems and act in society to promote change. They also need to use their expertise to influence governing and regulatory bodies.

Early Interventions

Worldwide, children and adolescents are disproportionately represented among the poor. Chronic exposure to poverty increases adolescents' risk for depression, substance use, early sexual debut, and criminal activity. The most effective and cost-efficient time to prevent inequalities is early in life before trajectories have been firmly established. Action or lack of action will have lifetime consequences for adult functioning, for the care of the next generation, and for the well-being of societies. Society should invest in interventions for early child development because this is the most cost-effective period in the human lifespan to intervene. Events starting from fetal development influence child's behavior, learning ability, and productivity throughout the course of their lives, including adulthood and later years. Fortunately, there are known effective strategies to reduce stress, poverty, and other risks factors and increase brain development, executive functions, wellness, schooling, and productivity. Comprehensive interventions have the capacity to be sustainable because parents and families may carry these changes over to subsequent children, and the children may carry this progress onto following generations.

Programs That Work

There is a strong evidence base for effective interventions from early childhood to very old adulthood. Current neuroscientific findings suggest that the brain continues to grow well into older adulthood. Many programs have demonstrated efficacy in improving the developing brain of children who develop under very stressful conditions, and in preventing declines promoted by aging. Intervention programs increase academic achievement in disadvantaged populations and salient factors in successful intervention programs within and across age groups have been identified. Furthermore, research suggests that interventions promoting reading proficiency may foster neuronal plasticity.

Research and Feedback

Research is currently available that supports psychologists' and social justice leaders' professional endeavors and provides relevant knowledge for practice (e.g., Grawe, 2007; Ivey & Zalaquett, 2011; Lipina & Columbo, 2009). Despite this significant progress, much research is needed to determine the effects of many neuroscientific contributions. Furthermore, there is a need for reliable measures across countries to properly evaluate intervention designs and analyses. Thus, it is important to participate in multidisciplinary teams to ensure a coordinated and appropriate delivery of services and advocacy for economic resources to support these services. Programs and practitioners may engage in or collaborate in the development of such measures and in research projects using fMRI and other neuroscientific tools to assess the outcomes of their interventions. The results of such research can be used as feedback to improve and advance practices and policies.

Inequalities

Reducing inequalities requires early-integrated interventions that target the many risks to which children in a particular setting are exposed. Studies done in many developed countries suggest that as income increases, the proportion of families reporting poor health declines. The decline in health by income becomes steeper as children age, suggesting the cumulative effect of poverty. Stress from inequalities negatively impacts brain development and wellness. Thus, it is imperative for psychologists to advocate for and act on behalf of social justice. Neuroscience clearly points out that environmental contingencies can harm human development, and helping professionals should incorporate this information into their daily professional activities. Social justice leaders and psychologists need to remain active participants in the provision of mental health services to adolescents in poverty and advocate increasingly for the creation of policy changes that address the mental health needs of this population.

Stigmatization

Those affected by stress, unjust conditions, and threats are frequently stigmatized. The stigma associated with poverty, for example, places children and adolescents at risk for bullying and isolation. Society should change its views of these children's learning styles as deficits and recognize that they are simply differences in approach—an environmental and neurological adaptation that, under certain conditions, allows these children to cope with challenging and environmental stressors. Neuroscience research suggests that people should avoid pity and embrace empathy, as pity leads teachers to hold lowered expectations for their students, resulting in self-fulfilling prophecies of failure. In contrast, empathy leads to an understanding of challenges as differences and demonstrates respect for students with alternative learning styles—in lieu of stigmatization. Society should not lower its expectations of poor children's achievement and behavior or view their learning styles as deficits. Evidence suggests that with appropriate level of social, cognitive, and environmental stimulation and the support of their families and schools, these children can perform at the same level as their higher SES peers. Furthermore, providing culturally sensitive and socially appropriate care and education can reduce the stigmatization of children and adolescents who live in poverty.

Access

Research has identified numerous economic barriers that limit access to mental health services: barriers to evidence-based practice prevent the use of effective treatments; critical mental health provider shortages limit available services; and the inappropriate allocation of limited resources often leads to an uncoordinated provision of multiagency services. Psychologists and social justice leaders should continue offering effective multidisciplinary and comprehensive frameworks (e.g., those affecting individual's micro-, meso-, and exo-systems) to those affected by stress and unjust conditions of living, especially children. In addition, they should promote programs that connect those in need with relevant resources. For example, they might find (and refer parents to) free or low-cost programs for children in the local community that stimulate learning as well as encourage parents to communicate with their child's school and teachers. Likewise, they should encourage parents to enroll their children in nutrition supplemental programs such as Women, Infants, and Children (WIC) and free or reduced school lunch programs, as needed.

Stress Management, Wellness, and Life Changes

Given the ubiquitous nature of stress and stress conditions, psychologists should make stress management an intervention of choice. Counseling and psychotherapy are clearly moving to more of a health and wellness orientation. Along with this comes the need to help clients make informed and wise decisions about taking care of themselves and their loved ones. For psychologists, this means increasing clients' awareness of stress management techniques, enabling them to make good use of therapeutic lifestyle changes, and educating them on recent neuroscience findings with regards to methods of stress reduction and the benefits of exercise and wellness plans.

Innovate

Psychologists should also develop or seek out innovative services, such as outreach teams, to increase access to mental health services for rural adolescents who live in poverty. Promising methods for addressing some of the cognitive effects of stress, poverty, and other threats focus on the training of basic cognitive skills, in some cases using fMRI and other neuroscience derived techniques to assess efficacy. We hope social justice leaders, clinicians, and educators will be inspired to consider the applicability of cognitive neuroscience to real-world problems and begin to guide the development of novel prevention and intervention models and strategies.

The Challenge

Psychologists and social justice leaders must apply the information learned to themselves and others. Exercise, meditation, social relationships, and a general wellness orientation for social justice and psychology are essential. How effective are psychologists at stress management? Moving beyond the personal, clients who experience social injustice need exactly the same orientation toward wellness as the professionals who advocate on their behalf. Another key application of recent neuroscience findings to clinical and social justice practice is the necessary awareness that oppression of all types, whether abuse, economic, racial, or otherwise, injures people and, if sustained, can be detrimental to their long-term mental and physical well-being.

In addition, social justice leaders need to remain active advocates and participants in the creation of policy changes that include neuroscientific knowledge to address societal problems. Furthermore, they should use advocacy as a tool to increase policymakers' awareness of how the combination of psychology, neuroscience, social justice, and other disciplines, reveals the ways in which unjust conditions and inadequate access to resources affects the central nervous systems of the world's most vulnerable individuals. We hope that social justice leaders will use this multidisciplinary approach to determine potential improvements to public policy as well as effective solutions to current social problems with the view of promoting a more just world.

REFERENCES

American Psychological Association. (2000). *Resolution on poverty and socioeconomic status*. Retrieved from http://www.apa.org/pi/urban/povres.html

Anthony, A. K., King, B., & Austin, M. J. (2011). Reducing child poverty by promoting child well-being: Identifying best practices in a time of great need. *Children and Youth Services Review, 33,* 1999–2009.

Arán-Filippetti, V., & De Minzi, M. C. R. (2012). A structural analysis of executive functions and socioeconomic status in school-age children: Cognitive factors as mediators. *The Journal of Genetic Psychology, 173*(4), 393–416.

Arehart-Treichel, J. (2001). Evidence is in: Psychotherapy changes the brain. *Psychiatric News, 36*(13), 33.

Bandy, R., & Ottoni-Wilhelm, M. (2012). Family structure and income during the stages of childhood and subsequent prosocial behavior in young adulthood, *Journal of Adolescence, 35,* 1023–1034. doi: 10.1016/j.adolescence.2012.02.010

Benson, H., & Proctor, W. (2010). *Relaxation revolution: Enhancing your personal health through the science and genetics of mind body healing.* New York, NY: Scribner.

Boles, D. B. (2011). Socioeconomic status, a forgotten variable in lateralization development. *Brain and Cognition, 76,* 52–57. doi: 10.1016/j.bandc.2011.03.002

Bronfenbrenner, U. (1979). *The ecology of human development: Experiments by nature and design.* Cambridge, MA: Harvard University Press.

Cacioppo, J. T., Berntson, G. G., & Decety, J. (2010). Social neuroscience and its relationship to social psychology. *Social Cognition, 28,* 675–685.

Cacioppo, J. T., & Decety, J. (2009). What are the brain mechanisms on which psychological processes are based? *Perspectives in Psychological Science, 4,* 10–18.

Cacioppo, J. T., & Decety, J. (2011). Social neuroscience: Challenges and opportunities in the study of complex behavior. *Annals of the New York Academy of Sciences, 1224,* 162–173. doi: 10.1111/j.1749-6632.2010.05858.x

Carter, R. (1999). *Mapping the Mind.* Berkeley, CA: University of California Press.

Clearfield, M. W., & Niman, L. C. (2012). SES affects infant cognitive flexibility. *Infant Behavior & Development, 35,* 29–35.

Corcoran, C., Walker, E., Huot, R., Mittal, V., Tessner, K., Kestler, L., & Malaspina, D. (2003). The stress cascade and schizophrenia: Etiology and onset. *Schizophrenia Bulletin, 29*(4), 671–692.

Dashiff, C., DiMicco, W., Myers, B., & Sheppard, K. (2009). Poverty and adolescent mental health. *Journal of Child and Adolescent Psychiatric Nursing, 22,* 23–32.

Davidson, R. J. (2000). Affective style, mood, and anxiety disorders: An affective neuroscience approach. In *Anxiety, Depression, and Emotion: The First Wisconsin Symposium on Emotion* (pp. 68–108). New York, NY: Oxford University Press.

Decety, J., & Jackson, P. (2004). The functional architecture of human empathy. *Behavioral and Cognitive Neuroscience Reviews, 3*(2), 71–100. Retrieved from http://home.uchicago.edu/%7Edecety/publications/Decety_CDPS06.pdf

Decety, J., & Jackson, P. L. (2006). A social-neuroscience perspective on empathy. *Journal of Association for Psychological Science, 15*(2), 54–58.

Diamond, A., Barnett, W. S., Thomas, J., & Munro, S. (2007). Preschool program improves cognitive control. *Science, 318,* 1387–1388.

Divino, C.L., Moore, M.S. (2010). Integrating neurobiological findings into psychodynamic psychotherapy training and practice. *Psychoanalytic Dialogues, 20,* 337–355.

Drevets, W. C., Savitz, J., & Trimble, M. (2008). The subgenual anterior cingulate cortex in mood disorders. *CNS Spectrum, 13*(8), 663–681.

Evans, G. W., & Rosenbaum, J. (2008). Self-regulation and the income-achievement gap. *Early Childhood Research Quarterly, 23,* 504–514.

Fiese, B. H., & Jones, B. L. (2012). Food and family: A socio-ecological perspective for child development. *Advances in Child Development and Behavior, 42,* 307–337.

Fiske, S. T. (2007). On prejudice and the brain. *Daedalus* (winter), 156–159.

Gazzaniga, M. S. (2008). *Human: The science behind what makes us unique.* New York, NY: Harper Collins Publishers.

Gornick, J. C., & Jäntti, M. (2012). Child poverty in cross-national perspective: Lessons from the Luxembourg Income Study. *Children and Youth Services Review, 34,* 558–568.

Grawe, K. (2007). *Neuropsychotherapy: How the neurosciences inform effective psychotherapy.* Mahway, NJ: Erlbaum.

Hackman, D. A., & Farah, M. J. (2009). Socioeconomic status and the developing brain. *Trends in Cognitive Sciences, 13*(2), 65–73. doi: 10.1016/j.tics.2008.11.003

Hackman, D. A., Farah, M. J. & Meaney, M. J. (2010). Socioeconomic status and the brain: Mechanistic insights from human and animal research. *Nature Reviews Neuroscience, 11,* 651–659.

Hatfield, E. Cacioppo, J. T., & Rapson, R. L. (1994). *Emotional contagion.* Cambridge, UK: Cambridge University Press.

Huston, A. C., & Bentley, A. C. (2010). Human development in societal context. *Annual Review of Psychology, 61,* 411–437.

Iacoboni, M. (2008). *Mirroring people: The new science for how we connect with others.* New York, NY: Farrar, Straus and Giroux.

Ivey A., Ivey, M., & Zalaquett, C. (2010). *Intentional interviewing and counseling: Facilitating client development in a multicultural world* (7th ed.). Belmont, CA: Brooks/Cole/Cengage.

Ivey, A. E., & Zalaquett, C. (2011). Neuroscience and Counseling. *Journal for Social Action in Counseling and Psychology, 3,* 103–116. Retrieved from www.psysr.org/jsacp/ivey-v3n1-11_103-116.pdf

Krugman, P. (2008, February 18). Poverty is poison. *New York Times.* Retrieved from http://www.nytimes.com/2008/02/18/opinion/18krugman.html

Lewis, B. L. (2011). Social justice in practicum training: Competencies and developmental implications. *Training and Education in Professional Psychology, 4,* 145–152.

Likhtik, E., Popa,D., Apergis-Schoute, J., Fidacaro, G. A., & Paré, D. (2008). Amygdala intercalated neurons are required for expression of fear extinction. *Nature, 454,* 642–645.

Lipina, S. J., & Colombo, J. A. (2009). *Poverty and brain development during childhood: An approach from cognitive psychology and neuroscience*. Washington, DC: American Psychological Association.

Mistry, R. S., & Wadsworth, M. E. (2011). Family functioning and child development in the context of poverty. *The Prevention Researcher, 18*(4), 11–15.

Mitchell, R. L. C., & Phillips, L. H. (2007). The psychological, neurochemical and functional neuroanatomical mediators of the effects of positive and negative mood on executive functions. *Neuropsychologia, 45,* 617–629.

Ramiro, L. S., Madrid, B. J., & Brown, D. W. (2010). Adverse childhood experiences (ACE) and health-risk behaviors among adults in a developing country setting. *Child Abuse & Neglect, 34,* 842–855. doi: 10.1016/j.chiabu.2010.02.012

Ratey, J. (2001). *A user's guide to the brain*. New York, NY: Vintage.

Ratey, J. (2008). *Neuroscience and the brain: Implications for counseling and therapy* (Video). Framingham, MA: Microtraining Associates.

Rhoades, B. L., Greenberg, M. T., Lanza, S. T., & Blair, C. (2011). Demographic and familial predictors of early executive function development: Contribution of a person-centered perspective. *Journal of Experimental Child Psychology, 108,* 638–662.

Santiago, C. D., Etter, E. M., Wadsworth, M. E., & Raviv, T. (2012): Predictors of responses to stress among families coping with poverty-related stress. *Anxiety, Stress & Coping: An International Journal, 25*(3), 239–258.

Sawyer, S. M., Afifi, R. A., Bearinger, L. H., Blakemore, S., Dick, B., Ezeh, A. C., & Patton, G. C. (2012). Adolescence: A foundation for future health. *Lancet, 379,* 1630–1640. doi: 10.1016/S0140-6736(12)60072-5

Schibli, K., & D'angiulli, A. (2011). The neuroscience of poverty: Implications for teaching. *Education Canada, 51*(2), 17–20. Retrieved from www.cea-ace.ca/educationcanada

Schwartz, J., & Begley, S. (2003). *The mind and the brain: Neuroplasticity and the power of mental force*. New York, NY: Regan.

Siegel, D. J. (2012a). *The developing mind, second edition: How relationships and the brain interact to shape who we are*. New York, NY: Guilford Press.

Siegel, D. J. (2012b). *Pocket guide to interpersonal neurobiology: An integrative handbook of the mind*. New York, NY: W.W. Norton & Company.

Toporek, R. L., & Vaughn, S. R. (2010). Social justice in the training of professional psychologists: Moving forward. *Training and Education in Professional Psychology, 4,* 177–182.

Walker, S. P., Wachs, T. D., Grantham-McGregor, S., Black, M. M., Nelson, C. A., Huffman, S. L., . . . Richter, L. (2011). Inequality in early childhood: Risk and protective factors for early child development. *Lancet, 378,* 1325–1338.

Wight, V. R., Chau, M., & Aratani, Y. (2011). *Who are America's poor children? The official story*. New York, NY: National Center for Children and Poverty, Columbia University.

Wight, V. R., Chau, M., Thampi, K. & Aratani, Y. (2010). *Examining the landscape of child poverty in the US today*. New York, NY: National Center for Children and Poverty, Columbia University.

World Bank. (2001). *World development report*. World Bank: Washington DC.

World Bank Group. (2012). *New estimates reveal drop in extreme poverty 2005–2010*. Retrieved from http://go.worldbank.org/4K0EJIDFA0

World Health Report. (2000). *Health systems: Improving performance*. Geneva, Switzerland: Author.

Chapter 11

Transforming Self and World: Achieving Justice through Socially Engaged Spiritual Psychology

Katherine E. Coder, Curtiss Paul DeYoung, and Harris L. Friedman

The major world religions have traditionally been concerned with social justice by dealing with humans' relationship to each other, as well as humans' possible relationship to supernatural forces, seen as manifestations of the divine or sacred. In fact, many of the world's religious traditions began as social movements aimed to build compassionate societies and to address human suffering (Armstrong, 1993, 2006; Hawken, 2007; Loy, 2003). For example, in the West, the Biblical Old Testament specifies laws presented as commandments from a supernatural being dictating how to live a just life while, in the East, the Bhagavad Gita presents guidelines through the story of a manifestation of a spiritual being giving similar advice. However, in an increasingly secularized world, religion has become separated into two components for many, namely religiosity and spirituality (Pappas & Friedman, 2004). In this context, religiosity refers to the exteriorized or institutionalized aspects of religion, such as shared rituals, beliefs, and ethics (Hill, 2000), whereas spirituality refers to the "doctrines and practices that help facilitate lived transformations of self and community toward fuller alignment with or expression of what is 'sacred'" (Rothberg, 1993, p. 105). In an increasingly secularized society, many claim to be spiritual but not religious, whereas traditionally, spirituality and religion were intertwined and did not exist apart conceptually.

Similarly, secularization has resulted in a perceived splitting of religion and spirituality from concerns about social justice (Rothberg, 2008), although some scholars have challenged this separation (Ferrer, 2008; powell, 2012). Even when devoid of traces of institutionalized religiosity, spirituality is not only concerned with the individual having isolated transcendent experiences, but can be transpersonal in the sense of going beyond or bridging (i.e., "trans") the individual (i.e., "personal") to an interconnectedness with a larger whole of which the individual is a part, including with others in a way that implies concerns about social justice (Friedman, 1983). These concerns from a spiritual vantage point often share commonalities, such as realizing a sense of interconnectedness toward all of humanity (McFarland, Brown, & Webb, 2013) and the recognition of the healing power of love (Boesak & DeYoung, 2012; powell, 2012). In fact, barriers between spirituality as solely an internalized experience and social justice as only an externalized concern crumble as many begin to realize the need for both (DeYoung, 2007; Rakoczy, 2006). In short, spirituality and social justice remain interdependent, even as religiosity and spirituality become increasingly separate (Coder, 2012). To be responsible, those concerned about spiritual psychology and social justice face profound intrapersonal and interpersonal developmental challenges that are needed to transform consciousness (powell, 2012; Vaughan, 2002). Combining both also is predicated on the mutuality of healing self and world, and on the power of actualizing human virtues and values in so doing.

For the purposes of this chapter, we explore the spiritual psychology and social justice nexus, which we approach from the perspective of what we call *socially engaged spiritual psychology*. Rothberg and Coder (2013) investigated a similar domain called transpersonal social engagement, which looked at emergent spiritual, psychological, and socially engaged phenomena. This chapter explores themes similar to those of Rothberg and Coder, and Coder (2011, 2012)[1] in her previous work. In this chapter, we define essential terms, offer a rationale for socially engaged spiritual psychology, examine its roots, and explore some of its current models and related empirical studies, as well as pose critical questions and suggest areas of future research and application. Throughout the course of this exposition, global threads of socially engaged spiritual psychology are offered.

DEFINING SPIRITUAL PSYCHOLOGY AND SOCIAL JUSTICE

Spiritual psychology is difficult to demarcate from related areas, especially as being distinct from both the psychology of religion and transpersonal psychology. There are wide variances in how religiosity and spirituality are understood and defined (Zinnbauer & Pargament, 2005). Sperry and Shafranske (2007) noted that both spirituality and psychology share a profound interest in the "fundamental perspectives on the nature of human existence" (p. 23), whereas Elkins (2007) suggested that spiritual psychology could be defined as a holistic psychological approach that describes human beings in terms of body, mind, emotions, and behavior—and that also attends to spirituality. Miovic (2004) explained that spiritual psychology includes many forms of religious expression, such as theistic psychology and Buddhist psychology, as well as more broad topics such as mind-body medicine and transpersonal psychology. Transpersonal psychology, which developed initially to explore spirituality and mystical experience, has been defined recently by Hartelius, Caplan, and Rardin (2007) as "an approach to psychology that 1) studies phenomena beyond the ego as context for 2) an integrative/holistic psychology; this provides a framework for 3) understanding and cultivating human transformation" (p. 11). Transpersonal psychology can also be seen as, among other things, an effort to present a secularized view of the interconnectedness of self with world, devoid of the supernatural connotations in the term spirituality (Friedman, 2013). Although some would argue that transpersonal psychology functions as a subset of spiritual psychology (e.g., Miovic, 2004), others see it as distinct from spiritual psychology (e.g., Pappas & Friedman, 2004). Thus, the term *spiritual psychology* overlaps with both the psychology of religion and transpersonal psychology, and retains considerable ambiguity.

Likewise, the term *social justice* contains considerable ambiguity, but it can be related to spiritual psychology. For example, powell (2012) explained that social justice "involves claiming a shared, mutual humanity" (p. xvii), which is a transpersonal notion, whereas Prilleltensky and Prilleltensky (2006) defined social justice more materially as "addressing the origins of inequality and supporting policies that distribute resources equitably" (p. 196). Edwards and Post (2008) expanded on powell's understanding by conceptualizing social justice as confronting through love "any factor that stands in the way of realizing the rights and dignity of every human being" (p. 4). Rothberg and Coder (2013) defined transpersonal social engagement as "a form of inquiry and action connecting psychological, social, and spiritual dimensions" (p. 626). Thus, similar to transpersonal social engagement, the term we use in this chapter, *socially engaged spiritual psychology*, focuses on a combination of psychology, spirituality, and social justice practices oriented to effect synergistic changes in self and world. Examples of this phenomenon originate from religious and spiritual traditions, as well as from social justice movements. These are also associated with transpersonal approaches, such as those of Ken Wilber and others' integral evolutionary psychology (e.g., Wilber, 1995), Jorge Ferrer and others' participatory turn (e.g., Ferrer, 2008), and Michael Lerner and *Tikkun's* emancipatory spirituality (e.g., Lerner, 2000), as well as of ecopsychology (e.g., Gottlieb, 2001) and women's spirituality (e.g., Starhawk, 1987).

THE NEED FOR SOCIALLY ENGAGED SPIRITUAL PSYCHOLOGY

The contemporary world is fraught with increasingly complex challenges involving economic, political, social, and environmental instabilities and crises, many of which relate to underlying religious ideologies. These present challenges that demand sophisticated personal and community-based engagement require solutions that recognize the religious and spiritual dimensions of people's worldviews and lived experiences. Psychospiritual development fosters a higher level of egoic maturation than most of the population has attained (Kegan, 1994). We believe that advocates of social justice must advance to such higher levels of egoic development through psychospiritual means to successfully engage within the contemporary intricate world, which implies a spiritual, rather than just religious, development—as religions differ across cultures, but spirituality can be seen as more universal. Through higher egoic development, one can develop the capacity to hold multiple perspectives and operate from greater levels of abstraction (Cook-Greuter, 2005), both of which can enable social justice change agents to engage with the complexities of contemporary challenges with increased agility. Psychospiritual development also offers the attainment of greater degrees of self-actualization with accompanying shifts in personal values, felt sense of interconnectedness, concern for humanity, intensification of reverence and gratitude, and expression of the highest forms of psychological maturity (Grof & Grof, 1993). Maslow (1970) wrote that "self-actualizing people . . . are also our most compassionate, our greatest improvers and reformers of society, our most effective fighters against injustice, inequality, slavery, cruelty, exploitation (and our best fighters for excellence, effectiveness, competence)" (p. xii).

The focus of spiritual psychology on psychospiritual development models and practices makes it a compelling partner for furthering social justice engagement. Social justice work requires a passionate desire to create shared community through expressions of equality, respect for difference, and attainment of a mature form of humanness (powell, 2012). powell explained that social justice work also offers many, often unrecognized, gifts to seekers of psychospiritual growth. As a form of spiritual practice, social justice work catalyzes significant developmental growth and provides an essential opportunity to open deeply to others by connecting through love and compassion. Just as social justice work offers spiritual psychologists a way to engage in social and community-based development to achieve community-based healing, it also benefits individuals in achieving psychospiritual growth.

Combining spiritual psychology with social justice thus offers many benefits toward balancing the differentiating and integrating tendencies of the contemporary challenges to social justice. It can provide a forum to highlight the importance of differentiating the subjective, objective, and intersubjective spheres, as well as provide attention to the integration and harmonizing of these spheres across cultural divides. With this harmonizing, spiritual psychology has the potential to engender appropriate approaches to address the complex challenges of modern times. The nexus of spiritual psychology and social justice offers the opportunity to practice an integrated postmodern discipline that combines science, spirituality, and social engagement. Integrated disciplines are needed as mechanisms to achieve significant, positive change and tackle the growing complexity of a multicultural world. Without such integration, Western psychology contains implicit underlying spiritual narcissism, consisting of cultural assumptions that are considered universal but are not. Mainstream psychology, devoid of a nuanced understanding of the importance of spirituality, contains unfortunate blinders that support an unjust status quo, while secular social change agents who lack appropriate spiritual grounding lose the vital benefits of inner development (Rothberg & Coder, 2013).

ROOTS OF SOCIALLY ENGAGED SPIRITUAL PSYCHOLOGY

Socially engaged spiritual psychology has roots in progressive social transformation movements, religious and spiritual traditions, and socially minded psychologies (Rothberg & Coder, 2013). Ruffing (2001) defined social transformation as "intentional attempts to change a particular social group or some aspect of an entire society for the better according to some kind of shared norms" (p. 18). Premodern and modern social movements inform socially engaged spiritual psychology. In premodernity, defined as the age before the Enlightenment, movements addressed the "development of the individual conscience" (Armstrong, 1993, p. 27) and produced many of the world's great religious traditions, such as the Eastern expressions of Buddhism, Hinduism, Confucianism, Taoism, Jainism, and the Western monotheistic traditions, such as Zoroastrianism, Judaism, Christianity, and Islam. All of these traditions, at least in part, confronted social justice issues, such as societal inequality and exploitation (Loy, 2003). These traditions were concerned with individual behavior and social justice, how to live the good life, and produced ethical and moral guidelines to that end (Armstrong, 2006).

Since time immemorial, spiritual and religious traditions have envisioned principles such as compassion, nonviolence, equality, interdependence, and justice, and provided structures and resources to support the actualization of those principles. Sages from a variety of religious traditions "preached a spirituality of empathy and compassion" (Armstrong, 2006, p. xviii), and religious practices developed to demand rigorous self-examination, being responsible for one's own behavior, and taking sensible effectual action. For example, social justice and service were mandated in the Western monotheistic religious traditions of Judaism, Christianity, and Islam, often through prophecy that combined contemplation with speech and action (DeYoung, 2007, 2012). The prophets saw that authentic spiritual development integrated religious experience with daily life, and, after enlightenment, men and women returned to the marketplace to "practice compassion for all living beings" (Armstrong, 1993, p. 45). In Islam, the prophet Muhammad serves as the archetypal example of a human being of highly developed character concerned with issues of morality, social justice, oppression, and humanitarianism. He was considered a moral and social reformer by his followers, teaching justice and equality and setting the example to be followed by all Muslims (Rothberg, 2011). In many traditions, saints and mystics served as living examples of the marriage of contemplation and action, and provided guidance and inspiration for others (Rakoczy, 2006).

Spiritual aspirants in premodern Hindu traditions proffered a goal of complete liberation that released the individual from *samsara*, the interminable cycle of birth, death, and rebirth (Armstrong, 2006). Intense yogic practices, moral training, and abidance of prohibitions were required of aspirants to maintain their liberatory path. Jainism and Buddhism developed in reaction to Hinduism as their respective founders, Mahavaira and Gotama, realized that the development of virtues was also essential for enlightenment. Compassion and service rose to supreme importance, and *bodhisattvas* emerged as beacons of inspiration. Bodhisattvas are spiritual masters in some Buddhist traditions who choose to help others awaken, instead of themselves merging into the so-called bliss of ultimate enlightenment (Armstrong, 2006). Within the Hindu communities, householders developed devotional *bhakti* practices to attain communion with a deity (Armstrong, 2006) and *karma yoga* practices to attain liberation through work (Banerjee, 1964), both vehicles outside of a path of renouncing the world.

The 20th century had many examples of faith-inspired movements for social justice, including those led by Mohandas Gandhi, Martin Luther King Jr., and Lech Walesa. These contributions to social justice activism from religious and spiritual traditions continue into the 21st century. In September 2007, Buddhist monks marched in the streets of cities across Burma protesting the actions of the military junta (Ostergaard, 2008). Many participants in the "Arab Spring" protests in 2011 were motivated by their religious faith. The work of the interfaith Jerusalem Peacemakers network is gaining some notice, in which Orthodox Jews, Sufi Muslims, Palestinian Christians, and Druids in the Holy Land prayed together in the "Old City of Jerusalem, the most contested religious 1/4 of a mile in the world" (Gopin, 2012, p. 72).

Apart from what are called the great world religions, a variety of indigenous traditions also place significant importance on developing harmony within the self and the community, and in which full humanity is seen as being achieved through the development of relationships with others (Mankiller, 2004). As Smith-Christopher (2007) wrote, indigenous spiritual traditions have been teaching about and honoring peace and nonviolence centuries before Christian and Islamic missionaries arrived in their homelands. For example, Tamihere (2007) explained that for the Māori, peace is the most commonly expressed value in its wisdom traditions. Many of the peacemaking and nonviolent traditions of indigenous peoples remain more or less unknown in Western and academic culture, which itself is a concern of social justice because of this marginalization of other vibrant traditions (Smith-Christopher, 2007).

However, it is also important to not romanticize either the great world religions or even the many indigenous traditions (Friedman, 2005, 2010). All of the great world religions have participated in various forms of social injustice, such as unjust conquests and wars that were often pursued under the highest religious ideals of these parochial traditions, but to disastrous results. From the conquistadores slaughtering the Aztecs in the name of Christianity in the West to the current Buddhist civilian attacks on Muslims in Burma in the East, all great traditions have promulgated their share of injustice meted out in the name of their religions (Kuhn, 2013; Stout, 2004). Likewise, indigenous traditions are particularly prone to being romanticized, despite that their traditions have similarly violent and exploitive aspects, such as the fact of the Māori's highly valuing peace being counterbalanced by this value being embedded within a highly warlike culture.

PSYCHOLOGICAL TRADITIONS

Modernity, in contrast with premodernity, produced more secularized expressions of social justice, such as "democratic, socialist, anarchist, feminist, ecological, and civil rights movements, among others" (Rothberg & Coder, 2013, p. 630). And modernity can be traced from the rational systems of Confucius in the East and those of the ancient Greeks in the West, all of which worked in some ways to further the realization of human and nonhuman rights (Martin, 2013; Wei-Ming, 1996). One expression of this trend in recent times is in some forms of contemporary psychology.

For example, Watkins and Shulman (2010) explained that certain depth psychologies were formed with an "acute consciousness of social inequalities" (p. 55) and that many early psychoanalysts practiced hoping for social and psychological liberation, which were often seen as intertwined (Jacoby, 1986). Depth psychology was also linked to social critiques, such as by the Frankfurt School critical social theorists, including Fromm and Marcuse (see Watkins & Shulman, 2010). Rothberg (2011) wrote that depth psychologies offer (1) the ability to identify the individual, interpersonal, sociocultural, and universal unconscious dimensions of human experience related to social justice, and (2) a wide variety of therapeutic methods that bring awareness and healing where consciousness is lacking and suffering exists. Liberation psychology, community psychology, ecopsychology, and transpersonal psychology all maintain a foundation in social and individual change, and their interdependence in terms of melding social justice and psychological concerns is reflected in the many models of socially engaged spiritual psychology (Rothberg & Coder, 2013).

Models of socially engaged spiritual psychology include liberation psychologies (Watkins & Shulman, 2010), engaged spirituality (Stanczak, 2006), consciousness-in-action (Quiñones Rosado, 2007), contemplation in action (Rohr, 2009), deep ecology (e.g., Gottlieb, 2001), the "Work That Reconnects" (Macy & Johnstone, 2012), ecofeminism (e.g., Diamond & Orenstein, 1990), integral ecology

(Esbjörn-Hargens & Zimmerman, 2009), integral international development (Hochachka, 2007), subtle activism (Nicol, 2010), mystic activism (DeYoung, 2007), socially engaged Buddhism and integrative spirituality (Rothberg, 2008), sacred activism (Harvey, 2009), transpersonal activism (Friedman, 2004; Machinga & Friedman, in press), and mature spiritual activism (Coder, 2012). We explore a few of these models to clarify how spirituality, psychology, and social justice can act in concert.

Liberation Psychologies

Watkins and Shulman (2010) defined liberation psychologies as "ideas, practices, and projects that nurture an imagination of alternative ways of thinking and acting together that can transform participation in social, economic, and ecological change and address psychological sufferings" (p. 3). Liberation psychologies find their bedrock in an interdependence paradigm and in hope for "peaceful, just, and ecologically vibrant communities that support psychologically well-being" (p. 10). Liberation of one is perceived as integral to the liberation of all. Although liberation psychologies do not include a strong explicit basis in spiritual teachings, the Watkins and Shulman model envisions liberation psychologies as restorative through both "*tikkun nefesh*, repair of our souls, and *tikkun olam*, repair of the world through our relations with others and nature" (p. 335).

Sacred Activism

Sacred activism is defined by spiritual teacher and mystical scholar Andrew Harvey (2009) as "the joy of compassionate service . . . married to a practical and pragmatic drive to transform all existing economic, social, and political institutions [in] a radical and potentially all-transforming holy force" (p. xviii). Sacred activism works toward a "humbling and amazing transfiguration" (Harvey, 2009, p. xix) of humanity. Harvey recommended that sacred activists serve the divine, serve oneself as sacred instrument, serve the local community, serve all sentient beings in one's life experience, and serve the global community. Sacred activism is made possible by surrendering to the divine, engaging in daily spiritual practices, committing to shadow work, transforming anger, and engaging in *networks of grace*. Networks of grace are groups of "like-minded, like-hearted beings brought together by passion, skill, serendipity in order to pool their energies, triumphs, grievances, hopes, and resources" (p. 209).

Integral Theory

Integral theory is the result of approximately 40 years of inter- and transdisciplinary scholarship in which Ken Wilber and others have integrated knowledge from a wide-ranging domains, including spirituality, psychology, philosophy, anthropology, biology, and sociology (see Brown, 2006). The integral framework consists of five major components—states, stages, lines, quadrants, and types—that can be examined in four major domains: interior-individual (e.g., psychological, spiritual), interior-collective (e.g., cultural), exterior-individual (e.g., behavioral), and exterior-collective (e.g., systems, societal structures). Integral theory offers a multiperspectival framework for empirical investigation and activism. Applications of integral theory connecting spiritual, psychological, and social dimensions include consciousness-in-action (Quiñones Rosado, 2007), integral international development (Hochachka, 2007, 2010), integral ecology (Esbjörn-Hargens & Zimmerman, 2009), and integral sustainability (Brown, 2006), and are being utilized in such countries as Peru, Sierra Leone, El Salvador, and Nigeria.

Transpersonal Activism

Friedman (2004) discussed how the transpersonal perspective provides a unitive framework for people quarreling over divisive religious traditions, illustrating this in terms of peace implications within Fiji and Israel that could inure from finding spiritual commonalities. Machinga and Friedman (in press) furthered this perspective toward designing intervention programs in Zimbabwe, in which people from both Christian and indigenous Shona traditions could pursue reconciliation after years of destructive conflict. Hoot and Friedman (2011) also showed how a transpersonal perspective could relate to environmental aspects of social justice.

Mature Spiritual Activism

Coder (2012) presented a potential form of socially engaged spiritual psychology based on an exemplar study of *mature spiritual activism*. Mature spiritual activism consists of interdependent dynamic processes of interior-individuality, exterior-individuality, and sociocultural milieus that potentiate healthy individual and sociocultural transformation (Coder, 2011). Coder's model highlights the importance of personal and spiritual development in social engagement, and notes its necessity in maintaining healthy interpersonal relationships, developing stamina and resilience for challenging situations, and mitigating stress effects. This model suggests that combining social activism with psychospiritual development is synergistic, and supports the validity of socially engaged spiritual psychology interventions.

EMPIRICAL STUDIES ON SOCIALLY ENGAGED SPIRITUAL PSYCHOLOGY

Although empirical investigations in socially engaged spiritual psychology are few (Coder, 2011), a number of studies reveal important findings for this field. DeYoung (2004), for example, used a combination of historical research, biography, and social science portraiture to examine the lives of three mystic activists. He uncovered four major themes:

> (1) They were motivated by their religious faith; (2) they had a worldview that emerged from the margins of society; (3) their identity was rooted in a belief that we share a common humanity; and (4) they embraced an ethics of revolution that demanded structural change. (DeYoung, 2004, p. 10)

This study revealed that the mystic-activists studied did not separate their faith from social justice or political action, remained hopeful, approached faiths outside their own, and found rest and renewal in spiritual practices.

Burdge (2006) studied four exemplary religious peace activists in Israel, utilizing psychological phenomenology to discern the essential experiences of spiritually oriented peace activists working within a region of cross-cultural conflict. She looked for a relationship between peace activism and religious or spiritual experience. Results revealed a common phenomenological structure that included:

> a heart-centered open receptivity to experiences of self, others, and the Divine; an inability to psychically compartmentalize memories or experiences; a yearning to learn from differing others as a path towards deeper spiritual and self understanding; a deep inner awareness and connection with an internal sense of self that is experienced as divinely infused with universal human understandings; a consistently active spirituality-based moral filter through which actions are evaluated; an ability to sense similarities across apparent orientational divides; and a nearly continuous connection with love as a motivation for and appraiser of potential actions. (Burdge, 2006, pp. iii–iv)

Walworth's (2008) research utilized biographical enquiry to study the lives of two contemporary spiritually based social activists in order to understand the phenomenon of engaged spiritual life. Relevant to transpersonal social engagement are Walworth's findings that socially engaged spirituality is "an interconnected, multifaceted, cross-cultural movement" (p. 356), which points to the "indivisibility of spirituality and social transformation" (p. 357).

Coder (2011, 2012) studied three exemplary spiritually mature social change agents from Sri Lankan, Hopi-Havasupai, and American backgrounds using a hybrid methodology of constructivist grounded theory and multiple case studies. In addition to the findings aforementioned, the cross-case analysis suggested that personal change was being catalyzed as the individual experiences and personality traits of change agents met outward actions in social contexts. Catalyzing personal change was identified as an intrinsic process, which when combined with catalyzing sociocultural change seemed to lead to a dynamic, living macro-process that yielded ongoing individual and sociocultural transformations. The exemplars believed that combining spiritual and social engagement was critical for their own needs, and each supported this connection in the social movements in which they were involved. This analysis suggested that the exemplars mitigated stress and resisted experiences of compassion fatigue (and burnout) through resilience. Committed, long-term spiritual practice was a key component in the development of such resilience.

Brenner and Homonoff (2004) utilized grounded theory to explore the influence of Zen Buddhist meditation practice on clinical social work and examined the practitioners' "practice framework, clinical practice, and interactions within larger systems" (p. 261). The data analysis revealed themes of increased awareness and attunement, acceptance of varied perspectives in clients and colleagues with a nonjudgmental stance, and responsibility, which involved seeing clearly and taking appropriate action.

Golden, Piedmont, Ciarrochi, and Rodgerson (2004) studied burnout in clergy using a composite index of three questionnaires and a hierarchical multiple regression analysis. Results showed that spirituality, particularly the "individual's perceived relationship with God" (p. 123), "showed incremental significance in predicting burnout even when controlling for personality and work environment" (p. 115). Their study supports the tenet that spirituality can help social change activists handle stress and develop resilience.

Stanczak and Miller's (2002) qualitative research identified and examined the connection between social change and spirituality, showing that the conversation about spirituality was beginning in academia, catalyzed by some of the most recent advances in psychotherapy, psychology, and business. The study concluded that engaged spirituality affects the "personal, local, and everyday" spheres as well as social networks, and exists as "a latent social resource among larger constituencies that do not have a viable outlet for this personal commitment" (Stanczak, 2006, p. 162). Spirituality and social change were determined to be synergistic, but spirituality must be "enacted through practice, through others, through institutions, through social structures, and through direct action to produce change" (Stanczak, 2006, p. 174).

CONCLUSION

Akin to transpersonal social engagement, socially engaged spiritual psychology is an emerging phenomenon at a relatively early stage of development (Rothberg & Coder, 2013). As emergent, socially engaged spiritual psychology offers great potential for further theoretical, empirical, and practical development. More specifically, most of the expressions of socially engaged spiritual psychology have not yet been integrated with other psychological, social, and spiritual dimensions. Current research mostly involves a few qualitative studies of exemplars, and more scientific examination of this phenomenon is needed. Methodological, theoretical, and practical challenges remain, such as the following: How can one combine and integrate multiple methodologies (e.g., phenomenological and social analytical) to study inner development and outer action, while attending to larger social structures and ideologies? How is it possible theoretically to connect all three perspectives when it is not clear how to understand the relationship between the psychological and the social, the psychological and the spiritual, and the social and the spiritual? And, what examples of socially engaged spiritual psychology can be used to examine how progress might be made in creating innovative psycho-social-spiritual practices?

Concerns also exist about whether socially engaged spiritual psychology can fairly include theories, findings, and practices generated from traditionally marginalized communities, rather than emanating only from privileged or Western academic locations (Rothberg & Coder, 2013). The principle of interconnectedness that undergirds both transpersonal and spiritual psychology with social justice concerns mandates the development of a highly inclusive and equitable discipline. As this phenomenon is founded within traditions that embrace feminist, critical, postmodern, and other nontraditional methodologies, and one that studies marginalized communities, most of the extant research stems from the West and would benefit from adding a more global perspective.

Further concerns question how deeply the psychological, social, and spiritual dimensions can be integrated, both theoretically and practically. Is it possible to reach this depth in the dimensions combined, or is there a tendency to provide more superficial expressions of each of these areas when all three are integrated? The healthiest forms of socially engaged spiritual psychology flourish when "the resources from psychological forms of healing and inquiry, social analysis and action, and spiritual traditions, help practitioners . . . attain transformative depth" (Rothberg & Coder, 2013, p. 636). This positive transformation of self and world is one of the most profound goals of socially engaged spiritual psychology, although interventions based on this goal are needed, along with empirical studies that can help frame and assess its achievements and deficits.

Although the socially engaged spiritual psychology field is relatively new, the potential usefulness of its further development appears compelling, given the severity and scale of so many contemporary global challenges. The intersubjective, subjective, and objective worlds of social justice, spirituality, and psychology must function interdependently, as we believe only postconventional thought and action can engender adequate solutions in these complex times. This chapter is a call to remake self and world by co-creating an entirely new, shared space that is abundantly fertile and increasingly human in the holistic sense of being explicitly interrelated, mutual, and participatory. Psychology, no matter how much it might try to appear value-free, is always enmeshed within webs of evaluative assumptions, including spiritual values, that should be an important part of any conversation related to the interface of psychology and social justice.

NOTE

1. Parts of this chapter are based on the previously published work of Coder (2011, 2012) and Rothberg and Coder (2013).

REFERENCES

Armstrong, K. (1993). *A history of God: The 4,000-year quest of Judaism, Christianity, and Islam*. New York, NY: Ballantine Books.

Armstrong, K. (2006). *The great transformation: The beginning of our religious traditions*. New York, NY: Anchor Books.

Banerjee, G. R. (1964). Karma yoga and social case work practice in India. *The Indian Journal of Social Work, 24*(4), 229–234. Retrieved from http://www.tiss.edu/Academic/indian-journal-of-social-work.php

Boesak, A. A., & DeYoung, C. P. (2012). *Radical reconciliation: Beyond political pietism and Christian quietism*. Maryknoll, NY: Orbis Books.

Brenner, M. J., & Homonoff, E. (2004). Zen and clinical social work: A spiritual approach to practice. *Families in Society, 85*(2), 261–269. Retrieved from http://www. fami liesinsociety.org/

Brown, B. (2006). Theory and practice of integral sustainable development: Part 1-Quadrants and the practitioner. *AQAL: Journal of Integral Theory and Practice, 1*(2), 366–405.

Burdge, S. (2006). *The relationship between spirituality and peace activism: Phenomenological inquiry into the experience of peace activists in Israel*. Unpublished doctoral dissertation, Institute of Transpersonal Psychology, Palo Alto, CA.

Coder, K. E. (2011). *"Shaking the world awake": A multiple case study of spiritually advanced social change*. Unpublished doctoral dissertation, Institute of Transpersonal Psychology, Palo Alto, CA.

Coder, K. E. (2012). "Shaking the world awake": A constructivist cross case analysis of the phenomenon of spiritually mature activism. *The Australian Community Psychologist, 2*(24), 111–132.

Cook-Greuter, S. R. (2005). *Ego development: Nine levels of increasing embrace*. Retrieved from http://www.cook-greuter.com/

DeYoung, C. P. (2004). *Mystic-activists: Faith-inspired leaders working for social justice and reconciliation*. Unpublished doctoral dissertation, University of St. Thomas, St. Paul, MN.

DeYoung, C. P. (2007). *Living faith: How faith inspires social justice*. Minneapolis, MN: Fortress Press.

DeYoung, C. P. (2012). Christianity: Contemporary expressions. In M. D. Palmer & S. M. Burgess (Eds.), *The Wiley-Blackwell companion to religion and social justice* (pp. 61–76). West Sussex, UK: Wiley-Blackwell.

Diamond, I., & Orenstein, G. (Eds.). (1990). *Reweaving the world: The emergence of ecofeminism*. San Francisco, CA: Sierra Club Books.

Edwards, M., & Post, S. G. (Eds.). (2008). *The love that does justice: Spiritual activism in dialogue with social science*. Stony Brook, NY: Unlimited Love Press.

Elkins, D. N. (2007). A humanistic approach to spiritually oriented psychotherapy. In L. Sperry & E. P. Shafranske (Eds.), *Spiritually oriented psychotherapy* (pp. 131–151). Washington, DC: APA.

Esbjörn-Hargens, S., & Zimmerman, M. (2009). *Integral ecology: Uniting multiple perspectives on the natural world.* New York, NY: Random House/Integral Books.

Ferrer, J. N. (2008). Spiritual knowing as participatory enaction: An answer to the question of religious pluralism. In J. N. Ferrer & J. H. Sherman (Eds.), *The participatory turn: Spirituality, mysticism, religious studies* (pp. 135–169). Albany, NY: State University of New York Press.

Friedman, H. (1983). The self-expansiveness level form: A conceptualization and measurement of a transpersonal construct. *The Journal of Transpersonal Psychology, 15,* 37–50.

Friedman, H. (2004). Frameworks for peace: Reframing the conflict in Fiji. *International Journal of Transpersonal Studies, 23,* 118–124.

Friedman, H. (2005). Problems of romanticism in transpersonal psychology: A case study of Aikido. *The Humanistic Psychologist, 33,* 3–24.

Friedman, H. (2010). Is Buddhism a psychology? Commentary on romanticism in "Mindfulness in Psychology." *The Humanistic Psychologist, 38,* 184–189.

Friedman, H. (2013). The role of science in transpersonal psychology: The advantages of middle-range theory. In H. Friedman & G. Hartelius (Eds.). *The Wiley-Blackwell handbook of transpersonal psychology* (pp. 300–311). Oxford, UK: Wiley-Blackwell.

Golden, J., Piedmont, R. L., Ciarrochi, J. W., & Rodgerson, T. (2004). Spirituality and burnout: An incremental validity study. *Journal of Psychology and Theology, 32*(2), 115–125. Retrieved from https://wisdom.biola.edu/jpt/

Gopin, M. (2012). *Bridges across an impossible divide: The inner lives of Arab and Jewish peacemakers.* New York, NY: Oxford University Press.

Gottlieb, R. S. (2001). The transcendence of justice and the justice of transcendence: Mysticism, deep ecology, and political life. In J. K. Ruffing (Ed.), *Mysticism & social transformation* (pp. 179–194). Syracuse, NY: Syracuse University Press.

Grof, S., & Grof, C. (1993). Transpersonal experiences and the global crisis. In R. Walsh & F. Vaughan (Eds.), *Paths beyond ego: The transpersonal vision* (pp. 251–253). New York, NY: Jeremy P. Tarcher/Putnam.

Hartelius, G., Caplan, M., & Rardin, M. A. (2007). Transpersonal psychology: Defining the past, divining the future. *The Humanistic Psychologist, 35*(2), 1–26. doi: 10.1080/08873260701274017

Harvey, A. (2009). *The hope: A guide to sacred activism.* New York, NY: Hay House.

Hawken, P. (2007). *Blessed unrest: How the largest social movement in history is restoring grace, justice, and beauty to the world.* New York, NY: Penguin.

Hill, J. (2000). A rationale for the integration of spirituality into community psychology. *Journal of Community Psychology, 28(2),* 139–149.

Hochachka, G. (2007). An introduction to integral international development. *Journal of Integral Theory and Practice, 2*(1), 102–119. Retrieved from http://aqaljournal.integralinstitute.org/public/Issues.aspx

Hochachka, G. (2010). Integrating spirituality in a post-secular approach to development. *Trialog, 107*(4), 27–59.

Hoot, R., & Friedman, H. (2011). Sense of interconnectedness and pro-environmental behavior. *International Journal of Transpersonal Studies, 30*(1–2), 89–100.

Jacoby, R. (1986). *The repression of psychoanalysis.* Chicago, IL: University of Chicago Press.

Kegan, R. (1994). *In over our heads: The mental demands of modern life.* Cambridge, MA: Harvard University Press.

Kuhn, A. (2013). Are Buddhist monks involved in Myanmar's violence? *National Public Radio, May 17*, n.p. Retrieved from http://www.npr.org/blogs/parallels/2013/05/17/182904712/ Are-Buddhist-Monks-Involved-In-Myanmars-Violence

Lerner, M. (2000). *Spirit matters*. Charlottesville, VA: Hampton Roads.

Loy, D. (2003). *The great awakening: A Buddhist social theory*. Boston, MA: Wisdom.

Machinga, M., & Friedman, H. (in press). Developing transpersonal resiliency: An approach to healing and reconciliation in Zimbabwe. *International Journal of Transpersonal Studies.*

Macy, J., & Johnstone, C. (2012). Active hope: How to face the mess we're in without going crazy. Novato, CA: New World Library.

Mankiller, W. (2004). *Every day is a good day: Reflections by contemporary indigenous women*. Golden, CO: Fulcrum.

Martin, T. (2013). *Ancient Greece: From prehistoric to Hellenistic times* (2nd ed.). New Haven, CT: Yale University Press.

Maslow, A. H. (1970). *Motivation and personality* (2nd ed.). New York, NY: Harper and Row.

McFarland, S., Brown, D., & Webb, M. (2013). "Identification with all humanity" as a moral concept and psychological construct. *Current Directions in Psychological Science, 22*, 192–196.

Miovic, M. (2004). An introduction to spiritual psychology: Overview of the literature, East and West. *Harvard Review of Psychiatry, 12*(2), 105–115, doi: 10.1080/10673220490447206

Nicol, D. (2010). *Subtle activism: The inner dimension of social transformation*. Unpublished doctoral dissertation, California Institute of Integral Studies, San Francisco, CA.

Ostergaard, A. (2008). Burma VJ: Reporting from a closed country. (Film released 2008)

Pappas, J., & Friedman, H. (2004). Scientific transpersonal psychology and cultural diversity: Focus on measurement in research and clinical practice. In W. Smythe & A. Baydala (Eds.), *Studies of how the mind publicly enfolds into being: Mellen studies in psychology* (Vol. 9, pp. 303–345). Lewiston, NY: Edwin Mellen Press.

powell, j. a. (2012). *Racing to justice: Transforming our conceptions of self and other to build an inclusive society*. Bloomington, IN: Indiana University Press.

Prilleltensky, I., & Prilleltensky, O. (2006). *Promoting well-being: Linking personal, organizational, and community change*. Hoboken, NJ: John Wiley & Sons.

Quiñones Rosado, R. (2007). *Consciousness-in-action: Toward an integral psychology of liberation & transformation*. Caguas, Puerto Rico: Caguas: Ilé Publications.

Rakoczy, S. (2006). *Great mystics & social justice: Walking on two feet of love*. New York, NY: Paulist Press.

Rohr, R. (2009). *The naked now: Learning to see as the mystics see*. New York, NY: Crossroad.

Rothberg, D. (1993). The crisis of modernity and the emergence of socially engaged spirituality. *ReVision: A Journal of Consciousness and Transformation, 15*(3), 105–114. Retrieved from http://www.revisionpublishing.org/

Rothberg, D. (2008). Connecting inner and outer transformation: Toward an extended model of Buddhist practice. In J. N. Ferrer & J. H. Sherman (Eds.), *The participatory turn: Spirituality, mysticism, religious studies* (pp. 349–370). Albany, NY: State University of New York Press.

Rothberg, D. (2011). The spirit of change: Spiritual and religious resources for peace and social justice movements. In M. Pilisuk & M. Nagler (Eds.), *Peace movements worldwide: History, psychology, and practices* (pp. 113–128). Santa Barbara, CA: Praeger Greenwood.

Rothberg, D., & Coder, K. (2013). Widening circles: The emergence of transpersonal social engagement. In H. Friedman & G. Hartelius (Eds.). *The Wiley-Blackwell handbook of transpersonal psychology* (pp. 626–639). Oxford, UK: Wiley-Blackwell.

Ruffing, J. K. (2001). Introduction. In J. K. Ruffing (Ed.), *Mysticism & social transformation* (pp. 1–25). Syracuse, NY: Syracuse University Press.

Smith-Christopher, D. L. (2007). Indigenous traditions of peace: An interview with Lawrence Hart, Cheyenne peace chief. In D. L. Smith-Christopher (Ed.), *Subverting hatred: The challenge of nonviolence in religious traditions* (pp. 76–85). Maryknoll, NY: Orbis Books.

Sperry, L. & Shafranske, E. P. (Eds.) (2007). *Spiritually oriented psychotherapy.* Washington, DC: APA.

Stanczak, G. C. (2006). *Engaged spirituality: Social change and American religion.* New Brunswick, NJ: Rutgers University Press.

Stanczak, G. C., & Miller, D. E. (2002). *Engaged spirituality: Spirituality and social transformation in mainstream American religious traditions.* Los Angeles, CA: Center for Religion and Spiritual Culture, University of Southern California. Retrieved from http://crcc.usc.edu/ docs/EngagedSpirituality2.pdf

Starhawk. (1987). *Truth or dare: Encounters with power, authority, and mystery.* San Francisco, CA: Harper & Row.

Stout, M. (2004). *Aztec.* Milwaukee, WI: Gareth Stevens.

Tamihere, D. S. (2007). The struggle for peace: Subverting hatred in a Māori context. In D. L. Smith-Christopher (Ed.), *Subverting hatred: The challenge of nonviolence in religious traditions* (pp. 86–106). Maryknoll, NY: Orbis Books.

Vaughan, F. (2002). What is spiritual intelligence? *Journal of Humanistic Psychology, 42*(2), 16–33, doi: 10.1177/0022167802422003

Walworth, C. L. (2008). *Crossing borders with Elias Amidon and Elizabeth Roberts: A biography of engaged spiritual lives.* Unpublished doctoral dissertation, Union Institute & University, Cincinnati, OH.

Watkins, M., & Shulman, H. (2010). *Toward psychologies of liberation.* Houndsmills, UK: Palgrave Macmillan.

Wei-Ming, T. (1996). *Confucian traditions in East Asian modernity.* Cambridge, MA: American Academy of Arts and Sciences.

Wilber, K. (1995). *Sex, ecology, spirituality: The spirit of evolution.* Boston, MA: Shambhala.

Zinnbauer, B. J., & Paragment, K. I. (2005). Religiousness and spirituality. In R. F. Paloutzian & C. L. Park (Eds.), *Handbook of the psychology of religion and spirituality* (pp. 21–42). New York, NY: The Guilford Press.

Chapter 12

Shifting the Tide: Psychology's Role in Addressing Human Rights Violations

Thema S. Bryant-Davis, Pamela A. Counts, and Anthea A. Gray

Human rights represent the legal and social obligations societies adopt to ensure that systems are in place to provide for the basic needs of people (Kinderman, 2007). The Universal Declaration of Human Rights was adopted by the UN General Assembly on December 10, 1948. The rights covered by the declaration include equality, dignity, and freedom. People from diverse legal and cultural backgrounds came together to make this document a common standard for all peoples and all nations. It sets out, for the first time, fundamental human rights to be universally protected. The Geneva Convention consists of four treaties, and three additional protocols, that establish the standards of international law for the humanitarian treatment of war. These include the standards for basic, wartime rights of prisoners (civil and military); established protections for the wounded; and established protections for the civilians in and around a war zone. An increasing number of research and interventions have been developed by psychologists to prevent and address human rights violations, such as human trafficking, mistreatment of immigrants/refugees, torture, sexual violence, war, mistreatment of people with disabilities, political oppression, discrimination, genocide, and denial of resources. Psychologists have focused efforts on attempting to understand causes, effects, and solutions to these global issues. Interdisciplinary approaches have included attending to individual, interpersonal, and systemic factors (Melton, 2010). Solutions have included psychologically informed prevention activities, intervention programs, and advocacy initiatives. The following review provides an overview of some of the work psychologists have undertaken to address human rights violations.

HUMAN TRAFFICKING

The term *trafficking* is defined by the UN Protocol to Prevent, Suppress, and Punish Trafficking in Persons as the "recruitment, transportation, transfer, and harboring of persons by the threat or use of force such as fraud, coercion, deception, and the abuse of power" (p. 2). As indicated, individuals are forced to work in adverse conditions with little or no compensation, and are subjected to physical force, debt bondage, and psychological and physical terror. Given that trafficked persons are involuntarily entered into the labor force and sex industry, and are coerced into working in poor conditions that violate labor and human rights, it is considered a form of modern-day slavery. According to the International Labor Organization (ILO) (2012), nearly 21 million individuals are in forced labor, with numbers rising. Out of those subjected to forced labor, the ILO (2012) estimated that 4.5 million (22%) are sexually exploited. The United Nations Office of Drug and Crime (UNODC) (2012) reported that women and young girls account for 75% of those trafficked for sexual exploitation. In addition to sexual exploitation, others are trafficked and placed in indentured servitude in activities involving agriculture, construction, domestic work, or manufacturing (ILO, 2012; UNODC, 2012). Trafficked persons often sustain physical and psychological injuries as a result of the assaults—verbal, physical and sexual—commonly associated with trafficking. Psychologists can serve a particularly important role in helping trafficked individuals recover from these injuries. Psychologists can also offer preventative interventions that help reduce trafficking in high-risk populations.

According to the ILO (2007), at least 2.4 million women and children are trafficked worldwide, with as many as 1.2 million under the age of 18. Gender, poverty, and political unrest in their country of origin especially place low-income women and children living in rural or war-torn nations at higher risk for being trafficked (Chung, 2009; Crawford & Kaufman, 2008). Women and children are more likely to seek and consent to adverse employment conditions to improve their family's economic status and quality of life (Bryant-Davis, Tillman, Marks, & Smith, 2009; Sossou & Yogttiba, 2009). For example, in northwestern countries of Africa, specifically Ghana, Nigeria, and Togo, Sossou and Yogttiba (2009) have documented the parent's role in the trafficking of children. The authors noted that parents in these developing countries are likely to transfer their child's care to relatives who were more financially secure or childless to maintain kinship expectations and responsibilities, and also to overcome economic hardship. However, upon transfer to their kinsmen, the parents sometimes know that their child will be sent to industrialized cities where they will be subjected into indentured servitude, work as domestic servants in well-to-do homes or as physical laborers in plantations and fish farms. Similar cases were documented in Vietnam in which Vijeyarasa (2010) documented the culture's emphasis on familial piety, and how it helped to create justification for impoverished families to sell the bodies of their daughters into sex trafficking. Like the case in northwestern Africa, expectations of familial duty contributed to the parents' deliberate entry of young women and girls in the family into sex trafficking. These cases indicated that young women and children become more vulnerable to traffickers and organized crime networks that hide behind the guise of employment agencies promising education opportunities and economic prosperity. However, once removed from familiar networks, they are stripped of their identity (e.g., passports and visas) and are subjected to debt bondage where they are coerced into labor and sex work to repay their debt. For example, Gabriella, the eldest child of a fatherless family in Columbia, sought work in the United States to support her family. She agreed to move to the United States after a friend convinced her that he would be able to help her find work in a restaurant. Upon arriving to the United States, however, she was held in debt bondage of $10,000, and traffickers threatened to harm her family if she sought help. She was forced into prostitution in brothels and moved from different brothels every week so that she would not know her location (Polaris Project, 2012). Gabriella's case is one of many in which traffickers utilize the victim's vulnerability to assert control and power in limiting the victim's choice and freedom.

High levels of physical force and sexual coercion (e.g., rape) that lead to numerous physical injuries (e.g., broken bones, burns, and concussions), health problems (e.g., sexually transmitted diseases and birth complications), and even death are prevalent in cases of human sex trafficking. In addition to physical and sexual assaults, traffickers employ psychological terror to incite submission and compliance to their demands (Gjermeni et al., 2008; Kotrla, 2010; Raymond & Hughes, 2011; Wilson & Dalton, 2008). Thus, survivors of human sex trafficking sustain long-term psychological consequences such as depression, anxiety, posttraumatic stress disorder (PTSD), substance use problems, malnutrition, and self-destructive behaviors (Kotrla, 2010; Raymond & Hughes, 2001; Yakushko, 2009) as a result of being subjected into these deplorable conditions. They are also likely to be suspicious of others and lack knowledge of where and how to seek help. The lack of awareness about the nature of trafficking and the victims' experience also leads to the tendency of victims and survivors to be criminalized by law enforcements, which further minimizes their supports.

Between 2007 and 2010, the UNODC (2012) reported that trafficking cases were detected in 118 countries worldwide. It is described as the third largest international crime industry, following the trafficking of illegal drugs and arms. The generation of large sums of profit creates global routes similar to the trafficking of drugs, or arms, highlighting the extent to which vulnerable populations are dehumanized and transformed into commodities in our current and historical systems of trade. In most cases, emergency and crisis interventions are necessary to ensure safety and begin the recovery process for those victims unable to exit on their own. In other cases, psychologists play an important role in treating survivors clinically, educating the community to prevent trafficking, and advocating for survivors' rights as a person.

REFUGEES

Refugees are individuals who have been granted international protection as a result of persecution in their country of origin. Unlike immigrants who migrate to foreign countries with desire and intention to improve their economic livelihood, refugees are often forced to suddenly evacuate their homes and relocate to an unfamiliar country due to threat to their physical safety. Although most immigrants may have established networks or access to resources in their country of destination, most refugees enter countries that are unfamiliar to them and have very limited to no resources available. In addition, negative political and social messages about refugees transmitted through the dominant culture's media perpetuate discrimination and maltreatment of refugees. Language barriers exacerbate this discrimination, which lead refugees to isolate themselves instead of seeking safety from authorities. As a result of these adverse pre- and postmigration encounters, refugees are likely to experience elevated levels of acculturation stress and traumatization (Cox, 2011; Renner, Laireter, & Maier, 2012; Weine, 2011).

The United Nations High Commissioner for Refugees (UNHCR) (2011) estimated that 15.2 million of forcibly displaced persons are refugees. In 2011, the UNHCR reported that 800,000 people were displaced as refugees across international borders. Developing countries hosted four-fifths (8.4 million) of the refugee population worldwide, and 45% of the world's refugees reside in countries where the GDP (PPP) per capita is below $3,000. Pakistan hosted the largest number of refugees worldwide (17 million) with the Islamic Republic of Iran following second, and the Syrian Arab Republic following third. The UNHCR (2011) reported that 22 countries admitted refugees for resettlement, and it noted that the United States admitted the highest number of refugees for resettlement (51,500). In the Middle East and South Asia, political discord contributes to the largest number of refugees; in Africa, local wars, famine, and political upheavals motivate refugee movements across and within the region; in Europe, East Asia, Latin America, and the Caribbean, individuals flee for political unrest, and limited economic opportunities to settle in neighboring or distant countries. In 2011, it was noted that approximately 17,700 applications for asylum were submitted by unaccompanied or separated children (UNHCR, 2011). According to Martin and Yankay (2012), 34% of those refugees who were admitted to the United States in 2011 were under 18 years of age.

Acculturation barriers, such as lack of knowledge of the dominant culture's language, customs, and beliefs, make it difficult for refugees to navigate in their new setting. According to Renner et al. (2012), refugees have a tendency to rely on social security because of difficulties securing well-paying jobs which, in turn, exacerbate socioeconomic challenges. In addition, they have lost important social networks and are isolated, which can worsen anxiety and depression among refugees (Renner et al., 2012). This acculturation distress can also harm family relationships as it can reduce time and attention spent in caring for children. Thus, children of refugees are also likely to experience symptoms of anxiety, depression, and trauma (Henley & Robinson, 2011). As a result, children and adolescents of refugees may have learning and behavioral difficulties, which include early delinquency, drugs, alcohol, early pregnancy, and HIV risk (United Nations Population Fund, 1999). In a music program in New York, Choi (2010) observed that distrust of others led refugee students from North Korea to behave in ways that tested limits, demonstrated aggression without reason, and expressed distrust toward other students, necessitating the need for increased psychological interventions and services for this group. These behaviors illustrate the importance of a clinician's ability to seek information and understand the social and political climate from which displaced persons originate and are moved into, as well as the necessity of culturally based interventions in the treatment setting.

VICTIMS OF TORTURE

Acts of torture test the limits of suffering, pain, and tolerance of victims. In contrast, acts of torture test the bounds of human goodness, decency, and morality of perpetrators. By definition, torture is a psychologically or physically obtrusive act, used as a means to collect a piece of information or punish an individual, often based on identifying features, such as prescribed race, ethnicity, religion, political affiliation, or social economic status (SES). If any of these identifying markers are sought after as a means to persecute, the perpetrator usually possesses identifying features characterized as the antithesis. Perpetrators of torture may or may not be associated with their respective government and acts of torture may or may not be endorsed by the government at large. The torturer's profile is further expanded by characteristics unconstrained by faith, gender, ethnicity, or SES (Campbell, 2007).

International humanitarian law L categorizes torture as either a war crime or a crime against humanity. To be classified as a war crime, the torture would have occurred during the time of conflict, coupled with the constructs of torture, mentioned prior. To be classified as a crime against humanity, the torture can be directed at any individual, but is usually directed toward a group of people in times of peace or conflict. It is also likely that the perpetrator's respective government sanctioned acts of torture considered as crimes against humanity.

The United States promotes total intolerance toward torture and confessions obtained through means of psychological or physical coercion, but following the

September 11, 2001, attacks on America, the U.S. government's public, moral high ground on torture began to publically unravel. "The War on Terror" provided the ultimate justification for using the Central Intelligence Agency's (CIA) "enhanced" interrogation techniques, which lasted from 2002 to 2009. Such techniques included grabbing the detainee by the shirt and shaking, open-handed slaps to evoke fear and pain, slaps to the belly, preventing detainees from sitting down or forcing them to stand in awkward, uncomfortable positions, exposing detainees to extreme temperatures, and waterboarding. Outside of these enhanced interrogation techniques—conducted at detainment camps such as Abu-Gharib and Guantanamo Bay—detainees were also subjected to unsanctioned torture as well, which civilians saw firsthand via images distributed by major news outlets across the globe. Some of the most infamous acts of torture caught on film were committed by Lynndie England, former U.S. Army Reserve soldier, who famously dragged detainees on dog leashes and forced masturbatory behavior.

The CIA's interrogation methods were duplicitous in nature: scientific research by means of human torture. The effects of sleep deprivation, susceptibility and tolerance to pain, and new techniques in waterboarding were some of the offshoots of these studies, which were monitored by medical and mental health professionals (Physicians for Human Rights, 2010). Following the publication of these reports, the American Psychological Association (APA) issued a statement that barred psychologists from participating or having knowledge of interrogations that,

> mock execution; water-boarding or any other form of simulated drowning or suffocation; sexual humiliation; rape; cultural or religious humiliation; exploitation of phobias or psychopathology; induced hypothermia; and the use of psychotropic drugs or mind-altering substances for the purpose of eliciting information. In addition, the following acts were banned for the purpose of eliciting information in an interrogations process: hooding; forced nakedness; stress positions; the use of dogs to threaten or intimidate; physical assault including slapping or shaking; exposure to extreme heat or cold; threats of harm or death; and isolation and/or sleep deprivation used in a manner that represents significant pain or suffering or in a manner that a reasonable person would judge to cause lasting harm; or the threatened use of any of the above techniques to the individual or to members of the individual's family. (APA, 2007, para. 2)

Torture—a potentially traumatic event—in civilians of war may not only leave physical reminders of the trauma, but also lasting psychological impressions (Basoglu et al., 1994; Campbell, 2007; Goldfield, 1988). Pathology and torture are not mutually exclusive; however, a significant proportion of victims suffer from PTSD (Basoglu, Jarenson, Mollica, & Kastrup, 2001) as well as anxiety and depression (Basoglu,1992, 2001; Kira, Clifford, Wiencek, & Al-Haidar, 2003). Current literature also mentions the presence of complex–PTSD, which though currently unrecognized by the *DSM IV-TR* (American Psychiatric Association, 2000), these symptoms are included in the dimensions of *DSM-V*'s (American Psychiatric Association, unknown) classification of PTSD.

Using unmatched research designs for a number of studies, Basoglu et al. (2001) found a wide range of prevalence in those who suffered range from 15% to 85%. This vast variance is accounted for by the prevalence of not only PTSD but also stand-alone features, such as sexual dysfunction, memory loss, trouble in memory recollection, insomnia, and disorientation. In the same set of studies, Basoglu et al. (2001) found symptom expression far differing from orthodox Western trauma symptoms, most commonly personality change. Within the same vein, Gaithri Fernando's research conceptualized the Sri Lankan definition of trauma, the symptoms, and the ways in which Sri Lankans expressed their profound distress in response to a traumatic event—in a culturally appropriate manner (Fernando, 2005a, 2005b). In the case of Sri Lankans, Fernando (2005a, 2005b) found primary symptoms, which presented in a somatic nature, and attitudes and behaviors that stifled social relations as well as community and family duties, which might in part be reflective of the Sri Lankan collectivist society. These findings highlight the importance of recognizing cultural differences in symptomatology for those survivors of torture.

GENOCIDE

Genocide, recognized by the IHL as an intentional and deliberate act, is used to eliminate a specific group of people. Targets of such violence are often targeted because of their race, ethnicity, gender, or political affiliation. IHL recognizes the following as acts of genocide: killing members of the group, inflicting bodily harm to members of the group, intentionally coercing or creating conditions that are intended to bring destruction to the group, imposing measures intended to prevent births within the group, and forcibly transferring children of the group to another group.

The pages of history are marred by the horrors of genocide. Following such acts, survivors are left to grapple with the paradoxical trauma of survival. In the wake of survival, the deluge of interdialog, "Why did I survive?" begins to pour, with ethereal answers such as luck, faith, and destiny surfacing. Genocide survivors are essentially casualties of war in a fight for which they never enlisted, which defies all that is logical and fair—both in the world and interpersonally.

The psychological complexity of trauma related to genocide is compounded by the relationship the perpetrators had to the victims. More often than not, victims were not violated or killed by strangers. They were attacked by people they most likely knew, as in Nazi Germany, where friends, romantic partners, business associates, and neighbors were forced to cut off ties from those who were Jewish in fear of being persecuted themselves (Staub, 1989, 2006). Also, it was far from uncommon for the perpetrators of murder to be children, such as the boy soldiers of Sierra Leone who fought for the rebel Revolutionary United Front (RUF; Denov & Maclure, 2006).

The violence of genocide is not restricted to traditional weapons of war. Rape can also serve a genocidal function of "ethnic cleansing" (Milillo, 2006). There is no more effective way for a perpetrator to eliminate the perceived enemy's population than to impregnate women with the "good" seed or damage women's reproductive organs, so that they can no longer produce progeny of their own ethnic background. In comparison to rape outside of the context of war, typically rape in wartime is more violent, sadistic, and carried out by more than one person at a time, occurring in the presence of witnesses (e.g., families), and happening over an extended period of time (e.g., women held in rape camps or are held captive for a number of hours or days) (Milillo, 2006).

The communal execution of rape serves as a protective barrier against one's own sense of self (Tajfel & Turner, 1986), offering a safe emotional distance from the perpetrator's psyche and the victim. Felson (2002) explains the former in a twofold model. The first part of the model holds rape as a "retributive justice." It is the perpetrating groups' way of conquering the perceived enemy for any grievances (e.g., social, political, and economic) for which they hold the victims responsible. For example, the Tutsi ethnic group was considered socially superior to the Hutu ethnic group within Rwandan society. Though Tutsi and Hutu did intermarry, it was not commonplace. Outside of this example and within the context of genocide, rape is often a way to obtain vengeance for socioeconomic and class disparity (Mukamana & Brysiewicz, 2008). The second part of the Felson's model views war rape as a "desired identity." In times of war, teamwork, collectivist mentality, and displaying a united front (Milillo, 2006) are enforced and considered key elements of winning a war.

Long thought of as merely one of the rotten fruits war bares upon its civilians (Tomaseli & Porter, 1986), the civil unrest that occurred in Rwandan and Bosnian wars of the 1990s sent an earth-shattering message to the international community: sex acts are devastating weapons of genocide. Because of the formerly mentioned civil wars, rape and various other acts of sex are now recognized by international humanitarian law as crimes against humanity (e.g., rape, sexual slavery, enforced prostitution, forced pregnancy, enforced sterilization) or acts of genocide (e.g., imposing measures intended to prevent births within the group, sex acts in war). Staub (2007) cites the basic need for security, feelings of effectiveness, control over important events in one's life, positive identity, positive connections to other people and communities, and a comprehension of reality of one's own place in the world as essential components of emotionally surviving genocide. Without these components, which create a secure sense of self, the opportunity for psychopathology is present. Though PTSD, anxiety, and depression are common disorders related to trauma, it is important to keep in mind the cultural variables that might affect expression of symptomatology (Campbell, 2007). One example of this can be found in Cambodian refugees. Abe, Zane, and Chun (1994) found significantly high rates of expressed and experienced anger when using the Anger Reaction Index on Southeast Asian refugees. In another study sampling Cambodian psychiatric clinic refugees, Hinton, Hsia, Um, and Otto (2003) found an increased rate of anger and 58% of patients with PTSD experienced somatic arousal symptoms so great that they qualified for panic attacks. These findings necessitate the psychologist's role in adapting existing models and interventions to match the needs and cultural context of survivors.

CLINICAL INTERVENTIONS

In regard to provision of mental health services, psychologists have an important role in preventing and addressing human rights violations, such as human trafficking, mistreatment of immigrants/refugees, torture, and genocide, by educating individuals who are susceptible to these offences about their fundamental human rights to equality, dignity, and freedom. For individuals who have experienced a violation of human rights, it is not only important for psychologists to help the survivor build coping resources but also to connect them with networks that will help to build financial, political, and medical autonomy. Based on diverse backgrounds of survivors of human trafficking, refugees, and survivors of torture and genocide, psychologists also need to be familiar with culturally competent interventions for survivors as well as with the social and political contexts that impact the countries and communities from which they originate. Psychologists may also need to undertake advocacy and outreach roles to expand awareness about these human rights violations, and collaborate with other service providers to promote and facilitate healing and integration for survivors within their communities.

The negative and deleterious consequences of acts against human rights are well documented in the literature. These include depression, anxiety, PTSD, substance dependence, and even death. In addition to psychological effects, cognitive impairment has been found. For example, survivors of war torture might have trouble with recall, due to the heightened emotional, physical, and sensory awareness endured in captivity and the activation of protective defense mechanisms (Campbell, 2007; Mollica & Caspi-Yavin, 1991). The use of an evidenced-based symptom checklist has been suggested to aid in the assessment of memory loss in survivors of torture (Campbell, 2007). For instance, the Structured Clinical Interview for Diagnosis of Axis I Disorders (SCID-1; First, Spitzer, Gibbon, & Williams, 1996) is considered an effective means of gathering symptoms for a proper diagnosis (Allodi, 1991; Campbell, 2007). Though this symptom checklist and the SCID-1 are both empirically reliable and valid in Western society, it may not be valid for individuals from international countries. Thus, psychologists have an important role in adapting diagnostic instruments to match the cultural context of survivors when identifying assessment tools and interpreting results (Hooberman, Rosenfeld, Lhewa, Rasmussen, & Keller, 2007).

On a similar note, several evidence-based interventions have been found to be effective with trauma survivors. For example, Paunovic and Ost (2011) found that cognitive behavioral therapy (CBT) was an effective treatment for trauma survivors, yielding a 50% decrease in PTSD symptoms in an unmatched, controlled study. In his work with survivors of torture, Basoglu (1998) complemented the cognitive aspect of CBT with in vivo exposure and implosive therapy (Basoglu, 1998; Campbell, 2007). Shauer (2005) used Narrative Exposure Therapy (NET) to allow survivors of torture to verbally recount, transcribe, and edit their experiences (Campbell, 2007; Schauer, 2005). Staub (2006) used psychoeducation to help survivors of genocide recognize their experience as a tactic of persecution rather than a personal attack. Though survivors of trafficking, torture, and genocide are likely to originate from developing and war-torn countries, there is a very limited amount of research that specifically adapts existing models to match the diverse populations encountering these human rights violations. Based on diverse backgrounds of survivors, psychologists need to be familiar with culturally competent interventions as well as the social and political contexts that impact clients' countries and communities of origin. Therefore, psychologists have an ethical responsibility to adapt and modify clinical interventions to meet the needs and context of survivors of trauma in the treatment setting.

One intervention that was developed to include cultural components is the HEARTS model (Campbell, 2007; Hanscom, 2001), which was designed to include community involvement in interventions for survivors of torture. According to the author, there are six components of the model: hearing the history of the victim, focusing on emotions and reactions, asking about symptoms, explaining the reason for symptoms, teaching relaxation techniques and coping skills, and helping with self-change (Hanscom, 2011). Given that many torture survivors have been separated from their families and social support systems (Mollica et al., 1998) as a result of war casualties or diaspora (forced or pressured by violence), we posit that building community networks was a critical piece of recovery for this group. Like those who have survived human sex trafficking, displacement, and genocide, individuals who have experienced torture are isolated and left with a distrust of other human beings. To mend these scars, it is often helpful for survivors to meet with other survivors and reconnect with people going through similar difficulties (Proceedings, 2002; Staub & Gibson, 2004; Yakushko, 2009). Using communal support as a tool for recovery can be useful in offering a space for survivors of trauma to share their stories (Staub, 2006).

Integration of religion and spirituality has also been described as an essential part of treatment. For example, in a randomized clinical trial of refugees from Chechnya and Afghanistan, Renner et al. (2012) found that sponsorship by a church-based nongovernmental charity organization helped to reduce anxiety, depression, and other psychological problems for refugees with high levels of trauma when compared to the control group. This finding suggests that psychologists can play a fundamental role in identifying culturally congruent protective resources that will aid in the adaptation and reintegration into the communities in which the survivors reside. Similarly, in an ethnographic participant-observation study of three Buddhist mutual assistance associations in the United States and Canada, Canda and Phaobtong (1992) found that Buddhist temples afforded South East Asian refugees cultural links by providing language and art classes to refugee children, recreational activities congruent with culture, liaisons with agencies and personnel who are bilingual and familiar with South East Asian culture, and spiritual support. In these temples, monks provided mental health services similar to those found in Western culture, but incorporated Buddhist principles that may be familiar and customary among some East Asian refugees, including meditation and bereavement rituals. Supporting refugees places an added strain on countries that do not have enough resources to provide for their own native populations; therefore, the provision of services in excess of the refugee's basic needs (e.g., shelter and food) is limited. Hence, psychological services are often not available to refugees who have been moved to a host country. Nevertheless, the aforementioned findings suggest that the use of spiritual- and faith-based organizations may be useful in providing psychological and social support for individuals and families residing in refugee camps in developing countries.

Modifications for language differences have also been recommended. For example, Lykes (2000) developed the PhotoVoice program to help indigenous women in Guatemala use photography as a medium to articulate the lives and stories of those who survived war crimes.

Given the global scale of acts that violate human rights, psychologists must be able to collaborate with lawmakers, community officials, and medical personnel to design policies that safeguard the safety and rights of individuals worldwide. Promoting available and accessible mental health resources for low-income groups vulnerable to human rights violations may reduce the strain of financial hardship. Similarly, working toward a framework that promotes fundamental human and labor rights, such as adequate opportunities for education and employment, may also decrease social and gender disparities that place individuals at risk for human rights violations (Limoncelli, 2009). This may include educating lawmakers and social agencies about human rights violations, such as trafficking, torture, genocide, mistreatment of refugees, and the basic needs of survivors such as safety, shelter, legal, and economic resources (Yakushko, 2009; Farley, 2003). For example, in Rwanda, Staub (2006) trained 35 Rwandans (two-thirds Tutsi and one-third Hutu) to teach the community about the origins of genocide, effects of trauma, how to heal trauma, and basic human needs. The treatment included writing their stories (50% were illiterate and could not write), a technique of narrative therapy, reflection, and then sharing in small groups (Staub, 2006; Staub & Pearlman, 2001). The interethnic groups created an audience of sympathizers, which was described as an essential component to victim relief as it likely prevented feelings of victimization among survivors.

Since refugees, survivors of trafficking, torture, and genocide, are likely to have been moved to unfamiliar towns, regions, and even countries, they are unaccustomed to the traditions and customs of the areas to which they are relocated. They have little or no ability to communicate, have minimal or no knowledge of their legal rights, are unfamiliar with the host country's customs, and are susceptible to mistreatment and discrimination. As they enter countries that are unfamiliar to them, mistreatment during their migration/relocation experience is likely to contribute to fear of authorities and underutilization of mental health services. For example, refugees may not ask for additional details to clarify and fully understand legal policies and procedures and how and where to access support. Trafficking victims are coached by their traffickers to avoid law enforcement. Therefore, providing psychoeducation has been found to be an effective intervention in raising awareness and understanding of legal policies and procedures for these individuals.

In addition to dealing with loss of human rights and adjusting to a new culture, survivors of trauma who have children have to learn to overcome challenges in parenting, wherein they are forced to balance between the traditions of the dominant culture in which they reside and those of their country of origin. Psychologists have an important role in providing culturally sensitive treatment that enhances clients' knowledge and skills of parenting by fostering positive communication and interactions with their children (Henley & Robinson, 2011).

Psychologists have an important role in linking survivors of trauma with the community by raising awareness about the survivors' culture and migration experience through advocacy and outreach campaigns (Weine, 2011). In doing so, doctors, social workers, and law enforcement can understand the personal context that shapes the survivor's experience and minimize the discrimination and alienation they experience when seeking medical or legal assistance. In refugee and relocation camps, where there may be very minimal resources allocated for psychological services, this may include educating government agencies in the host country to advocate for increased mental health support for refugees and survivors of trafficking, torture, and genocide. Within the realm of psychology, it is important to be cognizant of political and social factors that affect the client's life as these factors may affect case conceptualization as well as the treatment plan. Sensitivity to cultural factors, such as language, can reduce the likelihood of pathologizing the client and lessen the survivor's apprehension of seeking assistance from health care providers.

The multitier programs, in which counseling, home visits, and community support are incorporated into the intervention, have also been developed to meet the needs of various survivors of trauma. For example, Khamphakdy-Brown, Jones, Nilsson, Russel, and Klevens (2006) discussed the development of a multitiered empowerment program for refugee women in the United States in which collaboration with the individuals' native and host country, lawyers, nurses, interpreters, and case workers are sought to provide women with information and support that is comprehensive and culturally sensitive. The authors recommended becoming mobile and adaptive (e.g., home visits), and utilizing bicultural and bilingual advocates to gain credibility and accessibility among women in need. These findings indicate that comprehensive care that targets individual, community, legal, health, and psychological needs is necessary to improve the well-being of refugees during and after their relocation.

Overall, psychologists play an important role in reducing distress associated with entering an unfamiliar country, and can highlight strengths that promote resilience and integration into society. Additionally, psychologists can collaborate with other disciplines to reduce stigma and discrimination and foster positive well-being.

CONCLUSION

Although there have been significant steps taken by psychologists to address human rights violations (Kinderman, 2007), the influence of these efforts requires further examination. Some evaluations have been completed but much more is needed on a global scale to determine the pathways through which psychological research, practice, and policy interrupt or reduce the perpetuation of human rights violations. The prevalence of these assaults reflects the continued need for sustained efforts for interdisciplinary collaboration to end human rights violations. Multiple disciplines within psychology need to work together, and likewise further collaboration with disciplines outside of psychology is needed to maximize the benefits of efforts to resist human rights violations. By building on best practices from multiple domains that are based in the best science, global citizens can act to ensure the preservation of human dignity across and within borders.

REFERENCES

Abe, J., Zane, N., & Chun, K. (1994). Differential responses to trauma: Migration-related discriminants of post-traumatic stress disorder among Southeast Asian refugees. *Journal of Community Psychology*, 22(2), 121–135.

Allodi, F. (1991). Assesment and treatment of torture victims: A critical review. *Journal of Nervous and Mental Disorders, 179,* 4–11.

American Psychiatric Association. (2000). *Diagnostic and statistical manual of mental disorders* (4th ed., rev). Washington, DC: Author.

American Psychiatric Association. (unknown). *Diagnostic and statistical manual of mental disorders* (5th ed.). Washington, DC: Author.

American Psychiatric Association. (2007, August 20). American Psychological Association calls on U.S. government to prohibit the use of unethical interrogation techniques. Retrieved from http://www.apa.org/news/press/releases/2007/08/council-res.aspx

Basoglu, M. (1992). Introduction. In M. Başoğlu (Ed.), *Torture and its consequences: Current treatment approaches* (pp. 1–22). New York, NY: Cambridge Press.

Basoglu, M. (1998). Behavioral and cognitive treatment of survivors of torture. In J. M Saranson and M. K. Popkin (Eds.), *Caring for victims of torture* (pp. 131–148). Washington, DC: American Psychiatric Press.

Basoglu, M. J., Jaranson, J. M, Mollica, R., & Kastrup, M. (2001). Torture and mental health: A research overview. In T. K. E. Garrity (Ed.), *The mental health consequences of torture* (pp. 35–62). New York, NY: Plenum.

Basoglu, M., Paker, M., Paker, O., Ozmen, E., Marks, I., Incesu, C., & Sarimurat, N. (1994). Psychological effects of torture: A comparison of tortured with nontortured political activists in Turkey. *American Journal of Psychiatry, 151*(1), 76–81.

Bryant-Davis, T., Tillman, S., Marks, A., & Smith, K. (2009). Millennium abolitionists: Addressing the sexual trafficking of African women. *Beliefs and Values: Understanding the global implications of human nature.* International Beliefs and Values Institute.

Campbell, T. (2007). Psychological assessment, diagnosis, and treatment of torture survivors: A review. *Clinical Psychology Review, 27,* 628–641.

Canda, E. R. & Phaobtong, T. (1992). Buddhism as support system for South East Asian refugees. *Social Work, 37*(1), 617–667.

Choi, C. (2010). A pilot analysis of the psychological themes found during the CARING at Columbia—Music therapy program with refugee adolescents from North Korea. *Journal of Music Therapy, XLVII*(4), 380–407.

Chung, R. C. (2009). Cultural perspectives on child trafficking, human rights & social justice: A model for psychologists. *Counseling Psychology Quarterly, 22*(1), 85–96.

Cox, P. (2011). Issues in safeguarding refugee and asylum-seeking children and young people: Research and practice. *Child Abuse Review, 20,* 341–360.

Crawford, M., & Kaufman, M. R. (2008). Sex trafficking in Nepal: Survivor characteristics and long-term outcomes. *Violence against Women, 14*(8), 905–916.

Denov, M., & Maclure, R. (2006). Engaging the voices of girls in the aftermath of Sierra Leone's conflict: Experiences and perspectives in a culture of violence. *Anthropologica, 48*(1), 73–85.

Farley, M. (2003). Prostitution and the invisibility of harm. *Women & Therapy, 26*(3), 247–280.

Felson, Richard B. (2002). *Violence and Gender Reexamined.* American Psychological Association.

Fernado, G. (2005a). Interventions for survivors of the tsunami disaster: Report from Sri Lanka. *Journal of Traumatic Stress, 17,* 267–268.

Fernando, G. (2005b, November). Differential impact of traumatic events on the psychosocial well being of Sri Lankans. Paper presented at the Annual meeting of the International Society of Stress Studies, Toronto, Canada.

First, M. B., Spitzer, R. L., Gibbon, M., & Williams, J. (1996). *Structured clinical interview for DSM-IV Axis I Disorders—Patient Edition (SCID-I/P, Version 2.0.* Biometrics Research Department. New York, NY: New York State Psychiatric Institute.

Gibson, J. L. (2004). Does truth lead to reconciliation? Testing the causal assumptions of the South African Truth and Reconciliation process. *American Journal of Political Science, 48*(2), 201–217.

Gjermeni, E., Van Hook, M. P., Gjipali, S., Xhillari, L., Lungu, F., & Hazizi, A. (2008). Trafficking of children in Albania: Patterns of recruitment and reintegration. *Child Abuse & Neglect, 32*(10), 941–948.

Goldfield, A. M. (1988). The physical and psychological sequelae of torture: Symptomatology and diagnosis. *Journal of the American Medical Association, 259,* 2725–2729.

Hanscom, K. (2001). Treating survivors of war trauma and torture. *American Psychologist, 56,* 1032–1039.

Henley, J., & Robinson, J. (2011). Mental health issues among refugee children. *Clinical Psychologist, 15,* 51–62.

Hinton, D., Hsia, C., Um, K., & Otto, M. W. (2003). Anger-associated panic attacks in Cambodian refugees with PTSD; a multiple baseline examination of clinical data. *Behaviour Research and Therapy, 41*(6), 647–654.

Hooberman, J. B., Rosenfeld, B., Lhewa, D., Rasmussen, A., & Keller, A., (2007). Classifying the torture experiences of refugees living in the United States. *Journal of Interpersonal Violence, 22*(1), 108–123.

International Organization of Migration (IOM). (2007). The IOM handbook on direct assistance for victims of trafficking. Retrieved from http://www.iom.int/jahia/webdav/site/myjahiasite/shared/shared/mainsite/published_docs/books/CT%20handbook.pdf [1 October 2010]

International Organization of Migration (IOM). (2012). The ILO 2012 global estimate of forced labor executive summary. Retrieved from http://www.ilo.org/wcmsp5/groups/public/—ed_norm/—declaration/documents/publication/wcms_181953.pdf

Khamphakdy-Brown, S. Jones, L. N., Nilsson, J. E., Russel, E. B., & Klevens, C. L. (2006). The empowerment program: An application of an outreach program for refugee and immigrant women. *Journal of Mental Health Counseling, 28*(1), 38–47.

Kinderman, P. (2007). Commentary: Human rights and applied psychology. *Journal of Community & Applied Social Psychology, 17*(3), 218–228.

Kira, I., Clifford, D., Wiencek, P., & Al-Haidar, A. (2003). Iraqi refugees in Southeast Michigan: *First report. Unpublished Manuscript.*

Kotrla, K. (2010). Domestic minor sex trafficking in the United States. *Social Work, 55*(2), 181–187.

Limoncelli, Stephanie A. (2009). The trouble with trafficking: Conceptualizing women's sexual labor and economic rights. *Women's Studies International Forum, 32*(4), 261–269.

Lykes, M. (2000). Possible contributions of a psychology of liberation: Whither health and human rights?. *Journal of Health Psychology, 5*(3), 383–397.

Martin, D. C., & Yankay, J. E. (2012). Refugees and Asylees: 2011. Office of Immigration Statistics, 1–7.

Melton, G. B. (2010). It's all about relationships! The psychology of human rights. *American Journal of Orthopsychiatry, 80*(2), 161–169.

Milillo, D. (2006). Rape as a tactic of war: Social and psychological perspectives. *Affilia, 21*, 196–204.

Mollica, R., & Caspi-Yavin, Y. (1991). Measuring torture and torture related symptoms. *Journal of Counsulting and Clinical Psychology, 3*(4), 581–587.

Mollica, R., McInnes, K., Pham, T., Smith-Fawzi, M., Murphy, E., & Lin, L. (1998). The dose-effect relationship between torture and psychiatric symptoms in Vietnamese expolitical detainees and a comparison group. *Journal of Nervous and Mental Disease, 189*(9), 543–553.

Mukamana, D., & Brysiewicz, P. (2008). The lived experience of genocide rape survivors in Rwanda. *Journal of Nursing Scholarship, 40*, 379–384.

Paunovic, N., & Öst, L. G. (2001). Cognitive-behavior therapy vs. exposure therapy in the treatment of PTSD in refugees. *Behaviour Research and Therapy, 29*, 1183–1197.

Physicians for Human Rights (2010). A White Paper. Experiments in torture: Evidence of human subject research and experimentation in the "Enhanced" Interrogation Program.

Polaris Project. (2012). Survivor Stories. [Web file]. Retrieved from http://www.polarisproject.org/what-we-do/client-services/survivor-stories

Proceedings of Stockholm International Forum: A Conference on Truth, Justice and Reconciliation, Stockholm (2002, April 23–24), Stockholm: Regeringskanliet.

Ramona, V. (2010). The State, the family and language of "social evils": Re-stigmatising victims of trafficking in Vietnam. *Culture, Health & Sexuality: An International Journal for Research, Intervention and Care, 12*(S1), S89–S102.

Raymond, J., & Hughes, D. (2011). Sex trafficking of women in the United States: International and domestic trends. Retrieved from http://www.catwinternational.org/Home/Article/99-sex-trafficking-of-women-in-the-united-states-international-and-domestic-trends

Renner, W., Laireiter, A., & Maier, M. J. (2012). Social support as a moderator of acculturative stress among refugees and asylum seekers. *Social Behavior and Personality, 40*(1), 129–126. doi: 10.2224/sbp.2012.40.1.129

Schauer, M. N. (2005). *Narrative exposure therapy: A short term intervention for traumatic stress disorders after war, terror, or torture.* Cambridge, MA: Hogrefe and Huber.

Sossou, M., & Yogtiba, J. (2009). Abuse of children in West Africa: Implications for social work education and practice. *British Journal of Social Work, 39*(7), 1218–1234.

Staub, E. (1989). *The roots of evil: The psychological and cultural origins of genocide and other forms of group violence.* New York, NY: Cambridge University Press.

Staub, E. (2006). Reconciliation after genocide, mass killing, or intractable conflict: Understanding the roots of violence, psychological recovery, and steps toward a general theory. *Political Psychology, 27*(6), 867–894.

Staub, E. (2007). Preventing violence and terrorism and promoting positive relations between Dutch and Muslim communities in Amsterdam. *Peace and Conflict: Journal of Peace Psychology, 13* (3), 333–361.

Staub, E., & Pearlman, L. A. (2001). Healing, reconciliation, and forgiving after genocide and other collective violence. In R.G. Helmick & R.L. Petersen (Eds.), *Forgiveness and reconciliation: Religion, public policy, and conflict transformation* (pp. 195–217). Radnor, PA: Templeton Foundation Press.

Staub, E., & Pearlman, L. A. (2006). Psychological interventions in times of crisis. In L. Barbanel & R. Sternberg (Eds.), *Advancing healing and reconciliation* (pp. 213–245). New York, NY: Springer-Verlag.

Tajfel, H., & Turner, J. C. (1986). The social identity theory of inter-group behavior. In S. Worchel & L. W. Austin (Eds.), *Psychology of intergroup relations* (pp. 7–24). Chicago, IL: Nelson-Hall.

Tomaselli, S., & Porter, R. (1986). *Rape*. Oxford, UK: Blackwell.

United Nations High Commisioner for Refugees (UNHCR). (2011). UNHCR Global trends. Retrieved from http://www.unhcr.org/4fd6f87f9.html

United Nations Office on Drug and Crime (UNODC). (2012). *Global Report on Trafficking in Persons 2012.* Retrieved from: http://www.unodc.org/documents/data-and-analysis/glotip/Trafficking _in_ Persons _2012_web.pdf

United Nations Population Fund. (1999). Reproductive health in refugee situations. New York, NY: Author.

Weine, S. M. (2011). Developing preventive mental health interventions for refugee families in resettlement. *Family Process, 50*(3), 410–430.

Wilson, J. M., & Dalton, E. (2008). Human trafficking in the heartland: Variation in law enforcement awareness and response. *Journal of Contemporary Criminal Justice, 24*(3), 296–313.

Yakushko, O. (2009). Human trafficking: A review for mental health professionals. *International Journal for the Advancement of Counseling, 31,* 158–167.

Part 2

Professional Issues

Chapter 13

Pedagogical Tools for Social Justice and Psychology[1]

Maurianne Adams, Maureen Perry-Jenkins, and Linda R. Tropp

This chapter brings together two academic disciplines—social justice and psychology—and explores whether the pedagogical tools developed in the interdisciplinary field of social justice education (SJE) are applicable to subfields in psychology. The three authors recognize the complexity of this linkage and have explored its challenge in their own classroom practice. The first author is a college and graduate-level social justice educator whose social justice practice was strongly influenced by counseling, developmental, and social psychology. The second author is a developmental psychologist in a clinical psychology program who has drawn intentionally on social justice in both research and teaching to examine how social inequities shape human development. The third author is a social psychologist whose research and training of students emphasizes quantitative methods that address socially relevant research questions and that are in many ways conceptually aligned with principles of social justice pedagogy.

We organize this chapter in keeping with the empirical research traditions of psychology and the value of situating ourselves professionally and personally in relation to our subject matter. We start with an overview of SJE as an interdisciplinary field primarily situated in schools of education within the academy, and present some principles of social justice pedagogical practice derived from several subdisciplines of psychology. We then describe our views regarding the role of social justice and its pedagogies in two specific subdisciplines within psychology, namely developmental psychology and social psychology. In this section, we describe our classroom practice with specific examples of social justice pedagogical tools in use in our classrooms, both at the undergraduate and graduate levels. We conclude by reflecting on the importance of founding principles from psychology to the development of SJE and suggest the implementation of these principles in the psychology classroom and the training of clinicians.

OVERVIEW OF KEY TERMS, ACADEMIC DISCIPLINES, AND PRINCIPLES OF PRACTICE

We start by clarifying what we mean by justice and social justice, and asking what a social justice approach has to offer the subdisciplines within psychology.

Traditions of Justice and Social Justice

For contemporary discussions of justice as well as *social* justice, the work of John Rawls (1971, 2001) is a good place to start, given its political and philosophical emphasis on "the basic structure[s] of society" and society defined as "a more or less self-sufficient association of persons who in their relations to one another recognize certain rules of conduct as binding and who for the most part act in accordance with them" (1971, p. 3). Justice is stipulated by Rawls to be "the first virtue of social institutions, as truth is of systems of thought" (1971, p. 3) "because the effects of the basic structure on citizens' aims, aspirations, and character, as well as on their opportunities and their ability to take advantage of them, are pervasive and present from the beginning of life" (2001, p. 10). He imagines social justice on the basis of a theoretical "original position," or shifting his metaphor, a "veil of ignorance," as if individuals were able to structure society without reference to how they might personally gain or lose based on the social structure they imagined (Rawls, 1971, pp. 12, 136–142). For these reasons, and to arrive at fair and impartial principles of justice despite the inherent and inevitable inequities derived from accidents of birth and fortune, Rawls asks that principles of justice start at a point at which all people are ignorant of their social location and can be imagined to agree upon impartial principles of justice.

Although Rawls presents an important starting point for contemporary discussions of social justice, equally important are the social movements of the 1960s that took issue with theories of the individual as the basis for justice and rights (as articulated, for example, by the French Revolution, the U.S Constitution, and the Rawlsian philosophical tradition). For the emergent movements of the 1960s, the accumulations of unaddressed social inequality, inequity, and injury became the basis for organized and sustained social protest. For example, the civil rights movement challenged race-based injustices in voting rights, *de jure* segregation, "separate but equal" schooling, and systemic political and economic disenfranchisement. The women's movement focused on gender inequity at home and in the workplace. Social justice claims characterized movements for gay, lesbian, bisexual, and transgender rights, for disability rights, against classism, and against age-based injustices. Native American peoples sought redress in the courts for their loss of access to sacred sites appropriated during the U.S. westward-expansion and Native American removals.

These claims for social justice—whether posed by Rawls or thinkers rooted in social movements—challenge structural patterns of advantage and disadvantage based on social group memberships as distinct from rights and privileges that accrue to citizens as individuals. The discourse on social justice emphasizes procedures, relationships, and social position; it asks for recognition, respect, a role in decision making, and access to power and opportunity. As articulated by Iris Marion Young (1990), social justice movements ask "who benefits and who is harmed" through analyses of social position and status as well as economic or political interests.

For these reasons, contemporary social justice literature explores the unconscious assumptions and structural features of social hierarchies that perpetuate inequalities, and the commonalities of social status, shared histories, and grievances that characterize members of marginalized social identity groups (Young, 1990). The concerns associated with social justice differ from those associated with individual justice concerns in that social justice focuses attention on the recognition of structural inequality in decision-making processes and procedures and in the division of labor and status hierarchies, and it regards these criteria as important for the redistribution of material goods such as things, resources, income, and jobs as well as the recognition of privileged or disadvantaged social groups and positions (Fraser 1997; Olson 2008; Young, 1990).

Disciplinary Roots of Social Justice Pedagogy in Psychology

Due to their social and cultural centrality, schools and college classrooms offer rewarding sites for exploring social justice questions. Accordingly, social justice scholars have asked whether K–12 schooling, higher education, and the array of academic disciplines inadvertently perpetuate and reproduce cultural and intellectual as well as material systems of advantage and disadvantage (Ayres, Quinn, & Stovall, 2009; Darder, Baltodano, & Torres, 2009). They explore the extent to which the voices and perspectives of students from marginalized social positions are included in classroom dynamics. In so doing, they document processes of curriculum transformation (Beyer & Apple, 1998; Schuster & Van Dyne, 1985) and principles of pedagogical practice rooted in different historical and disciplinary traditions that continue to nourish and influence each other in complex and beneficial ways (Adams, 2007, 2010).

Although the term *pedagogy* has been used broadly to refer to the total curriculum as it constrains, shapes, or offers opportunities for learning (Chapman & Hobbel, 2010; Freire, 1970), in this chapter, pedagogy refers to specific practices used by instructors to teach course content to a socially and culturally diverse group of students (Adams, 2007; Wink, 2000). The term pedagogy helps instructors to focus on the distinction (not always clear in the moment) between what is taught (subject matter, course content) and how it is taught (instructional designs and materials, including lectures, dialogue, small-group discussions, audio-visual materials to illustrate content or stimulate discussion).

Given the focus of this chapter on social justice pedagogies and psychology, it is important to note that some of the sturdiest roots of social justice pedagogy started as transplants from psychological research. Examples include the work of Gordon Allport (1954/79) and Kurt Lewin (1938); Bronfenbrenner's (1979) ecological theory in developmental psychology, research grounded in social identity and identity-based consciousness-raising (Sherif & Sherif, 1970); experiential, social-learning reforms identified with John Dewey (1916/1944); and the application of psychological research to challenging the "separate but equal" doctrine in *Brown v. Board of Education* (Pettigrew, 2004; Pettigrew & Tropp, 2005). Scholars within psychology have noted the impact of cognitive science and developmental theory on college learning theory (Nummedal, Benson, & Chew, 2002). The contribution of early-to-mid-20th-century psychological research with social justice principles of educational research offers a suggestive foundation for social justice pedagogical practice in the psychology classroom.

Three of the key frameworks for pedagogy developed by social justice educators during the past half-century draw explicitly from social, developmental, and counseling psychology. From social psychology, social justice theorists learned how social group differences are perpetuated, and how social inequalities are rationalized and reproduced in education as in other social institutions. Studies of group dynamics and intergroup processes reach back to Kurt Lewin's exploration of intergroup prejudice in 1940s community settings, where he observed how simulations and feedback within small-group interactions can elicit interpersonal and group awareness that "get into the shoes of the other" (Bradford, Gibb, & Benne, 1964; Lippitt, 1949). Lewin's basic principles of structured, facilitated group interactions enabled participants in SJE to achieve insight into themselves and each other in mixed group-based settings. Practices based on Lewin's initial research led to the fields of group dynamics, multicultural group process, and intergroup dialogue, all of which shaped social justice pedagogies (Adams, 2007, 2010).

In Lewin's spirit, social justice instructors have learned how to use films, discussions, simulations, or structured interactions as specific, socially situated prompts for discussion and interpretation of challenging abstractions about racism, classism, and other oppressions that can then be interpreted and analyzed (processed) from multiple perspectives, with varying degrees of feedback for individual classroom participants. Most recently, pedagogical tools associated with structured intergroup dialogue, which has a line of direct descent from the work of Pettigrew and others on the conditions that govern effective intergroup contact, have been used with considerable success in educational and community settings (Engberg, 2004; Schoem & Hurtado, 2001; Stephan & Vogt, 2004), and have benefitted from research linking specific outcomes to a range of social justice pedagogical tools (Engberg, 2004; Nagda, Gurin, Sorensen, & Zuñiga, 2009; Zúñiga, Lopez, & Ford 2012).

A second legacy from psychology to social justice starts from Piagetian cognitive development and Eriksonian social developmental legacy applied to development within social justice settings by educators who draw upon Vygotsky and cultural-historical psychology (Cole, 1996; Moll, 1990; Rogoff, 2003; Wertsch, 1985; Wertsch & Kanner, 1992). Cognitive development research enables social justice educators to understand pathways by which learners' meaning-making develops from simple, dichotomous, either-or thinking to complex, critical abstract thought that is capable of coordinating the contradictions, divergent perspectives, and challenges posed by inequality and injustice or by different perspectives based on different social contexts and experiences (Bidell, Lee, Bouchie, Ward, & Brass, 1994; King & Kitchener, 1994; King & Shuford, 1996). Social justice educators use principles of cognitive development to anticipate and plan for the dissonance that occurs in the classroom when familiar ways of thinking are challenged by information or perspectives that contradict students' current ways of thinking.

In teaching social justice issues as part of discipline-specific course content, it is important that instructors pay attention to their students' evolving capacities and skill to think abstractly and to coordinate abstract theories about social systems or human processes with the anecdotes or personal experiences that are part of their concrete thinking. Challenging classroom interactions, along with specific pedagogical tools for working with them, have been described in cognitive development literature on college students, female learners, and the development of what is generally called critical thinking or reflective judgment (Baxter Magolda, 1992; Belenky, Clinchy, Goldberger, & Tarule, 1986; King & Kitchener, 1994). Nummedal et al. (2002) call attention to "the problem of prior knowledge" by which they mean the preconceptions held by their college-level psychology students, preconceptions largely based on "personal psychologies, the overgeneralization of anecdotal evidence, or the reification of common stereotypes" (p. 170). These preconceptions present special challenges when dealing with social justice issues and course content.

A third social justice pedagogical tradition, rooted in developmental as well as clinical and counseling psychology, brings together the cognitive and social dimensions of identity development in a relatively new literature on social identity development (racial, gender, sexual). Exemplars of this work in psychology include approaches to Black identity (Cross 1991, 2001; Tatum, 1997) and other racialized identities (Wijeyesinghe & Jackson, 2012). Tatum's application of racial identity development to the college classroom (1992, 1994) offers an example of a psychology of race and racism classroom in which racial identity development is used pedagogically to anticipate and support student responses to the challenges posed by course content.

In addition to the psychological roots that have over many decades nourished and informed social justice pedagogy, several other key disciplines and communities of practice have been generative, most notably feminist and antiracist theory, Paolo Freire, and critical theory, experiential education, and learning theory, to name some but not all. The following principles of social justice pedagogical practice are derived from sources such as these (Adams, 2007, 2012), and provide an overlay for specific pedagogical tools that we will describe later in this chapter.

Social Justice Principles of Pedagogical Practice

The overview of social justice and social justice pedagogy describes the focus of social justice educators on how we do what we do. This approach assumes that faculty want to achieve congruence between course content that deals with justice and equity, and the course procedures through which students experience such a course. Anticipating that student reactions might be challenging, disconcerted, confused, this approach encourages faculty to think ahead about the instructional procedures they plan to use, as well their options when planning goes awry.

1. SJE pedagogies balance the emotional and cognitive components of the learning process.
2. SJE pedagogies acknowledge and support the personal (the individual student's) experience while illuminating the systemic theories of the interactions among social groups and social systems.
3. SJE pedagogies pay attention to social relations and dynamics within the classroom.
4. SJE pedagogies utilize reflection and experience as tools for student-centered learning.
5. SJE pedagogies value awareness, personal growth, and change as outcomes of the learning process.
6. SJE pedagogies acknowledge and seek to transform the many ways in which identity-based social position and power, and privilege and disadvantage, shape participant interactions in the classroom and everyday contexts.

In the next section of this chapter, we use a personal voice instead of the objective third-person to position ourselves in relation to our disciplinary practice and to illustrate the ways in which we draw upon social justice pedagogy in descriptions of our own teaching practice.

POSITIONED IN ACADEME: ENGAGEMENT WITH SOCIAL JUSTICE IN THE CLASSROOM

Maurianne Adams

I entered academe in the 1960s with a PhD in English Literature and by the 1970s was collaborating with colleagues across disciplines to develop pedagogical practices that embodied social justice course content. Although not a psychologist by training, I participated in faculty institutes directed by Robert Kegan, Gil Noam, and Lawrence Kohlberg, and through them came to the work of the cognitive development tradition noted earlier.

As a new faculty member, I was disciplinarily proficient but pedagogically an amateur. A half century later, too many of us still teach in ways we ourselves were taught rather than drawing upon a research-based literature on teaching and learning that attends to the social and cultural differences at play in our classrooms. Given the dramatically shifting demographics within higher education, faculty across disciplines are turning to the emergent literature on social justice teaching and learning and assessing their own social justice curricular and pedagogical approaches (Adams, Bell, & Griffin, 2007; Chapman & Hobbel, 2010; Skubikowski, Wright, & Graf, 2009).

In the undergraduate general education course on diversity and social justice that my doctoral students teach and I supervise, we draw upon the principles of social justice practice listed in the first section of this chapter. We introduce ourselves (including the instructor) by recounting the meaning or the story behind our first or last names. This name-exchange locates each one of us socially, culturally, religiously, and/or historically (by way of migrations) in relation to each other, but also within national contexts or global diasporas to be discussed later in the course, thus linking the students' family histories to components of course content. In the first week, we exchange the hopes and concerns that each of us brings to this class (using 3 × 5 cards, small-group discussions, or whole-group brainstorming sessions), and then develop clear and explicit norms and guidelines for the entire semester based on the hopes and worries we have heard from each other. We acknowledge we'll have good use for these guidelines throughout the semester. (Instructors participate in developing norms and guidelines, based on our own hopes for the semester.) Among these norms is confidentiality, which means that personal stories or examples that students share with the class stay within the class.

In the first week, we also talk about learning edges, noting that students should not confuse feeling "comfortable" with feeling "safe," especially when they experience a learning edge on challenging topics. We distinguish safety from comfort in the process of creating group norms and discussion guidelines, based on the airing of student hopes and concerns about the course. For example, we ask students to write their hopes for the course on one side of a 3 × 5 card, and their concerns about the course on the other. We then collect, scramble, and redistribute the cards so that students can read them off, one by one, while we keep track on chalkboard or newsprint. Typically, students will hope to learn from each other's experiences, to be honest in exploring issues, and want to probe deeply rather than being superficial. Normally, students will worry that they will offend someone, say the wrong thing, or they will decide not to speak up. It is powerful for them to hear each other's hopes and concerns, read one by one, and it is then more powerful to build guidelines that they can revisit throughout the semester, in their effort as a group to achieve their hopes while avoiding their concerns. One important guideline that often emerges is the belief that everyone is there to learn, and that in the process of learning, they are all likely to make mistakes. Another important guideline is that of confidentiality—that students will take their insights and new information outside the classroom, but not stories or experiences that are told to them by their classmates.

For us, as instructors and facilitators, how we respond to these learning edges and opportunities for new learning, while reminding students that they are all there to learn, is a way of balancing the excitement (or butterflies) of not feeling comfortable with a sense that the classroom norms and guidelines will keep them safe. Similarly, there are ample opportunities during classroom discussions to remind students of why we have a guideline for confidentiality.

We use films, film clips, YouTube selections, and an array of current AV materials to illustrate and personalize the conceptual frameworks and social phenomena. We present short lectures to provide manageable chunks of new information, concepts, or clarification. Most of what we might call curricular information is conveyed through homework assignments or presented on the course website rather than classroom lecture. Valuable classroom time is reserved for active learning, based on interactions that explore, dramatize, and personalize the core concepts or information on the syllabus for that day. We have students draw upon multiple sources of information, and use ourselves as instruments to support their active student learning (Adams & Love, 2005, 2010; Marchesani & Adams, 1992).

Maureen Perry-Jenkins

Issues of multiculturalism, social disparities, and social justice have come to the forefront of my teaching in the past 10 years. My undergraduate education was in a traditional psychology program where the prevailing notion was that humans grow and develop in similar ways and where the primary goal was to control for variability in any factors, such as social class, race, and ethnicity, that may muddy our understanding of human development.

This perspective, however, was completely upended during my graduate training in a human development and family studies program, steeped in the theoretical work of Urie Bronfenbrenner, a developmental psychologist who shocked the field of developmental psychology in the mid-1970s by suggesting that social context was not something to be controlled away but rather was critical to understanding differences in developmental processes. Bronfenbrenner's students, in later years, began to show how social contexts such as social class, neighborhoods, and racial and ethnic backgrounds were key moderators of family processes. Bronfenbrenner's (1979, 2006) contention that social context is critical to understanding human development was contentious in the field of developmental psychology where the primary focus had been on randomized controlled trials (RCTs) s in laboratory settings that focused on aspects of children's social and cognitive development. In contrast, Bronfenbrenner conducted his studies, often RCTs, in children's homes, schools, and neighborhoods believing that these and other contexts influence and shape children's development in unique ways.

It is useful to understand that a core question that has guided developmental psychology from its inception is to what degree human development is guided by intrinsic biological processes or guided by environment: the classic nature-nurture debate. The field of developmental psychology has cycled between the ascendance of nurture versus nature since the late 1800s, although of late, developmental science has moved toward a dialectical perspective emphasizing the interconnectedness of the individual and context (Sameroff, 2010).

For example, current research on brain development, genes, and heritability focuses attention on the notion of plasticity in human development across the life course, plasticity being the idea that change, and the potential for change, varies across the life course and across individuals as a function of contextual factors, with critical interactions between genes and environment (Lerner, 2002). In fact, new areas of study such as cultural neuroscience and culture and cognitive development (Cole 1995; Miller & Kinsbourne, 2011) have grown exponentially over the past decade, highlighting the wedding of culture, neuroscience, and genetics. Moreover, provocative new research by Belsky and Pleuss (2009) argues that more plastic individuals may not only be more susceptible to negative life stressors but also more able to benefit from supportive environments than less plastic individuals.

The idea that it is the interaction of organismic and experiential factors in concert that produce development, what Gottlieb (2007, p. 1–2) labeled "probabilistic epigenesis," has changed the very nature of questions that developmental psychologists are asking. Considering how social context can shape everything from gene expression and neural circuitry in the brain to attachment behaviors and psychological well-being places both nature and nurture on equal footing. Thus, our research has begun to explore how contextual factors across the life course—factors as broad as social class and race to contexts as proximal as hormone levels during pregnancy—shape gene expression, and brain development and behavior. These developments have not only focused a spotlight on what aspects of culture matter, such as language, food, rituals, routines, inequities, power, life stressors, but also how these dimensions of culture differentially shape aspects of human development at different points across the life course. This heightened attention to the role of environment in human development, by its very nature, has stimulated discussions about how the quality of these environments, such as the availability of resources and privileges, inequities based on race, social class or gender, and oppression inherent in our laws and social mores, shapes developmental trajectories. Accordingly, as the field of developmental psychology has developed over the past half century, issues of social justice and equity have come to the forefront of discussions about development. As research in developmental psychology has demonstrated, significant relationships between social context and human development constitute a call to action for the discipline of developmental psychology. It is through this pathway that my research led me to understand that social justice issues must permeate not only my research but also my teaching, mentoring, and outreach.

Issues of SJE have become paramount in both my graduate and my undergraduate training. Turning first to SJE issues in our doctoral program in clinical psychology, it is important to understand that the American Psychological Association (APA) has numerous course requirements for graduate training. Specifically, graduate students must take courses in 18 substantive areas spanning biological, social, cognitive psychology and neuroscience as well as psychopathology, assessment, statistics, methods, and theory. Much of the training for clinical graduate students focuses on what students need to know and less on how they come to know it.

To understand how social justice issues came to the forefront of my graduate teaching, it is instructive to describe a series of events that occurred around the multicultural psychology course in our graduate program, a required course for all clinical graduate students. We had a class from social psychology, titled *Prejudice and Stereotyping*, which fulfilled the APA multicultural requirement and did an excellent job educating students on research that examines the causes and consequences of prejudice and stereotyping. Our students liked the class but kept coming back to the faculty and asking for more help understanding their own prejudice and stereotyping, and for opportunities to explore their own blind spots around issues of race, ethnicity, gender, social class, religiosity, and ability. If they were going to be out in the world practicing as clinicians or doing research with groups of individuals vastly different from themselves, they felt they needed to understand who they were as diverse individuals and to prepare themselves for their own research and practice across social differences and positionalities.

As faculty, we were fairly resistant to this request for many years. Pragmatically, we already had a course on the books that covered the requirement and did not want to spend new resources for another class. In terms of pedagogy, many faculty felt that the research class was fine and were disinclined to create experiential or touchy-feely courses when our job was to teach about research. The prospect of experiential teaching made many of my colleagues and me very uncomfortable and nervous; it was far easier to simply ignore the issue. As it became clear, however, that our students not only had valid points but also were not going to let the issue slide, a clinical colleague and I, two White women, accepted the challenge of designing a new course that had an experiential component as well as a more traditional educational focus on multicultural issues. We spent hours conceptualizing the class and our goals and met with consultants who could offer resources to help us link substantive issues with practice and experience.

In keeping with a basic principle of social justice, we worked to balance the emotional and cognitive components of the learning process. We developed a class that not only taught about the theories of racial identity development but also had each student evaluate his or her own racial and ethnic identity. We split the class into groups based on how individuals self-identified (e.g., White, Latino, Black) and then each group read through and discussed models about their own group's racial identity development (e.g., Cross, 1991). Each person then tried to identify at what stage he or she was in his or her own development. In addition, we often showed video clips of Tim Wise discussing racial identity; given that he is a White man and a social activist, his direct commentary about White privilege is especially powerful. We also examined research on social class and its relationship to mental health, while incorporating in-class activities that explored our own perceptions of social class privileges and disadvantages. We examined research on racial and ethnic inequality and analyzed the types of research questions we typically ask out in the field (e.g., Are their racial and ethnic differences in depression?) as well as the ones we are less likely to pose (e.g., Are our measures and assessments of psychopathology ethnocentric and class bound?).

The first time, we found this class to be both incredibly exhausting and exhilarating. It also became quite clear that once we began to use these new pedagogical tools in our graduate teaching, it would be impossible to turn back. The growth our students—and we as instructors, mentors, and guides—experienced during this class has, no doubt, made us better researchers as well as more effective teachers and practitioners. For example, as our psychology students (female and male) examined their own racial identity development and understood how their privileges and constraints in our society had affected their development, the notion of racial identity became not simply a construct to be assessed in our research protocols but something to consider as we assessed our personal roles in the research process. For example, after conducting home interviews with low-income families in the field, we came to weekly project meetings and considered how our own race and class shaped our experience on the interview and the experience of our families as well. This weekly exercise kept issues of race, class, and ethnicity foremost in our minds as we conducted our research.

Changes in the field of developmental psychology that are described earlier, having to do with the role of context in shaping pathways of development, have directly affected the readings and discussion topics in both my graduate and my undergraduate seminars on human development. I begin each of these classes by having students consider the question: "Are there universals that guide human developmental processes, regardless of context, or can human development only be understood in context?" Whereas much of developmental psychology has attempted to describe and understand normal developmental processes, and to that end, aim to control for environmental factors in the hopes of defining some true process, there are developmentalists who argue that in lieu of one, uniform psychology framed as normal, there are multiple, diverse psychologies, or developmental pathways, that question any single norm (Shweder et al., 2006). I use this framing in all my classes to consider the empirical research that supports these differing viewpoints. I challenge students in short writing assignments and debate exercises to make a case for the role of biology, the role of environment, and the interaction of the two as they influence all aspects of development from face processing and locomotion to emotion regulation and psychopathology.

Turning to my undergraduate teaching, psychology majors are required to take a breadth of classes across the subdisciplines of psychology. Although issues of social inequities and social justice have become themes in many of our undergraduate classes in social psychology, developmental psychology and clinical psychology, by and large these issues are taught about in lecture formats with limited discussion. Over the years, I have worked to broaden my use of different teaching approaches in my undergraduate course titled *Child, Family and Community*, in which we examine how social contextual factors, such as social class, race, ethnicity, gender, and religion, shape children's developmental trajectories.

At the outset, I spend considerable time exploring with students the role of social context in children's lives. Since all the students in this upper-level seminar are psychology majors, they often conceptualize development and change at a very individual level. I see my first job as broadening their view of factors that shape child development to look past the family to consider how broader social conditions and inequities play out in a child's life. For example, we read Joanna Lipper's *Growing Up Fast* (2003), which documents the lives of 10 teenage mothers in Pittsfield, Massachusetts, in the late 1990s. It highlights how the shutting down of a large General Electric plant in Massachusetts that moved its operations to China for lower labor costs, devastated a whole community, caused high unemployment, and led to a drug trade moving in from New York. In small groups, we discuss the stories of these 10 young women and analyze the multiple levels of influence that shaped their development and that of their infants. On large poster paper, we sketch out the multiple levels of influence that are at work and link processes to cognitive, social, and emotional outcomes. Each small group then brainstorms about possible levels of intervention, from very macro-level policies and social movements to micro-level therapeutic interventions that could enhance development.

Using an ecological model, we continue to explore how broader social systems and policies (e.g., Title IX, gay marriage) affect family life and child development. Students are assigned to assess the impacts of micro-systems, such as family and peer groups, and macro-systems, such as social class and race, on their own development. While they prepare this assignment, I present in class the ways in which family, schools, communities, media, social class, race, ethnicity, and gender all have influences on human development. We talk about how racism and White privilege affect the development of not only children of color but White children as well. This assignment enables students to draw on their own experiences to evaluate how social systems affect lives in both positive and negative ways and to use the ecological model as a tool for understanding human development.

I place high value on my students' personal growth and increasing awareness of social justice issues and try to incorporate activities into my class to jumpstart that process. For example, in an effort to explore the role of race and racism in human development, I have the undergraduate class watch a clip from the movie *Crash*, which is an intense, disturbing movie about race relations in the United States. During one class, after showing a clip where police sexually molest an African American woman during a routine traffic stop, a White male spoke up and said, "Well, that was a bit over dramatic." An African American woman in the class turned to him, glaring, and said, "You don't know what the hell you are talking about." The class then turned to me to address the conflict—and although I was a bit shaken—it was obvious that this was one of the teachable moments, or learning edges, that Maurianne notes earlier. I asked the class to take a deep breath, grab a piece of paper, and write about what they were feeling. This gave me some time to collect my thoughts. I asked them to hand in their anonymous comments, sleep on what happened, and come back to class in two days ready to discuss what had happened and how they felt about it. Not surprisingly, students had many intense, emotional reactions to the incident, but the time to reflect and think about their feelings proved to be extremely important. They got past the intensity of the moment and were able to identify what triggered many of their responses. We ended up having a meaningful and insightful discussion about power, privilege, and disadvantage, and considered how these types of incidents shape the day-to-day realities of all of us.

Linda R. Tropp

As a social psychologist, my research, teaching, and mentoring come together in three core values and goals as a scholar. The first involves a commitment to rigorous research used to address social issues and promote social justice. The second involves the dissemination and translation of research findings for practitioners and policymakers as well as across disciplinary boundaries, to broaden the impact of social psychological work and to effectively reduce conflict and improve relations between groups locally, nationally, and around the world. The third involves a concern for training and mentoring younger generations of scholars, while encouraging them to maintain a commitment to social issues and policy-relevant work as their careers unfold.

Generally, social psychologists focus on understanding how social situations, environments, and structures impact individuals. Many scholars in this area establish links between basic social psychological mechanisms and processes (e.g., cognitive, affective, motivational, behavioral) and their implications for social justice issues (e.g., reducing prejudice, promoting equality). Conducting socially relevant research has been part and parcel of my professional training and is a defining feature of professional associations such as the Society for the Psychological Study of Social Issues (SPSSI), which brings together psychologists and other social scientists interested in "the application of research on the psychological aspects of important social issues to public policy solutions" (SPSSI, 2013). With Kurt Lewin as one of its founders in the 1930s (see Bargal, Gold, & Lewin 1992), SPSSI and its members have been leaders in conducting scientific, action-oriented research toward the resolution of social problems.

Although social psychologists are typically engaged in a quest to identify general principles that underlie human cognition, emotion, and behavior, there is increasing awareness of the need to attend closely both to the shared commonality of human tendencies and the ways in which psychological processes and mechanisms may manifest themselves differently across social contexts. My training took place within a tradition that adopts such a contextualized social psychological approach (Pettigrew, 1991). This approach seeks to understand how psychological processes are impacted by their sociohistorical contexts (Christie, 2006) and by social conditions at multiple levels of analysis, including both specific situations and societal structures (Pettigrew, 2006). Scholars in this tradition tend to believe that this approach may help to bridge gaps between scientific research and its practical application, because greater contextualization can establish links between abstract theoretical principles and the concrete social realities relevant to policy and intervention (Brewer, 1997; Pettigrew, 2006; Stephan, 2006).

Part of this contextualization often involves adopting a phenomenological approach (Allport, 1954), whereby researchers seek to identify processes and mechanisms that guide individuals' psychological responses to their social environments. As such, researchers in this tradition often seek to understand how people perceive and experience their social contexts, and the psychological motivations and needs that underlie their emotional and behavioral responses to those contexts. Ultimately, adopting this kind of approach has social justice implications, particularly in the areas of intergroup relations and prejudice reduction: the better we can understand the perceptions and motivations that fuel intergroup prejudice and inequality, the more effectively we can devise strategies to reduce prejudice and work toward sustainable, equal, and peaceful relations between groups.

Despite this long-standing legacy, each generation of social psychologists must also work to establish their scientific credentials by testing theory-driven hypotheses using rigorous research methods. Although career-oriented and policy-oriented goals are not necessarily at odds with each other, many social psychologists seek to find a balance between demonstrating their legitimacy as research scientists and engaging in social justice issues. As such, I find that many highly motivated younger scholars ask if, when, and how they should become involved in social justice issues. My view is that each individual needs to make his or her own decision; and, whereas others might recommend that they wait until after tenure,

I typically encourage my graduate students and other early career scholars to think deeply and strategically about their broader professional goals and how engagement in social justice issues may contribute to reaching those goals. As such, my graduate students and I often discuss how their experiences in field settings can inform how they frame and test basic research questions, and how these field experiences in turn can help them evaluate extant psychological research and the likely effectiveness of strategies designed to promote prejudice reduction, reconciliation, and social justice. In recent years, and consistent with Lewin's original call for action-oriented research, greater numbers of social psychologists are actively maintaining a dual commitment to research rigor and broad social relevance; many social psychologists are now forging partnerships with nongovernmental organizations and policy advocates, while greater value is being granted to socially relevant research within the mainstream of the field.

Here, a primary issue concerns whether our research is or should be value-free (see Crosby, Clayton, Downing, & Iyer, 2004; Tropp, Smith, & Crosby, 2007). Historically, social scientists have sought to demonstrate their objectivity both in the pursuit of rigorous scientific research and to remove the stigma of being a value-laden (i.e., soft) field of study (see Haney, 1980). Yet, more broadly, we must consider whether the conclusions drawn from social scientific research are ever truly value-free. Given that scientists, like other people, reside within communities and societies that have shared norms and standards for behavior (Merton, 1968), we must acknowledge that the pursuit of scientific knowledge cannot be entirely independent of the values and influences from our social and historical contexts. Even when we attempt to maintain the highest standards of scientific integrity in our work, the kinds of questions we ask, the ways in which we frame arguments, and the sources to which we refer for information, all are likely to be influenced by what we perceive to be of value. Yet, recognizing that there is some degree of subjectivity in research need not diminish the scientific rigor of our work or the sound reasoning that underlies the conclusions we draw (see Crosby et al., 2004; Smith, 2000; Vollhardt & Bilali, 2008). Indeed, our values may influence decisions regarding the topics we choose to pursue without necessarily affecting our judgment in testing and evaluating research hypotheses in light of gathered data (Vollhardt & Bilali, 2008).

These issues are not only crucial considerations for social psychologists, but also inform the strategies we use to teach courses relevant to social justice issues. Often, undergraduate students grow accustomed to viewing course material through the lens of their own experiences, such that they find it challenging to consider perspectives that do not relate directly to their own experiences, or to consider how their individual experiences can be situated within broader societal processes. I invite undergraduates to consider how individual experiences and broad theoretical models can mutually inform each other, inviting them both to look beyond their own experiences to understand systemic processes and to evaluate the extent to which theoretical frameworks resonate with their experiences, to identify gaps in the existing literature and develop directions for future research. I typically assign both empirical research articles and contemporary essays on racial and ethnic relations as required readings, and I reserve time during class meetings for viewing relevant film clips and engaging in group discussions, to facilitate these processes and help students make connections between academic research and lived experience.

It is also important to note that undergraduates are likely to enter classrooms with a variety of prior experiences and perspectives regarding group relations and patterns of social inequality that carry important implications for teaching courses relevant to social justice issues. As such, at the start of each semester, I review some basic ground rules and norms for classroom discussions—emphasizing the fundamental importance of mutual respect when both listening and responding, and offering guidance on effective communication strategies—in an attempt to establish an equal status and cooperative environment for all members of the class. In so doing, I also highlight that we may not always see things in the same way, we may not always agree, and that discussions of sensitive topics may not always be easy, but that everyone in the classroom has something valid to say, given that we all live in a society consumed by group differences in status. As such, I seek to distinguish between the recognition that all students have equal opportunities to participate and their expectations that all students will necessarily have similar things to say.

Course content then swiftly proceeds to the review of guiding principles in social science research and broad theories of prejudice and intergroup relations to prepare students for later exploration of divergent perspectives and application to social policy. My hope is that by introducing students to theoretical concepts and models early on, they will be equipped with a common knowledge base and language for discussing these issues, which will help them to feel less personally threatened, more open to listening to others' views and experiences, and better able to engage if and when more sensitive topics emerge later in the course. Establishing this common knowledge base also assists me in guiding classroom discussions and encouraging students to consider alternate points of view in a way that is one step removed from their personal experiences. For example, rather than setting up a potentially alienating situation wherein a teacher might challenge their views, the shared knowledge base provides scaffolding for students to consider their position in the social structure, and to investigate how people in different status positions within a social structure might have very different views of the same context.

CLOSING THOUGHTS

Across subdisciplines of psychology, the importance of social context, and by definition, social injustice, have taken on increased significance because of the large research base pointing to the negative effects of racism, sexism, and classism on social interactions and human development. Great attention has been focused on these issues in both empirical studies and intervention projects. In classrooms, these topics have also begun to receive attention, but efforts to bring these issues to life in courses and in students' lives are lagging behind. Principals of SJE have been instrumental in providing tools and frameworks for linking the cognitive components of teaching with the emotional experience of studying social inequality in all its forms, yet the actual practice of including these approaches is a work in progress.

The central tenets of social justice—the role of social structures, institutions, policies, and practices in the process of socialization—are clearly relevant to many subfields of psychology. Yet, there remains the challenge of whether, and how, to incorporate social justice theories, principles, and practices in the preparation and supervision of psychological researchers, clinicians, and mental health professionals. In his collection of essays, *Advancing Social Justice through Clinical Practice*, Etiony Aldarondo (2007) comments:

> Without a clear appreciation of the social justice dimension of our work, it is relatively easy to confuse harmful effects of social conditions with psychological and interpersonal deficits or to focus on interpersonal and intrafamilial dynamics without understanding how these dynamics reflect the influence of social factors. (p. 12)

It is becoming evident that many psychological researchers, theorists, and practitioners in the clinical, therapeutic, and health worker fields understand the importance of social position, privilege, and disadvantage in relationships between client and therapist, in the framing of research questions and weighing of research variables, and in the dynamics of social life that shape human life. Still, it is likely that these factors will become more visible in the next generation, as our students take our places in academia, and as the role and measurement of social context becomes more central in all aspects of our research, teaching and practice: the contexts in which social justice education can occur.

NOTE

1. Material describing justice and social justice frameworks, and material presenting social justice principles of pedagogical process are adapted from the following sources: Adams, M. (2010). Social justice education. In D. Christie (Ed.), *Encyclopedia of peace psychology*. 2 vols. Hoboken, NJ: Wiley-Blackwell; Adams, M. (2010). Roots of social justice pedagogies in social movements. In T. D. Chapman & N. Hobbel (Eds.), *Social justice pedagogy across the curriculum: The practice of freedom* (pp. 59–85). New York: Routledge; Adams, M. (2007). Pedagogical frameworks for social justice education. In M. Adams, L. A. Bell, L.A., & P. Griffin (Eds.), *Teaching for diversity and social justice* (2nd ed., pp. 15–34). New York: Routledge.

REFERENCES

Adams, M. (2007). Pedagogical frameworks for social justice education. In M. Adams, L. A. Bell & P. Griffin (Eds.), *Teaching for diversity and social justice* (2nd ed., pp. 15–34). New York, NY: Routledge.

Adams, M. (2010). Roots of social justice pedagogies in social movements. In T. K. Chapman & N. Hobbel (Eds.), *Social justice pedagogy across the curriculum: The practice of freedom* (pp. 59–86). New York, NY: Routledge.

Adams, M. (2012). Social justice education. In D. Christie (Ed.), *The encyclopedia of peace psychology* (3rd ed., pp. 333–336). New York, NY: Wiley-Blackwell.

Adams, M., Bell, L. A., & Griffin, P. (2007). *Teaching for diversity and social justice* (2nd ed.). New York, NY: Routledge.

Adams, M., & Love, B. J. (2005). Teaching with a social justice perspective: A model for faculty seminars across academic disciplines. In M. L. Ouellett (Ed.), *Teaching inclusively: Diversity and faculty development.* Stillwater, OK: New Forums Press.

Adams, M., & Love, B. J. (2010). A social justice education faculty development framework for a post-grutter Era. In K. Skubikowski, C. Wright, & R. Graf (Eds.), *Social justice education: Inviting faculty to transform their institutions* (pp. 3–25). New York, NY: Stylus.

Aldarondo, E. (2007). *Advancing social justice through clinical practice.* Mahwah, NJ: Erlbaum.

Allport, G. W. (1954). *The nature of prejudice.* Reading, MA: Addison-Wesley.

Ayres, W., Quinn, T., & Stovall, D. (Eds.) (2009). *Handbook of social justice in education.* New York, NY: Routledge.

Bargal, D., Gold, M., & Lewin, M. (1992). The heritage of Kurt Lewin: Theory, research and practice. *Journal of Social Issues, 48,* 3–14.

Baxter-Magolda, M. B. (1992). *Knowing and reasoning in college: Gender-related patterns in students' intellectual development.* San Francisco: Jossey-Bass.

Belenky, M. F., Clinchy, M. B., Goldberger, N. R., & Tarule, J. M. (1986). *Women's ways of knowing: The development of self, voice, and mind.* New York, NY: Basic Books.

Belsky, J., & Pluess, M. (2009). The nature (and nurture?) of plasticity in early human development. *Perspectives on Psychological Science, 4,* 345–351.

Beyer, L. E., & Apple, M. W. (Eds.). (1998). *The curriculum: Problem, politics, and possibilities* (2nd ed.). Albany, NY: State University of New York Press.

Bidell, T. R., Lee, E. M., Bouchie, N., Ward, C., & Brasa, D. (1994). Developing conceptions of racism among young white adults in the context of cultural diversity coursework. *Journal of Adult Development, 1*(3), 185–200.

Bradford, L. P., Gibb, J. R., & Benne, K. D. (Eds.). (1964). *T-Group theory and laboratory method.* New York, NY: John Wiley & Sons.

Brewer, M. (1997). The social psychology of intergroup relations: Can research inform practice? *Journal of Social Issues, 53,* 197–211.

Bronfenbrenner, U. (1979). *The ecology of human development.* Cambridge, MA: Harvard University Press.

Bronfenbrenner, U. & Morris, P. A. (2006). The bioecological model of human development. In. R. M. Lerner & W. Damon (Eds.), *Theoretical models of human development* (Vol. 1, pp. 793–828). Hoboken, NJ: Wiley & Sons.

Chapman, T., & Hobbel, N. (Eds.) (2010). *Social justice pedagogy across the curriculum: The practice of freedom.* New York, NY: Routledge.

Christie, D. (2006). What is peace psychology the psychology of? *Journal of Social Issues, 62,* 1–17.
Cole, M. (1995). Culture and cognitive development: From cross-cultural research to creating systems of cultural mediation. *Culture and Psychology, 1*(1), 25–54.
Cole, M. (1996). *Cultural psychology: A once and future discipline.* Cambridge, MA: Harvard University Press.
Crosby, F. J., Clayton, S., Downing, R. A., & Iyer, A. (2004). Values and science. *American Psychologist, 59,* 125–126.
Cross, W. E., Jr. (1991). *Shades of Black: Diversity in African-American identity.* Philadelphia, PA: Temple University Press.
Cross, W. E., Jr. (2001). Encountering nigrescence. In J. G. Ponterotto, J. M. Casas, L. A. Suzuki, & C. M. Alexander (Eds.), *Handbook of multicultural counseling* (2nd ed, pp. 30–44). Thousand Oaks, CA: Sage.
Cross, W. E., Jr., & Phagen-Smith, P. (2001). Patterns of African-American identity development: A life-span perspective. In C. Wijeyesinghe & B. W. Jackson (Eds.), *New perspectives on racial identity development: A theoretical and practical anthology* (pp. 243–270). New York, NY: New York University Press.
Darder, A., Baltodano, M. P., & Torres, R. D. (Eds.) (2009). *The critical pedagogy reader.* New York, NY: Routledge.
Dewey, J. (1916/1944). *Democracy and education.* New York, NY: Simon & Schuster.
Engberg, M. E. (2004). Improving intergroup relations in higher education: A critical examination of the influences of educational interventions on racial bias. *Review of Educational Research, 74*(4), 473–524.
Fraser, N. (1997). *Justice inerruptus: Critical reflections on the "postsocialist" condition.* New York, NY: Routledge.
Freire, P. (1970). *Pedagogy of the oppressed.* New York, NY: Continuum.
Gottlieb, G. (2007). Probabilistic epigenesis. *Developmental Science, 10,* 1–11.
Haney, C. (1980). Psychology and legal change: On the limits of a factual jurisprudence. *Law and Human Behavior, 4,* 147–199.
King, P. M., & Kitchener, K. S. (1994). *Developing reflective judgment: Understanding and promoting intellectual growth and critical thinking in adolescents and adults.* San Francisco: Jossey-Bass.
King, P. M., & Shuford, B. C. (1996). A multicultural view is a more cognitively complex view: Cognitive development and multicultural education. *American Behavioral Scientist, 40*(2), 153–164.
Lerner, R. M. (2002). *Concepts and theories of human development.* New York, NY: Random House.
Lewin, K. (1946). Action research and minority problems. *Journal of Social Issues, 2*(4): 34–46.
Lippitt, R. (1949). *Training in community relations.* New York, NY: Harper & Brothers.
Marchesani, L. S., & Adams, M. (1992). Dynamics of diversity in the teaching-learning process: A faculty development model for analysis and action. In M. Adams (Ed.), *Promoting diversity in college classrooms: Innovative responses for the curriculum, faculty, and institutions* (pp. 9–20, New Directions for Teaching and Learning, 52). San Francisco: Jossey-Bass.
Merton, R. K. (1968). *Social theory and social structure.* New York, NY: Free Press.
Moll, L. C. (Ed.). (1990). *Vygotsky and education: Instructional implications and applications of sociohistorical psychology.* Cambridge, UK: Cambridge University Press.

Nagda, Bj. A., Gurin, P., Sorensen, N., & Zuñiga, X. (2009). Evaluating intergroup dialogue: Engaging diversity for personal and social responsibility. *Diversity and Democracy, 12*(1), 4–6.

Nummedal, S. G., Benson, J. B., & Chew, S. I. (2002). Disciplinary styles in the scholarship of teaching and learning: A view from psychology. In M. T. Huber & S. R. Morreale (Eds.), *Disciplinary styles in the scholarship of teaching and learning: Exploring common ground* (pp. 163–180). Menlo Park, CA: Carnegie Foundation for the Advancement of Teaching and American Association for Higher Education.

Olson, K. (2008). *Adding insult to injury: Nancy Fraser debates her critics.* London, UK: Verso.

Pettigrew, T. F. (1991). Toward unity and bold theory: Popperian suggestions for two persistent problems of social psychology. In C. W. Stephan, W. G. Stephan, & T. Pettigrew (Eds.), *The future of social psychology: Defining the relationship between sociology and psychology* (pp. 13–27). New York, NY: Springer.

Pettigrew, T. F. (2004). Justice deferred: A half-century after *Brown v. Board of Education. American Psychologist,* 59(6), 521–529.

Pettigrew, T. F. (2006). The advantages of multilevel approaches. *Journal of Social Issues, 62,* 615–620.

Pettigrew, T. F., & Tropp, L. R. (2005). Allport's intergroup contact hypothesis: Its history and influence. In J. F. Dovidio, P. Glick, & I. Rudman (Eds.), *On the nature of prejudice: Fifty years after Allport* (pp. 262–277). Malden, MA: Blackwell.

Rawls, J. (1971). *A theory of justice.* Cambridge, MA: Belknap Press of Harvard University Press.

Rawls, J. (2001). *Justice as fairness: A restatement.* Kelley, E. (Ed.). Cambridge, MA: Belknap Press of Harvard University Press.

Rogoff, B. (2003). *The cultural nature of human development.* Oxford, UK: Oxford University Press.

Sameroff, A. (2010). A unified theory of development: A dialectical integration of nature and nurture. *Child Development, 81*(1), 6–22.

Schoem, D., & Hurtado, S. (2001). *Intergroup dialogue: Deliberative democracy in school, college, community and workplace.* Ann Arbor: University of Michigan Press.

Schuster, M. R., & Van Dyne, S. R. (1985). *Women's place in the academy: Transforming the liberal arts curriculum.* Totowa, NJ: Roman 7 Allanheld.

Sherif, M., & Sherif, C. (1970). Black unrest as a social movement toward an emerging self-identity. *Journal of Social and Behavioral Sciences, 15*(3), 41–52.

Shweder, R. A., Goodnow, J. J., Giyoo, H., Levine, R., Markus, H. R., & Miller, P. J. (2006). The cultural psychology of development: One mind, many mentalities. In W. Damon & R. M. Lerner (Eds.), *Handbook of child psychology: Theoretical models of human development* (6th ed., Vol. 1, pp. 716–792). Hoboken, NJ: John Wiley & Sons.

Skubikowski, K., Wright, C., & Graf, R. (Eds.) (2009). *Social justice education: Inviting faculty to transform their institutions.* Sterling, VA: Stylus.

Smith, M. B. (2000). Values, politics, and psychology. *American Psychologist, 55*(10), 1151.

SPSSI (2013). Home page. Retrieved from www.SPSSI.org.

Stephan, W. G. (2006). Bridging the researcher-practitioner divide in intergroup relations. *Journal of Social Issues, 62,* 597–605.

Stephan, W. G., & Vogt, W. P. (2004). *Education programs for improving intergroup relations.* New York, NY: Teachers College Press.

Tatum, B. D. (1992). Talking about race, learning about racism: The application of racial identity development theory in the classroom. *Harvard Educational Review, 62*(1), 1–24.

Tatum, B. D. (1994). Teaching white students about racism: The search for white allies and the restoration of hope. *Teacher's College Record,* 95(4), 462–476.

Tatum, B. D. (1997). *"Why are all the Black kids sitting together in the cafeteria?" and other conversations about race.* New York, NY: BasicBooks.

Tropp, L. R., Smith, A. E., & Crosby, F. J. (2007). The use of research in the Seattle and Jefferson County desegregation cases: Connecting social science and the law. *Analyses of Social Issues and Public Policy, 7,* 93–120.

Vollhardt, J., & Bilali, R. (2008). Social psychology's contribution to the psychological study of peace: A review. *Social Psychology, 39,* 12–25.

Wertsch, J. V. (Ed.) (1985). *Culture, communication and cognition: Vygotskian perspectives.* Cambridge, UK and NY: Cambridge University Press.

Wertsch, J. V., & Kanner, B. G. (1992). A sociocultural approach to intellectual development. In R. J. Sternberg & C. V. Berg (Eds.), *Intellectual development.* Cambridge, UK: Cambridge University Press.

Wijeyesinghe, C. L., & Jackson, B. W. (2012). *New perspectives on racial identity development: Integrating emerging frameworks* (2nd ed.). New York, NY: NYU Press.

Wink, J. (2000). *Critical pedagogy: Notes from the real world* (2nd ed.). New York, NY: Longman.

Young, I. M. (1990). *Justice and the politics of difference.* Princeton, NJ: Princeton University Press.

Zuñiga, X., Lopez, G. E., & Ford, K. A. (2012). *Intergroup dialogue: Engaging difference, social identities, and social justice.* Special Theme Issue of *Equity & Excellence in Education, 45* (1), 1–236.

Chapter 14

A Model for Integrating Social Justice Roles in Psychology Doctoral Training: The Case of Counseling Psychology[1]

Lisa A. Goodman, Belle Liang, Pratyusha Tummala-Narra, Angela M. Borges, Milena Claudius, and Julie Woulfe

Over the last several decades, scholars, practitioners, and activists across subdisciplines of professional psychology have called for a greater focus on social justice in graduate programs, training the next generation of practicing psychologists (e.g., Arredondo & Rosen, 2007; Fox, Prilleltensky, & Austin, 2009; Hage et al., 2007). This call has been especially pronounced in counseling psychology (Baluch, Pieterse, & Bolden, 2004; Caldwell & Vera, 2010; Fouad, Gerstein, & Toporek, 2006; Goodman et al., 2004; Ivey & Collins, 2003; Kiselica, 2004; Lewis, Toporek, & Ratts, 2010; Singh et al., 2010). In 2001, for example, at the conclusion of the National Counseling Psychology Conference in Houston, 88% of attendees voted to support the idea that counseling psychologists should reclaim a social advocacy agenda (Fouad et al., 2004); and in 2007, *The Journal for Social Action in Counseling and Psychology* was established.

In response, a growing body of scholarship on social justice training in counseling psychology has demonstrated graduate students' hunger for such training (e.g., Beer, Spanierman, Greene, & Todd, 2012; Singh et al., 2010), identified factors that contribute to the development of a social justice orientation and commitment (e.g., Caldwell & Vera, 2010; Miller & Sendrowitz, 2011), described the importance of a developmental framework for teaching and learning about social justice (e.g., Lewis et al., 2010), offered a range of overarching principles to guide social justice training (e.g., Goodman et al., 2004), and argued for teaching strategies that cross content areas and pedagogical techniques (didactic courses, experiential learning, clinical and community practice) (e.g., Burnes & Singh, 2010; Nilsson, Schale, & Khamphakdy-Brown, 2011; Talleyrand, Chung, & Bemak, 2006).

Although there has been widespread support for social justice training at the doctoral level, scholars have also pointed out the lack of cohesive practice models that integrate traditional counseling approaches with social justice (e.g., Burnes & Singh, 2010; Pieterse, Evans, Risner-Butner, Collins, & Mason, 2009; Speight & Vera, 2008). Despite a handful of descriptions of practice innovations in counseling psychology programs across the country, few attempts have been made to integrate these descriptions into a model of graduate training. Following a brief overview of our conceptualization of social justice in the context of training, we describe a three-pronged model of training that integrates some of the inspiring examples of innovative teaching practices emerging from the counseling psychology literature. We conclude with a discussion of some of the common themes that emerge across teaching practices.

It is important to note that although this chapter focuses on the case of counseling psychology doctoral programs in particular, many have called for social justice training within other subdisciplines of the field of psychology—in this country and beyond (e.g., Diaz & Kirkel, 2012; Wilson & Meyer, 2011). Where applicable, we will comment on how our model can be applied in other types of graduate programs.

CONCEPTUALIZATION OF SOCIAL JUSTICE

Counseling psychologists have offered a wide variety of conceptualizations of social justice training (e.g., Lewis, Arnold, House, & Toporek, 2003; Pieterse et al., 2009; Ponterotto, Casas, Suzuki, & Alexander, 2009). Common across conceptualizations is the recognition that the individual struggles experienced by many communities are rooted in oppressive social, political, and cultural forces. Supporting mental health in those communities may therefore entail working to change those systems and structures (Goodman et al., 2004). Conversely, supporting people to make changes in their immediate contexts and larger communities may involve helping them address internal psychological barriers (Goodman et al., 2007; Moane, 2003). Neither part of this equation is possible without the other. Thus, social justice training in counseling psychology can be defined as supporting students to develop the capacities and skills necessary to work toward external, contextual change as well as internal, psychological change. Whereas traditional counseling psychology training tends to focus on the latter, a social justice–oriented training model focuses equally on both.

INTEGRATING SOCIAL JUSTICE INTO COUNSELING PSYCHOLOGY DOCTORAL TRAINING

Building on this conceptualization of social justice training, we offer the beginnings of a potential training model—developed based on a combination of our own experience as faculty and students in the counseling psychology program at Boston College and a review of innovative social justice training practices emerging from the counseling psychology literature. The model gives equal weight to (1) helping students increase awareness of their own social positions, especially in relation to the concepts of oppression and privilege (Adams, 2007), illustrated here through the example of learning through teaching; (2) teaching students how to integrate external context-change into traditional clinical practice, illustrated here through the example of advocacy training; and (3) training students to target community-level or systemic change, illustrated here through the example of service learning courses.

Expanding Social Justice–Related Self-Awareness through Teaching

An important aspect of social justice training—perhaps the first and foundational step—involves helping students increase awareness of their own social identities and how these identities shape their views of others as well as other's views of them (Adams, 2007). This kind of awareness is a necessary precursor to any attempt to intervene in people's contexts in ways that are built on a clear set of values and goals. Although all mental health providers are called on to engage in ongoing self-evaluation, a social justice framework stresses the need for self-reflection on how one's various social locations confer power or disempowerment (Moe, Perera-Dilitz, & Sepulveda, 2010). Referring to feminist therapy, but equally applicable to social justice–oriented practice, Brabeck and Brown (1997) wrote:

> [We] attend to hierarchies of power and dominance among and between people in all practice settings. We notice the ways in which we are both oppressed and oppressor, dominant and marginal, as well as the interactive relationships that emerge from these different positions of power. (p. 25)

Extending the idea of purposeful self-examination outside the bounds of the therapy office to the community, social justice scholars have introduced the term *multiple selves* to describe the ways that practitioners may interact with community members in different ways as they draw on different roles over time (Fine, 1992; LeCompte, 1995; Reinharz, 1997). Each of the multiple selves that emerge over the course of the work should be acknowledged and explored in terms of how they shape practitioners' interactions and how they create specific perceptions of practitioners' roles and intentions among community members (see Goodman et al., 2004 for a more detailed discussion of this idea).

Students can learn to do this kind of ongoing self-exploration in a variety of contexts, including seminars, lecture courses, counseling practica, and community work. This section illustrates the use of doctoral student teaching as one such context. Specifically, we describe the impact on doctoral students of the Boston College counseling psychology program's psychotherapy skills training model. This model requires all doctoral students to teach and supervise master's-level mental health counseling students as these students learn and practice helping skills. This teaching role (common to many graduate psychology programs that include doctoral and master's programs) provides fertile training ground for doctoral students to explore the idea of multiple selves in vivo. On the following pages, we describe briefly the counseling skills lab model and then illustrate how the lab provides doctoral students opportunities for self-examination and then transformation in relation to social location, privilege, and oppression.

The Counseling Skills Lab

The lab itself consists of a weekly meeting of 10 master's students and a doctoral student lab instructor, during which the master's students practice counseling skills they learn in an accompanying didactic course and explore personal challenges relevant to developing their professional identity. Lab instructors develop and implement their own curriculum for the weekly group sessions using multiple learning modalities, including counseling skills role plays, experiential exercises, small- and large-group discussions, and training videos. Outside the lab, students meet with the lab instructor in pairs for a dyadic supervision session in which they share recordings of role played counseling sessions and provide feedback to each other. Doctoral lab instructors, in turn, meet with a supervisor (as a group) every week to describe their experience of teaching and the observations about self and others that emerge from the experience.

A core feature of the lab is the integration of social justice–related knowledge and traditional counseling skills. Thus, doctoral student instructors and master's students are engaged in a parallel process: while doctoral students are engaging in the self-examination necessary for good teaching from a social justice perspective, they are providing opportunities for self-reflection to the master's students through their teaching and supervision. To illustrate this process, we next provide one telling example, drawn from the experience of Julie Woulfe.

Case Example

Julie, a White woman who identifies herself as queer (bisexual), described how teaching the lab helped her examine her multiple intersecting identities.[2] Julie was teaching a lab with a racially diverse group of nine women and one man (reflecting the gender demographics of the program). During the second semester of the course, the man, who was Black, spoke with her in supervision about his feelings of disengagement from the lab. He felt that he was an outsider in the lab group because (1) the counseling styles used in the lab represented the way women would counsel women; he did not see the therapy as representing how he might counsel male clients; and (2) when the group did counseling role plays, the clients were mostly White, women, and sexual minority clients. Julie recognized this moment as a learning opportunity for herself. With the help of a supervisor and her peer lab instructors, she identified four specific insights she gained from her conversation with the student and her own reflection on her multiple selves in the role of lab instructor.

First, Julie realized that she had been basing the clients she played in role-plays on herself, in part because she felt uncomfortable representing identities and experiences she did not hold. However, in the process, she realized that she may have "whitewashed" the role-play experiences by always playing a young White woman, a queer White woman, or someone with a similar identity to herself. Although she was well meaning, she recognized that this expression of White privilege was likely contributing to this student's disengagement. Second, she realized that this man's experience in her lab was inseparable from his broader experience of counseling psychology, which systematically overrepresented White people and White people's experience. This was underlined for her when, after her conversation with the student, she went to look for therapy videos that had more racial diversity and had a difficult time finding them. As a result, she began to think about ways to revise the curriculum so that she was not just using her own frames of reference in the role-plays.

Third, because Julie had been open with her lab group about her sexual identity as a queer woman, several other members of the lab had become interested in issues of sexual and gender diversity; so she and many students had chosen to role-play LGBTQ individuals in class and in their individual dyads. Given the marginalization of LGBTQ identified individuals both in society and in the field, she admitted she very much enjoyed the students' enthusiasm and encouraged it. In retrospect, she wondered whether she used her privileged positions as the instructor and as a White person to gratify a need coming from her experience of heterosexism; and in turn, whether that decision was unintentionally made at the expense of the Black man in her group.

Fourth, this teaching moment caused her to consider what it means to do therapy as a raced, classed, gendered being. In particular, she reflected on the gendered aspect, wondering whether she had chosen to emphasize skills that come more naturally to her, having been socialized as a woman. She said, "I found myself wondering if I was teaching a 'White Lady' version of therapy." Whatever the answer to these challenging questions, this is exactly the type of inquiry that instructors must undertake in order to investigate their positionality vis-à-vis their students; and it is the kind of investigation that psychologists must undertake in both individual- and community-level work.

Since many graduate programs outside of counseling psychology engage doctoral students in teaching undergraduate or graduate students courses, this strategy for incorporating social justice into doctoral training can be readily adapted for other types of graduate programs. For example, doctoral student instructors can infuse literature on privilege and oppression into their course curricula and can engage with peers in supervision groups to talk about the way their own social identities inform their teaching.

Bringing Advocacy to Traditional Clinical Practice

Armed with skills in self-examination, doctoral students are ready to engage in the second prong of the social justice training model proposed here: bringing context change to traditional clinical practice. Scholars and practitioners have identified a variety of ways of accomplishing this (e.g., Arredondo & Rosen, 2007; Burnes & Manese, 2008; Burnes & Singh, 2010; Goodman et al., 2004; Weintraub & Goodman, 2010). All share two unifying characteristics: first, as with multicultural and feminist approaches to practice, they highlight the interconnectedness between people's psychological well-being and the contextual factors that shape their experience. Second, moving a step beyond recognition of that interconnection, they underscore the need to help clients change oppressive conditions. This is often accomplished through advocacy (Lewis, Ratts, Paladino, & Toporek, 2011). In the next section, we provide a brief description of the nature of advocacy in the context of clinical practice, and then highlight three examples of how doctoral programs have begun to incorporate advocacy training into their curriculum.

Advocacy in Clinical Practice

Advocacy can be defined as actions taken to facilitate the removal of external barriers to opportunity and well-being (Toporek, 2000). Although advocacy may take a variety of forms, its goals appear to span a continuum ranging from expanding access to services and opportunities for individuals and families (micro-level advocacy) to system change (macro-level advocacy). Given this section's focus on the intersection of advocacy and clinical practice, it focuses on micro-level advocacy that takes place in conjunction with traditional psychotherapy rather than macro-level advocacy, although the two levels are often intertwined and inseparable. (Macro-level advocacy is described in the next section.)

At the micro level, advocacy usually involves identifying obstacles to clients' health and well-being, identifying both client strengths and potential allies for confronting those obstacles, and collaborating with clients and allies to gain access to the resources needed to improve well-being (Green, McCollum, & Hays, 2008). Mental health practitioners can use advocacy in different ways and for different purposes depending on a variety of contextual factors. For example, to determine whether to advocate on behalf of clients versus simply supporting clients to advocate for themselves, a counselor might consider the client's mental health status, relative access to resources, or power dynamics within the therapist–client relationship and between the client and a particular system (Toporek, Lewis, & Ratts, 2010).

Regarding what to advocate for outside the mental health context, micro-level advocacy is often conducted within agencies focusing on a particular issue (e.g., housing, domestic violence, legal issues, medical treatment), wherein advocates usually target specific problems (Goodman & Epstein, 2008). However, in the context of mental health counseling, clients may present with multiple and interdependent external needs and difficulties that should be addressed. Indeed, the line between internal and external needs may be entirely blurred. For example, a therapist may help a client obtain food stamps, then explore with her the shame she feels when the manager at her grocery store tells her loudly that her food stamps do not cover the type of food she tries to buy, and then perhaps work with her to change the way this and other managers speak to people using food stamps (Goodman, Pugach, Skolnik, & Smith, 2013. Advocating for low-income, multicultural students in an urban school may involve working directly with a student and then collaborating with a teacher to address the classroom dynamics that shape that student's experience and behavior.

Indeed, advocacy is complex work and raises a host of pragmatic, ethical, and conceptual challenges (see Liang, Glenn, & Goodman, 2005 for a discussion of these). Not surprisingly, then, advocacy often goes unrecognized and unreimbursed—and may even be criticized as inappropriate to the role of therapist. In an attempt to remedy this situation, in 2003, the American Counseling Association (ACA) endorsed the ACA advocacy competencies (Lewis et al., 2003) to guide counselors interested in advocacy as a component of traditional clinical practice. Nevertheless, organized attempts to train professional psychologists in advocacy skills remain few and far between. Acknowledging the complexities of providing advocacy within a clinical context, a number of recent efforts have attempted to teach doctoral students more systematically how to engage in advocacy skills in the context of traditional clinical practice. The next section describes efforts underway at Seton Hall University, the University of Missouri-Kansas City, and Ball State University.

Seton Hall

At Seton Hall, first-year doctoral trainees participate in a year-long, twice weekly practicum in which they engage in counseling and advocacy at two distinct settings: an elementary school in a poor, urban part of New Jersey and an assisted living program for older adults (L. Palmer, personal communication, July 12, 2012). Doctoral trainees working at the elementary school learn that sometimes the best way to advocate for their student clients is to offer support and training directly to teachers—helping them understand the contextual factors influencing their students, and cope with the secondary traumatization they themselves are experiencing. By contrast, trainees at the assisted living site learn about the experience of older adults who may be isolated, disabled, and dealing with mental illness, family issues, and trauma histories. Just as trainees in the elementary school advocate for students by working with teachers, students in this setting advocate for their older clients by teaching caregivers (family members and health care providers) about the complex mental health needs of older adults.

Through their exposure to these two community settings, trainees learn how to address both individual and systematic factors that shape well-being as they shift from counseling to advocacy and back again. This is intensive work requiring a great deal of close supervision. Two faculty members and a group of third-year doctoral students work closely with first-year trainees on-site on a weekly basis. Indeed, both the strength and challenge of the Seton Hall training model is its labor intensiveness. Due to limited funding, there is no external supervision from the site staff for students, only internal supervision from the doctoral program (L. Palmer, personal communication, July 12, 2012).

University of Missouri-Kansas City

At the University of Missouri-Kansas City, doctoral students can opt to be part of an advocacy and counseling program working with and for immigrant and refugee women from all over the world, including Somalia, Sudan, Vietnam, Mexico, and Pakistan (Nilsson et al., 2011). Students help clients navigate language barriers, acculturation issues, unemployment, domestic violence, and other challenges through psycho-educational workshops, home visits, and/or traditional counseling.

As part of their involvement in this program, students also receive ongoing didactic training on the unique challenges faced by immigrant and refugee populations, including pre- and postmigration trauma, acculturation, and domestic violence. They learn about the range of community resources available to refugee and immigrant women (e.g., domestic violence programs, legal aid, tutoring services, subsidized housing) and how to work with community agencies to help their clients obtain needed resources. As one student noted:

> I got real creative with her to try not to get her deported, and there was somebody that I worked with who worked in [name of senator's] office at the time so he worked with him and we had a lot of phone calls back and forth.

> We actually got paperwork pushed through Washington to get her to stay, so it made me be a lot more resourceful than I ever would have imagined I could get. (as cited in Nilsson et al., 2011, p. 417)

A recent qualitative study indicated that students who participated in the program came to understand more deeply the lived experience of refugees and immigrants as well as the many roles counseling psychologists can play beyond that of traditional counselor (Nilsson et al., 2011).

Ball State University

Ball State University offers counseling psychology doctoral students several social justice–oriented courses that provide students with a foundation in advocacy skills and an opportunity to practice them (Niegocki et al., 2012). For example, the final class assignment for one course involves developing a project that aims to address a social justice issue. One year, the product of this final assignment was a university-wide campaign to address racially motivated harassment (Alexander et al., 2010). Another year, students developed a community resource guide and advocacy tip sheet for therapists working at the university's practicum clinic, described next (Niegocki et al., 2012).

Building on the ACA advocacy competencies (Lewis et al., 2003), students in the class decided that their practicum clinic, which serves community members at low cost, needed to move beyond traditional counseling to facilitate clients' access to and use of needed community resources. Yet, because counseling trainees at the clinic lacked training on the nature of community resources and how to talk to clients about contextual needs, they were unable to advocate effectively. For their final assignment, the students decided to remedy this situation: they conducted a two part needs assessment in which they surveyed clients and clinicians about knowledge of and access to community resources. Findings from this needs assessment then informed the content of the resource guide they developed, which included information about child care services, financial services, legal services, recreation and leisure opportunities, volunteer opportunities, mental health services, health care services, substance abuse services, housing assistance, employment services, spirituality, and services for special populations (e.g., American Indians, LGBT individuals, individuals with disabilities). In addition, they developed a tip sheet that described how counselors should go about referring clients to community resources. This project served as an enormously important method for teaching students in the clinic to integrate advocacy into their clinical practice.

Despite many calls for the infusion of advocacy into clinical training as a core dimension of social justice practice, this is a complex undertaking. These programs demonstrate various possibilities for teaching advocacy skills to early doctoral trainees, each of which emphasizes training on how clients' mental health issues are influenced by context and how to address contextual factors directly to improve clients' well-being. They also illustrate how advocacy training can be tailored to fit within a variety of program structures and faculty and student interests.

Targeting Systemic Change through Service Learning

The third prong of the social justice training model proposed here involves moving beyond the bounds of clinical practice to helping students address context-change at the systems level (also called macro-level advocacy). This prong can be distinguished from the one before it, in that there is no longer a specific target client. Rather, a community consisting of a group of people with a shared identity, such as an organization, institution, or geographic locality (e.g., city, state, or country) is the focus of interest. At this level, practitioners work directly with systems to address the needs or challenges of a specific community.

Of course, a system is not an abstract set of disembodied structures. Individuals comprise a system and shape policies, cultural practices, and social norms. So working at a systemic level means working with people, which in turn means that students can harness the clinical skills they have learned in the context of traditional counseling work to address community-level problems. Students can use a variety of concrete strategies in their work to shift contexts, including community consultation, community organizing and community building, policy analysis and advocacy, psychoeducation of various types, and social change-oriented prevention.

Service learning is one effective vehicle for training students to address community-level issues (e.g., Ali, Liu, Mahmood, & Arguello, 2008; Nilsson et al., 2011). At its best, service learning is a pedagogical tool in which students do coursework on a particular topic, participate in related volunteer work in the community, and then reflect on how these two sets of experiences inform each other (Conway, Amel, & Gerwien, 2009). Thus, it allows students to learn about social justice from a scholarly and theoretical perspective while engaging in community work that informs and is informed by that perspective. Next, we provide two examples of how doctoral programs in the field are adopting a service learning approach to train counseling psychology students to address community-level change.

Boston College

The First Year Experience (FYE), developed by Boston College counseling psychology faculty over 10 years ago, is a combined course and field experience that enables first-year doctoral students to utilize clinical and counseling skills toward working directly with systems and communities (see Goodman et al., 2004, for a more detailed description). As a foundation for their fieldwork, students take a year-long biweekly seminar in which they immerse themselves in social justice–related literature across subdisciplines of psychology (e.g., community, feminist, multicultural, liberation, critical, and counseling psychology). The course uses an ecological model to investigate the rapidly growing empirical research on how oppression of all sorts fundamentally shapes health and well-being, and how practitioners can build on their clinical skills to address that oppression directly. Some major areas of study in this seminar include the role of power and privilege in mental health intervention, how context shapes psychological growth and access to opportunities, ethical guidelines for and dilemmas arising from meso- or macro-level work, and implementation of a range of social justice practices at the systemic or community level. Students have the opportunity to listen to guest speakers in the seminar who have vast experience in implementing social justice principles in their own community work, and to receive peer supervision from each other as they engage in such work themselves.

For their fieldwork, students in the course spend four to six hours per week throughout the year in community-based sites (e.g., schools, courts, community agencies, public health department), where they work in partnership with an organization, coalition, system, or political entity to initiate and implement an intervention that leads to sustained systemic (rather than individual) change. The intervention they choose may take a variety of forms, including psychoeducation, community consultation, community outreach, or advocacy for specific policies at the organizational, city, or state level. Students have, for example, developed a series of trauma awareness workshops for public school teachers and YMCA staff, worked to strengthen gay-straight alliances across the state; helped to develop programs for the children of new immigrants within community health centers, worked in a grassroots political-action organization for the rights and empowerment of Chinese immigrants, collaborated with a department of public health to investigate the needs of immigrant survivors of intimate partner violence, and worked on a community-organizing project for low-income women with depression. Irrespective of the particular activity, students learn to think about the community or institution as the locus of change rather than individuals or families.

University of Tennessee

The counseling psychology program at the University of Tennessee also emphasizes service learning as a tool for teaching about systems-level intervention. Typically, during their third year of study, as part of a social justice colloquium that explores the theoretical underpinnings of a social justice oriented approach, students are introduced to individuals and agencies engaged in social justice work in the surrounding community (B. Mallinckrodt, personal communication, July 12, 2012). On the basis of these introductions, students then choose to work with one of a variety of community organizations for the next academic year as part of a two semester social justice practicum. Organizations may include homeless shelters, domestic violence or sexual assault agencies, the criminal justice system, LGBT community outreach projects, or agencies serving immigrants, Although students are free to choose among these organizations, they are discouraged from committing to individual client service provision because, as with Boston College, the training specifically aims to help students create systemic change through work with groups, organizations, and communities.

The didactic portion of the social justice practicum sequence involves training in advocacy skills across micro-, meso-, and macro-levels, including how to convince others of the importance of a specific topic, prepare an action presentation for a community group, write a letter to the editor of a newspaper to advocate for a topic of interest, and persuade political decision makers in regards to changing policies.

For the practice portion of the social justice practicum sequence, students spend half a day weekly in their previously chosen agency participating in three activities: (1) a needs' assessment in which students interview staff and clients at their agencies to determine the needs of the target group, (2) a program development activity in which they develop an intervention to address the identified needs, and (3) an evaluation to determine the effectiveness of their intervention (B. Mallinckrodt, personal communication, July 12, 2012). To date, students have engaged in a variety of social justice projects, including collaborating with undergraduate students to develop campus mental health initiatives, developing a psychoeducational training about PTSD for staff at a placement agency for Iraqi refugees, and working with Iraqi women to sew crafts and sell them in the community (B. Mallinckrodt, personal communication, July 12, 2012).

Together, the Boston College and University of Tennessee examples illustrate methods for teaching students how to build on emerging clinical skills to work toward systemic, as well as individual, change. Psychology programs outside of counseling psychology could similarly create opportunities for doctoral students to address social issues and problems through service learning. For example, the Boston College Applied Developmental Psychology program offers an applied practicum experience in which doctoral students taking an academic course are placed in a community-based agency where they learn practical skills in community consultation and policy advocacy.

COMMON THEMES

Over the past 15 years, calls for social justice training in professional psychology have become louder and more frequent, and programs across the country have come forward to implement such training in innovative and inspiring ways. Based on our own experience at Boston College in combination with our reading of the literature emerging from other universities, we have proposed a model for training doctoral students to engage in social justice–oriented practice. This model has three goals: (1) to increase trainees' awareness of their own social identities, particularly related to oppression and privilege; (2) to increase students' knowledge of how to integrate external context change into traditional clinical practice; and (3) to increase students' skills in addressing community-level or systemic change directly. The model aims to accomplish these goals through a set of corresponding strategies, though we acknowledge that there are many others. These include using their role as teachers as a vehicle for helping doctoral students explore their own positionality, training doctoral students to bring advocacy into their traditional clinical practice, and engaging doctoral students in service learning as a mechanism for teaching about community or systems-change work. We conclude with a brief discussion of several overarching themes that emerge from the training examples offered here. These themes are also reflected in the broader literature on social justice–oriented psychology doctoral training.

Immersive Learning

The first theme is that *immersive learning*—learning that takes place experientially through immersion in contexts of interest—is a key tool for social justice training (Green et al., 2008). We have illustrated here, for example, how teaching may be a powerful strategy for developing social justice–oriented self-awareness. A classroom or small group of students represents a mini-community in which social justice–oriented group dynamics inevitably arise, and where community members can be encouraged to recognize, reflect on, and provide here-and-now feedback to each other and to the instructor. It therefore immerses both teacher and students in a context where they can test out their observations about how their own positionality shapes the experience of others.

Similarly, a service learning approach to social justice training enables an immersive learning experience in which students enter and work with real communities, moving from a purely academic understanding of theoretical concepts into settings where they can test out those concepts. Research indicates that such exposure, as long as it is grounded in a social justice framework and guided by a process of ongoing critical reflection, increases students' awareness of how systems of privilege and oppression shape their own and others' lives, reduces negative stereotypes about the individuals with whom they work, and improves helping skills (Mitchell, 2007; Rice & Pollack, 2000; Rosenberger, 2000; Weintraub & Goodman, 2010).

Developing Intellectual Foundations

A second theme is the importance of helping students to develop an intellectual or theoretical foundation for their social justice practice. Without such a foundation, students run the risk of approaching communities in ways that can disempower rather than empower. For example, without a basic understanding of social justice theory, doctoral students acting as teachers may not consider how their relative power vis–à-vis their students may shape their perceptions and responses to the students, and the other way around. As a result, they may unwittingly shame or diminish students by exerting power in destructive ways. Similarly, students may approach their role as advocates and community change agents with any one of a number of orientations—as service providers, experts, or collaborators, depending on their framework. Again, a basic understanding of social justice principles may enable them to keep central the need to prioritize client and community needs.

Building Bridges between Traditional and Social Justice–Oriented Practice

A third key theme is the importance of working with students to bridge the gap between traditional counseling practices with which students are more familiar (e.g., individual counseling) and social justice–oriented practices with which they are less familiar (e.g., advocacy, community building, or policy work). Watts (2004) describes this process as conceptual scaling, arguing that in our efforts to conceptualize the nature of social justice work, we should preserve traditional concepts and interventions but make them scalable by linking them to similar ideas at levels of analysis beyond the micro level. Indeed, in each of the three prongs of the social justice training model proposed here, students built upon earlier training experiences to understand and respond to the dynamics involved in social justice–oriented work. For example, Julie, the lab instructor, built on her awareness of psychodynamic processes and sharing power in the clinical context to understand her own responses to the community of her classroom (Liang, Tummala-Narra, & West, 2011). Students learned to integrate external context change into their clinical practice by building on their knowledge of feminist and multicultural counseling ideas such as giving voice, focusing on strengths, and leaving individuals with the tools for personal and social change. In targeting communities and systems through service learning, students built on an ecological model of human development and well-being, learning how to address community health through broader interventions.

CONCLUSION

Through the combined experiences gleaned from the proposed three-prong training model, students have the opportunity to benefit from a variety of roles and strategies. They are simultaneously instructors, clinicians, and social justice agents engaging in immersive learning and building upon the intellectual foundations of social justice–oriented work. They are gradually bridging the gap between traditional and social justice–oriented practice. These learning strategies may bring them one step closer to being able to work as counseling psychologists who can intervene on behalf of both individuals and communities toward the goal of social justice for all.

NOTES

1. Acknowledgments: We are enormously grateful to our colleagues at Boston College for their collaboration on thinking about bringing social justice to counseling psychology training over the last decade. We also deeply appreciate the willingness of our colleagues at other universities to be interviewed for this project. Unfortunately, we interviewed many more inspiring scholars and activists than we had space to include, but their thoughtful innovations continue to inform our own work.

2. The MA student involved in this vignette, Damon Pryor, gave permission to tell this story in this chapter. We are grateful for his sensitivity and courage, as revealed both in the vignette and in his decision to use his name here.

REFERENCES

Adams, M. (2007). Pedagogical frameworks for social justice education. In M. Adams, L. A. Bell, & P. Griffin, (Eds.), *Teaching for diversity and social justice* (pp. 15–33). New York, NY: Routledge/Taylor & Francis Group.

Alexander, C., Ægisdóttir, S., Gerstein, L. H., Snyder, E., Kirkpatrick, D., O'Heron, M., & Gordon, T. (2010). Responding to hate on a college campus: The Stop Hate Campaign and a multicultural climate assessment. In J. G. Ponterotto, J. M. Casas, L. A. Suzuki, & C. M. Alexander (Eds.), *Handbook of multicultural counseling* (pp. 577–590). Thousand Oaks, CA: Sage.

Ali, S. A., Liu, W. M., Mahmood, A., & Arguello, J. (2008). Social justice and applied psychology: Practical ideas for training the next generation of psychologists. *Journal of Social Action in Counseling and Psychology, 1*(2), 1–13.

Arredondo, P., & Rosen, D. C. (2007). Applying principles of multicultural competencies, social justice, and leadership—in training and supervision. In E. Aldorando (Ed.), *Advancing social justice through clinical practice* (pp. 443–458). Mahwah, NJ: Lawrence Erlbaum Associates.

Baluch, S. P., Pieterse, A. L., & Bolden, M. A. (2004). Counseling psychology and social justice: Houston . . . we have a problem. *The Counseling Psychologist. Special Issue: The Fourth National Counseling Psychology Conference: Houston 2001, 32*(1), 89–98.

Beer, A. M., Spanierman, L. B., Greene, J. C., & Todd, N. R. (2012). Counseling psychology trainees' perceptions of training and commitments to social justice. *Journal of Counseling Psychology, 59*(1), 120–133.

Brabeck, M., & Brown, L. (1997). Feminist theory and psychological practice. In J. Worell & N. G. Johnson (Eds.), *Shaping the future of feminist psychology: Education, research, and practice* (pp. 15–35). Washington, DC: American Psychological Association.

Burnes, T. R., & Manese, J. E. (2008). Social justice in an accredited internship in professional psychology: Answering the call. *Training and Education in Professional Psychology, 2*(3), 176–181.

Burnes, T. R., & Singh, A. A. (2010). Integrating social justice training into the practicum experience for psychology trainees: Starting earlier. *Training and Education in Professional Psychology, 4*(3), 153–162.

Caldwell, J. C., & Vera, E. M. (2010). Critical incidents in counseling psychology professionals' and trainees' social justice orientation development. *Training and Education in Professional Psychology, 4*(3), 163–176.

Conway, J. M., Amel, E. L., & Gerwien, D. P. (2009). Teaching and learning in the social context: A meta-analysis of service-learning's effects on academic, personal, social, and citizenship outcomes. *Teaching of Psychology, 36*(4), 233–245.

Diaz, J., & Zirkel, S. (2012). Globalization, psychology, and social issues research: An introduction and conceptual framework. *Journal of Social Issues, 68(3),* 439–453.

Fine, M. (1992). Passions, politics, and power: Feminist research possibilities. In M. Fine (Ed.), *Disruptive voices: The possibilities of feminist research.* Ann Arbor: University of Michigan.

Fox, D. R., Prilleltensky, I., & Austin, S. (2009). *Critical psychology: An introduction.* London, UK: Sage.

Fouad, N. A., Gerstein, L. H., & Toporek, R. L. (2006). Social justice and counseling psychology in context. In R. L. Toporek, L. Gerstein, N. A. Fouad, G. Roysircar, & T. Israel (Eds.). *Handbook of social justice in counseling psychology: Leadership, vision, and action* (pp. 1–16). Thousand Oaks, CA: Sage.

Fouad, N. A., McPherson, R. H., Gerstein, L., Blustein, D. L., Helledy, K. I., & Metz, A. J. (2004). Houston, 2001: Context and legacy. *The Counseling Psychologist, 32,* 15–77.

Goodman, L. A., Bohlig, A., Litwin, A., Weintraub, S. R., Green, A., Walker, J., . . . & Ryan, N. (2007). Applying feminist theory to community practice: A multi-level empowerment intervention for low-income women with depression. In E. Aldorando (Ed.), *Promoting social justice through mental health practice* (pp. 267–290). Florence, KY: Lawrence Erlbaum Associates.

Goodman, L. A., & Epstein, D. (2008). *Listening to battered women: A survivor-centered approach to advocacy, mental health, and justice.* Washington, DC: American Psychological Association.

Goodman, L. A., Liang, B., Helms, J. E., Latta, R. E., Sparks, E., & Weintraub, S. R. (2004). Training counseling psychologists as social justice agents: Feminist and multicultural principles in action. *The Counseling Psychologist, 32*(6), 793–837.

Goodman, L. A., Pugach, M., Skolnik, A., & Smith, L. (2013). Poverty and Mental Health Practice: Within and Beyond the 50-Minute Hour. *Journal of Clinical Psychology: In Session, 69*(2), 182–190.

Green, E. J., McCollum, V. C., & Hays, D. G. (2008). Teaching advocacy counseling within a social justice framework: Implications for school counselors and educators. *Journal for Social Action in Counseling and Psychology, 1* (2), 14–30.

Hage, S. M., Romano, J. L., Conyne, R. K., Kenny, M., Matthews, C., Schwartz, J. P., & Waldo, M. (2007). Best practice guidelines on prevention practice, research, training, and social advocacy for psychologists. *The Counseling Psychologist, 35*(4), 493–566.

Ivey, A. E., & Collins, N. M. (2003). Social justice: A long-term challenge for counseling psychology. *The Counseling Psychologist, 31*(3), 290–298.

Kiselica, M. S. (2004). When duty calls: The implications of social justice work for policy, education, and practice in the mental health professions. *The Counseling Psychologist, 32*(6), 838–854.

LeCompte, M. D. (1995). Some notes on power, agenda, and voice: A researcher's personal evolution toward critical collaborative research. In P. L. McLaren & J. M. Giarelli (Eds.), *Critical theory and educational research* (pp. 91–112). Albany, NY: University of New York.

Lewis, J., Arnold, M. S., House, R., & Toporek, R. (2003). ACA Advocacy Competencies. Retrieved from www.counseling.org/resources/ . . . /advocacy_competencies.pdf

Lewis, J. A., Ratts, M. J., Paladino, D. A. & Toporek, R. (2011). Social justice counseling and advocacy: Developing new leadership roles and competencies. *Journal for Social Action in Counseling and Psychology, 3*(1), 5–16.

Lewis, J. A., Toporek, R. L., & Ratts, M. J. (2010). Advocacy and social justice: Entering the mainstream of the counseling profession. In M. J. Ratts, R. L. Toporek & J. A. Lewis (Eds.), *ACA advocacy competencies: A social justice framework for counselors* (pp. 239–244). Alexandria, VA: American Counseling Association.

Liang, B., Glenn, C. & Goodman, L. A. (2005). Feminist ethics in advocacy relationships: A relational vs. rule-bound approach. *The Community Psychologist, 38*(3), 26–28.

Liang, B., Tummala-Narra, P., & West, J. (2011). Revisiting community work from a psychodynamic perspective. *Professional Psychology: Research and Practice, 42*(5), 398–404.

Miller, M. J., & Sendrowitz, K. (2011). Counseling psychology trainees' social justice interest and commitment. *Journal of Counseling Psychology, 58*(2), 159–169.

Mitchell, T. D. (2007). Critical service-learning as social justice education: A case study of the citizen scholars program. *Equity & Excellence in Education, 40*(2), 101–112.

Moane, G. (2003). Bridging the personal and the political: Practices for a liberation psychology. *American Journal of Community Psychology, 31*(1/2), 91–101.

Moe, J. L., Perera-Diltz, D., & Sepulveda, V. (2010). Are consultation and social justice advocacy similar?: Exploring the perceptions of professional counselors and counseling students. *Journal for Social Action in Counseling and Psychology, 2*(2), 106–123.

Niegocki, K. L., Mastroianni, E. M., Hurley, E. J., Green, M. M., Gerstein, L. H., Richardson, D. R., & Miller, D. A. (2012). Making the social justice connection: Development of a community resource guide. *Journal of Social Action in Counseling Psychology, 4*(2), *41–58.*

Nilsson, J. E., Schale, C. L., & Khamphakdy-Brown, S. (2011). Facilitating trainees' multicultural development and social justice advocacy through a refugee/immigrant mental health program. *Journal of Counseling & Development, 89*(4), 413–422.

Pieterse, A. L., Evans, S. A., Risner-Butner, A., Collins, N. M., & Mason, L. B. (2009). Multicultural competence and social justice training in counseling psychology and counselor education: A review and analysis of a sample of multicultural course syllabi. *The Counseling Psychologist, 37*(1), 93–115.

Ponterotto, J. G., Casas, J. M., Suzuki, L. A., & Alexander, C. M. (2009). *Handbook of multicultural counseling.* Thousand Oaks, CA: Sage.

Reinharz, S. (1997). Who am I? The need for a variety of selves in the field. In R. Hertz (Ed.), *Reflexivity and voice* (pp. 3–20). Thousand Oaks, CA: Sage.

Rice, K., & Pollack, S. (2000). Developing a critical pedagogy of service learning: Preparing self-reflective, culturally aware, and responsive community participants. In C. O'Grady (Ed.), *Integrating service learning and multicultural education in colleges and universities* (pp. 115–134). Hillsdale, NJ: Lawrence Erlbaum Associates.

Rosenberger, C. (2000). Beyond empathy: Developing critical consciousness through service learning. In C. O'Grady (Ed.), *Integrating service learning and multicultural education in colleges and universities* (pp. 23–43). Mahwah, NJ: Lawrence Erlbaum Associates.

Singh, A. A., Hofsess, C. D., Boyer, E. M., Kwong, A., Lau, A. S. M., McLain, M., & Haggins, K. L. (2010). Social justice and counseling psychology: Listening to the voices of doctoral trainees. *The Counseling Psychologist, 38*(6), 766–795.

Speight, S. L., & Vera, E. M. (2008). Social justice and counseling psychology: A challenge to the specialty. In S. D. Brown & R. Lent (Eds.). *The handbook of counseling psychology* (pg. 54–67). Hoboken, NJ: John Wiley.

Talleyrand, R., Chung, R. C-Y., & Bemak, F. (2006). Incorporating social justice in graduate training programs: A case study example. In R. L. Toporek, L. Gerstein, N. A. Fouad, G. Roysircar, & T. Israel (Eds.). *Handbook of social justice in counseling psychology: Leadership, vision, and action* (pp. 44–58). Thousand Oaks, CA: Sage.

Toporek, R. L. (2000). Creating a common language and framework for understanding advocacy in counseling. In J. Lewis & L. Bradley (Eds.), *Advocacy in counseling, clients, and community* (pp. 5–14). Greensboro, NC: Caps.

Toporek, R. L., Lewis, J. A., & Ratts, M. J. (2010). The ACA advocacy competencies: An overview. In M. Ratts, R. Toporek, & J. Lewis (Eds.), *ACA Advocacy Competencies* (11–20). Alexandria, VA: American Counseling Association.

Watts, R. (2004). Integrating social justice and psychology. *The Counseling Psychologist, 32,* 855–865.

Weintraub, S. R., & Goodman, L. A. (2010). Working with and for: Student advocates' experience of relationship centered advocacy with low-income women. *American Journal of Orthopysychiatry, 80*(1), 46–60.

Wilson, J. L., & Meyer, K. A. (2011). A time and a place: Social justice in a doctoral program. *Journal of College Student Development, 52*(6), 752–758.

Chapter 15

Social Justice Research Methods: The Problems of Abstracted Empiricism and the Politics of Evidence

Alphia Possamai-Inesedy

The role that social scientists play in fostering social justice and tackling seemingly intractable issues in relation to concerns such as poverty, discrimination, child abuse, education, housing and health care is reliant not only on the ability to collect and interpret data accurately and communicate results effectively but also on the ability to place the very notion of social justice at the core of methodology and method. Globally, disciplines within the social sciences are grappling with social justice methodology and research methods in an environment constrained by research funding agendas and a resurgence of the politics of evidence. In this context, the established set of methodological techniques is often applied to the empirical problems of social justice—elevating the commitment to the methods over the area of research. In this sense, methods are determining the social problem (Mills, 1959).

The debate surrounding the politics and ethics of evidence and what value qualitative methods have in addressing matters of social justice is at play (Lather, 2004).

Social justice research should promote creativity and imagination within a critical frame of reference to challenge the status quo; it should invite the researcher into creative spaces for thinking about and researching "the social," wherein the processes of social justice research (methodology) and the presentation of the research (re-presentation) are seen as intertwined. Instead, the current political environment that the researcher is constrained by has led to a crisis of imagination wherein claims of a reemergence of scientism, even in the face of its criticisms (e.g., Pietroni, 1992), are escalating (see Torrance, 2011). This positivist evidence-based epistemology is presented to researchers as the only path to obtain reliable and valid knowledge. It appears that social scientists are faced with the debates and constraints of the past, as Denzin (2009, 139) argues—"this is like old wine in old bottles, 1980s battles in a new century." The following sections will provide an overview of this landscape and examine potential pathways forward for the researcher who wishes to engage with social justice research outside of the constraints of abstracted empiricism.

SOCIAL JUSTICE RESEARCH AND ABSTRACTED EMPIRICISM

The challenges of social justice research are multilayered. How does the researcher represent the realities of social life without robbing these phenomena of their socially situated meaning? Compounded further by the quest to produce verifiable scientific knowledge, researchers are instead producing an abstract knowledge about the social world—one that has been situated by the political role of methodology.

Mills (1959) anticipated these dangers in his classic sociological piece—*The Sociological Imagination*. Although Mills was addressing what he considered to be the crisis of sociology, his argument is one that could be shared across the social sciences. The discipline of sociology, was, for him, one torn between grand theory fetishism and abstracted empiricism—a dilemma witnessed across many disciplines. On the one hand, we have the theories of the day that fetishize its concepts to the extent that it outruns any specific and empirical problem (1959, p. 58), and on the other, social scientists have lost their grip on the problems of the empirical world by confusing "whatever is to be studied with the set of methods suggested for its study" (p. 61).

Both of these issues block the researcher from what Mills deemed to be a truly empirical methodology—one that is both innovative and flexible. He adamantly argues that "no method . . . should be used to delimit the problems that we take up, if for no other reason that the most interesting and difficult issues of method usually begin where established techniques do not apply" (p. 83).

THE EMERGENCE OF SOCIAL RESEARCH METHODS—QUALITATIVE METHODOLOGIES

The increased fragmentation of methodological approaches within the social sciences has resulted in an emergence of specializations within both traditions (Alastalo, 2008). This differentiation of methodological approaches has created a tolerance—demonstrated by the increase of mixed methodology textbooks and the call for the incorporation of qualitative methodologies into disciplines that have been historically quantitative. The unintended consequence, however, has been the difficulty to comprehend the multitude of methodological alternatives. It follows that limited comprehension of these various methodologies leads to a static and potentially superficial dialogue between the diverse approaches. The politics and ethics of evidence is the focus—often leading to questions of the value of qualitative work in addressing matters of social justice. This is even more apparent within psychology wherein qualitative research is often equated to unscientific subjectivity.

The links to abstracted empiricism and the reemergence of scientism are better understood by unpacking the emergence of qualitative methodologies. A number of historical frameworks have been developed, and the following will focus on Denzin and Lincoln's (2011) sketch of the emergence of qualitative research in the social sciences. There are seven moments that Denzin and Lincoln distinguish, although they emphasize that these moments all circulate in the present, competing with and defining one another, and their ages are presented as follows: the traditional (1900–1950); the modernist or golden age (1950–1970); blurred genres (1970–1986); the crisis of representation (1986–1990); the postmodern, a period of experimental and new ethnographies (1990–1995); post-experimental inquiry (1995–2000); and, the future (2000—present).

The *traditional period* represents a time when qualitative researchers were firmly entrenched within the positivist paradigm. Accounts from these researchers were bound within the language and objectives of this paradigm. Denzin and Lincoln (2000) associate the traditional period with discussions of the scientific principles of objective ethnography espoused by researchers such as Malinowksi, as well as the urban ethnography practiced by the Chicago school. It was during this time period that the case study was developed beyond the confines of social work and clinical practice of medicine, yet its continued and separate development across a variety of disciplines—such as anthropology, sociology, and history—resulted in different methodological approaches and understanding of the method—a mirrored situation to current methodological developments.

The second moment, *the golden age*, is associated with the formalization of qualitative methods as a rigorous equal to its quantitative counterpart. Obviously, researchers within this period were still heavily engaged with the language of positivism and what became known as post-positivism. The gradual necessity for a bilingual dictionary of methodologies emerged with the onset of what Denzin and Lincoln call the "blurred genres," or the third stage of what Alasuutari (2004) critically terms their "progress narrative." Here the approaches of the human disciplines were slowly opening up to a more pluralistic, interpretative, and open-ended perspective. It was during this time period that the privileged voice of the observer and his or her interpretations were challenged.

Alasuutari's assertion that Denzin and Lincoln present the history of qualitative methodologies as a progressive one in which science is assumed to develop through comprehensive paradigms is demonstrated through the abstracted empiricism critique of Mills (1959), which was written during this time period—an argument that contradicts the age of the reflexive scholar.

According to the authors, *the crisis of representation* involved research that called into question the issues of class, race, and gender, and the notion of reflexivity. Books such as *Writing Culture* (Clifford & Marcus, 1986), *Works and Lives* (Geertz, 1988) and *The Predicament of Culture* (Clifford, 1988) critiqued the premise of the objective ethnography, and accordingly new methods, models of truth, and representation were sought. It was during this period that "issues such as validity, reliability, and objectivity, previously believed settled, were once more problematic" (Denzin & Lincoln, 2000, p. 26).

We define the postmodern period as one characterized by experimental and new ethnographies that give rise to different ways of knowing and space for other voices. Denzin and Lincoln make reference to Ellis and Bochner's (1996) work *Composing Ethnography: Alternative Forms of Qualitative Writing* to highlight the triple crisis of representation, legitimation, and praxis with which researchers were grappling. Denzin and Lincoln discuss *the post-experimental stage* and *the future stage* together. The authors present a time period in which fictional ethnographies, ethnographic poetry, and multimedia texts are taken for granted. It is in the present, the authors argue, that the post-experimental writer seeks to "connect their writings to the needs of a free democratic society. The demands of a moral and sacred qualitative social science are actively being explored by a host of new writers from many different disciplines" (Denzin & Lincoln, 2000, p. 29).

The attempt to map qualitative research methods and situate them within historical moments is a useful tool when analyzing the various epistemologies that have developed over time, which in turn have impacted on research methodologies. Denzin and Lincoln's framework provides details of the different major directions that qualitative methodology debates have witnessed. The hesitancy in the application of this across the social sciences, regardless of the multiple disciplines and disciplinary framework presented, is representative of the disparate rate of change across the different areas of the social sciences.

This hesitancy is readily apparent when examining the development of qualitative methodologies in psychology wherein much of the literature surrounding its use is geared toward legitimization as well as the development of guidelines toward assessment. It appears that the need for a bilingual dictionary is only now emerging. Although pathways into the employment of qualitative methods within psychology are evident from as early as the 1930s, with Allport's introduction of the Kantian debate of idiographic and nomothetic (Allport, 1937) and the late 1960s through the debates of phenomenological and indigenous psychologists, it is only within the last two decades that there has been a dramatic increase in its use. Regardless of these developments, strongly witnessed in areas of social justice research such as health and indigenous psychology, much of the debate is bogged down in issues of quality control. Avenues of dissemination of qualitative psychological research are still in their infancy—wherein the cultural wars of quality evidence further impact on development. This is readily demonstrated across all subfields, yet particularly evident in indigenous psychological research, especially Asian indigenous psychology, which has been grappling with non-positivist approaches to the use of social science knowledge, and yet has found difficulty in disseminating its research outside of its geographical boundaries.

METHODS À LA CARTE

Social scientific research, the offspring of the Enlightenment, is rooted in science as a truth-bearing discourse. From this heritage, knowledge is an *a priori* given. Even in the face of the politics of evidence, the pursuits of explaining, predicting, and controlling have expanded to better grasp the changeable and fluid nature of reality. Knowledge is more readily appreciated as partial, and goals of research are increasingly moving toward more complex levels of understanding that can be dirty, messy, and as Denzin and Lincoln (2005) argue, in need of reworking from the ground up to be more praxis-oriented and democratizing.

The porous definitional borders of qualitative methodologies are all premised on the notion of social justice as practice (Denzin, 2003a; Horsfall & Higgs, 2007). The methodologies also attempt to bridge the divide between researcher and researched (Pink, 2001) wherein research is seen as an interactive and collaborative endeavor. The methodological practices themselves are many and varied, a menu à la carte. This section of the chapter examines a range of qualitative practices, with an emphasis on arts-based practices. The examination is not intended to be definitive, as the practices by their very nature are flexible, emerging, and adaptive. An emphasis should also be placed on the multimethod focus of qualitative research. The aim of capturing an objective reality is increasingly understood as not possible; however, the combination of multiple methodological practices, empirical materials, and perspectives in a single study can provide an alternative to validation through rigor, breadth, complexity, richness, and depth (Flick, 2002, p. 229).

VISUAL ARTS–BASED INQUIRY

The use of visual arts (drawing, painting, photography, video) in interpretive research methods tends to fall into two broad camps: visual art created by the researcher to provoke reflections that words alone cannot; and visual arts as a medium to engage with, stimulate, and support inquiry of an issue or a subject group (Simons & McCormack, 2007). Examples of the former include Herman's (2005) use of images of "evil events" like genocide to examine researchers' mediated experiences of human cruelty, whereas instances of the latter include Clark-Ibanez's (2007) use of "photo elicitation" to study children's experience of poverty; Holliday's (2007) research into queer sexualities using video diaries; and Sawyer, Drew, and Duncan's (2007) participant-generated photographic approach to self-management practices by young people with chronic conditions.

Arts-based inquiry is characterized as respectful, transformative, and collaborative. The marginalized and voiceless individual is allowed increased control over data generation illuminating aspects of the lived experience that is often hidden or overlooked by the constraints of epistemologies and methodologies. Fattore, Mason, and Watson (2007) refer to their use of arts-based inquiry in their study on children's conceptualization of their well-being as "task oriented methods":

> These projects included the use of photography, collage, drawing or journal keeping, and provided participants with alternative forms of knowledge creation, directed and controlled by them. (p. 15)

These task-oriented methods support the researchers' child-centered epistemology and methodology by positioning the children centrally as research participants and allowing them to inform the researchers of what they considered as important to their well-being, thus contrasting with research involving adult-centric findings. Crucially the researchers stress that children's interests may not be seen as congruent with the interests of adults, and this goes to the heart of the social justice orientation of the new methodologies, whereby scholars are informed and educated by struggling and silenced peoples. As Conde-Frazier (2006) acknowledges, "it is research that is attached to the humanisation of persons in communities. Unattached research tends to create policies that continue to oppress" (p. 324).

AUTOETHNOGRAPHY

Autoethnography originally referred to the ethnographic study of a group of which the researcher was an integral part. Minge (2007), however, notes that in recent times the method has come to focus on "the self-narrative, or autobiographical voice, within social context," and has been variably referred to as personal ethnography, self ethnography, reflexive ethnography, emotional sociology, ethnographic autobiography, and experiential texts (p. 254). Autoethnographic practice draws on a number of styles, including narrative, poetry (Furman, Langer, Davis, Gallardo, & Kulkarni, 2007), visual arts, and combinations of these. Minge herself uses a fusion method of narrative and "embodied art" in her cutting exploration of "life-crushing moments," and her experience of rape in particular. She uses the autoethnographic method "to uncover the complexity of rape as I felt it, lived it, and interacted within it. It allows you, the reader, to walk into my experience and to complexity your understanding the sexual-abuse situation" (Minge, 2007, p. 269).

Common to all autoethnographic styles is the valuing of self-knowledge (Peseta, 2007), a notion converse to scientifically styled research, which promotes the ideas of objectivity, detachment, and rational knowledge. Ellis and Bochner (2003) question why academics are "conditioned to believe that a text is important only to the extent it moves beyond the merely personal?" (p. 221). The methodological permutation of self-knowledge and narrative is used to invite readers into places unknown, even though it yields the researcher vulnerable. However, "when you write vulnerably, others respond vulnerably" (Peseta, 2007, p.16), allowing and encouraging alternative readings and multiple interpretations (Ellis & Bochner, 2003).

Nevertheless, autoethnography has ethical implications for others appearing in the narrative:

> When we write about ourselves, we also write about others. In so doing, we run the risk that other characters may become increasingly recognisable to our readers, though they may not have consented to being portrayed in ways that would reveal their identity; or, if they did consent, they might not understand exactly to what they had consented. (Ellis, 2007, p.14)

Although this is an issue for all ethnographic work, the fact of the researcher as the researched means that the identity of people related in some way to him or her is more difficult to disguise, and the issue of consent becomes more complex.

Autoethnography has been criticized as being self-referential and not generalizable; criticism takes autoethnographers' take on the chin (Furman et al., 2007). Emotionalism, however, is a more difficult issue. Although emotion is an important aspect of autoethnography, it is difficult to disagree with Dennis (2005, p. 476), himself an autoethnographer, that at times the reader has to "do a lot of wading through discussions of feelings before getting to the good stuff." Some of Ellis's personal narratives (2004; Scott-Hoy & Ellis, 2008), for instance, seem quite superfluousness at times, particularly her overt admiration for partner Art Bochner scattered through her writing, for instance:

> We enter a crowded room where a talk is about to begin. "That's Art, my partner, the good-looking guy sitting at the table," I whisper to Sylvia, as we take seats in the back. (Ellis & Bochner, 2003, p. 216)

Alternately, Minge's writing on rape and body knowledge would not be as powerful without it:

> After slipping from her embrace, he slithers upstairs and into my pussy as I sleep. I wake to him inside me. I wake to him beside me after her lips

> licked his dick. I wake from a deep dream into his hands gripped against my breasts. My CJ, the infamous sailing instructor, cannot hear me as I grumble the word, "No." (Minge, 2007, p. 258)

Treating emotion in qualitative research as data not only opens up new areas of research interest, but it can also establish new ways of conceptualizing old lines of enquiry (Kleinman & Copp, 1993). Autoethnography privileges the researcher's subjective experience. Although this is contrary to the "scientific" method, it actually presents a space for developing new knowledge and conceptions of social issues. Essentially, autoethnographic research demands more from the reader than scientific-based research that presents findings and conclusions, as it requires the reader to "feel" the research and to be actively engaged in the production of knowledge through responding to, critiquing, and interpreting the autoethnographic data.

PERFORMANCE ETHNOGRAPHY

According to Denzin (2003a), "As praxis, performance ethnography is a way of acting on the world in order to change it" (p. 262). The performance is not merely the dissemination stage of the research process. Rather, the idea of performative method is integral to each stage of the research—as the framework of research design, as a method of data collection and data analysis, as a transformative means of reflecting on research findings, and as the primary research output whether in physical performance or performance text. In explaining the difference between critical ethnography and ethnography that is pedagogical and performative, Denzin (2003a) goes beyond Goffman's (1959) dramaturgical thesis that all of life is a stage. He argues that when the divisions between "person and character, between the performer and actor, between stage and setting, between script and text, and between performance and performativity disappear," then critical ethnography becomes pedagogical and performative (Denzin, 2003b, p. 26).

Performance ethnography is an embodied form of creativity and interpretation, and draws more from the tradition of the Brazilian theater director Augusto Boal's (2000) *Theatre of the Oppressed* developed during the 1950s, than 20th-century avant-guard theater movements. Boal argues that mainstream theater (as "monologue") reflects ruling-class control, but that theater as "dialogue" has revolutionary potential for transforming the audience into actors and, hence, has the capacity to induce social action and transform society. Boal promotes the idea of theatre as a platform for social justice and grass-roots transformative action.

McCall (2000), for instance, developed *Not "Just" a Farmer and Not Just a "Farmers Wife"* in 1993. This performance script explored the loss of the family farm during the 1980s farm crisis in the United States. The script was drawn from the transcript of a workshop on the subject attended by women who had experienced farm loss. Becker, McCall, and Morris (1989) developed *Theatres and Communities: Three Scenes*, drawing on formal interviews with 70 theatre people, from actors through to critics, to examine the social organization of professional theater in the United States. McCall (200) rather explains the "text-based" performance style:

> In performance we carried and read from scripts, did not wear costumes or use props, sat in chairs or stood behind podiums, and moved only to exchange seats or to get from chairs to podiums and back. We played multiple characters: ourselves, as sociologists and various people one of us had interviewed. (p. 424)

Similarly, Horsfall et al. (2007) detail their research performance in the nine-scene *Walking Creative Edges*, at the biennial Australian *Pacific Edge* conference in December 2006:

> This script was performed in the style of a play reading or what Americans know as readers' theatre. There's some movement, scripts are held and all performers are focused on making contact with the audience in a relaxed conversational manner. Generally, speakers stood stage right of the large screen onto which images were projected and the rest of the group sat stage left of the screen. (p. 139)

Contiguous with Boal's dialogical theater, readers' theater liberates the performers and the audience from the physical limitations of conventional theater, encouraging a more intense level of critical imagination. Peseta (2007) describes this experience on reading an ethnographic script about the interaction between a young academic and a vice chancellor when they find themselves sitting next to one another on a train journey. The scene is set with both characters reading about the nature of leadership, change, and management within universities:

> Imagine the scene—the respectful fumbling around each other's position while aiming to enforce the credibility of their own. . . . Pritchard's chosen form (play script) allowed me to connect with my own experience of similar conversations. Plus, the account itself is amusing, insightful, and articulate, and I wanted to insert myself, my views, and my morality into their conversation. I wanted to be on that train journey with them. Research writing like this occupies me in ways that I find very hard to get rid of. (Peseta, 2007, p. 20)

According to "Women Out to Lunch," the researchers, writers, and performers of *Walking Creative Edges*, the purpose of their research performance was to demonstrate how their "research, teaching, community work and creativity inform each other and enable a rich and complex set of practices to both emerge and be supported" (Horsfall et al., 2007, p. 139).

QUALITATIVE METHODS AND THE POLITICS OF EVIDENCE

Reflecting on the emergence, perception, and employment of qualitative research, it is necessary to not only review the nature of that enquiry with its various historical, theoretical, and methodological underpinnings, but also to consider the conditions outside of academic walls under which this kind of research is possible. Social justice research has intrinsic ties with policy—and the debate on how this research can better serve policy has been invigorated by concurrent governments in the United States, Australia, the United Kingdom, and the European Union, questioning the value of qualitative research and cutting funding to a number of research areas. Over the past few decades, these countries have witnessed changing conditions under which qualitative research has been conducted, including political and economic contexts, which have impacted on the general perception of qualitative research as well as framing the work of researchers generally.

In regard to the political context, parallels can be drawn between Australia and the United States where the "culture wars" and neo-conservatism have attempted to undermine certain forms of research, particularly postmodern and qualitative research (Lincoln & Cannella, 2004), which try to establish alternative viewpoints and a diversity of ideas. Indeed, in 2006, the then-Australian Minister for Education, Brendan Nelson, personally vetoed seven projects from receiving funding from the Australian Research Council (ARC) (Haigh, 2006). Although information on the specific projects never became public knowledge, it was reported that five of the projects were from the humanities and two from the social sciences (Haigh, 2006). Information about the process of the review and possible basis of the vetoes was also leaked by one of the nonacademic panel members of the Quality and Standards Committee.[1]

The assault on academic freedom can be argued to represent a backlash against the social sciences and qualitative research methodologies. Macintyre (2007) argues that one of the main reasons for this assault was the abandonment by researchers in the humanities and social sciences to engage with the "scientific search for truth." He continues:

> Many in the humanities understand their disciplines as involving a process of inquiry that is necessarily interpretive, neither testing a hypothesis nor producing a verifiable result, but rather offering interpretations that are always partial, perspectival and contingent. Many in the social sciences would reject the notion of intellectual inquiry as a neutral and disinterested activity. These positions do not negate the need for honesty and rigour, nor do they lessen the adherence to the professional paradigm, but they might well have weakened the epistemological foundations of academic freedom. (p. 58)

Economically speaking, neo-liberalism has also impacted universities from across the aforementioned stated geographic locations. Within universities in Australia and the United Kingdom there is increased pressure to adopt a more commercial, entrepreneurial, and managerial environment (Harman, 2005; Marginson & Considine, 2000)—one which has been readily apparent with the U.S. higher education sector for decades. Within three decades, the university sector in Australia and the United Kingdom has moved from one of high dependence on annual commonwealth government grants to one where these same grants now support less than 50% of university income. This is a clear demonstration of the commercialization shift of the sector, which in turn has created a system that is increasingly characterized by pressure on academics to attract external research funding and to be more financially productive in research.

The university-wide push toward a commercially oriented research and development culture has led to a battle for scarce resources. Within Australia there are two major funding bodies from which academic researchers can apply for funding. In 2012, for instance, only 21.95 percent of projects submitted to the ARC received funding (Australian Research Council, 2011). This is in an environment that has few other sources of public or private research funding. The other major source of external funding for Australian researchers is the National Health and Medical Research Council (NHMRC). This funding body's success rate is marginally higher than the ARC, commencing projects in 2011 at 22.9 percent. In relation to researchers from the human-focused disciplines, many believe that they have been starved of research funds as well as being largely forgotten by policymakers. Indeed, Harman (2005) illustrates that 70 percent of surveyed social science researchers believe that they are undervalued by the operator of the National Competitive Grants Program, the ARC. Furthermore, the NHMRC is known to marginalize, if not outright reject qualitative methodologies. In 1995, the NHMRC rated evidence from qualitative research at the lowest level; this was soon followed by the removal of qualitative evidence from its quality of evidence scale[2] altogether (Geanellos, 2004). In essence, rather than a broadening of acceptance and inclusion of qualitative methodologies, it can be argued that based on the context presented, social scientists are excluded from one of the two peak funding bodies and marginalized from the other.

Social scientists are less successful in attracting support from national competitive grant schemes as well as from business and industry than their science and technology counterparts. In an analysis of comparative data for Go8[3] universities, Harman (2005) found that only 15 percent of social science researchers were successful in gaining an ARC discovery grant compared with 47 percent of their science and technology counterparts. Generalizing Harman's findings is problematic when evaluating the *Discovery Projects Selection Report* for funding commencing in 2012. The success rate for researchers stemming from the social, behavioral, and economic (SBE) disciplines was listed at 23.2 percent. The disciplines within SBE performed well, ranking at the top of the list in terms of success rates. The difference is marginal; however, what should be emphasized is that the biological sciences and biotechnology group and the physics, chemistry, and Earth sciences disciplines have a success rate greater than their representation among the total number of grant application proposals.

The politics and institutional forces that fund research, structure policies, and educate researchers, as well as reproduce forms of enquiry demonstrate how researchers are engaged and linked to a particular social moment that might well hinder the embracement of the qualitative, interpretive, and nondeterministic points of view that have developed in research methodologies (Denzin & Lincoln, 2000). As Krug and Hepworth (1997) argue:

> These structures determine to a large degree whether research shall take a stance that seeks to make statements about a research area based on a range of "positivist" approaches regarded as scientific, or whether research will take a stance that seeks, through "subjective, interpretive or naturalistic" approaches. (p. 51)

This sentiment is echoed by Torrance (2011) who argues that the impacts of the politics of evidence, although differing in origins, orientations, and specific national aspirations, will "reassert broadly empiricist and technicist approaches to the generation and accumulation of social scientific evidence for policy making" (p. 570). There appears to be a global concerted attempt to impose, or as Denzin (2009) alludes—reimpose—"scientific certainty" on an increasingly uncertain social world. The crisis of measurement that qualitative researchers are facing today echoes the calls against abstracted empiricism forwarded by Mills over a half century ago. In the face of expanding pressures for qualitative researchers to justify their approach, it is imperative to return to their promise. As Mills (1959) argued, one must not fetishize the ready-made, rather one must invent or re-forge analytical devices and techniques from the empirical problems found within the social world.

NOTES

1. In 2001 the ARC introduced this committee to aid in ensuring consistency of judgement across panels. In 2005 Brendon Nelson made three nonacademic additions to the board and broadened the responsibilities of the committee to include consideration of national benefit. The new lay members included the former High Court judge Sir Daryl Dawson, the then editor of *Quadrant* magazine Padraic McGuinness, and the television anchorman Ross Symonds. (Haigh, 2006; Macintyre, 2007).

2. Rates methodologies and ascribes values to their evidence.

3. The Group of Eight represents Australia's leading universities. It has been operating as an informal network of vice-chancellors since 1994 and was formally incorporated in 1999. The group consists of the University of Queensland, the University of New South Wales, the University of Sydney, the Australian National University, the University of Melbourne, Monash University, the University of Adelaide, and the University of Western Australia.

REFERENCES

Alastalo, M. (2008). The history of social research methods. In P. Alasuutari, L. Bickman, & J. Brannen (Eds.), *The Sage handbook of social research methods*. Thousand Oaks, CA: Sage.

Alasuutari, P. (2004). The globalization of qualitative research. In C. Seale, G. Gobo, J. F. Gubrium & D. Silverman (Eds.), *Qualitative research practice* (Vol. 595–608). London, UK: Sage.

Allport, G. W. (1937). *Personality: A psychological interpretation*. New York, NY: Holt.

Australian Research Council. (2011). *Discovery projects: selection report for funding commencing in 2012*. Retrieved from http://www.arc.gov.au/

Becker, H. S., McCall, M. M., & Morris, L. V. (1989). Theatres and communities: Three Scenes. *Social Problems, 36*(2), 93–116.

Boal, A. (2000). *Theater of the oppressed* (C. A. McBride, M.-O. L. McBride, & E. Fryer, Trans. 2nd, First Published in 1974 as *Teatro del Oprimido* ed.). London, UK: Pluto.

Clark-Ibanez, M. (2007). Inner city children in sharper focus: sociology of childhood and photo elicitation interviews. In G. C. Stanczak (Ed.), *Visual research methods: image, society, and representation* (pp. 167–196). Thousand Oaks, CA: Sage Publications.

Clifford, J. (1988). *The predicament of culture: Twentieth-century ethnography, literature and art* Cambridge, MA: Harvard University.

Clifford, J., & Marcus, G. E. (Eds.). (1986). *Writing culture: The poetics and politics of ethnography*. Berkeley, CA: Univ of California Press.

Conde-Frazier, E. (2006). Participatory action research: Practical theology for social justice. *Religious Education, 101*(3), 321–329.

Dennis, J. P. (2005). The social is the literary: Experiments in radical ethnography. *Qualitative Sociology, 28*(4), 475–478.

Denzin, N. K. (2003a). Peforming [auto] ethnography politically. *The Review of Education, Pedagogy and Cultural Studies, 25*(2), 257–278.

Denzin, N. K. (2003b). *Performance ethnography: critical pedagogy and the politics of culture*. Thousand Oaks, CA: Sage.

Denzin, N. K. (2009). The elephant in the living room: Or extending the conversation about the politics of evidence. *Qualitative Research, 9*(2), 139–160.

Denzin, N. K., & Lincoln, Y. S. (2000). *Handbook of qualitative research* (2nd ed.). Thousand Oaks, CA: Sage.

Denzin, N. K., & Lincoln, Y. S. (2005). Introduction: The discipline and practice of qualitative research.. In N. K. Denzin & Y. S. Lincoln (Eds.), *The Sage handbook of qualitative research* (3rd ed., pp. 1–32). Thousand Oaks, CA: Sage.

Denzin, N. K., & Lincoln, Y. S. (Eds.) (2011). *The Sage handbook of qualitative research* (4th ed.). Los Angeles, CA: Sage.

Ellis, C. (2004). *The Ethnographic I: A methodological novel about autoethnography*. Walnut Creek, CA: Altamira.

Ellis, C. (2007). Telling secrets, revealing lives: Relational ethics in research with intimate others. *Qualitative Inquiry, 13*(1), 3–29.

Ellis, C., & Bochner, A. (1996). *Composing ethnography: Alternative forms of qualitative writing*. Walnut Creek, CA: AltaMira.

Ellis, C., & Bochner, A. (2003). Autoethnography, personal narrative, reflexivity: Researcher as subject. In N. K. Denzin & Y. S. Lincoln (Eds.), *Collecting and interpreting qualitative materials* (2nd ed., pp. 199–258). Thousand Oaks, CA: Sage.

Fattore, T., Mason, J., & Watson, E. (2007). Children's conceptualisation(s) of their well-being. *Social Indicators Research, 80*(1), 5–29.

Flick, U. (2002). *An Introduction to qualitative research* (2nd ed.). London, UK: Sage.

Furman, R., Langer, C. L., Davis, C. S., Gallardo, H. P., & Kulkarni, S. (2007). Expressive, research and reflective poetry as qualitative inquiry: a study of adolescent identity. *Qualitative Research, 7*(3), 301–315.

Geanellos, R. (2004). Nursing based evidence: Moving beyond evidence based practice in mental health nursing. *Journal of Evaluation in Clinical Practice, 10*(2), 177–186.

Geertz, C. (1988). *Works and lives: The anthropologist as author*. Palo Alto, CA: Stanford University.

Goffman, E. (1959). *The presentation of the self in everyday life*. Harmondsworth, UK: Penguin.

Haigh, G. (2006, May). The Nelson touch. *The Monthly*.

Harman, G. (2005). Australian social scientists and transition to a more commercial university environment. *Higher Education Research and Development, 24*(1), 79–94.

Herman, L. (2005). Researching the images of evil events: An arts-based methodology in liminal space. *Qualitative Inquiry, 11*(3), 468–480.

Holliday, R. (2007). Performances, confession, and identities: Using video diaries to research sexualities. In G. C. Stanczak (Ed.), *Visual research methods: Image,society and representation* (pp. 255–279). Thousand Oaks, CA: Sage.

Horsfall, D., & Higgs, J. (2007). Boundary riding. In J. Higgs, A. Titchen, D. Horsfall, & H. Armstrong (Eds.), *Being critical and creative in qualitative research* (pp. 69–77). Sydney, Australia: Hampden.

Kleinman, S., & Copp, M. A. (1993). *Theory and methods—Emotions and fieldwork: Qualitative research methods* (Vol. 28). Newbury Park, CA: Sage.

Krug, G., & Hepworth, J. (1997). Poststructuralism, qualitative methodology and public health: Research methods as a legitimation strategy for knowledge. *Critical Public Health, 7*(1 & 2), 50–60.

Lather, P. (2004). This is your father's paradigm: Government intrusion and the case of qualitative research in education. *Qualitative Inquiry, 10*(1), 15–34.

Lincoln, Y. S., & Cannella, G. S. (2004). Qualitative research, power, and the radical right. *Qualitative Inquiry, 10*(2), 175–201.

Macintyre, S. (2007). Universities. In C. Hamilton & S. Maddison (Eds.), *Silencing dissent: How the Australian Government is controlling public opinion and stifling debate* (pp. 41–59). Sydney, Australia: Allen and Unwin.

Marginson, S., & Considine, M. (2000). *The Enterprise University: Power, governance and reinvention in Australia*. Melbourne, Australia: Cambridge University.

McCall, M. M. (2000). Performance ethnography: A brief history and some advice. In N. K. Denzin & Y. S. Lincoln (Eds.), *Handbook of qualitative research* (pp. 421–433). Thousand Oaks, CA: Sage.

Mills, C. W. (1959). The sociological imagination. Harmondsworth, UK: Penguin.

Minge, J. M. (2007). The stained body: A fusion of embodied art on rape and love. *Journal of Contemporary Ethnography, 36*(3), 252–280.

Peseta, T. (2007). Troubling our desires for research and writing within the academic development project. *International Journal of Academic Development, 12*(1), 15–23.

Pietroni, P. C. (1992). Alternative medicine: Methinks the doctor protests too much and incidentally befuddles the debate. *Journal of Medical Ethics, 18,* 23–25.

Pink, S. (2001). *Doing visual ethnography.* London, UK: Sage.

Sawyer, S., Drew, S., & R. Duncan. (2007). Adolescents with chronic disease—The double whammy. *Australian Family Physician, 36*(8), 622–7.

Scott-Hoy, K., & Ellis, C. (2008). Wording pictures: Discovering heartful autoethnography. In G. J. Knowles & A. L. Cole (Eds.), *Handbook of the arts in qualitative research* (pp. 127–140). Thousand Oaks, CA: Sage.

Simons, H., & McCormack, B. (2007). Integrating arts-based inquiry in evaluation methodology. *Qualitative Inquiry, 13*(2), 292–311.

Torrance, H. (2011). Qualitative research, science, and government: evidence, criteria, policy, and politics.. In N. K. Denzin & Y. S. Lincoln (Eds.), *The Sage handbook of qualitative research* (pp. 569–580). Los Angeles, CA: Sage.

Index

About the Editors and Contributors

ABOUT THE EDITORS

JEANNETTE DIAZ, PhD, is an assistant professor of psychology at the University of West Georgia. Dr. Diaz's scholarship focuses on globalization, social justice and community-based approaches to mental health with an emphasis on critical and humanistic approaches to praxis. She is involved as a community psychologist both in her local community, where she is engaged in asset-based approaches to community development, and in Haiti where she is assisting in the establishment of a community-based mental health program.

ZENO FRANCO, PhD, is assistant professor of community engagement at the Medical College of Wisconsin (MCW) in the Department of Family and Community Medicine's Center for Healthy Communities and Research. He is also faculty in MCW's NIH supported Clinical and Translational Science Institute Community Engagement group. His research focuses on improving mental health and community resilience outcomes in collaboration with veteran, Hispanic, and African American–serving organizations in the city of Milwaukee. Dr. Franco's recent publications include "Heroism: A Conceptual Analysis and Differentiation between Heroic Action and Altruism"—in *Review of General Psychology*; "The Dirty Dozen: Twelve Key Failures of the Hurricane Katrina Response & How Psychology Can Help"—in *American Psychologist*; and "Community Engagement for Translational Disaster Research: Fostering Public, Private & Responder Group Partnerships"—in the *Proceedings of the Ninth International Conference on Information Systems for Crisis Response and Management.*

HARRIS L. FRIEDMAN, PhD, is a Florida-licensed psychologist specializing in clinical psychology and organizational development/consulting. He recently retired as research professor of psychology at University of Florida, where he remains on the courtesy faculty, and he is also professor emeritus at Saybrook University. He has over 200 professional publications, mainly in the areas of clinical and organizational psychology, as well as research methodology, and he has special interest in transpersonal psychology. He is a fellow of the American Psychological

Association, and serves as senior editor of *The International Journal of Transpersonal Studies* and associate editor of *The Humanistic Psychologist.*

CHAD V. JOHNSON, PhD, is an associate professor of human relations, clinical assistant professor of psychiatry, and a project director in the Center of Applied Research for Nonprofit Organizations at the University of Oklahoma. His scholarship and clinical interests include spirituality and psychology, social justice, group psychotherapy, and humanistic/existential/transpersonal studies. He has participated in community-based participatory research projects with several organizations and community groups, such as Indian Health Care Resource Center of Tulsa, Oklahomans for Equality, the Oklahoma Center for Community and Justice, the YWCA, and the Johns Hope Franklin Center for Reconciliation. His scholarship and clinical work include social justice (e.g., LGBTQ rights, race relations), spirituality, and group psychotherapy. He serves on the editorial boards for *The Journal of Counseling Psychology* and *The International Journal for Transpersonal Psychology.* He is also a licensed psychologist and has a private psychotherapy practice in Tulsa, Oklahoma. Dr. Johnson holds a doctorate in counseling psychology from Pennsylvania State University.

BONNIE K. NASTASI, PhD, is an associate professor in the Department of Psychology at Tulane University. Dr. Nastasi's research focuses on the use of mixed-methods designs to develop and evaluate culturally appropriate assessment and intervention approaches for promoting mental health and reducing health risks, such as sexually transmitted infections (STIs) and HIV, both within the United States and internationally. She has worked in Sri Lanka since 1995 on the development of school-based programs to promote psychological well-being and is currently directing a multicountry study of psychological well-being of children and adolescents with research partners in 12 countries. She has worked in India since 2001 as one of the principal investigators of an interdisciplinary public health research program to prevent STIs among married men and women living in the slums of Mumbai. She is active in the promotion of child rights and social justice within the profession of school psychology, and is an associate of the International Institute of Child Rights & Development (IICRD), Centre for Global Studies, University of Victoria, British Columbia. She directed the development of a curriculum for training school psychologists internationally on child rights, *School Psychologist as Advocate for Child Rights*, a joint effort of International School Psychology Association, IICRD, and Tulane University's School Psychology Program. Her published works include the book, *School-Based Mental Health Services: Creating Comprehensive and Culturally Specific Programs*, published by the American Psychological Association in 2004. Dr. Nastasi is immediate past-president for Division 16 (School Psychology) of the American Psychological Association. She holds a doctorate in school psychology and early childhood education from Kent State University.

ABOUT THE CONTRIBUTORS

MAURIANNE ADAMS, PhD, in English Literature from Indiana University (Bloomington), is professor of education emerita in the Social Justice Education Concentration, College of Education at the University of Massachusetts, Amherst. She was an external fellow at the Clinical Developmental Institute (Belmont, Massachusetts) and at the Lifespan Clinical-Developmental Institute (Harvard). She is editor of *Equity & Excellence in Education*; co-editor of *Teaching for Diversity and Social Justice* (2nd edition, 2007), *Readings for Diversity and Social Justice* (3rd edition, 2013), *Strangers and Neighbors: Relations between Blacks and Jews in the United States* (1999), *Promoting Diversity in the College Classroom* (1992); and has published essays on social justice education, social justice pedagogy, faculty development, inclusive teaching, religious oppression, anti-Semitism, and classism.

BRUCE A. ARRIGO, PhD, is professor of criminology, law, and society in the Department of Criminal Justice and Criminology at the University of North Carolina at Charlotte. He holds additional faculty appointments in the Departments of Psychology and Public Health Sciences, as well as the Program in Public Policy and the Center for Professional and Applied Ethics. He is an elected Fellow of the Academy of Criminal Justice Sciences and the American Psychological Association, and is the 2012 recipient of the Lifetime Achievement Award from the Crime and Juvenile Delinquency Division of the Society for the Study of Social Problems. Arrigo holds a doctorate in the administration of justice from the Pennsylvania State University.

TYA M. ARTHUR, PhD, MPH, is a postdoctoral research associate in the Department of Psychology at the University of Florida in Gainesville, Florida. She received a master of public health in Health Policy and Management from the Texas A&M Health Science Center School of Rural Public Health and a doctorate in health education from Texas A&M University in College Station, Texas. Dr. Arthur co-directs grant funded community-engaged research to develop, implement, and evaluate community-based, culturally sensitive health promotion interventions.

KAREN J. BERTE, PhD, is manager of Mental Health Residential Rehabilitation Services at the Clement J. Zablocki VA Medical Center, and assistant professor of psychiatry and behavioral medicine at the Medical College of Wisconsin (MCW), both in Milwaukee. Her areas of clinical specialization include the treatment of stress disorders in combat veterans, and co-morbid PTSD and addictive disorders. Dr. Berte has overseen the development of a specialized residential treatment program focused on postdeployment readjustment to address the needs of newly returning combat veterans. She is the Zablocki VA consultant/liaison to DryHootch of America, with a focus on improving the communication infrastructure to facilitate access to care for veterans referred by community peer mentors.

She is codirector of the MCW/VA PTSD Residency Training Clinic at Zablocki VA and supervises the clinical work of psychiatry residents, psychology interns, and postdoctoral fellows. In addition to her local responsibilities, Dr. Berte is chair of the VISN 12 regional PTSD workgroup involving all VA medical centers in Wisconsin and northern Illinois.

ANGELA M. BORGES, MA, is a doctoral candidate in the counseling psychology program at Boston College and a predoctoral intern at Harvard Medical School/ Cambridge Hospital in Cambridge, Massachusetts. She is also a lead trainer for prevention innovations at the University of New Hampshire and has provided training and consultation on sexual assault prevention to universities and nonprofit organizations both nationally and internationally. Her research interests include innovative domestic violence interventions, sexual assault prevention, the intersection of domestic violence and poverty, psychotherapy with clients in poverty, and social justice training for psychologists.

DIANE BRETHERTON, PhD, is an honorary professor in the School of Political Science and International Relations at the University of Queensland and a visiting professor in the Zhou En Lai School of International Relations at the University of Nankai in Tianjin, China. She was the founding director of the International Conflict Resolution Centre, in the School of Behavioural Science at the University of Melbourne. During the lead-up to the International Year of a Culture of Peace in 2000 she was seconded to UNESCO Headquarters in Paris to help manage the Culture of Peace Program. She completed her PhD at the University of Keele in Staffordshire in the United Kingdom. She is a co-editor of *Community Resilience in Natural Disasters* (Palgrave Macmillan, 2011) and has extensive practical experience of conducting peace and conflict resolution programs in a number of countries. Her e-mail address is d.bretherton@uq.edu.au.

THEMA S. BRYANT-DAVIS, PhD, is an associate professor of psychology at Pepperdine University and director of the Culture and Trauma Research Lab. Dr. Bryant-Davis is a past president of the Society for the Psychology of Women. Dr. Bryant-Davis is also a former American Psychological Association representative to the United Nations. She is author of multiple peer-reviewed articles and chapters as well as the author of the book *Thriving in the Wake of Trauma: A Multicultural Guide* and editor of the book *Surviving Sexual Violence: A Guide to Recovery and Empowerment*. Her research and clinical work focuses on cultural considerations of recovery from traumatic experiences such as sexual assault, intimate partner violence, human trafficking, and racism.

MILENA CLAUDIUS is a third-year doctoral student in counseling psychology at Boston College. She completed her undergraduate studies in psychology at Boston University and her master's degree in mental health counseling at Boston

College. Her interests are in the areas of trauma, immigration, and topics at the intersection of psychology, social justice, and human rights.

KATHERINE E. CODER, PhD, is a community and transpersonal psychologist who counsels, consults, teaches, writes, and builds communities of healing and transformation. She serves as an adjunct faculty member at the University of Miami. Her research interests include mystic activism, holistic well-being interventions, and innovative models of social change.

PAMELA A. COUNTS, MA, is a doctoral student in clinical psychology at Pepperdine University. She is a research assistant at Pepperdine's Culture and Trauma Lab, and a founding co-chair of the university's Asian American Psychology Student Association. Her clinical and research interests include trauma, multicultural issues, women's rights, and children and families.

ROBERT CURRY is president/founder of DryHootch of America, a veteran-serving community-based organization based in Milwaukee, Wisconsin. Mr. Curry served in the U.S. Army from 1969 to 1972, co-piloting over 250 combat missions in Vietnam and Laos. In 2005, Robert was diagnosed as 100% permanently disabled with posttraumatic stress disorder (PTSD) as a result of these experiences. He founded DryHootch in 2008 as a means to help the younger generation of Iraq and Afghanistan veterans combat PTSD and drug/alcohol addiction. Mr. Curry oversees the organization's relationships with a variety of partners, including the VA, state veteran agencies, local governments, and health and mental health groups. He is chair of the Wisconsin Vietnam Veterans of America Committee on PTSD/Addiction. Mr. Curry obtained a BS in economics from UW Milwaukee in 1975, and worked for many years with major information technology firms, including IBM, AT&T, and Lotus.

CURTISS PAUL DEYOUNG, EdD, is the professor of reconciliation studies at Bethel University (St. Paul, Minnesota). He has written several books, including *Living Faith: How Faith Inspires Social Justice*. He regularly promotes the work of reconciliation and social justice in communities, institutional settings, and religious congregations.

AMARPREET K. DHAMI is a graduate student in the mental health counseling master's program at Long Island University–Brooklyn. Ms. Dhami is currently an intern at a mental health agency, which provides multidisciplinary mental health services for people living with HIV/AIDS who have severe mental illness and/or substance use disorders.

MARK FLOWER is the Director for Community Programs at DryHootch of America, a veteran-serving community-based organization based in Milwaukee,

Wisconsin. Mr. Flower is also veteran peer mentor at DryHootch. A veteran from the Cold War era, Mark joined the army in 1976, and served on active duty with the 25th Infantry Division through 1980. Later, he joined the 84th Training Division and served as an instructor/evaluator, and later as a medic and field sanitation NCO with the 452nd Combat Support Hospital. Mark struggled with alcoholism and drug addiction. He became involved in recovery in 1993. He has been sober since then and has helped other alcoholics by managing halfway houses, including the Manitoba House, the Alano Foundation, and Sals House Transitional Living Facility.

MARY A. FUKUYAMA, PhD, is a licensed psychologist and clinical professor at the University of Florida Counseling & Wellness Center, where she has worked for the past 30 years counseling students, supervising interns, teaching, and writing on multicultural topics. She is a graduate in counseling psychology from Washington State University. Her current interests include spirituality and counseling, and international initiatives such as promoting study abroad programs. She is a fellow in Division 17 (Counseling Psychology) of the American Psychological Association.

LISA A. GOODMAN, PhD, is a professor in the Department of Counseling and Applied Developmental Psychology at Boston College. She is the author of over 95 articles and chapters on the interaction between victims of intimate partner violence and the practices, systems, and policies that aim to help them; the psychosocial effects of intimate partner violence; innovative mental health practices for low-income communities; and bringing social justice to counseling psychology. She has also consulted extensively with community-based organizations that work with survivors and is the cofounder of the Massachusetts Domestic Violence Program Evaluation and Research Collaborative. Dr. Goodman holds a doctorate in clinical-community psychology from Boston University

ANTHEA A. GRAY is currently a PsyD student at Pepperdine University and a student therapist at the Union Rescue Mission. She also works as a research assistant in Pepperdine's Culture and Trauma lab and is the Advisory Board secretary for the Georges Malaika Foundation, a nonprofit organization that educates Congolese girls. Gray holds an MA from Teachers College at Columbia University.

INGRID HUYGENS, PhD, holds the position of research leader in the Centre for Health and Social Practice, Waikato Institute of Technology. She also coordinates a national decolonisation project, *Treaty People*. Her social justice scholarship has theorized feminist and antiracist activism, particularly for culturally dominant groups working in alliance with indigenous peoples. She is past Chair of the Institute of Community Psychology Aotearoa. She completed her masters in social psychology at University of Auckland, and her PhD at University of Waikato.

GAZI ISLAM completed his PhD in organizational behavior at Tulane University, where his research focused on organizational identity, voice, and power relations. He has served as a faculty member at Grenoble Ecole de Management, Insper, Tulane University, and the University of New Orleans. His current research interests include the organizational antecedents and consequences of identity, and the relations between identity, group dynamics, and the production of group and organizational cultures. His work has been published in journals such as *Organization Studies*, *Leadership Quarterly*, *Organization*, *Human Relations*, *The American Journal of Public Health*, *Journal of Business Ethics*, and *American Psychologist*.

ALLEN E. IVEY, EdD, is distinguished university professor (emeritus), University of Massachusetts, Amherst, and professor of counseling at the University of South Florida, Tampa (courtesy appointment). He is president of Microtraining Associates, an educational publishing firm. A diplomat in counseling psychology, Dr. Ivey was honored as a multicultural elder at the National Multicultural Conference and Summit. He is author and coauthor of more than 40 books and 200 articles and chapters, translated into 18 languages. He is the originator of the Microskills approach to counseling.

BELLE LIANG, PhD, is a licensed psychologist and associate professor at the Lynch School of Education in Counseling, Developmental, and Educational Psychology at Boston College. Her research focuses on relational interventions, especially youth mentoring and innovative social media–based interventions for diverse youth. Liang holds a doctorate in clinical psychology from Michigan State University.

ANISSA L. MOODY is a counseling psychologist and assistant professor of psychology at City University of New York, Queens borough Community College in Flushing, New York. She has published papers and given talks on the practice of mental hygiene and the intersections of race, health, and gender in underserved populations. Dr. Moody also has a private practice in New York City where she specializes in treating trauma and anxiety using holistic interventions.

POONAM OBEROI is a PhD candidate and an affiliate professor of Marketing at the Grenoble Ecole de Management. Poonam holds a Licence de Lettres Modernes from the Université de Rennes II and a BA(hons.) in business administration from the Open University, Milton Keynes. After completing a master of science in innovation and technology management at Grenoble Ecole de Management she joined the school's PhD program in 2009 with a research focus on inter-organizational collaborations and open innovation. Poonam was a visiting PhD at the London Business School for the academic year 2011–2012. Besides work, she is passionate about writing short stories and traveling.

MAUREEN PERRY JENKINS, PhD, is a professor in clinical psychology at the University of Massachusetts, Amherst. Her research focuses on the ways in which sociocultural factors such as race, gender, and social class shape the mental health and family relationships of employed parents and their children. Her current research involves a 10-year, longitudinal study funded by the National Institute of Mental Health that examines the transition to parenthood and transition back to paid employment for working-class, low-wage couples and for African American, Latino and European American single mothers.

DYNORA PIERRE-LOUIS, BS, is an administrative and research associate in the Department of Psychology at the University of Florida where she conducts community-engaged research to promote culturally sensitive health care. She has previously conducted biomedical research as a research intern in the Department of Pharmacology at Vanderbilt University Medical Center in Nashville, Tennessee, and in the Department of Cardiology at the University of Chicago, Pritzker School of Medicine in Chicago, Illinois. Dynora received a bachelor of science in health education from the University of Florida in Gainesville, Florida.

ALPHIA POSSAMAI-INESEDY, PhD, is a senior lecturer in sociology at the University of Western Sydney. She is the editor in chief of *The Journal of Sociology* (2013–2016) as well as the co-creator of the Risk Societies Thematic Group within the Australian Sociological Association. Her recent work includes *Sociology: A Down-to-Earth Approach* (with Henslin and Possamai, 2010, Pearson) and *New Methods in Social Justice Research for the Twenty-First Century* (with Gwyther, 2009, Taylor & Francis). Alphia is currently involved in ongoing research that focuses on risk society, religion, spirituality, and methodologies.

ISAAC PRILLELTENSKY, PhD, is professor and dean of Education and Human Development at the University of Miami, where he holds the Erwin and Barbara Mautner Chair in Community Well-Being. His scholarship deals with critical and community psychology, wellness, and fairness. Prilleltensky holds a doctorate in psychology from the University of Manitoba.

ANOUK RIDE is based in the Solomon Islands and is a writer, researcher, and film producer with 10 years' experience working in the Pacific Islands region on social and environmental issues (www.anoukride.com). She was editor of the *New Internationalist* magazine. She studied at the Australian National University in Canberra and at the University of California in San Diego and is currently a PhD candidate with the School of Political Science and International Relations at University of Queensland. She is the author of *The Grand Experiment* (Hachette Livre, 2007) and co-editor of *Community Resilience in Natural Disasters* (Palgrave Macmillan, 2011).

MANUEL RIEMER, PhD, is an associate professor of community and environmental psychology at Wilfrid Laurier University and the director of the Centre for Community, Research, Learning and Action and the Community, Environment and Justice Research Group. His current research focuses on using community and critical psychology principles, theories, and tools to address issues related to global climate change mitigation and adaptation with a special focus on environmental justice and youth. He received his PhD in psychology from Peabody College at Vanderbilt University, Nashville, Tennessee (USA).

BRENT DEAN ROBBINS, PhD, is coordinator of the Psychology Program, director of the MA Program in Clinical-Community Psychology, and associate professor of psychology at Point Park University, as well as a therapist at Mercy Behavioral Health, in Pittsburgh, Pennsylvania. He has a doctorate in clinical psychology from Duquesne University, and is president of Division 32 of the American Psychological Association—the Society for Humanistic Psychology. He co-edited the book *Drugging Our Children: How Profiteers Are Pushing Antipsychotics on Our Youngest and What We Can Do Stop It* (Praeger, 2012), he is editor-in-chief of the interdisciplinary, academic journal, *Janus Head* (www.janushead.org), and he was coauthor of the "Open Letter to the DSM-5 Task Force" which was signed by over 50 mental health organizations and over 14,000 mental health professionals and other individuals.

JULIA RONCORONI, MS, is a graduate research associate on Dr. Carolyn M. Tucker's Behavioral Medicine Research Team at the University of Florida in Gainesville, Florida. Julia conducts community-based, patient-centered culturally sensitive health care and health promotion research. She received a master's degree in psychology from the University of Florida. She is currently a doctoral student in the counseling psychology program at the University of Florida.

JACKELINE SANCHEZ, MS, is a graduate research associate on Dr. Carolyn M. Tucker's Behavioral Medicine Research Team at the University of Florida in Gainesville, Florida. Jackeline received a master's degree in mental health counseling from the University of Miami and is currently a doctoral student in the counseling psychology program at the University of Florida. Her research involves conducting community-based interventions focused on patient-centered culturally sensitive health care and health promotion.

TASIA M. SMITH, MS, is a graduate research associate on Dr. Carolyn M. Tucker's Health Psychology Research Team at the University of Florida in Gainesville, Florida. She received a master's degree in human development and family studies from the University of North Carolina at Greensboro. Tasia is a doctoral student in the counseling psychology program at the University of Florida. She conducts community-engaged research focused on culturally sensitive approaches to health promotion.

LINDA R. TROPP, PhD, is professor of psychology and director of the Psychology of Peace and Violence Program at the University of Massachusetts, Amherst. Her research concerns how members of different groups approach and experience contact with each other, and how group differences in status affect cross-group relations. She has worked with international organizations to present social science evidence in U.S. Supreme Court cases on racial integration, on state and national initiatives to improve interracial relations in schools, and with international organizations to evaluate applied programs designed to reduce racial and ethnic conflict.

CAROLYN M. TUCKER, PhD, is the Florida Blue Endowed Chair in Health Disparities Research at the University of Florida (UF) and the Richard and Thelma O. C. Barney Endowed Term Professor of Health Disparities in the UF College of Medicine. She also is a distinguished alumni professor, professor of psychology, professor of community health and family medicine, affiliate professor of pediatrics, research foundation professor, and a fellow in the American Psychological Association. She has spent most of her academic career conducting interdisciplinary, community-based participatory research programs with the goal of promoting individual and community health empowerment to promote health and prevent disease in at-risk communities. Dr. Tucker received a doctorate in clinical psychology from the State University of New York at Stony Brook.

PRATYUSHA TUMMALA-NARRA, PhD, is assistant professor in the Department of Counseling, Developmental and Educational Psychology at Boston College. Her research and scholarly work focuses on the topics of immigration, trauma, and cultural competence in psychotherapy practice. Dr. Tummala-Narra has served as the chair of the Multicultural Concerns Committee for Division 39 (Psychoanalysis), as a member of the Committee on Ethnic Minority Affairs (CEMA) in the American Psychological Association, and as a member of the APA Presidential Task Force on Immigration.

COURTE VAN VOORHEES is a clinical assistant professor in the Department of Education and Psychological Studies at the University of Miami. His research focuses on the physical and social contexts of community well-being. He primarily conducts community-based participatory action research to promote social justice, environmental justice, and sustainability. He earned his doctorate in Community Research and Action from Peabody College of Vanderbilt University.

WHITNEY WALL, MPH, MS, is a graduate research associate on Dr. Carolyn M. Tucker's Behavioral Medicine Research Team at the University of Florida in Gainesville, Florida. She received her master's degree in public health from the Arnold School of Public Health at the University of South Carolina and a master of science, with a concentration in psychology, from the University of Florida. She is currently a doctoral candidate in the counseling psychology program at the University of Florida. Whitney conducts community-engaged research and interventions focused on patient-centered culturally sensitive health care and health promotion.

JEFF WHITTLE, MD, MPH, is director of Health Services Research at the Clement J. Zablocki VA Medical Center and professor of medicine at the Medical College of Wisconsin, both in Milwaukee. His research focuses on common chronic conditions affecting the physical and mental health of older adults. He and veteran colleagues have developed and tested several interventions that use the existing social support present in community veterans organizations (e.g., the Veterans of Foreign Wars, the Vietnam Veterans of America, and the American Legion) to encourage healthy lifestyles. Dr. Whittle's recent publications include "Ethical Challenges in a Randomized Controlled Trial of Peer Education among Veterans Service Organizations" in *The Journal of Empirical Research on Human Research Ethics*; "What Can the VA Teach Us about Implementing Proven Advances into Routine Clinical Practice?" in *The Journal of General Internal Medicine*; and "Location and Organizational Features: What Type of Veteran Communities Participate in Health Programs?" in *Progress in Community Health Partnerships: Research, Education, and Action.*

CHRISTOPHER R. WILLIAMS, PhD, is professor and chairman of the Department of Criminal Justice Studies at Bradley University. Dr. Williams is a dedicated teacher who has created, developed, and taught a wide range of courses within criminology and criminal justice. Since 2000, he has taught over 20 different courses on topics such as criminological theory, ethics and criminal justice, criminal profiling, psychology and the legal system, crime and music, drugs and culture, and social justice. Dr. Williams is also an accomplished scholar, having published four books, over 25 academic journal articles and book chapters, and numerous essays and reviews, most confronting issues and controversies in social and criminological theory, the sociology of deviance, the philosophical foundations of crime, law, and justice, and the sociological and legal dimensions of mental health and illness.

WENDI S. WILLIAMS, PhD is counseling psychologist and associate professor and coordinator of counseling programs at Long Island University–Brooklyn. She is a graduate of the counseling psychology program at Georgia State University. Her work centers on health and wellness programming for urban youth and relational concerns of women of color, as well as the development and evaluation of culturally relevant curriculum for counselor-trainees.

JULIE WOULFE, MS, is a PhD student in Boston College's Counseling Psychology program. Her scholarship and clinical work focus on integrating social justice into counseling psychology and community mental health, LGBTQ communities, and the intersection of intimate partner violence and oppression. She received her MS in counseling psychology from the University of Wisconsin, Madison.

CARLOS P. ZALAQUETT, PhD, is professor and coordinator of the Clinical Mental Health Counseling Specialization in the Psychological and Social Foundations Department, University of South Florida, Tampa.

THE PRAEGER HANDBOOK OF SOCIAL JUSTICE AND PSYCHOLOGY

THE PRAEGER HANDBOOK OF SOCIAL JUSTICE AND PSYCHOLOGY

Volume 3

Youth and Disciplines in Psychology

Chad V. Johnson and Harris L. Friedman, Set Editors
Jeannette Diaz, Zeno Franco, and Bonnie K. Nastasi, Volume Editors

Foreword by Mary A. Fukuyama

Social Justice and Psychology

PRAEGER

AN IMPRINT OF ABC-CLIO, LLC
Santa Barbara, California • Denver, Colorado • Oxford, England

Copyright 2014 by Chad V. Johnson and Harris L. Friedman

All rights reserved. No part of this publication may be reproduced, stored in a retrieval system, or transmitted, in any form or by any means, electronic, mechanical, photocopying, recording, or otherwise, except for the inclusion of brief quotations in a review, without prior permission in writing from the publisher.

Library of Congress Cataloging-in-Publication Data

The Praeger handbook of social justice and psychology / Chad V. Johnson [and five others].
volumes cm. — (Social justice and psychology)
Includes index.
Contents: volume 1. Fundamental issues and special populations
ISBN 978-1-4408-0378-9 (hardcopy : alk. paper) — ISBN 978-1-4408-0379-6 (ebook)
1. Social psychiatry. 2. Social justice—Psychological aspects. 3. Psychology, Pathological—Social aspects. I. Johnson, Chad (Chad Vernon) II. Title: Handbook of social justice and psychology.
RC455.P6962 2014
616.89'071—dc23 2014000218

ISBN: 978-1-4408-0378-9
EISBN: 978-1-4408-0379-6

18 17 16 15 14 1 2 3 4 5

This book is also available on the World Wide Web as an eBook.
Visit www.abc-clio.com for details.

Praeger
An Imprint of ABC-CLIO, LLC

ABC-CLIO, LLC
130 Cremona Drive, P.O. Box 1911
Santa Barbara, California 93116-1911

This book is printed on acid-free paper ∞

Manufactured in the United States of America

Dedicated to the Memory of George Albee (1921–2006)

George was a pioneering psychologist whose path was to envision "a world free from exploitation and domination of one group by another, a world in which each person has the freedom and the resources to develop her or his potential to the fullest, a world in which the highest goal would be one person's concern and regard for others" (Kessler, Goldston, & Joffe, 1992, p. 19). And he worked ceaselessly toward these ends. When I first met him in the late 1990s, he and I were keynote speakers at a conference on psychology and juvenile justice. Having my attitudes and values toward professional psychology profoundly shaped by reading many of his contributions, I excitedly blurted out, "you are my hero." Unabashedly George responded, "We all must be heroes."—Harris L. Friedman

Kessler, M., Goldston, S., & Joffe, J. (1992). George Albee: An appreciation. In M. Kessler, S. Goldston, & J. Joffe (Eds.), *The present and future of prevention: In honor of George W. Albee* (pp. 3–32). Newbury Park, CA: Sage.

Contents

Acknowledgments

We would like to thank the contributing authors for their highly informative chapters, diligence, and responsive to requests for revision. We are deeply indebted to our editorial assistant, Lindsay Plott-Buckner, who worked tirelessly, superbly, and without complaint throughout the editing process. We are also grateful for additional editorial assistance provided by Heather Threadgill and Eamon Slattery. Finally, we acknowledge all those, both within and outside psychology, who struggle with oppression and injustice and work toward social justice and peace.

Introduction to Volume 3

Bonnie K. Nastasi, Zeno Franco, and Chad V. Johnson

Volume 3 addresses social justice and psychology applied to youth in the context of schools, and to various disciplines in psychology—counseling and clinical, community, industrial-organizational and consulting, and school. Here, we provide an overview of the volume and examines major themes across chapters in the volume. Part 1 of the volume addresses the roles of schools and other child-serving systems (families, communities) in promoting and protecting social justice and child rights for children as well as their roles in preparing children to participate in social justice action. Part 2 focuses on the role of specific applied disciplines of psychology in ensuring social justice through ethical foundations, research, practice, training, and policy. The chapters in Part 2 take both a present-oriented perspective (what can we do now to promote social justice?) and a future-orientated perspective (how do we make sure that the profession continues to ensure social justice?). In both parts, the authors provide historical perspective, review current status, and provide recommendations for enhancing and advancing the work of psychology in the social justice realm. Next, we provide an overview that summarizes key points of each section and chapter. We conclude with future directions and final thoughts for psychologists.

YOUTH AND SCHOOLS

The chapters in this part address the role of schools, families, and communities in promoting social justice among children and youth. In doing so, the authors acknowledge the importance of an ecological-developmental perspective and draw from a range of psychological theories and research (e.g., developmental, community, school). Several themes emerge in this section: (1) the interconnection of social justice and child rights, initially articulated by Hart and Shriberg; (2) the importance of thinking beyond a single system (e.g., school) and the essential involvement of stakeholders across systems (school, family, community);

(3) the responsibility of adults and organizations for promoting and protecting child rights and social justice, and for preparing children as socially responsible individuals; and (4) the centrality of the child's well-being to development of socially just communities and societies.

In Chapter 1, Hart and Shriberg explore the relationship between social justice and child rights, emphasizing their integrated nature, that is, one cannot exist without the other. They discuss the reflection of both social justice and child rights in professional ethics of psychology and current work of professional psychology organizations. The authors also examine five central themes of human nature that are foundational to both justice and rights: human needs, existential choice making, moral development, social relationships, and realization of self. Furthermore, they emphasize the importance of facilitating well-being as central to both social justice and child rights. Hart and Shriberg also note the absence of human (child) rights in social justice literature, despite the apparent overlap in goals and agendas for advocates. The authors provide a heuristic for guiding our perspectives, research, practice, and policy that is grounded in three interrelated issues that reflect both social justice and child rights—full development of the personality, eliminating violence, and attaining solidarity. Hart and Shriberg conclude the chapter with a call for serving the best interests of all children through action that encompasses the principles of child rights and social justice.

In Chapter 2, Naser, Nastasi, and Mulser discuss the roles and responsibilities of schools for promoting both social justice and child rights. The authors contend that schools can best meet these goals by incorporating system-wide behavioral management and social-emotional learning programs as basic to education for all children. They review school-based programs with substantial empirical support for building child resilience and identify key components for effectiveness. Of particular importance to success are the integration of program values and goals into school culture and system-wide practices, and participation of key stakeholders within (e.g., students, teachers, administrators) and outside (e.g., parents and community organizations) of the school. Furthermore, such programs are based on social justice and child rights principles, recognize the interrelationships of systems in which children live (e.g., family and school), and attend to cultural and historical background of individuals and systems. Naser and colleagues also emphasize the importance of assessing the specific needs and resources of the child and the system in order to provide appropriate services that promote resilience and ensure development to full potential for each child.

The Lewis and Swift chapter addresses the development of prosocial behavior through the family relationships as a means to promote social justice orientation among children and prepare them to be advocates for social justice (Chapter 3). The model proposed by the authors adopts an ecological family systems and strengths-based "relationship" approach, grounded in developmental psychology theories. The core components of the model are developing emotional and social skills, learning to value diversity and everyday conflict, and promoting social justice through service to others. The authors contend that the family relationship can provide the basis for recognizing and accepting humanity of others outside of one's own family and ethnic group, and respecting the needs and rights of others to resources for basic survival. The family relationship provides the context for developing empathy and intersubjectivity, understanding conflict as a normal aspect of relationships and learning to resolve conflict successfully and peacefully, and acquiring individual and family self-efficacy as change agents for social justice. Moreover, the authors contend, teaching these elements of social justice through social, particularly family, relationships is fundamental to the development of individuals who are socially connected and responsible and can engage in social justice action.

Siegel in Chapter 4 focuses on promoting social justice in urban communities characterized by neighborhood disorder. The author describes the integration of developmental theories (ecological and psychosocial) and community psychology research (neighborhood research) as foundations for promoting social justice for urban youth. Neighborhood research links social disorganization and consequent social alienation with poor psychological outcomes, and identifies components of social alienation as mistrust, powerlessness, normlessness, and social isolation. Drawing on Positive Youth Development program research, Siegel advocates for sustainable interventions that support development of multiple prosocial competencies through structured activities in multiple contexts (e.g., family, school, community). Such programs, when implemented with integrity, have documented effectiveness for preventing negative outcomes of neighborhood disorder and social disorganization. Siegel thus illustrates the potential for promoting social justice through evidence-based practice that draws on transdisciplinary foundations in psychology.

In Chapter 5, Nastasi proposes the integration of a child rights perspective into psychological research, with a particular focus on research as a mechanism for promoting and protecting *child participation* rights (e.g., right to express one's viewpoints, to be listened to by adults, and to have a voice in decisions affecting one's life). The chapter summarizes the articles of the UN Convention on the Rights of the Child (1989), describes the nature of child participation in research, and proposes five levels of research activity devoted to the promotion and protection of participation rights with examples from research in social science, education, and global development. The five levels are (1) examining child perceptions, (2) examining child experiences, (3) facilitating child-adult communication, (4) informing decisions that affect children (e.g., development of interventions or policies for children), and (5) performing participatory research (i.e., engaging children as co-researchers). The chapter also discusses methodological, ethical, and practical challenges related to child participation in research, as wells as the necessary researcher competences. Finally, the author calls for psychological researchers to consider their role as promoters and protectors of child participation rights.

In a special commentary (Chapter 6), 99-year-old esteemed psychologist Milton Schwebel makes a passionate plea for addressing long-standing injustices in education that have affected school children in the past and continue to threaten current and future generations. He begins by making the case that education begins at birth and it is incumbent upon political, social, and educational policymakers and advocates to ensure a just beginning for our nation's and the world's children. Research has established great disparities in opportunity and access to quality education for many children, particularly those from racial/ethnic minorities or living in poverty. He urges actions sooner rather than later. Schwebel argues that, unfortunately, what has been attempted by the past three presidential administrations has failed. He proposes four essential components for radical change in educational policy and practice: (1) a social safety net that ensures low-income and disadvantaged families adequate health care, prenatal care, early education, and other supports; (2) accessible quality parent education that helps prepare families for child-rearing and educational attainment, and promotes enriching environments and experiences for children; (3) high-quality free early education (nursery and preschool) for low-income families with instruction tailored to the cultural and educational needs of their children; and (4) school systems with highly trained and compensated teachers who are equipped to work in culturally competent ways with a diversity of students. Furthermore, those schools that serve predominantly poorer communities should receive per capita support greater than or equal to more affluent communities, including equal educational resources such as technology, buildings in good condition, and quality intracurricular and extracurricular programming. Schwebel concludes his chapter with encouraging words, suggesting social changes can be accomplished as have social transformations in the past—through the power of growing social consciousness and mass movements for change.

DISCIPLINES IN PSYCHOLOGY

This part addresses the role of social justice in several disciplines of psychology, including clinical and counseling, industrial-organizational (I-O) and consulting, community, and school psychology, what psychologists might describe as the applied disciplines, as well as research psychology. What best characterizes these disciplines is the diversity in values and action related to social justice, ranging from minimal to maximal integration (as characterized by the chapter authors), I-O/consulting, clinical/counseling, school, and community. Why is that the case? One reason might be the client base and primary goals; for example, the primary clients of I-O/consulting are organizations and corporations rather than individuals, with priority given to performance outcomes and organizational well-being rather than equality and diversity of their employees. In contrast, community psychology was developed with social justice as primary to its mission and focuses on the integral well-being of the personal, interpersonal, and collective. Clinical and counseling focus on the individual as client; although valuing nondiscrimination and equality, these disciplines, particularly clinical, have been less concerned with social justice as primary to their mission and more concerned with the health of individuals. In Chapter 7, Toporek and Suyemoto, however, do acknowledge that counseling psychologists are more explicitly concerned with social justice issues compared to clinical psychologists. Finally, school psychology has as clients individual children embedded in schools, families, and communities. As a function of legal attention to inequity (e.g., special education legislation in 1970s) and the increasing attention to disparities in education and health care, the discipline of school psychology has more explicitly focused on social justice in recent years. Despite these variations in commitment and action, all of the applied specialties struggle with internal and external challenges to promotion of and advocacy for social justice. These include differences in priorities within the discipline, need for more innovative research and practice methods, and need for integration of social justice mission and advocacy into graduate training programs.

Toporek and Suyemoto summarize the history of social justice perspectives in counseling and clinical psychology, present a current snapshot of the respective fields, review challenges to integrating social justice approaches in these disciplines, and make an important call to action for counseling and clinical psychologists. The authors begin with definitions that distinguish between clinical and counseling psychology, which perhaps share more similarities than differences. Historically as well as currently, each discipline has advocated for and promoted social justice, although with stronger emphasis and integration in counseling psychology. The authors also acknowledge several important challenges to effectively integrating social justice into clinical and counseling psychology. For instance, they contend that counseling psychology may demonstrate hubris and overidentify with social justice that in turn ironically results in lack of serious reflexivity and action. On the other hand, clinical psychology often views social justice as something separate and addressed in other disciplines, thus not necessitating its integration. Finally, the authors call clinical and counseling psychologists to action, recommending that social justice be integrated into the fabric of these disciplines lest they inadvertently perpetuate an oppressive status quo within psychology and society at large.

In Chapter 8, Evans, Rosen, and Nelson emphasize social justice as a central value and goal of community psychology, illustrate applications in the field through research and action, and discuss challenges to fulfilling this central mission. The authors provide definitions of social justice; distinguish between distributive and procedural social justice; and delineate social justice as a multilevel construct concerned with interpersonal relationships, organizations, and communities/societies (drawing on the work of Prilletensky and colleagues). Despite the centrality of social justice since the inception of community psychology, challenges still exist in its realization in practice, research, training, and action. The authors attribute these challenges to discrepancies in the values of community psychology and critical community psychology. Critical community psychology practice, in particular, is committed to empowerment, liberation, and transformation through broad social movements, and requires transformative-emancipatory and participatory action research approaches. They conclude the chapter with recommendations for theory, research, education, training, and practice that are grounded in critical community psychology.

Lowman in Chapter 9 focuses on the challenges for industrial-organizational (I-O) and consulting psychologists in promoting a social justice agenda. The primary challenges noted by the author are the potential conflict between value systems of business and psychology, and the "organization" as a client rather than individuals within the organization. However, Lowman also notes more recent corporate agendas of social responsibility that include advocacy. Acknowledging that I-O/consulting psychologists are less likely than psychologists from other disciplines to be aggressive in advocacy efforts (because of the aforementioned challenges), Lowman discusses how social justice issues might impact the work of these psychologists and how I-O/consulting psychologists can influence social justice agendas of organizations. For example, in reference to employee selection, Lowman states that I-O/consulting psychologists are uniquely qualified to help organizations balance concerns about job performance (selection outcome) and goals of creating diversity in the workplace (social justice outcome). Ultimately, the author reminds psychologists of the power of influence that comes from using research evidence and evidence-based practice in ways that ensure or foster social justice, and of engaging in what he calls "quiet advocacy" by raising issues that have implications for ensuring socially responsible and just organizations. One aspect of this quiet advocacy is raising social justice issues in relevant contexts without necessarily using the term *social justice*, but rather speaking in the language of the organization and its leaders. Finally, psychologists can be influential in helping to promote ethical responsibility within organizations through their consulting and advising roles.

Tracing the history of psychology and youth education, and school psychology and social justice, Shriberg in Chapter 10 points to (1) psychology's historical lack of interest in schools and (2) school psychology's lack of interest in social justice and related "missed opportunities" to advance justice causes. He discusses the changing priorities in school psychology in the 21st century, exemplified by advocacy efforts within major professional organizations (APA's Division of School Psychology, National Association of School Psychologists) related to the needs of LGBTQ students and child rights. Despite the explicit focus on social justice within the purview of school psychology in the past, the history of school psychology has been influenced by social justice movements in United States, most notably, the special education rights movement and related legislation of the 1960s and 1970s. Shriberg presents findings of recent research supporting the commitment of today's school psychologists to social justice, and concludes the chapter with descriptions of evolving models of "socially just school psychology practice."

CONCLUSION

This volume is devoted to the examination of the role of various disciplines within psychology and natural systems—schools, families, and communities—in promoting social justice and human rights for children. Both sections of the volume highlight contributions from psychology theory and research and emphasize the critical role of adults (psychologists, parents, teachers, community members, policymakers) in society for ensuring social justice in the present and the future. While acknowledging the past and current contributions of psychology to social justice action, all the authors stress a futuristic perspective. Across the chapters in the volume, several themes for future directions emerged. These include making social justice and child rights more explicit as underlying values, collaborating across disciplinary and systems boundaries to strengthen collective action, and recognizing the importance and responsibilities of all stakeholders (professional and nonprofessional) in ensuring socially just societies. Moreover, all authors recognize the important role of psychology in understanding how to best promote social justice, examining mechanisms that contribute to human injustices, and developing interventions for addressing current injustices while preparing both children and adults (including psychologists) to be active in promoting social justice for all.

REFERENCE

United Nations (UN). (1989). *Convention on the rights of the child.* Retrieved from http://www2.ohchr.org/english/law/crc.htm

Part 1

Youth and Schools

Chapter 1

Human Rights and Social Justice for Children

Stuart N. Hart and David Shriberg

The essential purposes of psychology are undergirded by values oriented toward respect for the human condition and promotion of human fulfillment. Human rights (including children's rights) and social justice provide essential guidance for promoting these values in the best interests of persons, their families, communities, and societies. Although particular emphasis is given by human rights to dignity and well-being, and by social justice to fairness, sanctity of life, and solidarity, their meanings and purposes are more wide-ranging and overlap significantly. Neither is likely to be fully achieved without commitment to the other.

Human rights and social justice are crucial elements of the very bedrock of psychology. They express, in part, the foundational why, or the essential purposes, over and about which the multiple layers of psychological knowledge, interests, techniques, and activities are rooted, refined, and applied. Fidelity to human rights and social justice is fundamental to the nature, value, and contributions of psychology.

Recognition and appreciation of the importance of human rights and social justice has been infused into the ethical principles and practice codes of psychology. Using the Code of Ethics of American Psychological Association (APA, 2010) as an example, the Preamble states that psychologists "respect and protect civil and human rights" (p. 3); and the General Principles include the phrases: "safeguard the welfare and rights of those with whom they interact professionally" (p. 3); "recognize that fairness and justice entitle all persons to access to and benefit from the contributions of psychology and to equal quality in the processes, procedures and services being conducted by psychologists" (p. 3); and "respect the dignity and worth of all people, and the rights of individuals to privacy, confidentiality, and self-determination" (p. 4). The preeminence of human rights is specifically established in the introduction to the Code of Ethics, which states that all ethical conflicts are to be resolved "in keeping with the basic principles of human rights" (p. 3), and in standards 1.02 and 1.03, which adamantly proclaim that "under no circumstances" may these standards be used to "justify or defend a violation of human rights" (p. 4). APA's *Guidelines for Multicultural Education, Training, Research, Practice and Organizational Change for Psychologists* (2003) adds numerous points of support framed particularly in social justice terms, that is, "Psychologists are uniquely able to promote racial equity and social justice" (p. 382). Societies of psychologists who work primarily with and for children, particularly within school communities, also have committed formally and publically to respect and serve human rights and social justice. Examples can be found in activities, documents, and publications of the International School Psychology Association (ISPA; see mission statement, available at www.ispaweb.org; and in *School Psychology International*, 2001), the National Association of School Psychologists (NASP; see NASP's *Position Statement on Children's Rights*, available at www.nasponline.org; and in *School Psychology Review*), and APA's Division 16 (Nastasi, 2010).

Social justice and human rights principles deserve further elaboration to facilitate their applications by psychology in the interests of all persons and particularly for children who depend on respectful stewardship in their best interests. This chapter is intended to further clarify the nature of social justice and human rights, with primary emphasis on the human rights of children toward inspiring and advancing psychology's service in early and particularly sensitive periods of human development. In the following sections human nature is explored, social justice and the human rights are clarified individually and in their relationships, and, in the final major section, an heuristic exploration is undertaken of their potential for beneficial employment by psychology in dealing with three key aspects of the human being and becoming.

HUMAN NATURE—JUSTIFICATION FOR HUMAN RIGHTS AND SOCIAL JUSTICE

Arguably, psychology has no higher purpose than to serve the full healthy development and functioning of human beings, individually and collectively. This responsibility is enormous when it is recognized that human beings have shown themselves capable of achieving nearly all, possibly all, that they imagine, for good and evil (Hart, 2010). This requires that we understand the essential nature of human beings. Here we briefly explore five central themes of human nature: (1) human needs, (2) existential choice making, (3) moral development, (4) social relationships, and (5) realization of self. This is undertaken to clarify further the justification for investment in human rights and social justice in ways that provide guidance for their application. These themes are dynamic both individually and across the set, and overlap at some points.

Human Needs

Primary human needs, including the realization of potentials, have been identified as the core of what should be respected about human beings. Adler (1997) considered the fulfillment of essential human needs that promote and assure well-being to deserve standing as human rights. Recent research in this area, building on Maslow's (1970) earlier constructions, has identified the following conditions as necessary to support happiness and satisfaction for human beings.

> Connectedness to other humans (i.e., affiliation and social support), competency (i.e., practical coping skills, critical thinking and problem solving), self-determination (i.e., independence, empowerment towards self-management and self-direction) and self-esteem (i.e., senses of worth, being valued by others, capable of and recognized for making constructive contributions). (Power & Hart, 2005, p. 97; for supportive research see Ryan & Deci, 2000; Sheldon, Elliott, Kim, & Kasser, 2001)

Existential Choice Making

The choices human beings make and the actions they take are expressions of attempts to fulfill human needs and can be judged as relatively positive or negative in regard to their influences on the actor's own status and future as well as that of others and the larger animate and inanimate environment. The quintessential characteristic of human beings, which most clearly establishes humans as special among all others, is existential thought and choice: rather than opposable thumbs, tool making, and even language, which are strongly supportive of existential processes (Kamii, 1984, 1991). No other living entity has shown itself capable of stepping out of the time stream to consider and evaluate past, present, and possible futures in support of choice making and creative acts that are well beyond instinctual behavior. It has been suggested by a respected futurist that it is improbable that this level of intelligence and behavior would be found anywhere else in the universe (Kurzweil, 2010). Existential thought and choice are primary contributors to the enormous potential of human beings. They formulate and direct social justice and human rights constructs, principles, and applications.

Moral Development

The moral development of human beings, making choices based on right and wrong, good and bad, is of unquestionable importance. Moral development for individuals and collectives seems best understood as needs and potentials fulfillment, which progresses to greater or lesser degrees: (1) through early stages of adjustment to strong external control/power, (2) on to increasingly formalized structured group regulation, (3) next to adherence to standards voluntarily contracted with others, and (4) eventually toward the possibility of internal personal management in respect to abstract universal principles acquired and formulated throughout the developmental process (Kohlberg, 1984). Appreciation of this basic progression has been augmented by recognition of (1) gender differences in the degree to which caring and relationships (in contrast with rules, justice, and principles) are given priority in moral reasoning and choice making (Gilligan, 1982), (2) the influences of emotion, social, and cultural factors on moral judgments (Haight, 2001), and (3) relationships between identity, personality, and moral functioning (Blasi, 1993). A recent exploration of the reasons for significant reductions in violence during that last 5,000 years has identified changes in the ways persons live and behave that seem to express this basic paradigm and noted gender associated emphases, giving prominent explanatory credit to progressive respect for human rights and increases in reason, empathy, moral sense, and self-control (Pinker, 2011). Further enlightenment in this regard, including that provided by applying emerging theories of moral development, may help humans deal with the unacceptably high levels of violence that continue around the world.

Social Relationships

Humans are social beings. Their need fulfillment and their cognitive, affective, volitional, and moral development and behavior all are strongly influenced by the affordances of their social environments and experiences (Bandura, 1986; Feuerstein & Hoffman, 1982; Goleman, 1995, 2006). Social support is strongly linked to physical and mental health (Vaillant, 1997, 2002). Relationships between human beings can range from strongly positive to strongly negative, including a mixture of the two and their gradations that promote health and well-being or limitation, corruption, and degradation (Hart, Brassard, Davidson, Rivelis, & Diaz, 2010).

Realization of Self

What is the superordinate condition served by the fulfillment of needs and of potentials, including social support, high levels of critical thinking, existential choice, and moral goodness? Popular and expert opinions tend to converge here. "I wish I'd had the courage to live a life true to myself not the life others expected of me" was found to be the number one human regret by Ware (2011, p. 37) through the experience of spending years tending to the needs of persons approaching death. Shakespeare's dictum on living the proper life is "this above all: to thine own self be true, and it must follow, as the night the day, thou canst not then be false to any man" (*Hamlet* Act 1, scene 3, 78–82). According to Joseph Campbell, "The privilege of a lifetime is being who you are." Herman Hesse states, "Each man has only one genuine vocation—to find the way to himself." And Soren Kierkegaard has made it clear that not to be oneself is "exactly" despair (2004). Appreciating these views, Hart (2010) postulated, "The essence of true respect for the dignity of a person is expressed in active appreciation and support for the actualization of his/her particular nature and possibilities at each period of existence and development" (p. 38).

As psychology seeks to apply these understandings of the nature of human beings to serve their best interests, it should find social justice and human rights principles and frameworks illuminating and supportive. Their inherent promotion and elucidation of human dignity, sanctity of life, well-being, and what is required in their support can significantly expand psychology's potential for constructive intervention. In the next three sections, we attempt to provide helpful clarification in their regard.

SOCIAL JUSTICE

Whereas modern scholarship focuses on the application of social justice to such diverse fields as psychology, sociology, education, law, political science, and economics, the first known use of the term *social justice* as it is presently understood comes from Roman Catholic writings in the mid-19th century (Zajda, Majhanovich, Rust, & Sabina, 2006). From these writings, and subsequent Catholic teachings, social justice is viewed as a way of thinking and behaving that covers a wide range of constructs such as sanctity of life, dignity, solidarity, charity, distribution, family, community, participation, religious conscience-freedom, preference to the vulnerable, responsibility, and choice.

As described throughout this volume, within psychology, social justice is a term that has many definitions and applications. For example, some may see social justice primarily as a process (e.g., the idea that all individuals should be treated respectfully and without prejudice), whereas others are more focused on outcomes (e.g., the idea that everyone should have an equal opportunity for economic success; Bell, 2013). Sander et al. (2011) describe social justice as an advocacy-related construct that centers on the core areas of access, respect, and fairness. In an extensive review of various definitions of social justice as applied to education, North (2006) indicates that common definitions of social justice include the dual ideas that individuals and groups must be treated with fairness and respect and that all are entitled to the resources and benefits that a system or society has to offer. Additionally, she notes that some social justice advocates and researchers tend to emphasize more micro-level components of social justice, whereas others tend to emphasize more macro-level concerns. Shriberg et al. (2008), based on a Delphi study of multicultural experts in school psychology, recommended a definition of social justice that emphasizes the protection of rights and opportunities for all and behaving in a nondiscriminatory, inclusive manner. The experts in this study recommended advocacy strategies that combined extensive knowledge with a commitment to action. In terms of bringing social justice ideas to practice, in a seminal work, Lisa Goodman and her colleagues (Goodman et al., 2004) identify six core components of social justice training: ongoing self-examination, sharing power, giving voice, facilitating consciousness-raising, building on strengths, and leaving clients the tools to work toward social change.

Much scholarship has focused on identifying core social justice definitions and advocacy strategies that can be applied to all levels from micro to macro. Simultaneous to the movement within psychology and related fields to define and better understand the implications of a social justice framework to practice has been an international movement to recognize and advance human rights. Indeed, often the terms social justice and human rights (or children's rights) are paired or used interchangeably in psychology committees or platforms. For example, in 2008, a Working Group on Social Justice and Children's Rights was created within Division 16 (School Psychology) of the American Psychological Association (Nastasi, 2010). Similarly, the Association for Counselor Education and Supervision established a Social Justice and Human Rights Committee in 2006 (Chang, Crethar, & Ratts, 2010).

However, despite the largely overlapping goals and agendas of social justice and human rights advocates, a human rights framework is largely absent from social justice scholarship. As Johnston (2009) notes:

> Human rights have a powerful role to play in any account of what it means to be socially just, because they have a major role to play in the justification of claims made on behalf of those seeking social justice. . . . I think that due attention to human rights as the ground of socially just practices makes something that is not obvious, more so. (p. 120)

If social justice cannot be achieved without a fundamental commitment to human rights, and vice versa, so also human rights cannot be achieved without an accompanying commitment to child rights. In most societies, it is only within the past 200 years that children have been viewed as distinct human beings and not miniature adults (Hart, 1991). If, as Goodman et al. (2004) state, social justice practice involves sharing power and giving voice, given the dependence of children on adults for basic needs, are not child rights an exceptionally good metric to analyze social justice? Additionally, as noted by Gutkin and Song (2012), from a prevention perspective, if one is seeking to advance social justice, focusing on children is a logical place to begin.

Given the dependent position that children hold in relation to adults, the rights extended to children directly reflect the extent to which adults in that society view children as deserving of these rights. Affirming the idea that children are human beings and not property, the 1989 United Nations Convention on the Rights of the Child (UN General Assembly, 1989) set the universal standards for the fundamental rights of children. This document, to be more fully explored in the next section, provides extremely fertile ground to enrich a social justice perspective. Social justice represents the broad themes and brushstrokes of respect and caring for the dignity and quality of life of persons, which are supported, defined, and detailed by human rights.

HUMAN RIGHTS—WITH CHILD RIGHTS EMPHASIS

Historically, growing awareness and appreciation of the nature of persons, their needs and potentials, has stimulated a wave of support for human rights. Advances initially focused on protection from exploitation and cruelty by persons in power have more recently and progressively moved toward assuring the protections, entitlements, and the opportunities necessary for persons to live fully and to experience well-being or good quality of life. Some might argue that Kohlberg's model of moral development (1981, 1984), fitting both individuals and their informal and formal collectives, and generally applicable across cultures with some caveats (Snarey, 1985), largely explains the path of enlightenment for human rights. Rights that initially focused on fear of power beyond the person, primarily emphasizing protection and acquisition of necessities, eventually came to focus on securing the conditions and possibilities of the good life for others that we wish for ourselves. Rights have come to be framed as golden rule and universal principles, undergirded by empathy, mutual respect, reflection, and judgment. This suggests that Rawls's (1982) "original position," acting and choosing for the good of all persons from the perspective of the "non-specific," universal "any person," has been intuitively and informally applied—with more and more persons wanting what is good or right for all persons judged from the perspective of any person.

Internationally, the most important milestones achieved on this path toward respect for the rights of human beings are the Universal Declaration of Human Rights (UDHR) and the UN Convention on the Rights of the Child (UNCRC). Hart (2007a, 2007b) has provided brief overviews of each. The Universal Declaration and the Convention on the Rights of the Child were established by the United Nations, in 1948 and 1989, respectively. The Universal Declaration is widely considered "the primary international statement" of human rights imperatives, which in some cases have been incorporated into national laws (Hart, 2007a). Although the Universal Declaration is not in itself legally binding, it has been divided into two international legal treaties, the International Covenant on Civil and Political Rights (United Nations General Assembly, 1996) and the International Covenant on Economic, Social and Cultural Rights (United Nations General Assembly, 1996).

The UN Convention on the Rights of the Child was preceded by two additional child-oriented, nonlegally binding international documents, both titled the Declaration of the Rights of the Child, first adopted by the League of Nations in 1924, and later expanded and upgraded by the United Nations in 1959. The Convention, unlike its predecessors, is a legally binding treaty, ratified by all but two nations of the world, Somalia and the United States. The United States has signed the Convention, an action that indicates intention to move toward ratification.

Compliance is encouraged through transparent national reporting, making information on status and progress available, and through moral persuasion, encouragement, and technical assistance toward advances.

The Universal Declaration and Convention embody comprehensive, coherent, and holistic frameworks of principles and standards providing essential guidance toward respect for the dignity of persons. Physical, psychological, social, spiritual, and moral domains are addressed. The document covers issues of health, education, work, leisure, liberty, and freedom with respect to individual, family, community, and societal contexts. The Declaration, and the two Covenants it produced, is intended to cover adults and children, but gives very little specific attention to children. Although much of the Convention is drawn from the Declaration, it is clearly the stronger and more comprehensive guide to fulfilling obligations to children. In addition to official commitment by the nations of the world, and its legally binding nature, it was written specifically for and about children, and gives attention to their developmental possibilities, vulnerabilities, and sensitivities.

Primary attention in the remainder of this chapter is given to the Convention wherein rights are considered. It is the most recent human rights expression of enlightenment regarding the necessities, aspirations, and dignity of human existence and fulfillment from a developmental perspective. The only elements included in the Universal Declaration that are not specifically mentioned in the Convention deal with rights generally reserved for adults: freedom of movement in residence and country, marriage, property ownership, involvement in government, right to work, and duties to community.

The Convention was adopted by the United Nations General Assembly without dissent on November 20, 1989. It is the most successful human rights treaty in history in terms of both the number of nations committing to it and the quickness with which these commitments accrued to achieve entry into force (9½ months). It includes 54 articles; the first 41 deal with substantive rights and the remainder focus on mechanisms and processes supportive of implementation. The rights articles of the Convention represent officially recognized obligations to children—a bedrock of universal values to be applied to all children, sectors of life, by all persons, at all times. This is the world's positive ideology of the child (Hart, 1991).

All articles of the Convention are given equal status and are to be implemented in a holistic and synergistic fashion according to the nature of conditions at issue. Four of the articles are considered general principles of basic relevance to the implementation of all other articles. They focus on the child's right to freedom from discrimination (Article 2); to have the child's best interests considered in all decisions of relevance to him/her (Article 3); to life, survival and development (Article 6); and to be listened to and taken seriously (Article 12). Article 29, the aims of education, is the Convention's best single statement of respect for the nature and potential of human beings, and support for their full, healthy and socially responsible development. We present it here to illustrate its meaningful relationship with other rights. Its significance for psychology is self-evident.

ARTICLE 29 OF THE U. N. CONVENTION ON THE RIGHTS OF THE CHILD

1. *States Parties agree that the education of the child shall be directed to:*
   - (a) *The development of the child's personality, talents and mental and physical abilities to their fullest potential;*
   - (b) *The development of respect for human rights and fundamental freedoms, and for the principles enshrined in the Charter of the United Nations;*
   - (c) *The development of respect for the child's parents, his or her own cultural identity, language and values, for the national values of the country in which the child is living, the country from which he or she may originate, and for civilizations different from his or her own;*
   - (d) *The preparation of the child for responsible life in a free society, in the spirit of understanding, peace, tolerance, equality of sexes, and friendship among all peoples, ethnic, national and religious groups and persons of indigenous origin;*
   - (e) *The development of respect for the natural environment.*
2. *No part of the present article or article 28 shall be construed so as to interfere with the liberty of individuals and bodies to establish and direct educational institutions, subject always to the observance of the principle set forth in paragraph 1 of the present article and to the requirements that the education given in such institutions shall conform to such minimum standards as may be laid down by the State.*

Source: http://www2.ohchr.org/english/law/crc.htm

Article 29 expects a universal commitment to the "full realization of each child's personality and its possibilities, in a manner which promotes socially responsible autonomy in a free society, respecting others, individually and collectively, and the environments in which they might flourish" (Hart, 2010, p. 36). The relevance of the full Convention for Article 29 can be illustrated by reference to the general principles: this commitment is to be applied to all children without discrimination (Article 2); it embodies and clarifies the best interests of the child (Article 3) and the nature of development desired for the child (Article 6); and its achievement is promoted by the child's evolving participation and agency (Article 12). Furthermore, one can make the case that fulfilling virtually all the articles of the Convention is necessary to and serves its aims for education and development, that is, children are protected from violence (Article 19), exploitive or dangerous work (Article 32), and given opportunities for play, leisure, and cultural experiences (Article 31), are better able to learn quantitatively and qualitatively. Respect for the human rights of children does advance their quality of life.

SOCIAL JUSTICE AND CHILDREN'S RIGHTS—RELATIONSHIPS FROM DEEPLY SHARED MEANING

Here, we argue that social justice and child rights share meanings and purposes derived from their service to the well-being of human beings, wherein well-being is understood to be a fundamental expression of *good*. According to Adler (1997), in the scheme and stream of life, good in the ontological sense trumps justice and rights and gives them their meaning. Adler argues that, of the living things on earth, human beings represent the highest level of perfection, in existence and possibility, and that good for a human being is achieved through meeting needs (not wants). He concludes that these needs deserve translation into rights and can be served by justice. Meeting of human needs, respect for human rights, and promotion of social justice in their regard, protect and promote the fulfillment of the being and becoming of the person—the good.

One can translate the word *good* to mean well-being in its broadest and deepest meanings. The term *well-being* appears to be rising toward zeitgeist level and to be sustainable as the shorthand phrase for fulfillment of human being and becoming. For the Convention on the Rights of the Child, the good to which it aspires is implicitly identified as well-being for the physical, mental, social, spiritual, and moral domains of human existence (UN General Assembly, 1989). Additionally, UN guidelines on child protection and prevention of violence establish child well-being as their major goal (United Nations Committee on the Rights of the Child, 2011), and accountability to child rights and well-being has been established by the Committee on the Rights of the Child to be of highest priority (IICRD, 2012). Social justice orientations strongly respect and promote wellness and well-being (Prilleltensky, 2011; Prilleltensky & Prilleltensky, 2006). Social justice and child rights standards and applications should and can advance child well-being.

In considering the relationships and distinctions between child rights and social justice, the following points are helpful. All social justice themes are represented in and expressed by human rights tenets. According to Miller (2003), "A central element in any theory of justice will be an account of the basic rights of citizens" (p. 13). Social justice champions rights and it is failed primarily by their violation. The circles of human rights and social justice nearly completely overlap. Their common ground is particularly strongly expressed in their promotion of the fundamental rights believed to be necessary for a just society (e.g., sanctity of life, dignity of persons, non-prejudiced based discrimination, and solidarity). Both call for active and accountable implementation. However, they do embody differences worthy of note. Social justice concentrates on in-depth consideration and promotion of fairness, nondiscrimination and equity, and in psychology, it is largely expressed through multicultural formulations and imperatives. Child rights (and human rights) more comprehensively deal with the human condition, the importance of establishing assurances for all persons regardless of culture, including respect for personal culture, the holistic nature of human needs and well-being, and support for the full and healthy development of the talents and personality of the individual.

Application of Child Rights and Social Justice in Psychology

Psychologists are professionals capable of applying the principles, knowledge bases, and evolving tools of their profession with high levels of discretionary power to fit the quite diverse and varying opportunities for service they encounter. With this in mind, a largely heuristic endeavor is undertaken here to explore the application of child rights and social justice concepts to three critical issues of the human condition. The three critical issues, strongly related to one another, are the full development of personality, elimination of violence, and attainment of solidarity. The first is a primary goal, possibly the primary goal of life and psychology; the second deals with a threat to that goal and to all aspects of quality of life; and the third is essential to achieving the first and second. For each theme, four application dimensions are given attention: perspective, research, policy, and practice. Themes and application dimensions are dynamic within and across one another. (Table 1.1 shows the relationship among the three critical issues and the four dimensions.). Material presented in text and Table 1.1 represents only a small sample of greater possibilities selected by the authors as useful for the purpose of this exploration. Although emphasis is given to the relevance of this information in the school community, largely defined, it has bearing across all sectors of the lives of children and applications of psychology. In the sections that follow, the four application dimensions are described in the context of each of the three goals.

Table 1.1
Four Child Rights and Social Justice Applications by Three Major Themes

Theme	Perspective	Research	Policy	Practice
Full development	• Significance of each child • Dignity of person • Superordinate purpose for persons, societies, and psychology	• Human potential • Existential choice	• Best interests of child • Holistic development • Character	• Prospective human development (PhD) • Critical thinking and choice-making • IEPs for all • Mastery approach augmented
Freedom from violence	• Well-being as goal • WHO definition of health augmented • Sanctity of life • CRC General Comment 19 • Causes and cures	• Nature of violence • Violence reduction • Resiliency • Gender characteristics	• Promotion of well-being • Constructive child discipline • Preparation for good parenting	• Promotion of wellness • Well-being periodic examination and tracking • Prosocial skill development • Parenting education

(Continued)

Table 1.1 (*Continued*)

Theme	Perspective	Research	Policy	Practice
Solidarity/ Equity	• Respect for cultures of others • Shared superordinate goals • Responsible life in a free society • Nondiscrimination • Social support • Happiness	• Empathy • Altruism • Honesty • Social support • Social contracts	• Superordinate goals • Community/ small-town environment • Participatory governance • Wellness promoted through social support	• Just Community schools • Shared school governance • Continuity of social network (the 'village') • Danish Class Teacher model • "No Child Left Behind" plus

Full Development of Personality

Perspective

Full development of the person, with high aspirations for personality at its apex, is expressed in Article 29 of the Convention on the Rights of the Child, embodied in the dignity construct inherent in rights and social justice constructions, and expected to be promoted by psychology. Each person's singular, unique, holistically framed personality is at stake here—this realization is the goal of human life according to Kierkegaard, Hesse, and many others.

Research

If the ultimate purpose of psychology, human rights, and social justice is promotion of full healthy development of the person, then research on human potential, well-being, and existential choice making, the quintessential human characteristic, must be given high priority. In particular, a case can be made for research to (1) operationally define well-being (including well-becoming) for the domains set forth by the UNCRC, physical, mental (i.e., psychological), social, spiritual, and moral; (2) provide instrumentation and systems for determining related status and progress (Huebner & Hills, 2013); (3) provide viable interventions for its promotion; and (4) hold the stewards of children (e.g., society, government, media, school community, church, family, and child) accountable for contributions and advances.

Policy

Promotion of the best interests of the child, a primary expectation of the CRC, which inherently requires support for holistic development, should be the hallmark of expectations set for society's stewards of children (see related arguments for development of physical, psychological, and spiritual anchors; Garbarino,

1999). This can include monitoring and applying relevant research on development, for example, moral and performance character development (Tough, 2012). The policies of national, religious, and school community institutions and service providers should express these commitments.

Practice

Researchers have recommended the prospective human development model to promote the sustainable full healthy development of the uniqueness of each person (Hart & Glaser, 2012). It builds on the history of prospective medicine (Robbins & Hall, 1970; Snyderman & Williams, 2003; Strohecker, 2011) and places the child client in full partnership with professional stewards, such as psychologists, to determine and pursue a course of full healthy development desired by children and their supporters. The psychologist, in this case, acts as a consulting detective, coach, and educator who provides information to the child and progressively assumes the responsibility for choosing the course of action to be taken. This orientation benefits significantly from the application of individual educational (developmental) plans for each child, now possible through application of technology, and a mastery approach that designs, allows, and respects paths to development that vary according to time and route, respecting the nature of the person (Bloom, 1974; Carroll, 1989). Implementation is particularly promising through partnerships that include the child, psychologists, parents, and educators.

Elimination of Violence

Perspective

According to Schweitzer (1993), all life is precious and sacred. Children's rights and social justice highly prioritize sanctity of life and require protection from and prevention of harm. UNCRC Articles 6, 19, and 29 combine to champion the right to life, full healthy development, and protection in their regard. The UNCRC, through the Committee on the Rights of the Child, takes the position that elimination of violence, including related primary proactive intervention, is superior to but also necessary in combination with reactive correction (Hart, Lee, & Wernham, 2011). This is a major paradigm shift embedded in General Comment 13, for Article 19 of the UNCRC, titled "the right of the child to freedom from all forms of violence" (United Nations Committee on the Rights of the Child, 2011). Well-being for the CRC is probably best represented by an expansion of WHO's definition of health as "a state of complete physical, mental and social well-being and not merely the absence of disease or infirmity" (WHO, 1948, p. 100) to include spiritual and moral well-being.

Research

Guidance toward interventions requires respect for research clarifying the nature of violence and viable interventions. Pinker (2002, 2011) shed light on the causes of violence and the influencing conditions of the 5,000-year trend line of lessening violence for human beings. He identified competition for limited goods and protection from threat, particularly loss of identity and humiliation as major aspects of human nature that promote aggression and violence, assisted by the "five inner demons" of predatory or instrumental violence, dominance, revenge, sadism, and ideology. He cites and elucidates the following characteristics as influential in the reduction of violence over the last 5,000 years: (1) six trends, that include the shift away from anarchy toward civilization, the civilizing process, the humanitarian revolution, emergence of great powers and long periods of peace, and the end of the cold war; (2) five historical forces: Leviathan—the powerful and punitive government or bureaucracy, commerce, feminization, cosmopolitanism, escalation of reason; and (3) the "four better angels" of empathy, self-control, moral sense, and reason.

The UNCRC, through General Comment 13, recognizes that the three major types of violence, physical, psychological, and sexual, are expressed in a wide variety of abuse, neglect, and exploitation forms, often together. Research has established that psychological maltreatment, alone and combined with other maltreatment related forms, is the most destructive to healthy development if the child is not killed outright (Hart et al., 2011). All maltreatment is in opposition to healthy human needs fulfillment. Proactive promotion of human needs fulfillment can reduce the likelihood that persons become antisocial (Hart et al., 2011), that is, as perpetrators of maltreatment, and it is meaningfully related to resiliency in the face of adversity (Garmezy & Rutter, 1983; Liebenberg & Unger, 2009; Luthar, 2003; Unger, 2005; Werner & Smith, 1987). Researchers have established identifiable genetic vulnerability to developing antisocial and violent behavior, in persons who were subjected to maltreatment as children (Caspi et al., 2002). Corporal punishment of children, an affront to the dignity of the person in child rights and social justice terms, has been found to be destructive to the interests of children and society, without redeeming qualities, and unnecessary in light of the availability of effective constructive discipline alternatives (Hart, Durrant, Newell, & Power, 2005). Finklehor (personal communication, August 25, 2010) identified three factors as contributing to violence prevention: rising normative standards promoting prosocial behavior and condemning violence, bystander mobilization, and child agency. This research knowledge has child rights and social justice implications and provides fertile ground for applications and extensions by psychology.

Policy

Policy at all levels should reflect the perspectives and research base just described. Laws and policies to decrease violence against children and embodying respect for and application of child rights exist (Hart et al., 2011; United Nations Committee on the Rights of the Child, 2011). Promotion of child well-being, constructive discipline, preparation for good parenting and child caregiving, and respecting the child's dignity have been formulated and are available in child rights and social justice terms (Hart et al., 2005, 2011).

Practice

Increases in empathy, prosocial values and skills, moral reasoning, agency, character, and solidarity for young persons (in fact, any age and reference group) can help reduce all forms of violence in all settings. These capacities are all embodied in and supported by human rights and social justice principles and frameworks; they and their underpinnings are primarily psychological in nature and proper areas for concentration toward advancing knowledge and applications. For young persons in the school community, regular, periodic well-being evaluations and close tracking and support of status and progress (such as embodied in the prospective human development model) enable children and their social support systems to correct and promote influencing conditions in the best interests of the children and the community. Preparation for good parenting (e.g., respect for child rights and dignity, child development knowledge, positive discipline, character development, coping skills, emotional stability, access to social support) should be provided through the school community to its students, in developmentally appropriate ways, and to pre-child bearing adults and parents of young children in the larger community. Violence against children is often found in discipline efforts gone wrong. Child psychologists in all major cultures of the world have identified effective, constructive child discipline strategies, which should be offered to child caregivers (Power & Hart, 2005). All these potential advances, including Finkelhor's three factors for violence prevention, supported by child rights and social justice principles, can benefit from the contributions of psychology and psychologists, and they hold genuine promise for reducing human tragedy from violence (see Dr. Michael Welner, *The best solution to prevent another Newtown*).

Attainment of Solidarity

Perspective

Solidarity (e.g., cohesion, commonality, harmony) within a population can provide the rationale and support needed to increase and secure the well-being of persons and their communities. It is advanced by knowledge of and respect for diversity in persons and cultures, shared superordinate goals, social support to deal with adversity and achieve happiness, and respect for fairness that reduces/eliminates discrimination based on prejudice. As noted in earlier sections, social justice and child rights orientations provide implicit and explicit encouragement for solidarity and benefit from achievement of solidarity.

Research

Numerous conditions, characteristics, and competencies promote solidarity and well-being. Research has found many that can be enhanced and applied. They include, but are not limited to, empathy (Eisenberg & Miller, 1987; Hoffman, 2000), which encourages understanding and appreciation of the circumstances and views of others; altruism (Post, 2007), which leads to caring and giving for the benefit of others; and honesty (Kelly, 2012), which provides a basis for trust and cooperation between and among persons (see also Goleman, 1995, 2006). Research evidence provides the rationale for supporting and achieving solidarity based on the nature and need for social support (Maslow, 1970; Ryan & Deci, 2000; Sheldon et al., 2001), moral development at the social contract stage (Kohlberg, 1984), the incorporation of sensitivity and caring in relationships (Gilligan, 1982), and the establishment of shared, superordinate goals (Sherif, Harvey, White, Hood, & Sherif, 1961).

Policy

Neither distress nor corrupting deviance can reach critical levels in a small town that embodies strong, positive, social networking (Karlson, H., personal communication, repeated over period of years). Similar to the African proverb "it takes a village to raise a child," Rich (1998) recommended that parents create a small town social environment in their children's interests wherever they might live. These perspectives, and supporting empirical evidence, should be translated into policy at all levels, and certainly in the school community to promote involvement in participatory governance and the development of shared goals and standards of care, respect, allegiance, social networking, and continuity of relationships to achieve mutual respect and social support.

Practice

Psychologists working with and for children have the expertise and opportunity to influence policies such as those just described and related practices. In promoting solidarity among young persons the school environment embodies particularly good opportunities, as the following examples validate. The Just Community Schools model provides direction for empowering young persons to establish and implement standards for student caring and conduct (Power, 1988). The Danish schools involve students, parents, and teachers jointly in their school boards and create families and communities of caring and support through their class-teacher model. The class-teacher model gives particular emphasis to close long-term relationships between professionals and children, which should be emulated by psychologists, counselors, and educators. Even a good idea that seems to have gone wrong, such as the No Child Left Behind Act (*Pub.L. 107–110*, 115 Stat. 1425, enacted January 8, 2002), might be reformulated in the service of well-being supported by solidarity. Although intended to raise achievement for all students, and particularly the disadvantaged or distressed, this law has been widely criticized for significantly narrowing the scope of school achievement and degrading student motivation and learning (Kolodziej, 2011; Ravitch, 2010). If its standards and accountability framework were to embody the holistic development required to respect the dignity, potential, and needs of children and incorporate a mastery approach, it would be much more likely that students, teachers, parents, and the larger community would rally their resources to commit and sacrifice for the success for all children.

CONCLUSION

Psychology has a major role in advancing the best interests of the persons. Proactive promotion of well-being is preferable to reactive correction of distress and distortion, providing good reason for psychology to give particular emphasis to working with and for children. Psychology's effectiveness in serving children, each child and all children, is best directed and most powerful if it is infused with the values, principles, and standards of children's rights and social justice. Successful application of this paradigm can significantly strengthen the moral capital of psychology.

REFERENCES

Adler, M. (1997). *Six great ideas.* New York, NY: Touchstone.

American Psychological Association (APA). (2003). Guidelines on multicultural education, training, research, practice, and organizational change for psychologists. *American Psychologist, 58*(5), 377–402. doi: 10.1037/0003-066X.58.5.377

American Psychological Association (APA). (2010). *Ethical principles of the psychologists and code of conduct* (Adopted 2002, effective 2003, amended 2010). Washington, DC: Author.

Bandura, A. (1986). *Social foundations of thought and action: A Social Cognitive Theory.* Englewood Cliffs, NJ: Prentice-Hall.

Bell, L. A. (2013). Theoretical foundations. In M. Adams, W. J. Blumenfeld, C. Castañeda, H. W. Hackman, M. L. Peters, & X. Zúñiga (Eds.), *Readings for diversity and social justice* (3rd ed., pp. 21–26). New York, NY: Routledge.

Blasi, A. (1993). The development of identity: Some implications for moral thinking. In G. G. Noam & R. E. Wren (Eds.), *The moral self* (pp. 99–122). Cambridge, MA: MIT Press.

Bloom, B. S. (1974). Time and learning. *American Psychologist, 29*(9), 682–688. doi: 10.1037/h0037632

Carroll, J. B. (1989). The Carroll model: A 25-year retrospective and prospective view. *Educational Researcher, 18*(1), 26–31. Retrieved from http://ejournals.ebsco.com/direct.asp?ArticleID=42439CA9FCDC39E78024

Caspi, A., McClay, J., Moffitt, T. E., Mill, J., Martin, J., Craig, I. W., . . . Poulton, R. (2002). Role of genotype in the cycle of violence in maltreated children. *Science, 297*(5582), 851. doi: 10.1126/Science.1072290

Chang, C. Y., Crethar, H. C., & Ratts, M. J. (2010). Social justice: A national imperative for counselor education and supervision. *Counselor Education & Supervision, 50,* 82–87.

Eisenberg, N., & Miller, P. A. (1987). The relation of empathy to prosocial and related behaviors. *Psychological Bulletin, 101*(1), 91–119. doi: 10.1037/0033-2909.101.1.91

Feuerstein, R., & Hoffman, M. B. (1982). Intergenerational conflict of rights: Cultural imposition and self-realization. *Viewpoints in Teaching, 58*(1), 44–63.

Garbarino, J. (1999). *Lost boys: Why our sons turn violent and how we can save them.* New York, NY: Free Press.

Garmezy, N., & Rutter, M. (1983) *Stress, coping and development in children.* New York, NY: McGraw-Hill.

Gilligan, C. (1982). *In a different voice: Psychological theory and women's development.* Cambridge, MA: Harvard University Press.

Goleman, D. (1995). *Emotional intelligence: Why it can matter more than IQ.* New York, NY: Bantam Books.

Goleman, D. (2006). *Social intelligence: The revolutionary new science of human relations.* New York, NY: Bantam Books.

Goodman, L. A., Liang, B., Helms, J. E., Latta, R. E., Sparks, E., & Weintraub, S. R. (2004). Training counseling psychologists as social justice agents: Feminist and multicultural principles in action. *The Counseling Psychologist, 32,* 793–837. doi: 10.1177/0011000004268802

Gutkin, T. B., & Song, S. Y. (2012). Social justice in school psychology: A historical perspective. In D. Shriberg, S. Y. Song, A. H. Miranda, & K. M. Radliff (Eds.), *School psychology and social justice: Conceptual foundations and tools for practice* (pp. 15–28). New York, NY: Routledge.

Haight, J. (2001). The emotional dog and its rational tail. A social intuitionist approach to moral judgment. *Psychological Review, 108,* 814–834. doi: 10.1037/0033-295X.108.4.814

Hart, S. N. (1991). From property to person status: Historical perspective on children's rights. *American Psychologist, 46*(1), 53–59. doi: 10.1037/0003-066X.46.1.53

Hart, S. N. (2007a). The Universal Declaration of Human Rights. *Encyclopedia on Moral Education.* Oxford, UK: Greenwood.

Hart, S. N. (2007b). The United Nations Convention on the Rights of the Child. *Encyclopedia on Moral Education.* Oxford, UK: Greenwood.

Hart, S. N. (2010). Be true to thyself. In S. Bennett & M. Pare (Eds.), *20th anniversary of the Convention on the Rights of the Child* (3rd ed., pp. 34–39). Ottawa: University of Ottawa.

Hart, S. N., Brassard, M. R., Davidson, H. A., Rivelis, E., Diaz, V. & Binggeli, N. (2010). Psychological maltreatment. In J. E. B. Myers (Ed.), *The APSAC handbook on child maltreatment* (pp. 125–144). Thousand Oaks, CA: Sage.

Hart, S. N., Durrant, J., Newell, P., & Power, F. C. (2005). *Eliminating corporal punishment: The way forward to constructive child discipline.* Paris: UNESCO.

Hart, S. N., & Glaser, D. (2011). Psychological maltreatment-Maltreatment of the mind: A catalyst for advancing child protection toward proactive primary prevention and promotion of personal well-being. *Child Abuse & Neglect, 35,* 758–766.

Hart, S. N., Lee, Y., & Wernham, M. (2011). A new age for child protection—General comment 13: Why it is important, how it was constructed, and what it intends? *Child Abuse & Neglect, 35,* 970–978.

Hesse, H. (2000). *Demian.* Mineola, NY: Dover Publications.

Hoffman, M. L. (2000). *Empathy and moral development.* Cambridge, UK: Cambridge University Press.

Huebner, E. S., & Hills, K. J. (2013). Assessment of subjective well-being in children and adolescents. In D. H. Sasklofske, V. L. Schwean, & C. R. Reynolds (Eds.), *Oxford handbook of child psychological assessment.* Oxford, UK: Oxford University Press.

IICRD (2012). *Report of the CRC accountability technical meeting.* Victoria, BC: Author.

Johnston, J. S. (2009). Prioritizing rights in the social justice curriculum. *Studies in Philosophy and Education, 28,* 119–133. doi: 10.1007/s11217-008-9100-8

Kamii, C. (1984, February). Autonomy: The aim of education envisioned by Piaget. *Phi Delta Kappan,* 410–415.

Kamii, C. (1991). Toward autonomy: The importance of critical thinking and choice making. *School Psychology Review, 20*(3), 382–387.

Kelly, A. (2012, August). *The science of honesty*. Presentation to the Annual Conference of the American Psychological Association, Orlando, Florida.

Kierkegaard, S. (2004–original 1849). *A sickness unto death: A Christian psychological exposition for edification and awakening by Anti-Climacus*. London, UK: Penguin.

Kohlberg, L. (1981). *Essays on moral development, Vol. I: The philosophy of moral development*. San Francisco, CA: Harper & Row.

Kohlberg, L. (1984). *Essays on moral development, Vol. II: The psychology of moral development*. New York, NY: Harper and Row.

Kolodziej, Theresa. (2011). The benefits and detriments of the No Child Left behind Act, *ESSAI: 9*, Article 21. Retrieved from http://dc.cod.edu/essai/vol9/iss1/21

Kurzweil, R. (2010). *10 questions for Ray Kurzweil*. New York, NY: *Time Magazine*.

Liebenberg, L., & Ungar, M. (Eds.). (2009). *Researching resilience*. Toronto, ON: University of Toronto Press.

Luthar, S. (2003). *Resilience and vulnerability: Adaptation in the context of childhood adversities*. Cambridge, UK: Cambridge University Press.

Maslow, A. (1970). *Motivation and personality*. New York, NY: Harper & Row.

Miller, D. (2003). *Principles of social justice*. Cambridge, MA: Harvard University Press.

Nastasi, B. K. (2010). President's message. *The School Psychologist, 64*(3), 4–6.

North, C. E. (2006). More than words? Delving into the substantive meaning(s) of "social justice" in education. *Review of Educational Research, 76*, 507–536. doi: 10.3102/00346543076004507

Pinker, S. (2002). *The blank slate: The modern denial of human nature*. New York, NY: Penguin Putnam Inc.

Pinker, S. (2011). *The better angels of our nature: Why violence has declined*. New York, NY: Viking.

Post, S. G. (Ed.) (2007). *Altruism and health: Perspectives from empirical research*. New York, NY: Oxford University Press.

Power, F. C. (1988). The just community approach to moral education. *Journal of Moral Education, 17* (3), 195–208.

Power, F. C., & Hart, S. N. (2005). The way forward to constructive discipline. In S. N. Hart, J. Durrant, P. Newell, & F. C. Power (Eds.), *Eliminating corporal punishment: The way forward to constructive child discipline* (pp. 91–128). Paris: UNESCO.

Prilleltensky, I. (2011). Wellness as fairness. *American Journal of Community Psychology*, doi: 10.1007/s10464-011-9448-8; published online

Prilleltensky, I., & Prilleltensky, O. (2006). *Promoting well-being: Linking personal, organizational, and community change*. Hoboken, NJ: Wiley.

Ravitch, D. (2010). *The death and life of the great American school system: How testing and choice are undermining education*. New York, NY: Basic Books.

Rawls, J. (1982). *A theory of justice*. Cambridge, UK: Cambridge University Press.

Rich, D. (1998). *MegaSkills: Building children's achievement for the information age*. New York, NY: Mariner Books; Houghton Mifflin Harcourt.

Robbins, L., & Hall, J. (1970). *How to practice prospective medicine*. Indianapolis: Methodist Hospital of Indiana.

Ryan, R. M., & Deci, E. L. (2000). Self-determination theory and the facilitation of intrinsic motivation, social development, and well-being. *American Psychologist, 55*(1), 68–78. doi: 10.1037/0003-066X.55.1.68

Sander, J. B., Sharkey, J. D., Groomes, A. N., Krumholz, L., Walker, K., & Hsu, J. Y. (2011). Social justice and juvenile offenders: Examples of fairness, access, and respect in educational settings. *Journal of Educational & Psychological Consultation, 21,* 309–337. doi: 10.1080/10474412.2011.620816

Schweitzer, A. (1993). *Reverence for life: The words of Albert Schweitzer.* New York, NY: HarperCollins.

Sheldon, K. M., Elliot, A. J., Kim, Y. & Kasser, T. (2001). What's satisfying about satisfying events? Comparing ten candidate psychological needs. *Journal of Personality and Social Psychology, 80,* 325–339. doi: 10.1037/0022-3514.80.2.325

Sherif, M., Harvey, O. J., White, B. J., Hood, W., & Sherif, C. W. (1961). *Intergroup conflict and cooperation: The Robbers Cave Experiment.* Norman, OK: The University Book Exchange.

Shriberg, D., Bonner, M., Sarr, B., Walker, A., Hyland, M., & Chester, C. (2008). Social justice through a school psychology lens: Definitions and applications. *School Psychology Review, 37,* 453–468.

Snarey, J. R. (1985). Cross-cultural universality of social-moral development: A critical review of Kohlbergian research. *Psychological Bulletin, 97*(2), 202–232. doi: 10.1037/0033-2909.97.3.411

Snyderman, R., & Williams, R. S. (2003). Prospective medicine: The next health care transformation. *Academic Medicine, 11,* 1079–1084.

Strohecker, J. (2011). *Wellness inventory: A brief history of wellness.* http://www.mywellnesstest.com/certResFile/BriefHistoryofWellness.pdf

Tough, P. (2012). *How children succeed. Grit, curiosity, and the hidden power of character.* New York, NY: Houghton, Mifflin, Harcourt.

Ungar, M. (2005). *Handbook for working with children and youth: Pathways to resilience across cultures and contexts.* Thousand Oaks, CA: Sage.

United Nations Committee on the Rights of the Child. (2011). *General Comment 13: The right of the child to freedom from all forms of violence.* Geneva, Switzerland: Author. http://www2.ohchr.org/english/bodies/crc/comments.htm

United Nations General Assembly. (1989). *Adoption of the Convention on the Rights of the Child.* New York, NY: Author.

United Nations General Assembly. (1996). *International Covenant on Economic, Social and Cultural Rights.* New York, NY: Author

Vaillant, G. E. (1977). *Adaptation to life.* Boston: Little, Brown.

Vaillant, G. E. (2002). *Aging well.* Boston: Little Brown.

Ware, B. (2011). *The top five regrets of the dying: A life transformed by the dearly departing.* Bloomington, IN: Balboa Press.

Werner, E., & Smith, R. (1987). *Vulnerable but invincible: A longitudinal study of resilient children and youth.* New York, NY: Adams, Bannister and Cox.

World Health Organization (WHO). (1948). *Preamble to the Constitution of the World Health Organization as adopted by the International Health Conference, New York, 19–22 June, 1946; signed on 22 July 1946 by representatives of 61 States (Official Records of the World Health Organization, no. 2, p. 100) and entered into force on 7 April 1948.* Geneva, Switzerland: Author.

Zadja, J., Majhanovich, S., Rust, V., & Sabina, E. M. (2006). *Education and social justice.* New York, NY: Springer.

Chapter 2

Social Justice in Schools: Building Child Resilience

Shereen Naser, Bonnie K. Nastasi, and Rosa Maria Mulser

Though the concept of justice has been discussed as far back as Plato's *The Republic,* the use of the term social justice is relatively new. The term social justice was coined in 1840 by a rather obscure Jesuit priest, Luigi Tapparelli. Tapparelli posited that social justice concerned the way that different levels of society interacted, and argued for the common good (Ayers, Quinn & Stovall, 2008). The concept of social justice being the direct result of society's interactions was reflected in the work of American education reformer Horace Mann. Mann argued that education was the most efficient and effective tool for closing the social schisms in society by providing each individual with the knowledge and skills they need to succeed and interact with others. In *Report No. 12 of the Massachusetts School Board* (1848), Mann wrote "Education, then, beyond all other devices of human origin, is the great equalizer of the conditions of men—the balance-wheel of the social machinery." Like Tapparelli, Mann went on to say that the inability to navigate social strata and the lack of education is what creates the great divides in society. With this logic, a sound argument can be made that education is the tool by which a society can close this divide and promote social justice.

In the past decade, significant gains have been made in simply promoting social justice by ensuring access and equity in education for children around the world.

Latest estimates have noted that almost 90% of the worlds' 4–12 year olds are attending primary schools, and 60% of children ages 12–15 years are attending secondary school (United Nations International Emergency Children's Fund, 2012). However, social justice for children goes beyond the provision of services. Educational philosophers and theorists, including German philosopher Georg Wilhelm Friedrich Hegel (1770–1831), have argued that it is the basic right of a child not only to receive an education but also to be educated in the skills needed to participate in dialogue (Butler, 2012). This philosophy is echoed in one of the main guiding principles of the United Nations Convention on the Rights of the Child (UNICEF, 2011), the child's right to participation, and reinforced by the articles related to universal access to education. It could be argued that promoting child growth and development and priming them for engagement and participation in their society should be one of the main social justice issues on which schools and educational systems focus.

This focus on engaging children at all level of society reflects the work of community psychologists Nelson and Prilleltensky (2011) who argue that social justice has to be the simultaneous working of practices that promote and protect the well-being of the individual while also creating systems change aimed at removing oppressive power structures and changing power relationships in order to create a sustainable system that protects and promotes child rights. Nelson and Prilleltensky (2011) categorize these two different types of social justice promotion as *ameliorative* and *transformative*. Ameliorative goals include advancing the well-being of individuals, whereas transformative goals focus more on systems change.

In an educational setting the ameliorative and transformative promotion of social justice may be translated as equipping students with the skills they need to succeed, empowering them through participation in their school and community, and creating school cultures that reinforce and always act in accordance with those values. Unfortunately, schools that create full systems of care and develop a school culture that values student participation are not the norm. For example, discipline systems used in schools, such as zero tolerance policies, often directly ignore a child's right to participation, instead relying on blanket rules without consideration for the individual's needs or perceptions. We believe that understanding how to build school-wide behavioral systems that respect student dignity and promote student resiliency is important to the promotion of social justice through the protection and promotion of child rights in the school setting. This chapter outlines potential problems in current school systems and makes the case for school-wide systems that promote child resiliency and child dignity as a way to realize social justice.

UNDERSTANDING THE RANGE OF CHILD NEEDS

From an ecological perspective, children's future success in school and life is most affected by the community in which they live, their school and family lives, and the resources that are available to them personally or otherwise (Elias & Haynes, 2008). In 1977, Urie Bronfenbrenner accused sterile laboratory settings as being devoid of external validity, noting that truly understanding human development requires looking at individuals within the context of their environment. Bronfenbrenner defined four different systems in which an individual is embedded: the *microsystem*, which represents the relationship between the child and those systems he or she directly interacts with such as the child's home and school; the *mesosystem*, the interrelations between these different systems; the *exosystem*, those systems that indirectly influence the child, and their interactions among each other and the mesosystem; and the *macrosystem*, the overarching, distal cultural structure around a child such as economic, social, or educational systems that influence institutions in the more proximal systems.

Children plagued by poverty and living in lower-income communities experience multiple stressors that tax each of the aforementioned systems. For example, children in low-income communities may be exposed to disproportionately high rates of violence and other traumatic events in their communities (i.e., exosystem; Elias & Haynes, 2008; Garbarino, Dubrow, Kostelny, & Pardo, 1992). In a study of African American youth living in Chicago, one-third of children reported witnessing a homicide, and two-thirds reported witnessing a serious assault. In a survey of 6th-, 8th-, and 10th-grade students in New Haven, Connecticut, 40% of the children reported witnessing one or more violent crimes in the prior year (Groves, Zukerman, Marans, & Cohen, 1993). Similarly, interviews conducted with 53 African American mothers of children ages 9–12 revealed that 51% of New Orleans fifth graders had been victims of violence, and nearly 91% had witnessed some type of violence (Fick, Osofsky, & Lewis, 1997). Children who live in inner cities also are more likely to be exposed to other life stressors brought about by poverty, including malnutrition, unsuitable housing, maladaptive child-rearing practices, inferior medical care, and inadequate schools (Garbarino et al., 1992). Research has shown that schools can act to buffer some of the effects of stressful communities; however, children who attend school in these settings are more likely to endure unimaginative curricula, overcrowded classrooms, poor school facilities, and negative teacher expectations (Owens & Shaw, 2003).

Constant stressors can take a toll on the mental health of children. Exposure to community violence and political strife can lead to difficulty concentrating due to intrusive thoughts, memory problems, and trouble sleeping (Elias & Haynes, 2008; Garbarino et al., 1992; Osofsky, 1995). School-age children who have experienced high rates of violence also show severe constriction in play and activities, showing less motivation to explore and master their environment in an attempt to avoid reminders of the event (Elias & Haynes, 2008). Furthermore, children exposed to these stressors display aggressive play, anxiety, anger, sadness, and uncaring attitudes (Garbarino et al., 1992; Osofsky, 1997). Family life often acts as a buffer against these mental health outcomes. However, students in inner-city communities are less likely to receive these family supports. In fact, parents experience additional burdens and receive less support due to overwhelmed services in their communities such as schools and churches (Osofsky, 1997).

Students who attend public school in low-income areas consistently show lower academic achievement and social skill development than their peers in suburban or rural schools (Owens & Shaw, 2003). For example, the national graduation rate is 68%; however, graduation rates for students who attend school in high poverty, racially segregated, and urban school districts lag from 15% to 18% behind their peers (Swanson, 2004). Low levels of school completion have lifelong economic implications. For instance, in the United States, the median income for adults 25 years of age and older with less than a high school diploma is about $471 a week, almost $200 less than those with a high school diploma (Bureau of Labor Statistics, 2012). Furthermore, a nationwide survey of reading scores revealed that fourth graders in urban schools performed lower than their peers in suburban or rural schools, and those students eligible for free lunch programs performed lower than those who did not (Swanson, 2004). In the same study, 46% of fourth-grade students in urban public schools were below the required reading achievement level compared to 32.5% in suburban schools and 34.1% in rural schools. In New Orleans, over half of fourth graders (51%) scored below proficient in English and Language Arts (The Cowen Institute, 2010).

Although the picture is bleak for students living in low-income, urban communities, it is certainly not a determining factor in child mental health and academic outcomes. Much research has been conducted to identify treatment and prevention programs to address specific academic and mental health issues. Some of the most intriguing developmental research in the past 25 years has explored risk and protective factors for children. This research takes a strengths-based approach to identify protective factors that promote resilience and help children to thrive despite the presence of risk factors. Risk factors, such as low socioeconomic status and parental psychopathology, are antecedent variables that usually predict dysfunction. It is important to note that risk factors are not inevitable predictors (Luthar, Cicchetti, & Becker, 2000). Protective factors, on the other hand, are those variables and processes that mitigate risk and generally help children thrive despite adverse situations (Beauchaine & Hinshaw, 2008).

Resilience refers to the dynamic process of interaction that encompasses positive adaptation (protective factors) within the context of significant adversity in a child's environment (risk factors; Luthar et al., 2000). This means that a child still meets societal norms for certain domains, including academic, social, and behavioral domains (Masten & Powell, 2003). For example, in the United States the school-age children are expected to do well in school (academic competence), be able to make friends and get along with them (social competence), and follow rules at school and at home (behavioral competence; Masten & Powell, 2003). These competencies then interact with risk factors to help combat maladaptive effects of adverse conditions.

An ecological perspective on developmental outcomes addresses two types of interactions. The first is the interaction between the child as a biological entity and the social environment. The second is the interaction of the different social environments around the child (Garbarino et al., 1992). This means that the interaction of protective factors to build resilience is both endogenous to the child and is found in the surrounding external environment. Internal resilience factors include good social and problem-solving skills (Luthar et al., 2000). School and school culture also play a role in resilience for at-risk youth. The World Health Organization (WHO, 2003) defined a healthy school environment as one in which there is interpersonal warmth, equity, cooperation, and open communication. Developmental resilience research provides important insight into the development of effective interventions to aid at-risk children (Baker, 2008).

Schools are in an incredibly unique and privileged position to impact the lives of children, and to provide resources to help children reach their full potential. Specifically, schools provide fertile ground for implementation of school-wide systems and organizational culture that promote resiliency for at-risk students by influencing both endogenous and exogenous factors that affect them. For example, school-wide social and emotional learning (SEL) programs help build resiliency by providing youth with the skills they need to navigate their social environment successfully and productively. When taught in a school that has a school-wide culture of positive behavioral support, SEL programs have been shown to increase both student behavioral and emotional well-being and academic outcomes (CASEL, 2005; Durlak, Weissberg, & Pachan, 2010).

BUILDING SCHOOL SYSTEMS THAT BUILD STUDENT RESILIENCY

Social and emotional competencies are critical to child well-being and resiliency. The presence of good social and problem-solving skills serves as a protective factor for at-risk youth (Luthar et al., 2000). Adequate social competence, including self-regulation, appropriate assertion, cooperation, and independence, among other social skills, aids in the development of mutually satisfying peer relationships (CASEL, 2005; Merrell, Gueldner, & Tran, 2008). The possession of these skills also aids in the development of academic and occupational success (Merrell et al., 2008). Children who grow up in extremely stressful environments, such as low SES urban communities, often are lacking in these skills. Deficits in these areas contribute to a failure to thrive, both in an academic and social sense, and launch a risky cycle of peer rejection, isolation, school failure, and school adjustment problems (Merrell et al., 2008). As noted earlier, social competence is one of the competencies found in resilient children and furthermore affects academic competence. For example, students are often asked to work in groups and their ability to engage in these group activities can facilitate how much they learn from them (Merrell et al., 2008). Also, the ability to regulate emotions is critical for behavioral and attentional control necessary to gain both academic competence and enhance social competence (Yates, Egeland, & Sroufe, 2003). This is especially important for at-risk youth who experience high rates of emotional dysregulation due to overwhelmed parents and high rates of trauma and exposure to community violence (Garbarino et al., 1991).

Social-emotional learning (SEL) programs seek to help children develop the fundamental social and emotional competencies they need to succeed in school and beyond. SEL programming is largely derived from research on risk and resilience (Zins & Elias, 2007). The Collaborative for Academic, Social and Emotional Learning (CASEL; http://casel.org/why-it-matters/what-is-sel/), an international collaborative organization of educators and researchers dedicated to social and emotional learning, has identified five core groups of social competencies. These include:

(1) *Self-awareness*: knowing what one is feeling in the moment.
(2) *Self-management*: handling one's emotions in a way that is adaptive and facilitates the task at hand rather than being disruptive.
(3) *Social awareness*: understanding what others are thinking and being able to take their perspective.
(4) *Relationship skills*: being able to build lasting, rewarding relationships based on cooperation, appropriate assertion, negotiating resolutions to conflict, and seeking help when needed.
(5) *Responsible decision making*: being able to make a decision based on consideration of all the relevant factors and consequences. This also includes the ability to take responsibility for one's own actions.

Although a considerable body of research has indicated the effectiveness of teaching these SEL skills (CASEL, 2005; Doll, Zuker, & Brehm, 2004; Zins & Elias, 2007), the research rarely includes recognition of core theories that explain learning. Instead, evaluation focuses on overall program effectiveness rather than effective components of SEL programs. Cognitive-behavioral theory (CBT), which is a central aspect of SEL programs, is a well-researched model that approaches treatment in a systematic way and emphasizes the relationship between cognitions, behaviors, and emotions (Kendall, 2000). CBT emphasizes the connection between changing thinking to affect behavior and emotion. Furthermore, the CBT model emphasizes practice both in and outside of the learning sessions. This reinforcement has been identified as a key component of SEL programs (Zins & Elias, 2007).

Another component of SEL programs found to consistently work is its comprehensive integration into the school system, and its inclusion of a family-school partnership (CASEL, 2005; Zins & Elias, 2007). For the past 25 years, individual and small-group social skill programs have shown modest results. However, programs that aim to promote SEL school-wide have yielded stronger, more effective results. An increasing amount of research promotes the use of school-wide, integrated systems of SEL, versus fragmented, topic-specific group approaches (Merrell et al., 2008). Therefore, the goal of schools should be to create a school climate that fosters and reinforces these cognitive-behavioral skills, as well as teaching them in a classroom context. Taking it one step further, the most effective SEL programs do not only integrate into the school, but also fully involve the families of the children with which they work (Zins & Elias, 2007). These extensions of systems provide an opportune area for future work with SEL programs.

School-Wide Programs to Support SEL

One approach that has gained much attention in recent years, and has successfully created positive school climates within which comprehensive SEL program may thrive, is School Wide Positive Behavioral Support (SWPBS). SWPBS is a systematic framework for reinforcing desired student behavior while decreasing rates of undesired student behaviors by eliminating unintended reinforcement of these behaviors (Bazelon Center for Mental Health Law, 2006). SWPBS has been widely researched and has gained support from the U.S. Department of Education and Individuals with Disabilities Education Act (IDEA). In 1997, amendments to the IDEA introduced SWPBS (Sugai et al., 2000). Current research shows that schools that employ SWPBS strategies to create a positive school climate have resulted in improved perceptions of school safety, improved academic success by students, and fewer office referrals and suspensions (Luiselli, Putnam, Handler, & Feinberg, 2005; Sugai & Horner, 2008).

SWPBS is mainly a process or overall approach and not a specific intervention, although behavioral theories and strategies are foundational to the approach. SWPBS acknowledges that student functioning both at school and at home requires a repertoire of behavioral skills that can be taught. SWPBS seeks to teach students desired behaviors to build their behavioral repertoire, to replace problem behaviors by positively reinforcing good behavior, and to break the reinforcement contingencies maintaining problem behaviors. Lastly, SWPBS emphasizes data-based decision making and data collection to monitor behavioral changes as a result of using positive support to reinforce replacement behaviors. SEL programming seeks to teach children the skills they need to be adaptive problem solvers and good citizens, and to act as a more specific intervention strategy that can accompany the building of a positive school climate.

Children in urban communities have a higher number of risk factors that interact to increase the chances these children will suffer from mental health problems and, subsequently, academic and work problems. Because schools are in constant contact with children and parents, schools are in a unique position to intervene using what is known about building resiliency in children. One way to build resiliency is by teaching the social-emotional skills children need to succeed. SEL programs have proven effective in providing these social-emotional skills, and are most effective when the school climate is warm and engaging, and the schools engage families in their efforts. A school-wide program that incorporates SEL learning in a positive school environment could go a long way in aiding children, especially at-risk youth in urban communities, in combating both endogenous and exogenous stressors effectively.

School Discipline Programs That May Preclude Resiliency and Child Rights

Students are more likely to be successful if a school environment offers high levels of engagement in productive activities, access to warm relationships, and guidance from adults, or access to responsive schools (Sugai & Horner, 2002). Furthermore,

SEL programs work best in school environments that are safe, well managed, caring, and participatory (McNeely, Nonnemaker, & Blum, 2002; Osterman, 2000)

Unfortunately, many of the breakdowns in providing these engaging and warm school environments happen when developing school discipline systems. Students with problem behaviors account for nearly 20% of the U.S. student population and 50% of behavioral incidents (Cohn, 2002). Being put out of class for problem behaviors can have a negative impact on the students' learning and academic achievement. Many resources are put into improving academic performance in schools; however, few of these interventions address the behavioral problems that are inextricably linked with academic achievement. Both teachers and the general public cite discipline problems as one of the main issues in public schools (Bazelon Center for Mental Health Law, 2006). According to the National Center for Educational Statistics (NCES), 1 in every 14 (7%) students was suspended at least once in 2006 (NCES, 2006). Generally, about 5% of the students in a school account for half or nearly half of all discipline referrals (Sprague, Sugai, Horner, & Walker, 1999).

A historically common response to behavioral problems is the punishment-based policy system called zero tolerance (APA, 2008; Sugai & Horner, 2002). Although there is no official definition of zero tolerance, policies based on zero tolerance rhetoric use predefined, mandatory, blanket consequences applied to the violation of school rules without regard to the seriousness of the behavior, mitigating circumstances, or situational context (APA, 2008). In general, zero tolerance policies arose from a desire to create concrete consequences for misbehavior that are generally severe, highly punitive, and intended to be applied regardless of the gravity of the behaviors or the situational context (Farmer, 1999). Furthermore, zero tolerance policies are based on the premise that removing disruptive students from the classroom leaves behind a better school climate for other students (APA, 2008). Zero tolerance policies have been used to explain the use of similar punishment for students who bring drugs to school and for those who are tardy. Such policies are incompatible with the principle that the punishment must fit the crime, and do not reflect the policies of society as a whole. Students are not given due-process treatment in which they are allowed to defend their behaviors or understand the reason for the punishment they are receiving.

In recent years, there has been an upsurge in the use of zero tolerance policies that espouse this philosophy (APA, 2008; Bazelon Center for Mental Health Law, 2006; Sugai & Horner, 2002). Reactive responses to incidences of antisocial behavior in schools tend to include establishing discipline structures based on zero tolerance policies (Sugai & Horner, 2002). The American Psychological Association Task Force on Zero Tolerance Policies notes that research does not support the efficacy of zero tolerance policies for any of these goals. Zero tolerance policies have failed to increase consistency of school discipline, create a better climate for well-behaved students, or reduce disruptive behaviors overall (APA, 2008). Furthermore, on top of failing to improve standards for well-behaved students, schools fail to teach students necessary replacement behaviors, or appropriate behaviors in lieu of the inappropriate ones (Sugai & Horner, 2002). This means that students might be told about behavioral instances that are wrong, but are not taught how to engage in correct behaviors. Research shows that those students who are suspended are at greater risk for misbehavior later on, and because they are never taught appropriate behaviors, they are also at risk for further suspensions (Farmer, 1999). This practice leads to the students who are repeatedly suspended being removed from continued access to services and quality education (Sugai & Horner, 2002). A recent review of Louisiana's suspension rates shows that not only have Louisiana's zero tolerance practices led to suspension rates almost double the national average, but that those students being repeatedly suspended are more likely to end up in the juvenile justice system and, later on, jail (Sullivan & Morgan, 2010); such practices raise serious concerns about social justice for these students. At present, schools are held to higher rates of accountability than in earlier times due to the instatement of the No Child Left Behind Act in 2001 (NCLB; Sugai & Horner, 2002). Removing students from services hinders a school's ability to adhere to NCLB. Furthermore, punitive measures are disproportionately applied to students of color (APA, 2002; Farmer, 1999). For instance, research demonstrates that African American students are consistently overrepresented in suspensions and expulsions (Buerkle, Whitehouse, & Christianson, 2009), another critical issue related to social justice for children and adolescents. This overrepresentation is not accounted for by socioeconomic status and persists despite the lack of data supporting the assumption that African American students exhibit any higher rates of disruption of violence than other students (APA, 2008).

Traditional forms of discipline may moderate behaviors for some students but can actually cause increases of misbehavior (Bazelon Center for Mental Health Law, 2006) and rates of suspension (Farmer, 1999; Miltenberger, 2008) among other students. Traditional forms of discipline that solely focus on punishment elicit emotional side effects (Mallot, 2008). These emotional side effects can include acts of aggression, which are then punished through suspension (Mallot, 2008; Miltenberger, 2008). Such cycles can cause a child to resent school (Sugai & Horner, 2002). Focusing solely on punishment also may result in inappropriate escape or avoidance behaviors by the person being punished. Often behaviors like lying are reinforced if it successfully results in avoidance of punishment, as well as avoidance of the person who delivers the punishment (e.g., a teacher or principal; Miltenberger, 2008). The use of punishment also may be negatively reinforcing for the person delivering the punishment. Delivering a punishment such as suspending a child removes the immediate disruption from the classroom, increasing the likelihood of the use of suspension in the future (Miltenberger, 2008). Lastly, punitive, reactive discipline strategies can model the very negative behaviors being warned against, instead of the desired behaviors (National Center for Mental Health in Schools [NCMHS], 2008).

These reactive responses also are often short-lived and do not produce long-term reductions in problem behaviors, generalization, or learning of more appropriate behaviors (Crone & Horner, 2003; Sugai & Horner, 2002). Reactive responses have been associated with short-term and immediate reductions in serious problem behaviors (Mayer, 1995), but they have failed to prevent the development of further problem behaviors and they often create a false sense of security (APA, 2008; Sugai & Horner, 2002). Numerous sources have called for more proactive approaches to remediating behavior, which break up the contingencies that maintain problem behaviors, increase academic success, and sustain positive school and classroom environments (Sugai & Horner, 2002).

Restorative justice programs are one potential answer to the problem of zero tolerance. The restorative justice model, unlike zero tolerance, emphasizes repairing harm done to relationships and the people involved due to offense, over and above laying blame. Those offended and those who have misbehaved collaborate to find a mutually accepted way to move forward (Hopkins, 2002). Restorative justice was first used in the school setting as a response to purely punitive systems of school behavior reform in Australia in 1990. Since then restorative justice practices have been used in schools around the world, including South Africa, the United Kingdom, and New Zealand as an alternative to punitive systems that employ zero tolerance or corporal punishment. Restorative justice provides an alternative to focusing on purely punitive reactions to misbehavior. Restorative justice challenges the idea that the threat of punishment is necessary to prevent wrongdoing and promotes a shift from retributive justice to one focused on reparation of social relationships and reentry into society. In the school setting, this is particularly suited to promoting practices of inclusion instead of exclusion. Students who commit the misbehavior are asked to work with trained personnel to understand why the misbehavior occurred and consider or generate alternative behaviors. Furthermore, restorative justice practices promote healing and building of social relationships instead of interrupting them, and thus reinforce community values (Wearmouth, McKinney, & Glynn, 2009).

Hopkins (2002) presents a model in which restorative justice in a school system includes establishing restorative justice practices that ensure development of skills among those implementing the program, promote collaboration with the local community, and establish shared ideology of repair versus retribution. It is important to keep in mind that restorative justice models are dependent on these skills and ideologies. This requires work at a systems level, including teaching students specific social and emotional skills, and creating a school environment where these skills can thrive. Although there is considerable evidence of the positive outcomes of restorative justice practices in the juvenile justice and criminal justice systems (see Sherman & Strang, 2007), fewer empirical research reports are available on how restorative justice works in addressing these issues in the school setting. The lack of empirical research articles available on restorative justice in schools is due to the relatively new emergence of a restorative justice system as a response to zero tolerance policies. However, schools across the world that have used restorative justice practices have provided micro-analyses and narratives on the effects of restorative justice practices and the positive outcomes that students experience as a result. For example, in Queensland, Australia, researchers followed multiple conferences between offenders and victims in a school setting and found that offenders had a high compliance rate with the terms of agreement set forth in the conferences, and that both parties expressed more positive feelings. The school administrators and staff also experienced these positive outcomes (Wearmouth et al., 2009). As the educational field moves forward in developing restorative justice–based school behavioral programs with positive outcomes for students that minimize punitive approaches, data collection is imperative for providing a fuller picture of outcomes and best practices.

Developing Sustainable Partnership-Based Approaches

Effective resiliency building for inner-city students integrates knowledge of SEL and creates a school climate that maximizes the effectiveness of SEL programs by being warm, engaging, and attentive to family and community functioning. However, any school program needs to be sensitive to and reinforced by the family and community systems around the child. This attention to the child's ecological context is critical; however, it does not stop at bringing different systems (like school and home) together. Rather, the goal should be to create a collaborative relationship through effective communication between the different systems (i.e., facilitating meso-system). For example, although parents in urban communities might not be involved in schools in a traditional sense (attending PTA meetings), there are ways in which they can be highly involved in their children's education (helping with child's homework; Lowie, Lever, Ambrose, Tager, & Hill, 2003). Developing an effective program means finding ways to recognize and use the strengths of all stakeholders.

Focus groups are one of the most effective ways to develop programming sensitive to the cultural context of the ecology surrounding the child, to assess the needs of the different groups, and to bring multiple groups into the conversation around program development (i.e., school, family, peers). Not only are focus groups a good way to involve parents and make them feel heard, but they also act as part of the formative research process, allowing parents to be part of implementation if they so choose, and helping identify parents who might want to play a greater role in implementation and research by acting as community liaisons.

These principles are congruent with the core components of a comprehensive school-based mental health program as defined by a Participatory Culture Specific Intervention Model (PCSIM) (Nastasi, Moore, & Varjas, 2004). PCSIM is an interdisciplinary model that emphasizes a culture-specific, recursive, and participatory process of program development. The different phases of program development outlined in PCSIM allow for the development of five main components of effective, comprehensive, school-based mental health programs. These include (Nastasi et al., 2004, p. 21):

(1) Integration of educational, mental health, and social services though interagency and interdisciplinary collaboration;
(2) A full continuum of services, including prevention, risk reduction, early intervention, and treatment;
(3) Focus on the ecological contexts of the child (school, family, peers, community, society);
(4) Systematically evaluate program process and outcome;
(5) Offer services that are based on empirical evidence of the complex array of factors that influence mental health of children and adolescents.

Addressing these five components helps to ensure program sustainability and institutionalization by increasing program buy-in from key stakeholders, thus assuring a culturally sensitive, adaptable program.

The PCSIM (Nastasi et al., 2004) involves several recursive stages for developing sustainable and institutionalized programs: (1) examining existing theory, research, and policy; (2) developing partnerships among stakeholders; (3) learning the culture of the school and community; (4) conducting formative research to understand the key psychological and social-cultural factors relevant to child well-being; (5) establishing goals endorsed by all stakeholders; (6) developing a culture- and context-specific conceptual model to guide program development; (7) implementing and evaluating culture- and context-specific programs (selecting, adapting or creating evidence-based programs); (8) disseminating program evaluation data to stakeholders and making relevant revisions; and (9) planning for sustainability and institutionalization. Implementation of PCSIM is a long-term process that typically involves system-wide change and requires commitment from stakeholders to the change process. The development of school-based programs that foster social justice and child rights requires attention to multiple factors that influence the various aspects of justice and rights (e.g., nondiscrimination, participation, protection from harm, promotion of well-being) and that are critical to meeting mission of education (e.g., academic achievement and learning). Thus, the school-specific conceptual model ideally incorporates all of these factors.

CONCLUSION

Children and youth spend a great portion of their day in school, which allows schools to play a key role in promoting social justice for children, youth, and their families. They provide children with important learning and coping resources and can help to ensure the rights of children and youth. However, schools sometimes fail to embrace student dignity and to promote student resilience, which are critical to ensuring child's rights and social justice. This chapter addressed several key factors that are crucial for schools to adopt to overcome many obstacles that prevent schools from building and fostering child resiliency, such as zero tolerance or corporal punishment.

For one, a child's entire environmental context should be taken into consideration when assessing children's needs and rights. More specifically, the various systems in which a child's life is embedded, the interrelationships between these systems, and the overarching historical and cultural background should be examined along with the personal risk and protective factors related to promoting resilience and ensuring children reach their full potential.

In addition, social-emotional skills, such as problem solving and the self-regulation, have been found to contribute to youth resilience. Therefore, schools should focus on adopting social-emotional learning programs with an emphasis on school-wide positive behavior support that not only helps children and youth improve their social competence but also can improve academic and life-long success. For any school effort or program to be effective, it needs to be sensitive to and reinforced by the family and community systems surrounding the child.

The overarching goal in advocating for youth's social justice should be to create collaborative relationships between the various systems. We introduced the PCSIM as a potential process for developing school programs that incorporate ecological and cultural considerations and empirical evidence, and involve a recursive participatory process across the key ecological systems (e.g., family, school, community). The development of school programs that promote social justice and child's rights can be effective only when all stakeholders take an active and collaborative role in program development and community building.

REFERENCES

American Psychological Association (APA) Task Force on Zero-Tolerance Policies. (2008). Are zero tolerance policies effective in the schools? An evidentiary review and recommendations. *American Psychologist, 63*(9), 852–862. doi: 10.1177/1053451212449735

Ayers, W., Quinn, T., & Stovall, D. (2008). *Handbook of social justice in education* (1st ed.). New York, NY: Routledge.

Baker, J. (2008). Assessing school risk and protective factors. In B. J. Doll & J. A. Cummings (Eds.), *Transforming school mental health services: Population-based approaches to promoting the competency and wellness of children* (pp. 1333–1347). Thousand Oaks, CA: Corwin Press with National Association of School Psychologists.

Bazelon Center for Mental Health Law. (2006). *Way to go: School success for children with mental health care needs*. Washington, DC: Author.

Beauchaine, T., & Hinshaw, S. (2008). *Child and adolescent psychopathology* (1st ed.). Boston: Wiley.

Bronfenbrenner, U. (1977). Toward an experimental ecology of human development. *American Psychologist, 32*, 513–531. doi: 10.1037/0003-066X.32.7.513

Buerkle, K., Whitehouse, E. M., & Christenson, S. L. (2009). Partnering with families for educational success. In T. Gutkin & C. Reynolds (Eds.), *The handbook of School Psychology* (pp. 655–680). Hoboken, NJ: John Wiley & Sons.

Bureau of Labor Statistics. (2012). *Earnings and unemployment rates by educational attainment.* Retrieved from http://www.bls.gov/emp/ep_chart_001.htm

Butler, C. (2012). *Child rights: The movement, international law, and opposition.* (1st ed.). New York, NY: Purdue University Human Rights Studies.

Cohn, A (2002). *Positive behavioral supports: Information for educators.* Retrieved from http://www.nasponline.org/resources/factsheets/pbs_fs.aspx

Collaborative for Academic, Social and Emotional Learning. (2005). *Safe and sound: Illinois edition.* UIC Series on Issues in Children's and Families' Lives. Retrieved from http://www.casel.org

Cowen Institute for Public Education Initiatives, Tulane University. (2010). *The state of public education in New Orleans 2010 report.* New Orleans, LA: Author.

Crone, D., & Horner, R. (2003). *Building positive behavior support systems in schools.* New York, NY: Guilford Press.

Doll, B., Zucker, S., & Brehm, K. (2004). *Resilient classrooms: Creating healthy environments for learning.* New York, NY: Guilford Press.

Durlak, J., Weissberg, R., & Pachan, M. (2010). A meta-analysis of after-school programs that seek to promote personal and social skills in children and adolescents. *Community Psychology, 45,* 495–309. doi: 10.1007/s10464-010-9300-6

Elias, M., & Haynes, N. (2008). Social competence, social support, and academic achievement in minority, low-income, urban elementary school children. *School Psychology Quarterly, 23*(4), 474–495. doi: 10.1037/1045-3830.23.4.474

Farmer, G. (1999). Disciplinary practices and perceptions of school safety. *Journal of Social Service Research, 26*(1), 1–38.

Fick, A. C., Osofsky, J. D. & Lewis, M. L. (1997). Perceptions of violence: Children, parents, and police officers. In J. D. Osofsky (Ed.), *Children in a violent society* (pp. 261–276). New York, NY: Guilford Press.

Garbarino, J., Dubrow, N., & Kostelny, K. (1991). *No place to be a child.* San Francisco, CA: Jossey-Bass.

Garbarino, J., Dubrow, N., Kostelny, K., & Pardo, C. (1992). *Children in danger.* San Francisco, CA: Jossey Bass.

Groves, B.M., Zuckerman, B., Marans, S., & Cohen, D. (1993, January 13). Silent victims: Children who witness violence. *Journal of the American Medical Association, 269* (2), 2.

Hopkins, B. (2002). Restorative justice in schools. *Support for learning, 17*(3). Retrieved from http://www.transformingconflict.org/system/files/libraryfiles/Doc 5—Restorative Justice in Schools 2002—Support for Learning 17.3.pdf

Kendall, P. C. (2000). *Child and adolescent therapy: Cognitive-behavioral procedures.* New York, NY: Guilford Press.

Lowie, J., Lever, N., Ambrose, M., Tager, S., & Hill, S. (2003). Partnering with families in expanded school mental health programs. In M. D. Weist, S. Evans, & N. Lever (Eds.), *Handbook of school mental health: Advancing practice and research* (pp. 386–396). New York, NY: Springer-Verlag.

Luiselli, J., Putnam, R., Handler, M., & Feinberg, A. (2005). Whole-School Positive Behaviour Support: Effects on student discipline problems and academic performance. *Educational Psychology, 25*(2), 183–198.

Luthar, S., Cicchetti, D., & Becker, B. (2000). The construct of resilience: A critical evaluation and guidelines for future work. *Child Development, 71*(3), 543–562. doi: 10.1111/1467-8624.00164

Malott, R. W. (2008). *Principles of behavior* (6th ed.). Upper Saddle River, NJ: Prentice-Hall.

Masten, A., & Powell, J. (2003). A resilience framework for research, policy and practice. In S. Luthar (Ed.), *Resilience and vulnerability: Adaptation in the context of childhood adversities* (pp. 1–28). New York, NY: Cambridge University Press.

Mayer, G. (1995). Preventing antisocial behavior in the schools. *Journal of Applied Behavior Analysis, 28*(4), 467–478.

McNeely, C. A., Nonnemaker, J. M., & Blum, R. W. (2002). Promoting student attachment to school: Evidence from the National Longitudinal Study of Adolescent Health. *Journal of School Health, 72*(4), 138–146. Retrieved from http://www2.gsu.edu/~wwwche/Promoting%20School%20Connectedness%20Evidence%20from%20the%20Natl%20Longitudinal%20Study%20of%20Adolescent%20Health.pdf

Merrell, K., Gueldner, B., & Tran, O. (2008). Social and emotional learning: A school-wide approach to intervention for socialization, friendship problems, and more. In B. J. Doll & J. A. Cummings (Eds.), *Transforming school mental health services: Population-based approaches to promoting the competency and wellness of children* (pp. 165–186). Thousand Oaks, CA: Corwin Press with National Association of School Psychologists.

Miltenberger, Raymond G. (2008). *Behavior modification: Principles and procedures* (4th ed.). Belmont, CA: Thomson Wadsworth.

Nastasi, B. K., Moore, R. B., & Varjas, K. M. (2004). *School-based mental health: Creating comprehensive and culturally specific programs.* Washington, DC: APA.

National Center for Educational Statistics (NCES). (2006). *The condition of education.* Retrieved from https://nces.ed.gov/programs/coe/

National Center for Mental Health in Schools (NCMHS). (2008). *Mental health in schools and school improvement: Current status, concerns and new directions.* Los Angeles, CA: Author.

Nelson, G., & Prilleltensky, I. (2011). *Community psychology, in pursuit of liberation and well-being.* (2nd ed.). London, UK: Palgrave MacMillan.

Osofsky, J. (1995). The effects of exposure to violence on young children. *American Psychologist, 50*, 782–788.

Osofsky, J. (1997). The effects of exposure to violence on young children. In J. M. Notterman (Ed.), *The evolution of psychology: Fifty years of the American Psychologist* (pp. 725–740). Washington, DC: American Psychological Association. doi: 10.1037/10254-050

Osterman, K. E. (2000). Students' need for belonging in the school community. *Review of Educational Research, 70*, 323–367. doi: 10.3102/00346543070003323

Owens, E., & Shaw, D. (2003). Poverty and early childhood adjustment. In S. Luthar (Ed.), *Resilience and vulnerability: Adaptation in the context of childhood adversities* (pp. 267–292). New York, NY: Cambridge University Press.

Sherman, L., & Strang, H., (2007). *Restorative justice: The evidence. Policy report from the Smith Institute.* London: Smith Institute. *http://www.iirp.edu/pdf/RJ_full_report.pdf*

Sprague, J., Sugai, G., Horner, R., Walker, H., (1999) Using office discipline referral data to evaluate school-wide discipline and violence prevention interventions. *OSSC Bulletin, 42*(2).

Sugai, G., Horner, R., Dunlap, G., Hieneman, M., Lewis, T., Nelson, C., et al. (2000). Applying positive behavior support and functional behavioral assessment in schools. *Journal of Positive Behavior Interventions, 2*(3), 131–143.

Sullivan, E., & Morgan, D. (2010). *Pushed out: Harsh discipline in Louisiana schools denies the right to education.* Families and Friends of Louisiana's Incarcerated Children and National Economic and Social Rights Initiative. Retrieved from http://www.nesri.org/fact_sheets_pubs/Pushed_Out_Report.pdf

Swanson, C. B. (2004, February). *Who graduates? Who doesn't? A statistical portrait of public high school graduation, Class of 2001.* Washington, DC: Education Policy Center, The Urban Institute. http://www.urban.org/publications/410934.html

UNICEF. (2011). *Rights under the Convention on the Rights of the Child.* Retrieved from http://www.unicef.org/crc/index_30177.html

United Nations International Emergency Children's Fund. (2012). *The state of the world's children.* Retrieved from http://www.unicef.org/sowc/index_61804.html

Wearmouth, J., McKinney, R., & Glynn, T. (2009) Restorative justice in schools: A New Zealand example. *Educational Research, 1*(49), 37–49.

World Health Organization. (2003). *Who information series on school health.* Retrieved from http://www.who.int/school_youth_health/media/en/sch_childfriendly_03_v2.pdf

Yates, T., Egeland, B., & Sroufe, A. (2003). Rethinking resilience: A developmental process perspective. In S. Luthar (Ed.), *Resilience and vulnerability: Adaptation in the context of childhood adversities.* New York, NY: Cambridge University Press.

Zins, J., & Elias, M. (2007). Social and emotional learning: Promoting the development of all students. *Journal of Educational & Psychological Consultation, 17*(2–3), 233–255. doi: 10.1080/10474410701413152

Chapter 3

Promoting Social Justice in Families

Marva L. Lewis and Allisyn L. Swift

The concept of social justice is typically thought of as an adult process or outcome often co-opted into an amorphous political adult mantra of rights of the individual. Children's rights are customarily addressed separately from a legal or social service perspective. Concepts of human rights originated in centuries-old religious doctrines and are often intertwined with terms of morality and ethics. When members of the same society who might hold different levels of social power define human rights, heated debates of what constitutes social justice are the usual outcome.

We define *social justice* as the equality of opportunity to exercise basic human rights. These rights include the right to life and resources needed for survival. The purpose of this chapter is to address how children learn the core elements of the broad construct of social justice that includes diversity and difference, human rights, children's rights, and the development of morality and prosocial behavior through relationships within their families and communities. To understand processes of how to promote the concept of social justice with children, one must think from the perspective of a child. A strengths approach to families from a global perspective links unique family, community, and cultural strengths to understand distinctive processes that may promote social justice in diverse families (Sullivan, 1992). Finally, an ecological family systems perspective provides further depth to the construct of family. The traditional nuclear family, composed of two parents with a child living in a separate household, is increasingly recognized as a social system—a whole composed of interrelated parts, each of which affects and is affected by the others (Ashford, LeCroy, & Lortie, 2006). Each part contributes to the functioning of the whole. As a dynamic social system each member has a specific role that maintains the integrity of the group as a family (Nichols, 2011). A family systems perspective helps with understanding the myriad of family relationships contributing to a child's development (Guadalupe & Welkley, 2012).

We propose a conceptual model with three key components: (1) emotional and social skills, (2) learning to embrace diversity and everyday conflict, and (3) promoting the value of social justice through service to others. The model is focused on the relationships within the family and the relationships of families with the larger community and global contexts in which they function. This conceptual framework uses a relationship-based approach that centers on family relational and emotional processes and maintains a focus on the developmental needs of children. As active learners the relationship lessons important to promotion of social justice become a central part of a child's family narrative and individual self-concept (Cole & Cole, 1989; Stern, 1985). Despite Western dominance in shaping world actions carried out in the name of social justice, there are two core elements of social justice applicable to cultural groups and countries around the world. These core elements, important to the socialization of children within families, and expressed in a variety of ways determined by culture, climate, and generation, comprise a universal construct of social justice (Healey, 2012). These elements are (1) the recognition of the common humanity with others and (2) the fundamental human right to equal access to the resources needed for basic survival, food, water, air, shelter, and human connection. As societies develop their unique standards, they begin to expand the core elements of social justice to include rights such as safety, education, or, as stated in the constitution of the United States, the right to "life, liberty and the pursuit of happiness."

Developmental psychologists have long studied how children learn and are taught prosocial behaviors but only recently are focused on the construct of social justice (Clark, 1963; Mays, 2000). Research findings document how children learn the elements of social justice from birth through late adolescence. The developmental trajectory of relationship behaviors begins with an infant's ability to recognize the emotions of their primary caregiver through social referencing (Emde, 1989). Babies are born to learn the critical behaviors that allow them to survive through their attachment and connection to parents and dedicated caregivers (Ainsworth & Bowlby, 1991; Newman & Newman, 2012). This relationship-focused learning continues with experiences in learning prosocial behaviors at daycare and early education centers or within the context of sibling and extended family relationships. A core goal of any preschool center is to teach children the patience required to wait their turn. Managing their urgent thirst expecting a sip of cool water while lining up for the water fountain or containing their excitement while waiting to take their turn on the playground see-saw provide opportunities to practice elemental behavioral skills critical to social justice. They then learn social perspective taking and rules for fairness in games and moral behaviors of their cultural group during middle childhood (Newman & Newman, 2012). As teenagers they begin to experience the consequences to their autonomy from their families of origin when they do not adhere to curfews or the rules for operating an automobile.

The dry throat of childhood thirst represents the insistent survival needs of any individual's basic needs for food, water, and air. The equitable achievement of these needs in the face of other humans' equally urgent needs is the fundamental illustration of social justice. Individuals are challenged with their common human social reality: "We both are human and need water to survive, so how can we both sufficiently drink the only water available to us?" Thus begins a young child's lessons in social justice on the playground with peers. At each developmental stage, children learn a variety of lessons focused on how to function within relationships with family, peers, and society.

Currently, there are many initiatives to teach children aspects of social justice within school and community settings (Cowan & Parker, 2008). Initiatives such as teaching tolerance, reducing bullying behaviors, and preparing curricula designed to promote cultural awareness in children are successful examples. Yet, the precursor to the earliest manifestation of what comprises social justice begins within a child's family.

Support for the components of the proposed conceptual model is drawn from diverse developmental and social theories. These theories frame the elemental factors needed for children to learn social justice in families and their communities. We briefly review these theories and how each informs our model for promoting social justice in families, and in turn within local and global communities.

We first examine concepts from John Bowlby's (1969) ethological theory of parent-child attachment to understand socialization processes and developmental outcomes that may or may not promote social justice. These concepts include Bowlby's formulation of the attachment relationship as a partnership. This early relationship becomes the psychological template, or internal working model, that directs the quality of future relationships throughout the child's lifetime.

Bronfenbrenner's (1989) ecological systems theory provides theoretical support for the third component of our model, service to others. This theory posits that interlocking environmental events and ecological conditions that surround an individual profoundly shape their behavior and development within their various social settings. The experience of particular importance for understanding group conflict and social injustice occurs at the ecological level of the *chronosystem*. This level includes the shared collective cultural-historical experiences of the family group associated with their ethnic or racial identities that create the everyday emotions accompanying the conflicts associated with that historical memory (Alexander, Eyerman, Giesen, Smelser, & Sztompka, 2004; Lewis, 2007).

A MODEL FOR A RELATIONSHIP-BASED APPROACH TO PROMOTE SOCIAL JUSTICE IN FAMILIES

The key to our model for promoting social justice hinges on the socio-emotional quality of relationships for young children and their families. The quality of the relationships with members from various subsystems within a family (parent-child, sibling, the executive parental subsystem), and relationships among extended family members with a nuclear family, all provide opportunities for children within that family to experience the core elements of social justice. These core elements are (1) the recognition and acceptance of the humanity of others and (2) respect for the rights of others to resources for their basic needs of survival.

How families nurture and discipline their children, the shared history of a brother and sister, the joyful experiences of connecting with grandparents, cousins, aunts, and uncles who share common cultural rituals and celebrations provide the relationship framework needed to promote social justice. Our thesis is that children's early family relationships provide the emotional, mental, and behavioral templates for their future interactions and potential conflicts with others from diverse groups. These early relationship experiences also prepare children to take leadership roles in areas where there is a critical need for social justice, for example, in fair employment and labor practices, or obtaining services from public and private agencies for health care, education, or mental health. Fair and just resolution of conflict can be a first step in a child's conceptualizing of social justice (Weinhold & Weinhold, 2000). Learning how to resolve a conflict with a sibling over mundane matters, such as who gets to use a coveted music iPod, provides a child with opportunities to practice the essential negotiation and conflict resolution skills that might be required in future advocacy for social justice.

Increasing developing children's knowledge of culture and history of their group and that of diverse other groups, their ability to critically reflect on the environmental systems that impact diverse families, and the skills learned through the resolution of everyday conflict are processes that most families can teach. These relationship experiences may result in the acceptance of the common humanity of others outside of their immediate family and ethnic group, recognition of the basic need of others' for survival resources, and ultimately promotion of social justice.

Social justice operates within three major contexts—the family, the community, and the global context. Elements within each component are expressed differently in the respective contexts. As previously noted, our model to promote social justice in families uses a strengths- and relationship-based approach and includes three core components: (1) developing emotional and social skills; (2) normalizing nontraumatic conflict and diversity; and (3) promoting the value of social justice through service to others. This relationship-focused model draws on developmental theories and concepts from ecological theories of development, attachment theory, and social learning theory to explain family socialization processes that promote social justice. Figure 3.1 presents the elements of each component of the model.

The emotional, cognitive, and behavioral skills needed to promote social justice may be achieved through the developing child's dynamic experience of what we propose is *family self-efficacy*. These skills include recognition of stereotypes; communication skills; critical analysis applied to groups, organizations, and systems; and empathic awareness of family values and the needs of others. An experience of a visiting aunt giving special presents and praise to one sibling and not the other

Figure 3.1
A Relationship-Based Model to Promote Social Justice in Families. This illustrates the three essential components: Emotional and Social Skills, Normalizing Non-Traumatic Conflict and Diversity, and Promoting the Values of Social Justice through Service as the basis for fostering social justice through relationships in the family, which is then extended to the community and the global contexts.

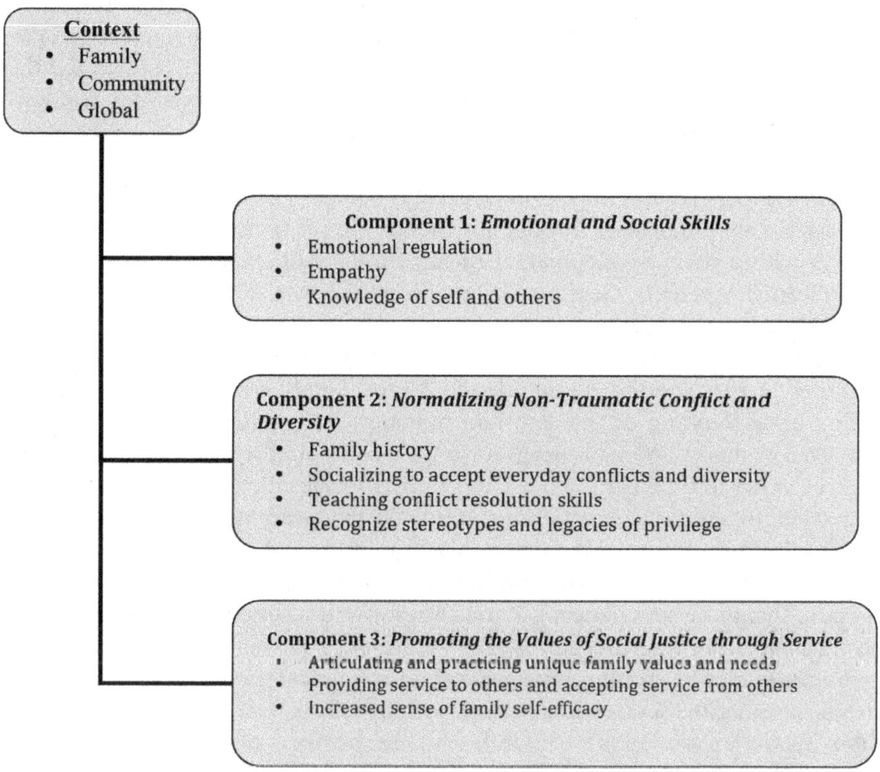

may provide an emotional template of the concept of fairness. When that same child realizes that his or her beloved baseball coach has never given a team member with a minor physical disability the opportunity to play in an actual game because of stereotypes the coach holds about people with disabilities, he or she may begin to better understand the concept of fairness.

This model normalizes conflict as a predictable, everyday occurrence in human relationships in family, community, and global contexts. Using an approach to interpersonal conflict as normal allows families to teach the skills needed to regulate the emotions inherent in conflicts. Subsequently, children should be able to generalize these skills to other settings. Before describing each component of the model in detail, we first discuss the centrality of the family for socializing children in the core tenats of social justice.

THE CENTRALITY OF THE FAMILY FOR PROMOTING THE CORE COMPONENTS OF SOCIAL JUSTICE

Individual families constitute the most emotionally powerful unit of any community. This strong emotional connection is true for families around the world (Ainsworth, 1977; Bowlby, 1988). We argue that children practice the core components of social justice—recognition of the common humanity with others and the rights of all to access to resources for survival—through their everyday relationships with family members. An emotional schema of acceptance or rejection of the humanity of others begins with unconditional or conditional acceptance by their family members (Bretherton, 1987). A child's concepts of worthiness, value, and self-esteem are established through interactions in relationships with attachment figures within their developmental niches throughout their childhood (Emde, 1989; Kerns, Aspelneia, Gentzler, & Grabill, 2001; Lewis, 2000; Newman & Newman, 2012; Rohner, 1986).

Sociologist Charles Cooley's (1902) seminal theory of the social looking glass provides further support to the idea that early family relationships establish a child's understanding of the common humanity with others. Cooley proposed that even as infants, human beings form their concept of self from the reflections and responses to their earliest behaviors during socialization by caregivers. Just as young children begin to experience emotionally the meaning of acceptance within the family, they also learn the emotional pain of inequality and rejection within the family (Rohner, 1986). They begin to learn what it feels like to be human. We propose that these experiences generalize to form the core component needed for social justice, that is, the recognition of the humanity of others.

Societies may be stratified along social class, political power, or some other indelible or inherited social characteristic such as culture, race, or ethnicity (Fanon, 1968; Pinderhughes, 1989). Children who are members of families at the lower levels of the social stratification may begin to experience social injustice over the course of their development. It is also within the earliest family relationships that children experience the emotionally charged experiences of inequality and invisibility (Lyons-Ruth, 2006). These early relationship experiences become imprinted on the brain of developing children (Schore, 2010). We next describe each component of our conceptual model and briefly review developmental theories that provide the foundation for the respective component.

COMPONENT 1: EMOTIONAL AND SOCIAL SKILLS

The first component of our relationship-based model begins with emotional and social skills, and includes learning to regulate emotions, empathic awareness, and knowledge of self and others. Each of these processes provides skills needed to promote social justice. Each cultural group provides the rules for their members to express and display emotions (Thoits, 1989). Yet there are universal characteristics of emotions recognized by humans around the world. Affect, the feeling tone that individuals experience in response to their circumstances, is critical to the survival of human beings. Emotions serve as motivators and alert people to information in their environments and prepare them to respond in particular ways. The well-known fight-or-flight response stems from the decades of research demonstrating the biological origins of these psychological responses. In situations of conflict that occur in human relationships, the regulation of emotional states is important to the resolution of those conflicts (Weinhold & Weinhold, 2000). Self-knowledge about emotional triggers, personality style, and habitual ways of responding to conflict prepare individuals to communicate their needs more effectively. Being aware of emotional responses also can help individuals identify experiences of invisibility and social injustices. Emotions or acting on emotional triggers can be the source of exacerbating and escalating conflict that could be better handled through respectful exchanges. Lack of emotional regulation can be the root of domestic violence or physical child abuse within the family, community violence, or even war in the global context. These forms of violence are all illustrations of emotional causes impinging on the basic human right to physical safety.

Children are in a better position to advocate for social justice beginning with empathic awareness. Empathic awareness is the emotional bridge needed to teach children to accept the humanity of others, a core element of social justice. Their knowledge of self includes the cognitive skills needed to regulate the emotions that arise in conflict with diverse others. "People must use the emotions attached to a conflict constructively rather than resolve them separately from the actual conflict" (Weinhold & Weinhold, 2000, p. 32).

Attachment Theory

Developed by John Bowlby and later by Mary Ainsworth, attachment theory is based on systematic observations of infant-parent dyads (Ainsworth & Bowlby, 1991; Bowlby, 1988). It provides an emotional and relationship-based framework for conceptualizing varying behavioral patterns between infant and caregiver. Bowlby proposed that infants are strongly predisposed to seek proximity to special individuals in their lives, under certain situations, based on the success of previously experienced interactions with these individuals. These attachment patterns are evident throughout the life span and preserved through what Bowlby termed internal working models of the relationship (Bowlby, 1988; Bretherton, 1987).

The concepts of intersubjectivity and attunement are intertwined with attachment theory, as they are both mechanisms and outcomes of secure attachments. Intersubjectivity has been described as a "condition of our humanity and essential function of the mind" (Lyons-Ruth, 2006, p. 602). Intersubjectivity is essentially the ability and capacity to read others' emotional states and exchange through show of affective and intentional cues (Lyons-Ruth, 2006). The quality of engagement and its capacity to regulate the child's fearful arousal has direct consequences on the development of the organizational processes involved in intersubjectivity. This is a function of neurobiological and social foundations of empathy. Intersubjectivity calls for a shared affective state; this enables the process of attunement. The neurobiological benefits of attunement are bi-directional. As a baby tunes in to the caregiver's speech, eye contact, voice, and touch, the right brain is activated, oxytocin is secreted, and cortisol and catecholamine are regulated (Schore, 2010). Simultaneously, as the caregiver tunes in to the baby, the right brain activates, oxytocin is secreted, and they experience heightened perception of attention and tactile information. As this exchange is taking place, the behavior of the caregiver is incorporated into the developing child's schema of behavior. Creating empathy in the child through family processes are the foundations of creating the core element of social justice recognition and acceptance of the common humanity of all.

Social Justice and Attachment

A key concept of attachment theory relevant to social justice is that the socio-emotional qualities of relationships have a pervasive effect on the acceptability of new knowledge and efforts to form effective partnerships (Bowlby, 1969). Bowlby viewed secure attachment conditions as optimal environments for learning because attachment is essentially a motivational system (Lyons-Ruth, 2006); an individual is motivated to seek proximity with a trusted individual who is more knowledgeable. Research in this area reveals that the quality of relationships and attachment styles between teachers, or school-based mental health practitioners, and students results in increased academic success, parent communication, and school attendance, and fosters resilience in diverse samples of students (Anderson, Christenson, Sinclair, & Lehr, 2004; Morris-Rothschild & Brassard, 2006). With strong family attachments children have the safety and protection of loving relationships to use as they form other relationships outside of their family. They feel safe to explore their environments. They have the foundation to recognize that primary core element of social justice, the common humanity of all.

Component 2: Normalizing Non-Traumatic Conflict and Diversity

The second component of the model normalizes diversity and everyday conflict. Every interpersonal relationship includes each person's family and group history (Nichols, 2011; Weinhold & Weinhold, 2000). To address discrimination and prejudice, children must be socialized to accept diversity and everyday conflict (Clark, 1963). When conflict resolution skills are taught as part of their required educational curriculum from the day they enter preschool to the day they graduate from college, individuals have many opportunities to practice the skills required to resolve conflicts.

An important process that children also must become aware of is the cognitive process of stereotyping individuals and groups who present as different (Clark, 1963; Cole & Cole, 1989). When children recognize stereotypes of other individuals and groups, they are better able to recognize the needs of others. They are able to regulate their emotional responses to difference and empathize with diverse others.

Understanding the normal processes of conflict as part of every human relationship prepares children and families to promote social justice (Weinhold & Weinhold, 2000). The core elements of social justice, recognition of the humanity of others and the rights of others to access to basic resources needed for survival, form a template for future conflict in individual and group relationships. An individual's perception of the scarcity of essential resources such as water rights, food security, and adequate shelter, and inherited group legacies of family or ethnic group may instill anger and resentment and potentially lead to violent outcomes. For example, children growing up in a Palestinian family on the Gaza strip may view the needs of families in Israel with strong emotions based on centuries of conflict between their ethnic groups.

Conflict resolution skills practiced in the family, such as talking through and problem solving, require recognition of the humanity of others and respect for their voices, opinions, and circumstances, even when there is disagreement. Thus, conflict resolution skills resonate on many levels and different contexts of social justice, such as negotiating needs when community or global resources are limited.

Cognitive appraisal skills also are needed for children to be able to discern the level of relationship conflict and instances of social injustice they encounter throughout their lives. We argue that for families to be able to advocate for themselves and others, they must be able to critically evaluate the level of justice within multiple systems in which their families function. Whether it is the education system, the health care system, the workplace, or community access to food and housing, each system impacts the quality of life and functioning of families. If families are members of oppressed minority groups within the larger social system, then the impact of larger systems on their everyday lives becomes more critical. To socialize the children within a family to promote social justice, family members must recognize these multiple forces. Ultimately, within diverse families from oppressed minority groups, we must build on both the strengths of individual members and their collective strengths to encourage their voices be heard.

Component 3: Promoting the Values of Social Justice through Service

The final component of our relationship based model requires the promotion of the value of social justice through service to others. This component includes learning the sense of family within the larger community and global contexts, learning to articulate expressed family values and needs, and increasing the value of parental and family self-efficacy through service to others. Helping those in need by performing services begins in the family, for example, helping to feed a younger sibling or bringing a cup of water to a medically fragile grandparent, volunteering in a soup kitchen to feed the homeless members of a community, or organizing to get food to other countries ravished by a natural disaster.

Bronfrenbrenner's Ecological Systems Theory and Service to Others

Bronfrenbrenner's (1979, 1989) theory is based on the recognition that the environmental events and ecological conditions that surround an individual have a profound effect on behavior and development. An understanding of Bronfrenbrenner's theory implies an understanding of how a person, or the family unit, perceives his or her ecological context. This requires a certain amount of self-reflection as the family acknowledges their presence as players in multiple contexts. The family's capacity to view themselves as change agents as they interact with other systems can afford them a dynamic role. Parents can be partners in their children's education in the context of the school system and strengthen relationships between the home and the school, thus affecting chances for success of the child. The family may also advocate for educational policies that will effect change on a broader level.

Bronfrenbrenner's theory identified "ecological transitions" as an instigator and consequence of developmental processes (Bronfenbrenner, 1979). For example, the biological transition from early childhood to school age involves a shift of role for the child and a physical environmental shift as well. These ecological transitions can occur at all or any level of ecosystems; a new baby at home, a move to a different neighborhood, parents changing jobs, hormonal/biological changes in adolescence, and political shifts in government ideology are all examples of ecological transitions that can have positive or negative effects on the developmental environment. Even if there is seemingly no effect, these changes and transitions could be discussed and used within the family as (1) a relational tool, that is, a parent displaying empathy and understanding for a child coping with difficulties, talking about the "we" as in "we can face this together"; and (2) a planning tool, that is, preparing for upcoming transitions and allocating resources or advocating for needed supports.

The biological and environmental shifts represent opportunities for families to teach children to give service appropriate to their developmental capacity. Teaching children to participate in community activities that benefit others, fund-raising events for charitable organizations, or cleaning up a playground lay a foundation for learning to provide service to others.

We next examine the individual concept of self-efficacy and then elaborate on what we call *family self-efficacy*. We propose that family self-efficacy is the key psychological process needed for young children to learn the core components of social justice within their family systems.

FAMILY SELF-EFFICACY

Bandura defined perceived self-efficacy as an individual's beliefs about "their capabilities to produce designated levels of performance that exercise influence over events that affect their lives" (1994, p. 33). A recent adaptation of this concept related to mobilizing communities to meet the needs of the elderly is called community efficacy (Newman & Newman, 2012). Building on Bandura's definition of self-efficacy we define *family self-efficacy* as the collective and unified efficacy of the family, that is, the extent to which the family perceives its collective effectiveness as a unit.

We propose it is the interrelationships of four individual processes leading to the development of self-efficacy that are the same sources that lead to the development of family self-efficacy. As a child develops throughout the life cycle, his or her identity as a family member will incorporate this sense of family self-efficacy. Figure 3.2 presents a unified concept of family self-efficacy based on four individual processes that lead to the development of individual self-efficacy: (1) vicarious experiences, (2) acts of social persuasion, (3) regulation of emotional-somatic states, and (4) mastery.

Figure 3.2
The Adaptation of Bandura's Individual Processes That Lead to Family Self-Efficacy. The four individual processes: Vicarious Experiences, Acts of Social Persuasion, Regulation of Emotional-Somatic States, and Mastery, are those that encourage development of self-efficacy. These same processes, when activated within and by the family unit, encourage the development of family self-efficacy.

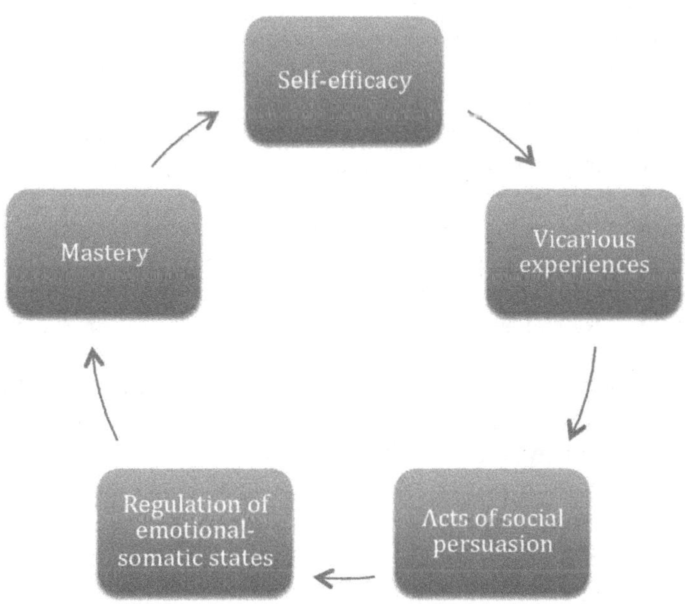

We propose that the four processes, when viewed from a family relationship perspective, provide the basis for a new conceptualization of family self-efficacy. Furthermore, the development of an individual's positive perceived self-efficacy aided by family processes may contribute to a unified optimistic perception of family self-efficacy. For example, parents may facilitate a sense of mastery in young children through recognition of individual accomplishments and structuring tasks that are developmentally appropriate, which in turn increase the likelihood of success and sense of personal power in the developing child. As a child develops, his or her identity as family member incorporates this sense of family self-efficacy.

The relational processes described in each of the three components of our model for promoting social justice in families contribute to family self-efficacy. The successes and failures of the resolution of conflicts at different stages of development contribute to individual member's sense of self-efficacy. Participating in the successful resolution of crises faced by the family, such as loss of employment, illness, or unexpected death of a family member, not only strengthens the resilience of individuals but also contributes to their collective family narrative of survival. The accomplishments of a family hero contribute to the pride of every family member (Nichols, 2011). New coping skills, family routines, and rituals may result from the family members' successful survival of a traumatic event (e.g., hurricane) experienced by the entire family (Salloum & Lewis, 2010).

Family self-efficacy reflects the individual and collective strengths needed to promote social justice in communities. Service to others becomes an outward manifestation of the family's self-efficacy. In addition, a sense of family self-efficacy forms a protective psychological umbrella for its members when they may experience social injustice.

The family unit becomes the target and recipient for various forms of social injustice (Markuly, 2008). Whether it is economic injustice in the form of poverty, unemployment or underemployment of the members of a family, or health disparities, these larger injustices impact both the physical and psychological well-being of individual family members. These injustices include inadequacies of urban public education that forecast the future of a community and society; injustices in the criminal justice system; high rates of community violence; and historic injustices of misogyny, patriarchy, racism, discrimination, and prejudice. Children experience the brunt of these injustices against families either directly or indirectly. Schools are a major context for children and families and may be one of the first places where a family has to advocate for social justice.

Many of the aforementioned injustices are associated with poverty. Infants and children experience social and environmental risk factors through the effect on their relationships (Zeanah, Boris, & Scheeringa, 1997). The infant and child experience risk factors such as poverty, maternal mental illness, and violence through the caregiver's coping mechanisms.

Wilkenson and Pickett (2009) have reconceptualized the construct of poverty as income inequality. They examined the relationship of income inequality to health and social problems such as education, teenage birth rate, homicides, social mobility, trust, and life expectancy, in countries around the world and individual states of the United States. Their systematic analyses of international databases revealed predictive relationships between income inequality and a host of social problems in societies around the world. For example, they found that as income inequality within a country increased, the life expectancy for members of the respective countries decreased. Or, stated another way, countries with the largest income differences among their members had on average lower life expectancy for those members at the lower end of the spectrum. The finding that is especially relevant to our discussion of social justice is the relationship between income inequality, child well-being, and sense of trust among members of a country. Wilkenson and Pickett (2009) reported that child well-being (as defined by the UNICEF index of child well-being) is better in countries where there is less income disparity. In their analysis of individual states within the United States, they found that levels of trust are higher in states with more equal income. The countries with better child-well-being included countries such as Sweden and Finland that have the lowest income inequalities. The countries with the highest level of income inequality and the worst child well-being indices were the United States and the United Kingdom.

The chronic overload of social injustices experienced by families of targeted social groups ranging from economic poverty to community violence provides the challenging context that many families must survive in order to rear their children. The psychic energy required to advocate for the basic needs of one's family in the face of disproportionality and racial disparities may preclude participation in advocating for the rights of others. Institutional services such as charities and social service agencies are provided by societies to protect its most vulnerable members. Yet these helping organizations teach passive coping such as skills to navigate the system. They do not routinely teach their clients the skills required to fight injustices and promote social justice for all. Among people of color and minority groups, distrust may be high for those social service agencies that proclaim their mission to assist these groups to cope with social injustices. The bureaucratic mission that may include language of social justice, in reality, teaches coping skills, and not skills required to change injustices and promote social justice (Ghosh-Ippen & Lewis, 2011).

Increasing family self-efficacy provides the psychological foundation for family members to begin to identify and communicate their survival and well-being needs and injustices they or others experience. A sense of family self-efficacy provides the emotional tools that can ultimately result in making visible those marginalized and forgotten groups and foster community advocacy to achieve social justice for all. The perception of one's family as an effective advocate for resources for family survival can enhance an individual member's sense of safety, security, and general well being. This increased positive perception of family self-efficacy can be the powerful driving force for individuals within the family social system to advocate for social justice for people within diverse societies.

Bandura's Social Learning Theory

Bandura's assertion that mastery, vicarious experiences, social persuasion, and emotional-somatic states are the sources of self-efficacy beliefs aligns with our model of how family processes can increase individual family member's perceived self-efficacy. A sense of mastery builds cognitive resources needed for the child dependent on the family group to successfully function in a broader social. A sense of mastery and autonomy enhances the developing child's ability to identify their moral values needed in conflict resolution. The vicarious experiences of social learning, as noted earlier regarding Cooley's (1902) social looking glass, contribute to the people's sense of how they perform the social rules for normative behavior within their social group. Finally, the individual's emotional-somatic states provide key information to the individual's sense of well-being.

Bandura conceptualized *social persuasion* as a method of strengthening people's beliefs in their own abilities to succeed by being verbally told so. Social persuasion contributes to positive perceptions of self-efficacy only if it is validated by accomplishments; however, the utility of social persuasion is in raising someone's beliefs in his or her own capabilities and strengthening motivation. Parents who provide many opportunities for a child to accomplish tasks and acknowledge the child's emerging competencies are scaffolding the child's developing sense of self-efficacy, while enhancing the likelihood that he or she will be motivated to persevere through more challenging circumstances (Vygotsky, 1997).

Vicariously experiencing others' successes can contribute to perceived self-efficacy (Bandura, 1994). The social role model must be perceived as similar to the person observing in order to increase this positive sense of self-efficacy ("if they can do it then I can do it too"). The strength of parent-child attachment relationships also contributes to the child's perception of family self-efficacy.

Bowlby defined attachment behaviors as "any form of behavior that results in a person attaining and maintaining proximity to some other clearly identified individual who is conceived as better able to cope in the world" (1988, pp. 26–27). Bowlby conceptualized the "other" as an individual who is perceived as having greater expertise. An individual is motivated to seek proximity to a wiser figure (Bowlby, 1975). This conceptualization of the attachment figure as the guiding expert in a relationship clearly speaks to the power of parents who can model effective advocacy on behalf of the family. The parent who has found a strong voice in advocating for the family is essentially exhibiting skills that effectively convey a sense of safety to the child and can strengthen attachment through creating a sense of security. Thus, a strong parental attachment figure contributes to family self-efficacy.

Vicarious experience may pose a distinct challenge for families of color, or same-sex parented families, and other marginalized and oppressed groups. In societies stratified along dominance and social power, there are likely few relevant, contemporary, and widely publicized examples of successes for social justice for these families. For people from groups that are marginalized and made invisible in their society, other strategies are required to ensure that individuals benefit from the proposed sources of self-efficacy in individuals. One rich source for social role models in marginalized and oppressed group is the history of survival and protective cultural traditions of that group, particularly the accomplishments of the group in acquiring rights or individual successes.

Bandura also noted that *mastery in self-regulation of somatic and affective states* is critical for the development of a positive sense of self-efficacy. Emotion regulation is the second component of the model to promote social justice in families. Individuals may judge their capabilities through the lens of temporary physical or emotional states, negative moods, or physical pain. Thus, they may perceive their inability to fight injustice as a sign of physical or emotional weakness that may cause self-doubt in their abilities. The final source needed by children to learn positive self-efficacy is self-regulation skills. Emotion regulation can decrease or modify stress reactions, giving the person a sense of control over his or her affective states. Knowledge of their emotional states allows individuals to learn not to misinterpret physical pain as a sign of impending failure. The goal here is to change perceptions of stress arousal to a motivating force rather than a debilitating one. Families that perceive stress arousal due to adversity as a motivational force can become advocates for social justice in spite of barriers. Healthy attachments and relationships within the family can promote emotional self-regulation processes within individual family members.

Vygotsky's Cultural-Historical Theory

Vygotsky's cultural-historical theory conceptualized developing human psychological processes as the result of continuous engagement and social interactions. He describes knowledge as a social process; that is, individuals cannot turn the mind off, so they constantly learn as they engage with other people and objects in their environment. Vygotsky also asserted that the mind is not individual, but socially shared (Wertch & Tulviste, 1992). Consequently, a person is the beneficiary of individual experiences that are available only to him or her because of accumulated cultural-historical experiences (Stetsenko & Vianna, 2010). These collective cultural-historical experiences contribute to the socially shared current body of knowledge. This means that one cannot separate people from their cultural-historical context; it is who they are and what they know.

The collective cultural-historical experience of the ethnic and racial group with which the family identifies provides a psychological template for values, emotion display rules, and family members' perception of what is just. These cultural-historical experiences shape the quality of the relationship between a family and the larger social context in which they rear and nurture children. For example, the history of institutionalized racism in the United States has instilled a sense of distrust of authority, especially the police, for many Black people (Reese, Vera, & Hasbrouck, 2003). A history of "separate but equal" social systems, and centuries of legal discrimination led Black communities to take care of social problems within the community themselves, rather than calling on help from authorities.

Vygotsky also viewed teaching and learning as a mutual process; the person in the role of a teacher, such as parents, must be a learner and observer of his or her child as a student. In turn, the child can display knowledge by teaching. In a practical sense, if the family is striving for social justice within a system of different cultural background the children may become the teachers, as they are living examples of the family culture and values.

We assert that the *historical and ecological context* includes the reframing of the families' narrative to reflect its values and strengths. This is a useful perspective for family advocates who are learning the cultures of various families; families must be allowed to be the teachers, as the advocates are the learners of their culture. Families who have found their voice and can articulate needs and values embedded in their unique history and cultures are contributors to social justice by imparting their original knowledge. Families who self-advocate are communicating their own sense of what is just, based on their cultural norms, beliefs, and values. Knowledge of others creates understanding that, in turn, leads to building respect for others in spite of inequalities.

The group's or family's history may prove beneficial as the source of examples of resilience within a historical context, and provide a wealth of contemporary models of successful families who have similar characteristics. Families who become models of advocacy for others in their community may increase the sense of their role as change agents both within their community and in the broader sociopolitical context. Parents also can provide examples of personal accomplishments for the family as children can witness their competence at advocating for the family. Thus, children must be taught the accurate history of their group and hear family stories of survival and bravery as well as "the good, the bad and the ugly" of their group's history. They may achieve the vicarious experience of learning from models from their family or group of previous generations or learn of contemporary actions of social justice by their family members. Oral traditions can convey the role that the family, community members, or people of similar economic standing, genders, ethnicity, or sexuality have played in larger social movements such as the civil rights movement, gay rights movement, farm laborers' strike with Caesar Chavéz, or the feminist movement. These narratives may provide sources of pride and models for children in oppressed families.

The concept of family self-efficacy provides the psychological tool needed for all members of the family, regardless of age or developmental stage, to promote social justice. A strengths perspective of diverse families allows one to identify specific family processes required to promote social justice, both within families and globally, in a variety of locations. These processes, first learned within the family, may later generalize to the larger community and globally.

CONCLUSIONS

In this chapter we have presented a developmentally based model of the family processes required to rear children to promote social justice. These family processes include three primary components: (1) developing emotional and social skills, (2) normalizing non-traumatic everyday conflict, and (3) promoting the values of social justice through service to others. The linchpin of these processes is what we call family self-efficacy, the collective perception of effectiveness to exercise influence over events that impact their lives both individually and as a family. We presented findings from an interdisciplinary set of theories to highlight the contributions from multiple contexts at the family, community, and global levels, and the interdependence of factors impacting family functioning.

Each component of this model to teach social justice to children in families is shaped by relationship theories of child development informed by an ecological and family systems conceptualization of family functioning. The first component includes a child's earliest relationship experiences of safety and security derived from acceptance and a healthy attachment relationship with a powerful primary caretaker. Within the nurturing confines of these earliest relationships, and the intersubjectivity with these caregivers, children learn to regulate their emotions, develop empathy for others, and expand knowledge of self and others. The behavioral skills that accompany these fundamental emotions related to survival are prerequisites for the recognition of the humanity of others and need for social justice.

The second component of our model highlights the need for families to normalize diversity and recognize stereotypes of diverse groups and everyday non-traumatic conflict that occurs in any human relationship. These complex factors begin with a nuanced appreciation of the cultural and historical relationship of the family's ethnic and cultural group to the dominant group. The legacies of group relationships include the cognitive use of stereotypes of minority groups as a means of justifying any form of social injustice and violence directed toward members of those groups. Structural racism, sexism, ageism, homophobia may further distance more powerful and dominant members of a society from recognizing systematic forms of oppression of members of diverse targeted groups (Healey, 2012; Pinderhughes, 1989).

The social landscape that the family must negotiate to socialize children includes ecological factors that shape institutional and systemic responses to families. The stark reality of income inequality within societies around the world is associated with a number of social maladies and indices of well-being, including poverty and trust. Lack of trust contributes to conflict among groups and the failure of fact-based experiences of injustice related to access to basic survival resources. When families belong to oppressed minority groups within those societies, their conflict resolution skills become critical to their ability to advocate for social justice for themselves and others. These factors separately, or in tandem, may serve as critical precursors to a need to take action for social justice. The families' self-efficacy can help shape individual and collective actions.

The final component of the theoretical model promotes the value of social justice through the provision of service to others. When children are taught to give as well as gracefully accept service when needed, they can be better members of any social group. The theoretical frameworks we provide highlight the contributions from multiple contexts and the interdependence of factors impacting family functioning.

Though we have presented a relationship model of promoting social justice, it is the individual within human relationships that will make the difference. The issues associated with injustice often appear chronic and intractable. The ability of people to find humor in the face of complex challenges and to draw on creativity to overcome the unpredictable pitfalls of any society may serve to maintain their courage as well as rally others to their cause. Using a sense of humor to arrive at creative solutions may be invaluable to promoting social justice for all.

Housing, clothing, and food are all the basic elements required for the survival and well-being of any developing child. Children need a loving, accepting caregiver to meet their basic emotional needs. The family unit must first meet these basic needs. Each of the various social injustices described earlier creates stress in family units that potentially interfere with the normal functioning of its family members. Conversely, chronic experiences of social injustices, oppression, or historical trauma of groups may also lead to the resilience of individuals within oppressed groups (Freire, 1970; Brave Heart, 1998). By processing social injustices, groups and individuals make their own meaning of their oppressive circumstances. One can learn from the rich cultural practices of diverse ethnic groups that contributed to his or survival from the horrors of injustices, from Native Americans to the Jewish survivors of the Holocaust. African Americans have used the cultural practices such as the creation and singing of spirituals and the informal adoption of children within extended family networks (Hill, 1972). These same spirituals became anthems of the civil rights movement (Carawan & Carawan, 1992). The musical legacy that was born in the crucible of slavery and Jim Crow segregation demonstrated how creativity fostered resilience in future generations of all Americans and oppressed groups around the world protesting and fighting for human rights.

The core elements of social justice occur with the recognition of a common humanity and the basic right of all to access the resources required for survival. Instilling these elements of social justice in children as part of their everyday social relationships is essential to their development as socially connected and responsible human beings. As outlined in the "drum major for social justice," by Reverend Martin Luther King Jr., it is the children of a society that will carry out the highest goals for its members' future survival (Mays, 2000).

REFERENCES

Ainsworth, M. D. S. (1977). Attachment theory and its utility in cross-cultural research. In P. H. Leiderman, S. R. Tulkin, & A. Rosenfeld (Eds.), *Culture and infancy: Variations in the human experience* (pp. 49–67). San Diego, CA: Academic Press.

Ainsworth, M. D. S., & Bowlby, J. (1991). An ethological approach to personality development. *American Psychologist, 46,* 333–341.

Alexander, J. C., Eyerman, R., Giesen, B., Smelser, N. J., & Sztompka, P. (2004). *Cultural trauma and collective identity.* Berkeley: University of California Press.

Anderson, A. R., Christenson, S. L., Sinclair, M. F., & Lehr, C. A. (2004). Check & connect: The importance of relationships for promoting engagement with school. *Journal of School Psychology, 42,* 95–113. doi: 10.1016/j.jsp.2004.01.002

Ashford, J. B., LeCroy, C. W., & Lortie, K. L. (2006) *Human behavior in the social environment: A multidimensional perspective* (3rd ed.). Belmont, CA: Thomson Brooks/Cole.

Bandura, A. (1977). Self-efficacy: Toward a unifying theory of behavioral change. *Psychological Review, 84,* 191–215.

Bandura, A. (1994). Self-efficacy. In V. S. Ramachaudran (Ed.), *Encyclopedia of human behavior* . New York, NY: Academic Press.

Bowlby, J. (1969). *Attachment and loss: Vol. I. Attachment.* New York, NY: Basic Books.

Bowlby, J. (1975). Attachment theory, separation anxiety, and mourning. In D. A. Hamburg & K. H. Brodie (Eds.), *New psychoanalytic frontiers.* New York, NY: Basic Books.

Bowlby, J. (1988). *Parent-child attachment and healthy human development.* London, UK: R.P.L. Bowlby/Basic Books.

Brave Heart, M. Y. H. (1998). The return to the sacred path: Healing the historical trauma response among the Lakota. *Smith College Studies in Social Work, 68*(3), 287–305. doi: 10.1080/00377319809517532

Bretherton, I. (1987). New perspectives on attachment relations: Security, communication and internal working models. In J. D. Osofsky (Ed.), *Handbook of infant development* (pp. 1061–1100). New York, NY: Wiley.

Bronfenbrenner, U. (1979). *The ecology of human development: Experiments by nature and design.* Cambridge, MA: Harvard University Press.

Bronfenbrenner, U. (1989). Ecological systems theory. In R. Vasta (Ed.), *Annals of child development* (Vol. 6, pp. 187–249). Greenwich, CT: JAI Press.

Carawan, G. & Carawan, C. (1992). *Sing for freedom: The story of the civil rights movement through its songs.* Bethlehem, PA: Sing Out Corporation.

Clark, K. B. (1963). *Prejudice and your child.* Middletown, CT: Wesleyan University Press.

Cole, M. & Cole, S. R. (1989). *The development of children.* New York, NY: Scientific American Books.

Cooley, C. H. (1902). *Human nature and the social order.* New York, NY: Scribner.

Cowan, M. A., & Parker, H. S. (2008). "We believe in one New Orleans": Embracing diversity post-Katrina. *The Seattle Journal for Social Justice, 7*(1), 139–162.

Emde, R. N. (1989). The infant's relationship experience: Developmental and affective aspects. In A. Sameroff & R. N. Emde (Eds.), *Relationship disturbances in early childhood: A developmental approach* (pp. 33–51). New York, NY: Basic Books.

Fanon, F. (1968). *The wretched of the earth.* New York, NY: Grove Weidenfeld.

Freire, P. (1970). *Pedagogy of the oppressed.* New York, NY: Continuum.

Ghosh-Ippen, C., & Lewis, M. L. (2011) A conceptual approach to understanding the cultural dynamics of client engagement. In J. D. Osofsky (Ed.), *Young children and trauma: What do we know and what do we need to know?* (pp. 131–157). New York, NY: Guilford Press.

Guadalupe, K. L., & Welkey, D. L. (2012). *Diversity in family constellations.* Chicago, IL: Lyceum.

Healey, J. F. (2012). *Race, ethnicity, gender, and class: The sociology of group conflict and change* (6th ed.). Los Angeles, CA: Sage.

Hill, R. N. (1972). *The strengths of Black families.* New York, NY: Emerson Hall Publishers.

Kerns, K. A., Aspelmeier, J. E., Gentzler, A. L., & Grabill, C. M. (2001). Parent-child attachment and monitoring in middle childhood. *Journal of Family Psychology, 15,* 69–81.

Lewis, M. L. (2000). The cultural context of infant mental health: The developmental niche of infant-caregiver relationships. In C. H. Zeanah (Ed.), *Infant mental health* (2nd ed., pp. 91–107). New York, NY: Guilford.

Lewis, M. L. (2007, December). *Nappy-haired ghosts in the nursery: The impact of racist legacies on relationships.* 22nd National Training Institute of the Zero to Three National Center for Infants, Toddlers, and Families, Orlando, Florida.

Lyons-Ruth, K. (2006). The interface between attachment and intersubjectivity: Perspective from the longitudinal study of disorganized attachment. *Psychoanalytic Inquiry, 26,* 595–615. doi: 10.1080/07351690701310656

Markuly, M. S. (2008). A terrible grace: Building a just society on the rubble of New Orleans. *The Seattle Journal for Social Justice, 7*(1), 1–10.

Mays, V. M. (2000) A social justice agenda. *American Psychologist, 55,* 326–327.

Morris-Rothschild, B. K., & Brassard M. R. (2006). Teachers' conflict management styles: The role of attachment styles and classroom management efficacy. *Journal of School Psychology, 44,* 105–121. doi: 10.1016/j.jsp.2006.01.004

Newman, B. M., & Newman, P. R. (2012). *Development through life: A psychosocial approach* (11th ed.). Belmont, CA: Wadsworth Cengage Learning.

Nichols, M. P. (2011). *The essentials of family therapy* (5th ed.). New York, NY: Allyn & Bacon.

Pinderhughes, E. (1989). *Understanding race, ethnicity and power: The key to efficacy on clinical practice.* New York, NY: The Free Press.

Reese, L. E., Vera, E. M, & Hasbrouck, L. M. (2003). Examining the impact of violence on ethnic and racial minority youth, their families, & communities: Issues for prevention, practice and science. In G. Bernal, J. E Trimble, A. K. Burlew, & F. T. L. Leong (Eds.), *Handbook of racial and ethnic minority psychology* (pp. 307–326). Thousand Oaks, CA: Sage.

Rohner, R. P. (1986). *The warmth dimension: Foundations of parental acceptance-rejection theory.* Newbury Park, CA: Sage.

Salloum, A., & Lewis, M. L. (2010). Parent-child coping and service needs post-Katrina. *Journal of Traumatology, 16,* 31–41. doi: 10.1177/1534765609348240

Schore, A. (2010). Relational trauma and the developing right brain: The neurobiology of broken attachments. In T. Baradon (Ed.), *Relational trauma in infancy: Psychoanalytic, attachment, and neuropsychological contributions to infant-parent psychotherapy* (pp. 19–47). New York, NY: Routledge.

Stern, D. N. (1985). The representation of relational patterns: Developmental considerations. In A. Sameroff & R. N. Emde (Eds.), *Relationship disturbances in early childhood* (pp. 52–69). New York, NY: Basic Books.

Stetsenko, A., & Vianna, E. (2010). Bridging developmental theory and educational practice: Lessons from the Vygotskian Project. In O. A. Barbarin & B. H. Wasik (Eds.), *Handbook of child development and early education* (pp. 38–54). New York, NY: Guilford Press.

Sullivan, W. (1992). Reclaiming the community: The strengths perspective and deinstitutionalization. *Social Work, 37,* 204–209.

Thoits, P. (1989). The sociology of emotions. *Annual Review of Sociology, 15,* 317–342.

Vygotsky, L. S. (1997). The historical meaning of the crisis in psychology: A methodological investigation. In R. W. Reiber & J. Wollock (Eds.), *The collected works of L.S. Vygotsk:. Problems of the theory and history of psychology* (Vol. 3, pp. 233–343). New York, NY: Plenum Press.

Weinhold, B. K., & Weinhold, J. B. (2000). *Conflict resolution the partnership way.* Denver, CO: Love.

Wertsch, J. V., & Tulviste, P. (1992). L.S. Vygotsky and contemporary developmental psychology. *Developmental Psychology, 28,* 548–557.

Wilkenson, R., & Pickett, K. (2009). *The spirit level: Why more equal societies almost always do better.* London, UK: Penguin.

Zeanah, C. H., Boris, N., & Scheeringa, M. (1997). Psychopathology in infancy. *Journal of Child Psychology, Psychiatry, and Allied Disciplines, 38,* 81–99.

Chapter 4

Promoting Social Justice for Youth in Urban Communities: Contributions from Developmental and Community Psychology

Christine Siegel

Since the mid-1980s increasing public and research attention has been given to the relationships among neighborhood, lived experience, and youth outcomes (Leventhal & Brooks-Gunn, 2010). *Savage Inequalities,* Jonathan Kozol's (1991) firsthand account of educational systems in differing but geographically proximal neighborhoods, chronicled the prevailing assumption that children may be either advantaged or disadvantaged by their community of residence. This thesis has been supported by scholarly investigations, collectively described as neighborhood research, which demonstrate that neighborhood of residence can positively or negatively influence youth's (1) academic achievement, (2) behavioral and emotional development, and (3) teen sexuality (e.g., Leventhal & Brooks-Gunn, 2000, 2010; Luthar & Becker, 2002; Luthar & Landtendresse, 2010).

According to UNICEF (2012), nearly half of all children and adolescents worldwide reside in cities, more than ever before in human history. Although some urban communities afford youth greater access to services that support their standard of living, health, and educational attainment, millions of children around the world live in low-income, ethnically diverse urban settings where they are confronted with daily challenges and denied basic rights. UNICEF (2012, p. 13) maintains that regardless of their place of residence, all children have the right to "development to the fullest." Although many agree with this aspiration, efforts to promote such social justice for youth in urban communities are currently hampered by ambiguous constructs and methodological debates (Zjada, Majhanovich, & Rust, 2006).

Integrating developmental theory with community psychology can provide a framework to guide social justice efforts for youth in urban communities. Within this integrated framework, understanding social justice rests on several assumptions. First, youth reside in a wide variety of communities (i.e., neighborhoods) that are unequal in social organization (e.g., degree of order, lawfulness, and cleanliness). Second, social inequities in neighborhoods directly and indirectly influence children and adolescents' interactions with parents, siblings, peers, and other adults in their homes, schools, and communities. Third, these interactions with significant others in immediate contexts form the foundation of human development, as they support the attainment of competencies (i.e., trust, hope, self-efficacy, and social connectedness) that establish one's identity. Fourth, disruptions to identity formation during childhood and adolescence have both immediate (e.g., school failure) and long-term (e.g., unemployment) consequences for youth. Based on these assumptions, *social justice for youth in urban communities* can be defined as those psychosocial practices that enable urban children and adolescents to participate in their neighborhoods in ways that allow them to develop identities as healthy, functioning, contributing members of society.

This chapter explores this definition of social justice for youth in urban communities by explicating the assumptions on which it is based. It begins with a review of two prominent developmental theories, ecological systems theory and psychosocial theory, which provide a foundation for the influence of context on youth development and detail the importance of early life experiences on later outcomes. It then reviews relevant findings from community psychology that describe differences in neighborhoods and how those differences impact the adults and children residing in them. Last, it reviews the research on *positive youth development*, the umbrella term for a set of interventions that attempt to help urban youth overcome the negative influences of their neighborhood by supporting experiences that promote healthy development in their home communities.

CONTRIBUTIONS FROM DEVELOPMENTAL PSYCHOLOGY

Developmental psychologists recognize childhood and adolescence as periods qualitatively distinct from each other and from adulthood, yet connected to other periods across the lifespan in meaningful ways. The physical, cognitive, social, and emotional growth that occurs during childhood and adolescence provides the foundation for a psychological identity that influences one's way of understanding and acting in the world throughout adulthood and into old age. Contemporary developmental theories recognize that development results from an interaction between the individual and his or her social contexts. Two well-known developmental theories, Bronfenbrenner's ecological systems theory and Erikson's psychosocial theory, emphasize the importance of context in development and thus are particularly relevant to a discussion of social justice for youth in urban communities.

Bio-Ecological Systems Model

Brofenbrenner's (2005) bio-ecological perspective explains how human development is influenced by the contexts in which it occurs. Initial formulations of his theory, termed Ecological Systems Theory (Bronfenbrenner, 1979a, 1979b), posited that all humans require active participation in increasingly complex interactions with persons, objects, and symbols in their immediate environments in order to develop intellectually, emotionally, and socially. Termed *proximal processes*, these reciprocal interactions need to occur on a regular basis and over extended periods of time. Within this theory, proximal processes are understood as transactions between the developing individual and his or her immediate and remote environments (Bronfenbrenner, 1979b). Bronfenbrenner developed a multilevel systems model to explain how these transactions contribute to the structure and maintenance of proximal processes.

At the primary level of this model, the *microsystem* consists of those immediate environments that serve as the child's main venues for learning about the world. Homes, schools, and communities constitute the microsystems in which children and adolescents interact with parents, siblings, peers, and significant adults. Research demonstrates that neighborhood of residence can directly impact interactions within these primary microsystems in ways that positively or negatively influence youth outcomes. In their study of approximately 1,400 urban minority adolescents, for example, Anderson, Sabatelli, and Koustic (2007) found that urban minority teens who maintained positive relationships with parents, friends, and adults at community centers and who regularly participated in community center programs had positive attitudes toward school, high levels of achievement motivation, high levels of social self-efficacy, and low levels of illegal substance use. In contrast, Luthar and Becker (2002) found that middle school students from affluent neighborhoods often experience isolation from parents, achievement pressure from teachers, and status pressure from peers resulting in higher than average rates of depression in girls and substance abuse in boys. Finally, DeCoster, Heimer, and Wittrock (2006) found that frequent interactions with delinquent peers increased the likelihood that youth in certain urban communities (i.e., those characterized by lawlessness and poverty) would engage in criminal behaviors.

Interactions (i.e., proximal processes) that occur within microsystems (i.e., immediate contexts) also are influenced by processes occurring in contexts that are removed from the developing child's immediate experience. Thus, *exosystems*, those environments that children experience vicariously through interactions with others in their microsystems, are also important to child development. One example of exosystem influence is the impact of neighborhood of residence on parenting practices and home environments. Compared to parents living in middle-class orderly neighborhoods, parents who live in urban, impoverished, crime-ridden neighborhoods are less likely to have support from other parents, are more likely to employ strict methods of behavior control to ensure children's safety, may be less available to their children due to their own mental or physical health needs, and are less likely to maintain regular household routines (Anderson et al., 2007; Evans, Gonnella, Marcynyszyn, Gentile, & Salpekar, 2005; Leventhal & Brooks-Gunn, 2000; Luthar & Becker, 2002). Thus in addition to the direct effects of neighborhood on their everyday experience, children contend with indirect effects via the impact of their neighborhood on their parents.

Within Bronfenbrenner's model, youth also are indirectly affected by connections between two or more microsystems that serve to sustain, support, or undermine the interactions that occur within their immediate contexts. These interconnections between microsytems, termed *mesosystems*, have been demonstrated to influence children's participation in community and school programs. For example, support from community mentors who maintain active communication with their mentees' home and school was found to foster achievement motivation, school attendance, and school completion for adolescents in urban, low-income, minority neighborhoods (Boussard, Mosley-Howard, & Roychoudhury, 2006).

Furthest removed from the immediate experience of the child is the *macrosystem*, comprising cultural attitudes, normative practices, and political trends present in the society at large that indirectly influence a child's everyday experiences. Social scientists have proposed that federal and local housing policies restrict residential choices, thus increasing the likelihood that poor, female-headed, minority families will reside in urban, impoverished, crime-ridden neighborhoods (e.g., DeCoster et al., 2006). Others have suggested that certain juvenile justice policies, including zero tolerance and lowered age-limits for juvenile offender status, contribute to the likelihood that young African American and Latino males who reside in urban areas will be incarcerated (Ginwright, Cammarto, & Noguera, 2005).

A bio-ecological model can inform understanding of social justice for youth in urban communities by demonstrating that neighborhoods influence children's experiences both directly and indirectly. For youth in some urban neighborhoods (i.e., those characterized by poverty, crime, and disorder), breakdowns in social organization appear to lead to maladaptive interactions with parents, peers, and other adults, and poor parenting practices that disrupt home routines. Further, limited interactions between adults across contexts of youth development (i.e., home-community) and larger social policies appear to contribute to maintaining the social alienation of urban youth. Proximal processes, interactions between children and others in their immediate contexts, influence youth development; and these processes are themselves influenced by interactions between children's immediate and remote contexts.

Psychosocial Theory

According to Erikson (1950, 1968), the interaction of people with their social contexts produces a series of eight identity conflicts that serve as developmental milestones across the lifespan. At each conflict, the developing person confronts a choice between two seemingly opposite psychosocial states of being, that is, *trust versus mistrust*, *autonomy versus shame*, *initiative versus guilt*, *industry versus inferiority*, *identity versus role confusion*, *intimacy versus isolation*, *generativity versus stagnation*, and *integrity versus despair*. Successful resolution occurs when the individual can reconcile the conflict in a way that gives rise to what Erikson called virtues (i.e., psychological competencies), including *hope*, *will*, *purpose*, *competence* (i.e., self-efficacy), *fidelity*, *love*, *care*, and *wisdom*. The collective acquisition of virtues across the lifespan provides the foundation for psychological well-being in the form of a stable identity or an integrated and consistent sense of self.

Psychosocial theory further proposes that although specific conflicts are dominant during specific age periods, individuals contend with all eight throughout their lives. Typically accomplished within the first year of life, for example, the resolution of trust versus mistrust is not fixed by age one (Erikson, 1950; 1968). Early damage to trust can be repaired in later years by subsequent interactions within a particularly trustworthy environment. Conversely, an initial basic sense of trust can be undermined during childhood or adolescence by repeated experiences with undependable people or unpredictable environments. Exposure to chronic violence in one's community, for example, undermines children's beliefs that the world is a safe place, resulting in mistrust and lack of hope altering identity development (Maschi, Perez, & Tyson, 2010).

As children proceed to school age, they practice and master culturally important skills. School-age children are driven by a desire to be productive and gain satisfaction through task completion (i.e., *industry*), resulting in a sense of competence or self-efficacy (Erikson, 1950). Research demonstrates that the impact of urban disadvantaged neighborhoods in the form of disrupted routines in the home and limited opportunities in the community can interfere with a child's skill attainment and developing sense of competence (Coulton & Korbin, 2007; Evans et al., 2005; Leventhal & Brooks-Gunn, 2000, 2010).

During adolescence, people's growing sense of self, based on competencies attained during younger years, is integrated with their perceptions of how others see them and societal norms, to achieve what Erikson (1968) termed *ego-identity*. Although the majority of research on the developmental impact of the neighborhood is correlational, a number of quasi-experimental and experimental studies provide strong support for the contention that neighborhoods set social norms that influence adolescent behavior and developing identity (Leventhal & Brooks-Gunn, 2000). These studies demonstrated that compared to youth who remained in urban, impoverished, crime-ridden neighborhoods, adolescents of families randomly assigned to middle-income or affluent suburban neighborhoods were less likely to be arrested for violent or nonviolent crime, engage in excessive drinking, or use marijuana. Furthermore, these adolescents were more likely to complete high school, go to college, and attain professional or managerial employment thus establishing an identity as a healthy contributing member of society.

In early adulthood, individuals transition from the search for identity to the establishment of intimate relationships (Erikson, 1950, 1968). Failure to achieve *intimacy* results in *isolation*. Successful resolution of the conflict of early adulthood is often defined as the establishment of a healthy monogamous relationship with an adult partner. Less well-known, but also important to forming intimate relationships, is Erikson's (1959) concept of *distantiation*, the readiness to defend an established identity and personal rights against attackers. In the face of "forces and people whose essence seem dangerous to one's own," an imbalance toward isolation over intimacy may constitute successful resolution of this conflict (Erikson, 1959, p. 95). However, if distantiation is generalized beyond those who truly present a threat to one's identity, an imbalance toward isolation can lead to feelings of loneliness and alienation. Distantiation helps explain how, in urban crime-ridden communities where threats of physical harm are present, distancing oneself from others serves a self-protective function. Although distancing can be protective, research suggests that generalized and sustained alienation from others in fact leads to psychological distress, physical illness, and maladaptive problem solving (Autry & Anderson, 2007; DeCoster et al., 2006; Hill, Ross, & Angel, 2005; Maschi et al., 2010; Ross & Mirowsky, 2009).

Psychosocial theory can inform one's understanding of social justice for youth from certain urban neighborhoods (i.e., those characterized by poverty, crime, and disorder). In such neighborhoods, unpredictable events, untrustworthy people, limited power, and lack of group norms may interfere with the successful resolution of psychosocial conflicts. Youth in these communities are thus disadvantaged by their circumstances and are unable to establish an ego-identity that is based on trust in others, a belief in one's own capacity to accomplish things, a continuous sense of self, and important connections to others that provide the foundation for success in life.

CONTRIBUTIONS FROM COMMUNITY PSYCHOLOGY

Community psychologists apply psychological theory, including developmental science, to study and intervene in the relationships among individuals, their communities, and society at large. Community psychology is rooted in the belief that "people affect and are affected by their environments, and that many human problems can be prevented" by an understanding of these mutual influences between people and their immediate and distal milieus (Shinn & Thaden, 2010, p. 2). Within the field of community psychology, *neighborhood research* examines the specific relationships between neighborhood of residence and developmental outcomes and thus has particular relevance to an exploration of social justice for youth in urban communities.

Research on Disordered Neighborhoods

Social scientists use the construct of *neighborhood* to describe the collection of socio-demographic characteristics that comprise specific communities of residence and the people who inhabit them (Leventhal & Brooks-Gunn, 2010). Location (e.g., urban, suburban, rural), economy, and ethnicity/race are among those characteristics most frequently used to describe neighborhoods, which are often delineated by census tracts (Leventhal & Brooks-Gunn, 2000). In community psychology research, for example, neighborhoods have been described as urban, impoverished, African American (e.g., DeCoster et al., 2006); rural, poor, White (e.g., Evans et al., 2005); and suburban, affluent, and primarily European descendant (Luthar & Becker, 2002).

Within the field of neighborhood research, a prominent line of inquiry has been the study of *neighborhood disorder*, which examines communities characterized by conditions of extreme disadvantage. According to neighborhood researchers, order in neighborhoods exists on a continuum from orderly, those clean, safe, quiet communities where buildings are in good condition, crime is low, and vandalism is rare, to disordered neighborhoods where poverty, dilapidated buildings, violent crime, and drug use are common (Ross & Mirowsky, 2009). Social scientists place neighborhoods along this continuum of order based on reported incidents of disorder by residents.

Although the majority of neighborhoods in the United States are orderly, some inner-city neighborhoods are disordered. Inhabitants of disordered neighborhoods are likely to be racial minorities, live in female-headed households, exist below the federal poverty line, and be welfare-dependent (DeCoster et al., 2006). Repeatedly, disordered neighborhoods are associated with negative experiences and outcomes for people who live in them, including but not limited to acute and chronic illness (e.g., Hill et al., 2005); psychological distress in the form of anger, depression, and anxiety (Ross & Mirowsky, 2009); exposure to crime and violence (DeCoster et al., 2000); academic failure (Leventhal & Brooks-Gunn, 2000); maladaptive problem solving (Maschi et al., 2010); and juvenile delinquency (Leventhal & Brooks-Gunn, 2000). Furthermore, these effects are not mediated by individual or family demographic characteristics alone, suggesting that other mechanisms moderate the relationships between neighborhood disorder and negative outcomes (DeCoster et al., 2006; Hill et al., 2005; Leventhal & Brooks-Gunn 2000, 2010).

Critical Mechanisms of Neighborhood Disorder

Neighborhood researchers have attempted to identify the critical mechanisms by which disorder in neighborhoods results in negative outcomes for individuals. Historically, these mechanisms have been examined in terms of five empirical models, including (1) limited availability of neighborhood resources, (2) competition among residents for scarce resources, (3) contagion of negative behaviors across peers in a neighborhood, (4) relative deprivation, and (5) breakdowns in social organization (Jencks & Mayer, 1990). Contemporary perspectives group these five models into three larger categories, and propose that, for children and adolescents, neighborhood influence on individual outcomes may be moderated by (1) availability and competition for resources, (2) neighborhood impact on parent-child relationships, and (3) disruptions to social organization (Leventhal & Brooks-Gunn, 2000). Among these factors, the strongest research evidence exists for those that relate limited social organization to negative outcomes (Leventhal & Brooks-Gunn, 2000).

Central to models of social organization is the construct of *social alienation*, feelings of being disconnected from the larger community, forgotten, and uncared for, which stem, in part, from the visible signs of social disorder (e.g., abandoned buildings, vandalism, noise, crime, violence). One set of neighborhood researchers, Ross and Mirowksy (2009), hypothesized that this breakdown in social organization leads to feelings of mistrust, powerlessness, normlessness, and social isolation that comprise the larger construct of social alienation. In addition to the findings of Ross and Mirowsky, results from other studies of disordered neighborhoods support this hypothesis.

Mistrust

Mistrust is the generalized belief that the intentions and behaviors of others are suspect. In neighborhoods where there are frequent fights between residents, crime is common, and threats of harm prevail, adolescents and adults are less likely to have confidence in the integrity of others (Ross & Mirowsky, 2009).

Perceived Powerlessness

Perceived *powerlessness* is the general expectation that one has little control over the meaningful circumstances in one's life (Ross & Mirowsky, 2009). Feelings of powerlessness have been attributed to adolescents and adults living in disordered neighborhoods. Adolescents growing up exposed to violence, feel powerless, anticipate harm to come their way, and subsequently engage in excessive risk-taking behavior (DeCoster et al., 2006; Ginwright et al., 2005; Maschi et al., 2010). Although residents may not want to live in a disordered neighborhood, individuals in these communities feel powerless about their ability to change their living circumstances (DeCoster et al., 2006).

Normlessness

Unlike powerlessness, in which individuals feel they have no control over their circumstances, *normlessness* refers to the condition in which people perceive there is no socially acceptable means to achieve their goals and instead resort to employing maladaptive behaviors (e.g., exploitation, victimization) for personal gain. In neighborhoods with high levels of disorder, the local culture does not promote respect for other people or their property (Ross & Mirowsky, 2009). Youth in disordered neighborhoods come to view robbery and violence as behavior that is acceptable in the community to solve problems and resolve conflicts (DeCoster et al., 2006; Maschi et al., 2010). Thus, children and adolescents who grow up in normless disorganized neighborhoods are more likely to become adults with maladaptive coping strategies, who often continue to live in the same neighborhood, contributing to its perpetual disorder (Shinn & Thaden, 2010).

Social Isolation

Social isolation is the lack of personal relationships that provide love, support, and care in ways that contribute to self-esteem (Ross & Mirowsky, 2009). In some disordered neighborhoods, the threat of harm and lawlessness contribute to strong social networks among long-term residents (e.g., Schieman, 2005). More often, however, the absence of trust, power, and social norms undermine an individual's capacity to connect, as neighborhood disorder has consistently been associated with high rates of social isolation (Autry & Anderson, 2007; DeCoster et al., 2006; Hill et al., 2005; Maschi et al., 2010; Ross & Mirowsky, 2009).

Integrated Perspectives on Social Justice for Youth in Urban Disordered Communities

Within the field of neighborhood research, specific attention has been given to the study of disordered neighborhoods, urban, impoverished, ethnic minority neighborhoods where the presence of crime, violence, structural disrepair, and drug use signals a breakdown in social organization. Compared to residents who live in orderly, peaceful neighborhoods, residents of disordered neighborhoods are more likely to experience a number of negative effects that cannot be explained by individual or family demographic characteristics alone. Neighborhood researchers have identified breakdowns in social organization and subsequent feelings of social alienation as the mechanism most likely to moderate the relationship between neighborhood disorder and poor psychosocial outcomes (Leventhal & Brooks-Gunn, 2000). One promising model explaining this mechanism further identifies mistrust, powerlessness, normlessness, and social isolation as essential components of social alienation (Ross & Mirowsky, 2006).

Applications of social organization models to promote social justice for youth in urban communities, however, are currently limited. Based on an extensive review of neighborhood research, Leventhal and Brooks-Gunn (2000) conclude that greater attention to theoretical explanations is needed in order to interpret research findings in ways that can guide community-based interventions for youth. Neighborhood research studies do not provide theoretical explanations that relate the experiences of growing up in disordered neighborhoods to the accomplishment of developmental tasks and subsequent long-term outcomes. Theories from developmental psychology, specifically Bronfenbrenner's bio-ecological perspective and Erikson's psychosocial theory, can be utilized to establish a conceptual link between disordered neighborhoods, limited social organization, and individual outcomes for children and adolescents in ways that can inform social justice interventions for youth in these communities.

Integration of these theories with neighborhood research findings suggests that disorder in neighborhoods negatively influences children's and adolescents' interactions with significant others via normlessness and social isolation in ways that undermine their development of psychosocial competencies, instead leading to feelings of mistrust and powerlessness. Failure to develop trust and a sense of efficacy in childhood can disrupt identity development during adolescence, leading to difficulties connecting with others, being productive, and having a sense of integrity during adulthood. Interventions to combat the negative effects of neighborhood disorder for urban youth, therefore, need to provide structures that foster feelings of trust in others and self-efficacy through the establishment of social connectedness and socially appropriate norms. Given the multilayered influence of context on the development of these competencies, those interventions that target homes, schools, communities, and the interactions between them are likely to have the greatest influence on urban youth.

POSITIVE YOUTH DEVELOPMENT: POTENTIAL INTERVENTION FOR SOCIAL JUSTICE

There is growing awareness among policymakers that promoting positive development through programmed intervention can help youth overcome community disadvantage and avoid negative outcomes (Catalano, Berglund, Ryan, & Hawkins, 2004). Consistent with this perspective, Positive Youth Development (PYD) programs funded by the U.S. Department of Health and Human Services have been implemented nationwide to prevent youth maladjustment. These programs are designed to accomplish one or more of the following objectives: (1) provide opportunities for prosocial interactions with adults and peers; (2) foster feelings of resilience, self-determination, and self-efficacy; (3) promote social, emotional, cognitive, and moral competence; (4) foster the establishment of prosocial group norms and positive individual identities; and (5) foster spirituality and belief in the future (Catalano et al., 2004).

The authors of a recent review of 161 PYD programs identified 25 as incorporating adequate evaluation methods (i.e., quasi-experimental design with comparison groups) with results (e.g., acceptable standard of statistical proof) that were deemed effective (Catalano et al., 2004). Examples of effective PYD programs from this review include Big Brothers-Big Sisters, Seattle Social Development Project, Success for All, and Midwestern Prevention Project. Effective programs were found to (1) incorporate multiple PYD objectives; (2) have a standard curriculum or structured activities to achieve their objectives; (3) implement the structured program for a period of nine months or longer; and (4) have methods to ensure fidelity to the program structure during implementation. Eight of the effective programs operated within one of the participants' immediate contexts (e.g., school or community); the remaining 17 implemented multicontext programs with activities in family, school, and community settings.

PYD Implementation

Successful implementation of PYD programs to promote social justice for youth in communities depends on both their effectiveness (i.e., ability to yield anticipated positive outcomes) and their sustainability (i.e., ability to be maintained over time). PYD research has consistently demonstrated that effectiveness depends, in part, on the use of a structured program and methods to ensure fidelity to program components during implementation. This line of research further demonstrates that sustainability depends on connections between members of the immediate contexts (e.g., family, school, and neighborhood) in which programs are implemented. In some studies, community mobilization efforts have been found to contribute to both intervention fidelity and inter-context connections in ways that support effectiveness of programs.

In their review of PYD programs, Catalano and colleagues (2004) identified adherence to a structured program protocol as an essential feature of effectiveness. Other research suggests, however, that similar types of prevention programs are often implemented without fidelity (Fagan, Hanson, Hawkins, & Arthur, 2008). In response to this weakness, methods have been developed to ensure program fidelity. The Communities That Care (CTC) framework, for example, is a prevention support system designed to increase the capacity of communities to implement evidence-based prevention programs. CTC includes the establishment of a planning board to assess community needs and select programs to meet those needs, as well as the use of multiple methods (e.g., fidelity checklists, program observations, participant surveys, staff training, and technical support) to ensure adherence to the selected programs during implementation. Use of the CTC framework has been demonstrated to yield high rates of adherence to PYD programs (Fagan et al., 2008).

Community mobilization has been defined as efforts that facilitate the engagement and explicit action of community members to address a specific community problem (Allison, Edmonds, Wilson, Pope, & Farrell, 2011). Community mobilization efforts have been shown to be effective in implementing and sustaining

PYD (Allison et al., 2011; Greenberg, Feinberg, Meyer-Chilenski, Spoth, & Redmond, 2007).

Given that members of disordered neighborhoods often feel powerless to change their situation, community mobilization for PYD programs may require supports from external partners. Indeed, two community mobilization projects designed to facilitate the implementation, effectiveness, and sustainability of PYD programs involved university partners for external support. The PROSPER (*PRO*moting *S*chool-university *P*artnerships to *E*nhance *R*esilience) project, a partnership between University of Pennsylvania and local communities, aims to mobilize communities in rural and small towns to implement evidence-based interventions to support positive youth development and reduce early substance abuse (Greenberg et al., 2007). PROSPER includes the establishment of strategic teams to select, implement, supervise, and sustain prevention programs. Results from a recent evaluation of PROSPER teams indicated that community demographics contributed significantly to team functioning six months after being established. Authors of this study conclude that in highly stressed, lower-resource, impoverished communities, external supports in terms of time and resources for team development may be necessary prior to program implementation. Similarly, results from a review of the multiple community mobilization projects, supported by the Clark Hill Institute at Virginia Commonwealth University, reveal that university support in the form of information about evidence-based programs, program evaluation methods, attention to treatment fidelity, and technical assistance are of benefit (Allison et al., 2011).

In sum, PYD programs aim to prevent negative outcomes for at-risk youth, including those from disadvantaged communities, by supporting the prosocial development of children and adolescents. Although PYD programs exist in many forms, those that are designed to promote multiple competencies through structured activities in more than one setting, and those that include methods to ensure adherence to program structure, have been shown to be the most effective. PYD implementation studies further demonstrate that, when implemented for social justice in disordered neighborhoods, effective and sustainable programs are those that also incorporate methods for community mobilization through the use of external partners.

SOCIAL JUSTICE FOR YOUTH IN URBAN DISORDERED COMMUNITIES: LESSONS FROM GLENVIEW PARK

Glenview is not unlike other inner-city neighborhoods in the United States where advocates for social justice attempt to organize community efforts to improve circumstances for youth in disordered communities. According to researchers Autry and Anderson (2007), Glenview (a pseudonym) consists of a federally funded housing complex, adjacent to several blocks of low-income housing and a neighborhood park. The housing complex, including 18 buildings each with

16 apartments, is designated for single mothers on welfare. It is surrounded by a nine-foot wrought-iron fence which itself is enclosed in an eight-foot cement block wall. Pedestrians, including children and adolescents, can access the outer neighborhood via a side gate that opens onto an alley leading to several streets of low-income housing. Many houses in this area have bars on the windows; other houses serve as places for drug sale and use. The side street off the alley also leads to Glenview Park, a recreation facility containing a track, basketball courts, playgrounds, and a sheltered picnic area. Although the park includes public restrooms, they are permanently locked to prevent use for drug and sexual activity by adolescents and adults. Adolescents who live in Glenview evidence high rates of truancy, drug use, violence, and teen pregnancy.

Due to concerns about the social condition of the Glenview neighborhood and the behavior problems of its youth, an advocacy group was formed to develop and implement a youth recreation program based on the assumption that structured recreation could combat neighborhood disadvantage (see Autry & Anderson, 2007, for full description). This group included members of several community and city agencies, who worked collaboratively throughout the course of one year, to plan, fund, and advertise the program prior to its implementation. Although initial interest was high, the program closed after one summer due to lack of participation by the youth. Paradoxically, failure of the program to remain open served to confirm beliefs about social disorder and contribute to feelings of hopelessness on the part of Glenview's children.

Following the closure of the Glenview recreation program, a qualitative study was undertaken to explore community member perceptions about the program specifically, and Glenview in general. Although the primary method of data collection for this study was interview, Autry and Anderson (2007) also employed participant observations and review of artifacts to triangulate their findings. Emergent themes from this inquiry centered around issues of social alienation related to (1) the physical and psychological separation between residents of the housing project and the surrounding community, (2) a lack of hope and trust between members of the community, which spread to members of the advisory board, and (3) the lack of parental involvement in the recreational program, which was viewed by many as the primary reason for its closure.

The failure of the Glenview Park recreation project serves to illustrate that there are multiple complexities to consider when promoting social justice for youth in urban communities with neighborhood disorder. Consistent with Ross and Mirowsky's (2009) hypothesis, the residents (adults and children alike) of Glenview experienced feelings of mistrust, powerlessness, normlessness, and social isolation related to living in a disordered neighborhood. Although it attempted to provide a forum for prosocial interactions between children and adults, the Glenview Park summer program failed to directly promote psychosocial competencies (e.g., self-efficacy), a characteristic of effective PYD programs.

Additionally, lack of attention to mesosytemic (i.e. home-community interaction) effects in the form of a community mobilization effort may have contributed to parental apathy toward the recreation program, which undermined youth attendance. Unfortunately, the subsequent closure of the program may have reinforced feelings of social alienation among the children and adolescents who reside in Glenview.

CONCLUSION

Contributions from developmental and community psychology, can aid psychologists in their attempts to promote social justice for youth in disordered urban communities. Developmental psychology demonstrates that interactions with significant others in immediate contexts support children and adolescent's attainment of psychosocial competencies (most importantly, trust, hope, self-efficacy, and social connectedness) that establish their identities. Within the field of community psychology, results of neighborhood research suggest that youth residing in poor, crime-ridden, inner-city neighborhoods may be at risk for failure to develop these competencies, as disorder in their communities directly and indirectly interferes with their interactions with others. Thus, interventions for inner-city youth (such as those known as Positive Youth Development programs) that promote positive interactions to explicitly foster psychosocial competencies across multiple contexts of child development can help children and adolescents achieve UNICEF's goal of development to the fullest potential regardless of their community of residence.

ACKNOWLEDGMENT

Author note: The author thanks Mollie Kimmel, Kathryn Min, and Don J. Siegel for their support of this work.

REFERENCES

Allison, K. W., Edmonds, T., Wilson, K., Pope, M., & Farrell, A. D. (2011). Connecting youth violence prevention, positive youth development, and community mobilization. *American Journal of Community Psychology, 48*(1–2), 8–20.

Anderson, S. A., Sabatelli, R. M., Koustic, I. (2007). Families, urban neighborhood youth centers, and peers as contexts for development. *Family Relations, 56*(4), 346–357.

Autry, C. E., & Anderson, S. A. (2007). Recreation and the Glenview neighborhood: Implications for youth and community development. *Leisure Sciences, 29*(3), 267–285.

Bronfenbrenner, U. (1979a). Contexts of child rearing: problems and prospects. *American Psychologist, 34*(10), 844–850.

Bronfenbrenner, U. (1979b). *The ecology of human development*. Cambridge, MA: Harvard University. Retrieved from http://books.google.com/books (Original work pub lished 1979)

Bronfenbrenner, U. (2005). *Making human beings human: Bioecological perspectives on human development.* Thousand Oaks, CA: Sage Publications. Retrieved from http://books.google.com/books (Original work published 2005)

Broussard, C. A., Mosley-Howard, S., & Roychoudhury, A. (2006). Using youth advocates for mentoring at-risk students in urban settings. *Children and Schools, 28*(2), 122–127.

Catalano, R. F., Berglund, M. L., Ryan, J. A. M., Lonzczak, H. S., & Hawkins, J. D. (2004). Positive youth development in the United States: Research findings on evaluations of positive youth development programs. *ANNALS of the American Academy of Political and Social Sciences, 591*(1), 98–124.

Coulton, C. J., & Korbin, J. E. (2007). Indicators of child well-being through a neighborhood lens. *Social Indicators Research, 84*(3), 349–361.

DeCoster, S., Heimer, K., & Wittrock, S. M. (2006). Neighborhood disadvantage, social capital, street context, and youth violence. *The Sociological Quarterly, 47*(4), 723–753.

Erikson, E. H. (1950). *Childhood and society.* New York, NY: Norton.

Erikson, E. H. (1959). *Identity and the life cycle in psychological issues* (monograph). New York, NY: International University. Retrieved from http://books.google.com/books (Original work published 1959).

Erikson, E. H. (1968). *Identity: Youth and crisis.* New York, NY: Norton.

Evans, G. W., Gonnella, C., Marcynyszyn, L. A., Gentile, L., & Salpekar, N. (2005). The role of chaos in poverty and children's socioemotional adjustment. *Psychological Science, 16*(7), 560–565.

Fagan, A. A., Hanson, K., Hawkins, J. D., & Arthur, M. (2008). Bridging science to practice: Achieving prevention program implementation fidelity in the community youth development study. *American Journal of Community Psychology, 41*(3–4), 235–249.

Ginwright, S., Cammarota, J., & Noguera, P. (2005).Youth, social justice, and communities: Toward s theory of urban policy development. *Social Justice, 32*(3), 24–40.

Greenberg, M. T., Feinberg, M. E., Meyer-Chilenski, S., Spoth, R. L., & Richmond, C. (2007). Community and team member factors that influence the early phase functioning of community prevention teams: The PROSPER project. *Journal of Primary Prevention, 28*(6), 485–504.

Hill, T. D., Ross, C. E., & Angel, R. J. (2005). Neighborhood disorder: Psychological distress and health. *Journal of Health and Social Behavior, 46*(2), 170–186.

Jenks, C., & Mayer, S. (1990). The social consequences of growing up in a poor neighborhood. In L. E. Lynn & M. F. H. McGeary (Eds.), *Inner-city poverty in the United States* (pp.111–186). Washington, DC: National Academy. Retrieved from http://www.nap.edu/openbook.php?record_id=1539&page=111

Kozol, J. (1991). *Savage inequalities.* New York, NY: Harper Collins. Retrieved from http://books.google.com/books (Original work published 1991).

Leventhal, T., & Brooks-Gunn, J. (2000). The neighborhoods they live in: The effect of neighborhood of residence on child and adolescent outcomes. *Psychological Bulletin, 126*(2), 309–337.

Leventhal, T., & Brooks-Gunn, J. (2010). Children and youth in neighborhood contexts. In M. Shinn & E. Thaden (Eds.), *Current directions in Community Psychology* (pp. 59–65). Boston, MA: Allyn & Bacon.

Luthar, S. S., & Becker, B. E. (2002). Privileged but pressured? A study of affluent youth. *Child Development, 73*(5), 1593–1610.

Luthar, S. S., & Landtendresse, S. J. (2010). Children of the affluent: Challenges to well-being. In M. Shinn & E. Thaden (Eds.), *Current directions in community psychology* (pp. 120–126). Boston, MA: Allyn & Bacon.

Maschi, T., Perez, R. M., & Tyson, E. (2010). Exploring the relationship between exposure to violence, perceptions of neighborhood safety, and children's adaptive functioning: Clinical and contemporary implications. *Journal of Human Behavior in the Social Environment, 20*(6), 744–761.

Ross, C. E., & Mirowksy, J. (2009). Neighborhood disorder, subjective alienation, and distress. *Journal of Health and Social Behavior, 50*(1), 49–64.

Schieman, S. (2005). Residential stability and the social impact of neighborhood disadvantage: A study of gender and race-contingent effects. *Social Forces, 83*(3), 103–1064.

Shinn, M., & Thaden, E. (Eds.). (2010). *Current directions in community psychology*. Boston, MA: Allyn & Bacon.

United Nations Children's Fund (UNICEF). (2012). *State of the world's children 2012: Children in an urban world*. Retrieved from http://www.unicef.org/sowc2012/

Zjada, J., Majhanovich, S., & Rust, V. (2006). Introduction: Education and social justice. *Review of Education, 52* (1), 9–22.

Chapter 5

Empowering Child Voices through Research

Bonnie K. Nastasi

INTRODUCTION

The Convention on the Rights of the Child (CRC/Convention, UN, 1989) provides for the promotion of child well-being (physical, psychological, spiritual, cultural), learning and development, and protection from harm. The CRC affords human rights to all children (birth to 18 years). The articles of the Convention address rights related to life, survival, development, best interests, nondiscrimination, participation, and protection (see Table 5.1; Nastasi, 2013). Moreover, the Convention holds governments and all adults (e.g., parents and other caregivers, teachers, community members, lawmakers) responsible for the promotion and protection of child rights. This chapter addresses the role of psychologists as researchers in promoting and protecting the rights of children.

Pertinent to this chapter are the articles that address children's right to participation or what we might describe as ensuring "child voice," specifically, Articles 4, 12–17, and 42 (Table 5.1). These articles ensure to children freedom of expression, thought, conscience, religion, association, and privacy. In addition, these articles make sure that children have access to information, including information about their rights, and have the opportunity to express their views and be heard relevant to decisions made about them. These rights come with responsibilities and caveats.

Exercising one's rights requires respecting the rights and freedoms of others. Expression of individual rights may be limited by law when doing so interferes with rights of others or with national security or public order, health, and morals. In addition, the Convention recognizes the importance of the child's developmental level; thus rights are afforded consistent with the child's capacity. Further, the Convention recognizes the rights and responsibilities of parents or caregivers to guide their children. Recognizing these caveats and related responsibilities, this chapter is focused on the meaning of child participation for psychologists as researchers, with participation ranging from children as research participants to children as researchers. The chapter also addresses researcher competencies and responsibilities with regard to research methods, ethics, and capacity to engage children as active agents. Drawing on examples of research that involves active participation by children (e.g., children's perspectives are reflected in data and findings, children participate as researchers), the chapter explores ways to contribute to the promotion and protection of child rights, particularly right to participation, through research activity.

CHILD PARTICIPATION IN RESEARCH

In this chapter child participation in research is envisioned within a child rights framework that necessitates consideration of child voices in decisions that affect children individually and collectively. Child rights also encompass considerations with regard to promoting the best interest of children, facilitating their well-being and development, and protecting them from all forms of harm (e.g., discrimination, oppression, violence, abuse). Thus, integrating a child rights framework into psychological research has implications for the questions asked, the methods used, and the interpretation and application of research findings. Moreover, a child rights approach necessitates the inclusion of child perspectives in research. Researchers, particularly in the social sciences and education, have advocated for redefining traditional approaches or developing new approaches to research and reconsidering the validity and criticality of child voices in research that will in turn affect children (Alderson, 2012; Hart, 1992). Such discussion has been minimal in psychology, although the experiences of researchers in social sciences, education, and global development can inform psychology. Alderson, for example, challenges current notions and practices related to child participation in research that attends to rights of protection (protection from harm) and provision (facilitating development) but fails to address participation rights (e.g., right to be heard and taken seriously). In response to these concerns, Alderson calls for the development of *rights-respecting* research consistent with child rights (and human rights) principles. Such research requires critical examination of our current research paradigms and methods (and inherent values), and development of new approaches to child research that involve children as active participants. So how do we accomplish this?

Murris (2013) suggests that active child participation in research requires that researchers view children as *knowers* (having the capacity for knowledge) and *sources of knowledge* (from whom adults can learn; see also Keat, Strickland, & Marinak, 2009). According to Bromstrom (2012), child advocacy through research requires that researchers (1) view the child as competent and having agency, (2) value the importance of the child's perspective, and (3) provide opportunities for active child participation and agency through research projects. Moreover, Mortari and Hartcourt (2012) cite ethical principles derived from Australia's National Health and Research Council as potential guidelines for child-respecting research:

> (1) The research must be important for the health and well-being of children; (2) the participation of children is indispensable because when the information is filtered by others it is not reliable; (3) the methods of inquiry must be suitable/right for children; and (4) the inquiry must be developed to guarantee the physical, emotional and psychological safety. (Mortari & Hartcourt, 2012, p. 235)

Finally, Kina (2012) calls for the transformation of adult researchers through critical reflexivity, that is, self-examination of actions, thoughts, and feelings as researcher.

Todd (2012) advocates for participatory approaches—child participants as active agents—that necessitate not only critical reflection but also critical dialogue with children. Moreover, Dalli and One (2012) advocate for research protocols that are culturally, contextually, and developmentally responsive. Thus, effectively engaging children as active agents in research requires reflection about our personal values and perspectives, conceptions of research, and the ways that researchers engage children as research participants. This has implications for all aspects of the research process, including theoretical foundations, research purpose and questions, data collection, analysis, interpretation, dissemination, and application.

THE NATURE OF CHILD PARTICIPATION IN RESEARCH

Active child participation in research can be characterized on several levels (see Table 5.2). Traditionally, researchers have attempted to include children as informants during data collection, for example, through the use of self-report measures such as surveys or questionnaires. Although such approaches reflect child responses, the extent of child participation is limited, as researchers create the measures, decide on questions from their own worldview, provide limited options of expression (e.g., respond using Likert scale), and interpret the data without necessarily reflecting the perspectives of children. Furthermore, such studies are limited typically to children who have sufficient cognitive and reading ability (typically ages eight years and older). Child participation that is consistent with a child rights approach requires research methods that capture children's perspectives or experiences in their own words, facilitate their communication with adults, provide opportunities to engage them in decision making, or facilitate their participation as co-researchers with adults.

For the purposes of this chapter, five levels of child participation in research are proposed (see Table 5.2). The levels vary with regard to purpose of child participation, degree of children's involvement as active agents, and representation of child voice at different stages of the research process. The stages of the research process, characterized by Nastasi, Hitchcock, and Brown (2010), include the following: (1) examining existing theory research, practice, policy; (2) articulating researcher's worldview; (3) formulating the purpose and research questions; (4) sampling; (5) collecting data; (6) analyzing data; (7) interpreting data (drawing inferences); (8) determining inference quality (e.g., reliability and validity); (9) representing data and disseminating findings; and (10) applying research findings to practice or policy. In this section, the five levels of child participation are described with examples drawn from the literature in social science, education, and global development.

Level 1: Examine Child Perceptions

The purpose at Level 1 is to capture child perspectives through the use of techniques such as structured or semistructured interviews that facilitate articulation of child voices. Such research can help us understand complex psychological or cultural phenomena from the child's viewpoint and in the child's words. To facilitate communication, researchers provide visual cues or offer nonverbal response options (e.g., Evans, Gayler, & Smith, 2001; Nicholls, Nelson, & Gleaves, 1995). Child voices are captured during data collection and preserved in analysis and interpretation of data (e.g., providing direct quotes from participants). For example, Thorkildsen and White-McNulty (2002) used structured interviews with children ages 6 to 14 years to elicit their perceptions of justice related to educational practices and curriculum (i.e., luck- versus skilled-based contests). Using cartoon drawings, the researchers described orally a science contest in which students win based on luck or skill. Participants were interviewed about their perceptions of fairness and effectiveness of the two approaches (luck versus skill) for enhancing learning. Interview transcripts were coded for perceptions of fairness, requirements for success in skill- versus luck-based contests, and perceived effectiveness of each for facilitating learning in different instructional settings (solitary work, peer tutoring, adult tutoring). Child voices were reflected in data collection, analysis, and interpretation. The authors noted that in addition to informing educational practice through child voice, the study procedures can facilitate development of children's vocabulary for engaging in dialogue with adults about justice.

Level 2: Examine Child Experiences

The purpose of these studies is to represent children's lived experiences, typically through qualitative or ethnographic methods such as participation observation, in-depth interviews, and focus groups. Data collection may be restricted to interviews and focus groups (Huang & Ayoub, 2011; Mudaly & Goddard, 2009; Sinha, 2010), although researchers might also observe children in their natural environments and/or interview them about those experiences (e.g., Kijo-Bisimba, 2010; Raittila, 2012). In some cases, researchers provide a range of options for expression of experiences, for example, through role play, drawing, diaries, or photography (Kijo-Bisimba). Studies of children's lived experiences provide an opportunity for researchers to represent child voices in data collection, analysis, interpretation, and dissemination. Furthermore, qualitative and ethnographic techniques typically require some form of member checking in which findings are presented back to informants to confirm accuracy of data and interpretation, and to ensure valid representation of child voice. Huang and Ayoub (2011) provide an excellent example of the use of ethnographic data collection (individual interviews, focus groups) and grounded theory analysis (i.e., inductive approach to explain life trajectories based on boys' life experiences) to examine the experiences of adolescent boys who successfully transitioned from living on the streets of La Paz, Bolivia. Using individual interviews, researchers collected life histories of 10 boys to understand the meaning of life on the streets, and the factors that contributed to entering life on the streets, deciding to leave, and transitioning to life off the streets through a residential program. Follow-up focus groups were conducted to examine the meaning of different (common) scenarios constructed from the life histories. The findings contributed to the existing literature by expanding the understanding of factors contributing to resilience (e.g., the role of structural as well as social supports). This group of boys identified "behavioral changes, spiritual transformation, academic achievement, rules and responsibilities, plans for the future, and being able to experience success and observe their own progress" (Huang & Ayoub, 2011, p. 24) as factors contributing to successful transition.

Level 3: Facilitate Child-Adult Communication

Level 3 studies are designed to enable effective child-adult communication and thereby ensure that children's voices are heard and that adults listen. Depending on the developmental level, researchers may employ innovative techniques. For example, Keat et al. (2009) provided preschool children with cameras so that they could take photos of their daily lives outside of school (e.g., people, contexts, events). Children then used the photos to facilitate video-recorded conversations with their teachers and thereby enhance teacher understanding of their experiences as recent immigrants. Authors reported a shift in child agency within the teacher-child relationship as a result of photo-narration, such that children directed the dialogue. Data analysis of conversation transcripts revealed several themes consistent with child agency and participation: (1) Here are persons, places, things that are important to me; (2) I know my life in a way that you do not; (3) listen to me and I will talk to you. As a result of this procedure, the participating school continued to use photo-narration at the beginning of each school year to facilitate child-teacher communication and enhance teacher understanding of children's lives, competencies, and voices.

Level 4: Inform Decision Making

Level 4 includes research designed to facilitate child participation in decision making that can in turn influence practice and policy. At this level, child voices are typically reflected in data collection, analysis, interpretation, dissemination, and application of research findings. For example, de Berry et al. (2003) conducted a series of focus group discussions with children (ages 7–18) and families affected by war in Afghanistan in order to inform development of culturally and contextually relevant intervention programs. These researchers used multiple strategies for data collection, including interviews, drawings, stories, recordings, charts.

Similarly, Nastasi, Hitchcock, Sarkar et al. (2007) used mixed-methods research in a series of studies for the purpose of developing and testing culture-specific assessment tools and mental health intervention programs to promote psychological well-being of adolescents in Sri Lanka. Nastasi and colleagues conducted focus groups, administered culture-specific measures of well-being, and examined student products from intervention activities. The voices of adolescents were evident in assessment tools, intervention protocols, evaluation results, and dissemination to stakeholders (e.g., educators, school and district administrators; Nastasi, Varjas, Sarkar, & Jayasena, 1998). For example, Nastasi et al. (2007) developed a culture-specific (ethnographic) measure of stress and coping for use with Sri Lankan adolescents. Based on analysis of focus group data, researchers incorporated stressful life situations (e.g., stress related to academic expectations, family conflict, absent parent) and reactions to stress (e.g., feelings, coping strategies, adjustment difficulties) in assessment items using the adolescents' language and experiences. In contrast, traditional nonchild participatory approaches rely on existing theory and research and existing measures from other cultures to develop or adapt instruments.

Findings from multiple studies in East Asia and the Pacific (UNICEF, 2011a) that involved children as research participants were used to inform decisions about children's vulnerability to climate change and development of child-sensitive policies. UNICEF (2012) used self-report measures to examine psychological well-being and related factors for students entering secondary school. Citing this as an example of child participation in research that can inform policy, the authors acknowledged the limitations of using structured self-report measures and the need for additional qualitative data collection. Most noteworthy from this study was the finding that children who are aware of their rights (i.e., CRC) reported higher levels of well-being.

Level 5: Participatory Research

The highest level of child participation in research is reflected in participatory action research and the engagement of children as active agents, that is, as researchers or co-researchers. At this level, children contribute to all aspects of the research process from generation of research questions to dissemination and application of findings. The work of Plotnik et al. (2013) reflects the most extensive participation of children in the research process. In this study, middle school children partnered with research scientists to explore elephant-human communication patterns. Students were involved in all aspects of the research process, including co-authoring the cited article.

Steffen (2010) demonstrated the application of CRC's Article 12 to research through the involvement of adolescents as active agents in participatory action research as a way to facilitate child advocacy. The purpose of the study was to explore children's/adolescents' roles in humanitarian crises (i.e., Children of Occupied Palestinian Territories). The study was conducted by Save the Children in collaboration with local nongovernmental organizations (NGOs). Adolescent researchers (ages 13–17) participated in the study process from design to application of findings, playing minor or major roles throughout. Adolescent researchers played an active role in managing the research process and collecting, analyzing, interpreting, and disseminating (presenting) data. They played a minor role in study design, writing dissemination reports, and using findings for advocacy. As the author notes, the level of child agency could be enhanced in future work through more active roles in study design, preparing dissemination reports, and using results for advocacy to facilitate change in practices and policies.

Level 5 studies not only promote child participation by representing their voices but also engage children as active producers of research and research guidelines. Hampshire et al. (2012), for example, engaged child researchers in developing an ethical code of practice based on their prior experiences as researchers. The ethical code addressed issues covered in the Convention on the Rights of the Child, specifically those related to child participation, best interests, and protection from exploitation. This study illustrates the potential contribution of children to our understanding of research ethics in light of child rights.

Perhaps the ultimate benefit comes from teaching children how to do research, thus providing them with tools for promoting and protecting their rights, influencing decisions made about them and other children, and engaging in the democratic process. The examples presented in this section are evidence that children can be active agents in research. However, as discussed in the next section, engaging children in research is not without its challenges.

ISSUES RELATED TO CHILD PARTICIPATION IN RESEARCH

Child involvement in research presents methodological, ethical, and practical challenges. The purpose of this section is to discuss these challenges and provide guidance for professionals interested in engaging children as active agents in research. Conducting research with children necessitates development of research protocols that take into account children's rights, capacities, and cultural background, the context of the study, and need for flexibility to address individual needs. These considerations have implications for how rapport is established and maintained, how children's rights are protected, how children are engaged effectively in research activities, what data collection methods researchers choose or develop, and how researchers adapt protocols to children's individual and developmental variations, while maintaining the study's integrity.

As the level of child involvement increases, researchers need to ensure that children have the competencies to communicate their viewpoints and experiences (Levels 1 and 2), engage in effective child-adult dialogue (Level 3), appreciate the potential impact of research on practice and policy decisions for themselves and others (Level 4), and participate as co-researchers (Level 5). In addition to ethical and methodological considerations, the issues delineated in this section necessitate critical reflection by adult researchers, critical dialogue with child researchers, professional development of adult researchers, and education and training for child participants and researchers (Kina, 2012; Todd, 2012).

Research Methodology

To ensure developmentally, culturally, and contextually appropriate research protocols, researchers must consider questions relevant to design and methods. Traditional designs and methods for psychological research may be inadequate for engaging children as active participants. The use of traditional structured surveys and questionnaires limit the extent to which child voice is reflected in responses (e.g., the questions and response options are framed by researchers and reflect their viewpoints) and restrict opportunities for young children or those with limited literacy to participate. Similarly, traditional positivist and post-positivist hypothetical-deductive research paradigms limit the choice of designs and methods, and can in turn preclude expression of authentic child voice. Solutions to these challenges come from nontraditional qualitative and mixed-methods research paradigms, referred to as second and third paradigms, respectively, for social and health sciences and educational research (the scope of this chapter prevents detailed discussion of these paradigms; for more detail, see Nastasi et al., 2010). Both qualitative and mixed-methods designs call for the use of inductive approaches, open-ended methods such as in-depth interviews and participant observation, development of grounded theory based in the perspectives and experiences of target populations (in this case, children), and participatory action research.

The studies cited in Table 5.2 provide excellent examples of innovative designs and methods for engaging children as active participants. Researchers have employed focus groups and/or in-depth interviews designed to capture the language and thinking of children (e.g., de Berry et al., 2003; Huang & Ayoub, 2011; Steffen, 2010); participant observation of children in their natural environments to understand the culture and context of their lives (e.g., Kijo-Bisimba, 2010; Raittila, 2012); and nonverbal methods (e.g., drawings, role play, and photography), sometimes in conjunction with interviews/dialogue, to facilitate expression of ideas (e.g., Hampshire et al., 2012; Keat et al., 2009; Kijo-Bisimba, 2010; Steffen,

2010). To further enhance child agency, some researchers have made children responsible for recording their life experiences (e.g., diaries, Hampshire et al., 2012; Steffen, 2010; mapping, UNICEF, 2011a; photo-narration, Keat et al., 2009; photo journaling, Hamsphire et al., 2012) to share with adult researchers. Finally, using participatory research approaches, researchers engage children as co-researchers (e.g., Hampshire et al., 2012; Plotnik et al., 2013; Steffen, 2010), thus equipping them with the tools necessary for child agency and advocacy. As illustrated in Table 5.2, researchers have developed innovative methods for eliciting child voice. The use of such methods, however, does not preclude systematic attention to inference quality (i.e., reliability, validity, integrity, trustworthiness, authenticity of data; see Nastasi & Schensul, 2005) and ethics.

Research Ethics and Child Rights

Regardless of paradigm or methods, psychologists are responsible for ethical conduct of research, which requires attention to issues of informed consent/assent and dissent (Dockett, Einarsdottir, & Perry, 2012), non-coercion (Mudaly & Goddard, 2009), and privacy, respect, beneficence, and nonmaleficence (Mortari & Harcourt, 2012). In the context of the UN Convention on the Rights of Child (1989; Table 5.1), research involving children necessitates promotion and protection of rights related to survival and development, best interests, nondiscrimination, participation, and protection from harm (Hampshire et al., 2012; Kijo-Bisima, 2010). As children become active agents (e.g., as co-researchers), adult researchers are responsible for promoting and protecting the rights of the broader population of children and ensuring that child researchers can effectively participate as supporters and defenders of the rights of other children (e.g., Bromstrom, 2012; Sinha, 2010; Steffen, 2010). Furthermore, research that addresses sensitive issues such as abuse or trauma demands additional considerations related to protection, beneficence, and nonmaleficence (Mudaly & Goddard, 2009; Steffen, 2010).

Engaging and Communicating with Children

Research with child participants can present challenges related to procuring and maintaining their interest and cooperation, building rapport and trust (Dalli & One, 2012), communicating expectations and responsibilities (Bromstrom, 2012; Mudaly & Goddard, 2009), managing power relationships and avoiding coercion (Kijo-Bisimba, 2010; Mudaly & Goddard, 2009), managing child behavior, and ensuring children have the necessary competencies to engage in research activities (Thorkildsen & White-McNulty, 2002). These issues need to be considered when developing the research protocol and determining if the researchers have the appropriate competencies and experiences. In addition, the context of research and prior experiences of the child warrant consideration (Nicholls et al., 1995). Prior negative experiences with adults or in the specific context (e.g., school, community center) could influence the child's initial response to researchers. These issues warrant consideration when determining if the researcher has the knowledge, experiences, and skills to work effectively with child participants, and to develop the research protocol. At a minimum, the research protocol must be culturally, contextually, and developmentally appropriate for the target population (whether children are participants or co-researchers; e.g., Dalli & One, 2012).

Potential challenges related to context should be considered. It is advisable to become familiar with the context in advance by spending time there (e.g., visiting school, participating in community activities); consulting with knowledgeable adults (e.g., key informants) about rules and regulations, cultural expectations, and population needs; and gaining necessary acceptance and permission to recruit children for research. Effective communication with child participants/co-researchers requires consideration of appropriate vocabulary, requisite level of cognitive and language capacities for planned research protocol, and need for nonverbal materials, directions, and response options (Thorkildsen & White-McNulty, 2002). Researchers should be prepared to explain and ensure understanding of the research protocol, expectations and responsibilities, the child's right to consent/dissent, and safeguards for privacy and confidentiality (including limits of confidentiality in cases of potential harm to self or others). Transparency about expectations and follow-through on promises (e.g., how data will be used) are critical to maintaining trust and ensuring ethical practice (Bromstrom, 2012; Dalli & One, 2012). Perhaps most critical is the researcher's flexibility and problem-solving skills to handle challenges with regard to child's cognitive, emotional, and behavioral needs. Researchers can plan for potential challenges but should be prepared that the unexpected may happen and situations may arise that call for making decisions in the best interests of the child at the expense of research protocol.

CONCLUSIONS

Research psychologists have unique opportunities to contribute to the promotion and protection of child rights by engaging children as research participants or co-researchers in ways that ensure child voice and prepare children as active agents. Five levels of research activity are proposed, ranging from developing research questions and methodology to capture the perspectives and experiences of children, to engaging children as researchers through participatory approaches; literature from social sciences, education, and global development provides example of research across the continuum. Such work can serve as models for psychologists interested in expanding their own research with children with the goal of promoting and protecting participation rights. Conducting research that ensures child voice and promotes child agency is not without challenges and we can learn from researchers in other fields about how to prepare for and meet those challenges. Ultimately, research for the purpose of promoting child participation can contribute to psychological science and enhance the lives of children and adult researchers.

Table 5.1
54 Articles of the Convention on the Rights of the Child (CRC, Nastasi, 2013)

Article 1: Definition of the child [GP]

Article 2: Non-discrimination [GP]

Article 3: Best interests of the child [GP]

Article 4: Protection of rights [PA, PR, SD]

Article 5: Parental guidance [SD]

Article 6: Survival and development [GP, SD]

Article 7: Registration, name, nationality, care [SD]

Article 8: Preservation of identity [SD]

Article 9: Separation from parents [SD]

Article 10: Family reunification [SD]

Article 11*: Kidnapping [PR]

Article 12: Respect for views of the child [GP, PA]

Article 13: Freedom of expression [PA]

Article 14: Freedom of thought, conscience and religion [PA, SD]

Article 15: Freedom of association [PA]

Article 16: Right to privacy [PA]

Article 17: Access to information; mass media [PA]

Article 18: Parental responsibilities; state assistance [SD]

Article 19: Protection from all forms of violence [PR]

Article 20: Children deprived of family environment [PR, SD]

Article 21: Adoption [PR]

Article 22: Refugee children [PR, SD]

Article 23: Children with disabilities [SD]

Article 24: Health and health services [SD]

Article 25: Review of treatment in care [SD]

Article 26: Social security [SD]

Article 27: Adequate standard of living [SD]

Article 28: Right to education [SD]

Article 29: Goals of education [SD]

Article 30: Children of minority/indigenous groups [SD]

Article 31: Leisure, play, culture [SD]

Article 32: Child labour [PR]

Article 33: Drug abuse [PR]

Article 34*: Sexual exploitation [PR]

Article 35*: Abduction, sale and trafficking [PR]

(Continued)

Table 5.1 (*Continued*)

Article 36: Other forms of exploitation [PR]
Article 37: Detention and punishment [PR]
Article 38*: War and armed conflict [PR]
Article 39: Rehabilitation of child victims [PR]
Article 40: Juvenile justice [PR]
Article 41: Respect for superior national standards [PR]
Article 42: Knowledge of rights [SD]
Article 43–54: Implementation measures

SD = Survival & Development; PA = Participation; PR = Protection; GP = Guiding Principles (SD, PR, PA are categories of rights, as outlined by UNICEF, 2011b. For details on all of the articles, see http://www.unicef.org/crc/.). Articles in **bold** are relevant to child participation in research as discussed in this chapter. For more detailed descriptions of the Convention and its articles, see websites for United Nations, http://www.un.org/en/index.shtml; and UNICEF, http://www.unicef.org/.

*The optional protocols were adopted by the UN on January 18, 2002, to further delineate and reinforce Articles 11, 34, 35 ("Optional Protocol on the Sale of Children, Child Prostitution, and Child Pornography"), and 38 ("Optional Protocol on Involvement of Children in Armed Conflict").

Note: This table was reprinted from B. K. Nastasi (2013). *The role of schools in promoting and protecting child rights.* White paper produced for the Institute for Democracy in Education (IDE), The Patton College of Education, Ohio University http://www.cehs.ohio.edu/centers-partnerships/centers/IDE/. Reprinted with permission.

Table 5.2
Research Studies Involving Child Voice at Different Levels of Participation

Citation	Purpose	Child Ages	Methods
	Level 1. Examine Child Perceptions		
Evans et al. (2001)	Perceptions	Ages 9–11	Present illustrated stories; children respond verbally and nonverbally
Nicholls et al. (1995)	Perceptions	Grades 1–8	Oral and pictorial presentation; children respond orally via interviews
Thorkildsen and White-McNully (2002)	Perceptions	Ages 6–14	Structured interviews
	Level 2. Examine Child Experiences		
Raittila (2012)	Experiences	Ages 4–6	Ethnographic tour (child-led tour of neighborhood; participation observation)
Mudaly and Goddard (2009)	Experiences	Ages 9–18	In-depth interviews
Sinha (2010)	Experiences	Grades 8 and higher	Interviews

Citation	Purpose	Child Ages	Methods
Kijo-Bisimba (2010)	Experiences	Ages 9–18	Ethnography, participant observation of daily life, drawings, diaries, interviews, focus groups, role play, songs, photography
Huang and Ayoub (2011)	Experiences	Ages 13–17	Ethnography using focus groups and individual interviews
	Level 3. Facilitate Child-Adult Communication		
Keat et al. (2009)	Communication	Ages 3–5	Photo-narration. Children take photos and describe orally.
	Level 4. Inform Decision Making		
de Berry et al. (2003)	Decision making	Ages 7–18	Focus groups using variety of techniques (interviews, drawings, stories, charts, tape recordings, etc.)
Nastasi et al. (2007)	Decision making	Grades 6–12	Series of studies; mixed methods using focus groups, culture-specific self-report measures, student products
UNICEF (2011a)	Decision making	Unspecified	Interviews, surveys, mapping; participatory risk assessment (across multiple studies)
UNICEF (2012)	Decision making	Age 12	Self-report measures of well-being, life satisfaction, perceptions and concerns
	Level 5. Participatory Research		
Hampshire et al. (2012)	Participatory action research	Ages 10–16	Child researchers using diaries, photo-journals, interviews, focus groups, accompanied walks. Produce book of findings.
Steffen (2010)	Participatory action research	Ages 13–17	Child researchers using workshops, role play, group discussion, drawings, diaries, photography, creative activities
Plotnik et al. (2013)	Co-researchers with scientists	Middle school children	Partners throughout the study process, including co-authoring academic articles

Note: This table is not meant to reflect an exhaustive review of the literature but as a representative of research involving active child participation. However, the inclusion of literature outside of psychology reflects the limited representation of such work in psychology research journals.

REFERENCES

Alderson, P. (2012). Rights-respecting research: A commentary on "the right to be properly researched: Research with children in a messy world." *Children's Geographies, 10* (2), 233–239. doi: 10.1080/14733285.2012.661603

Brostrom, S. (2012). Children's participation in research. *International Journal of Early Years Education, 20* (3), 257–269. doi: /10.1080/09669760.2012.715407

Dalli, C., & One, S. T. (2012). Involving children in educational research: Researcher reflections on challenges. *International Journal of Early Years Education, 20* (3), 224–233. doi: 10.1080/09669760.2012.715408

de Berry, J., Fazili, A., Farhad, S., Nasiry, F., Hashemi, S., & Hakimi, M. (2003). *The children of Kabul: Discussions with Afghan families.* Kabul, Afghanistan: Save the Children & UNICEF.

Dockett, S., Einarsdottir, J., & Perry, B. (2012). Young children's decisions about research participation: Opting out. *International Journal of Early Years Education, 20* (3), 244–256. doi: 10.1080/09669760.2012.715405

Evans, I. M., Galyer, K. T., & Smith, K. J. H. (2001). Children's perceptions of unfair reward and punishment. *The Journal of Genetic Psychology, 162* (2), 212–227. doi: 10.1080/09669760.2012.715408

Hampshire, K., Porter, G., Owusu, S., Mariwah, S., Abane, A., Robson, E., . . . Bourdillon, M. (2012). Taking the long view: Temporal considerations in the ethics of children's research activity and knowledge production. *Children's Geographies, 10* (2), 219–232. doi: 10.1080/14733285.2012.667921

Hart, R. (1992). Children's participation: From tokenism to citizenship. *Innocenti Essays* (#4). Florence, Italy: UNICEF International Child Development Centre.

Huang, K., & Ayoub, C. (2011). Crooked trees growing straight: The experiences of boys transitioning off the streets of La Paz, Bolivia. In H. E. Fitzgerald, K. Puura, M. Tomlinson, & C. Paul (Eds.), *International perspectives on children and mental health: Volume 1. Development and context.* Santa Barbara, CA: Praeger.

Keat, J. B., Strickland, M. J., & Marinak, B. A. (2009). Child voice: How immigrant children enlightened their teachers with a camera. *Early Childhood Education Journal, 37,* 13–21. doi: 10.1007/s10643-009-0324-1

Kijo-Bisimba, H. (2010). Conducting research with children: Capturing the voices of orphaned children heading households in Tanzania. *Law, Social Justice & Global Development Journal, 2.* http://www.go.warwick.ac.uk/elj/lgd/2010_2/kijo-bisimba

Kina, V. J. (2012). What we say and what we do: Reflexivity, emotions and power in children and young people's participation. *Children's Geographies, 10* (2), 201–218. doi: 10.1080/14733285.2012.667920

Mortari, L., & Harcourt, D. (2102). "Living" ethical dilemmas for researchers when researching with children. *International Journal of Early Years Education, 20* (3), 234–243. doi: 10.1080/09669760.2012.715409

Mudaly, N., & Goddard, C. (2009). The ethics of involving children who have been abused in child abuse research. *International Journal of Children's Rights, 17,* 261–281. DOI 10.1163/157181808X389920

Murris, K. (2013). The epistemic challenge of hearing child's voice. *Studies in Philosophy and Education, 32,* 245–259. DOI 10.1007/s11217-012-9349-9

Nastasi, B. K. (2013). *The role of schools in promoting and protecting child rights.* White paper produced for the Institute for Democracy in Education (IDE), The Patton College of Education, Ohio University. http://www.cehs.ohio.edu/centers-partnerships/centers/IDE/.

Nastasi, B. K., Hitchcock, J. H., & Brown, L. M. (2010). An inclusive framework for conceptualizing mixed methods design typologies: Moving toward fully integrated synergistic research models. In A. Tashakkori & C. Teddlie (Eds.), *Handbook of mixed methods in social and behavioral research* (2nd ed., pp. 305–338). Thousand Oaks, CA: Sage.

Nastasi, B. K., Hitchcock, J. H., Burkholder, G., Varjas, K., Sarkar, S., & Jayasena, A. (2007). Assessing adolescents' understanding of and reactions to stress in different cultures: Results of a mixed-methods approach. *School Psychology International, 28*(2), 163–178. doi: 10.1177/0143034307078092

Nastasi, B. K., Hitchcock, J., Sarkar, S., Burkholder, G., Varjas, K., & Jayasena, A. (2007). Mixed methods in intervention research: Theory to adaptation. *Journal of Mixed Methods Research, 1,* 164–182. doi: 10.1177/1558689806298181

Nastasi, B. K., & Schensul, S. L. (2005). Contributions of qualitative research to the validity of intervention research. *Journal of School Psychology, 43*(3), 177–195. doi: 10.1016/j.jsp.2005.04.003

Nastasi, B. K., Varjas, K., Sarkar, S., & Jayasena, A. (1998). Participatory model of mental health programming: Lessons learned from work in a developing country. *School Psychology Review, 27*(2), 260–276.

Nicholls, J. G., Nelson, J. R., & Gleaves, K. (1995). Learning "facts" versus learning that most questions have many answers: Student evaluations of contrasting curricula. *Journal of Educational Psychology, 87*(2), 253–260.

Plotnik, J. M., Pokorny, J. J., Keratimanochaya, T., Webb, C., Beronja, H. F., et al. (2013). Visual cues given by humans are not sufficient for Asian elephants (*Elephas maximus*) to find hidden food. *PLoS ONE, 8*(4), e61174. doi: 10.1371/journal.pone.0061174

Raittila, R. (2012). With children in their lived place: Children's action as research data. *International Journal of Early Years Education, 20* (3), 270–279. doi: 10.1080/09669760.2012.718124

Sinha, S. (2010). Child defenders for child rights. *Law, Social Justice & Global Development Journal, 2.* http://www.go.warwick.ac.uk/elj/lgd/2010_2/sinha

Steffen, B. (2010). Beyond child participation in the Occupied Palestinian Territories: The case for "protective solidarity." *Law, Social Justice & Global Development Journal, 2.* http://www.go.warwick.ac.uk/elj/lgd/2010_2/steffen

Thorkildsen, T. A., & White-McNulty, L. (2002). Developing conceptions of fair contest procedures and the understanding of skill and luck. *Journal of Educational Psychology, 94* (2), 316–326. doi: 10.1037//0022-0663.94.2.316

Todd, L. (2012). Critical dialogue, critical methodology: Bridging the research gap to young people's participation in evaluating children's services. *Children's Geographies, 10*(2), 187–200. doi: 10.1080/14733285.2012.667919

UNICEF. (2011a). *Children and climate change: Children's vulnerability to climate change and disaster impacts in East Asia and the Pacific.* Bangkok, Thailand: UNICEF East Asian and Pacific Regional Office. www.unicef.org/media/files/Climate_Change_Regional_Report_14_Nov_final.pdf

UNICEF. (2011b). *Rights under the Convention on the Rights of the Child.* Retrieved from http://www.unicef.org/crc/index_30177.html

UNICEF. (2012). *Children's well-being from their own point of view: What affects the children's well-being in the first year of compulsory secondary education in Spain?* Madrid: UNICEF Spain. http://www.unicef.es/sites/www.unicef.es/files/Childrens_subjective_well-being_Unicef_feb13.pdf

United Nations (UN). (1989). *Convention on the Rights of the Child.* Retrieved from http://www2.ohchr.org/english/law/crc.htm

Chapter 6

Special Commentary: The Injustice of Educational Deprivation[1,2]

Milton Schwebel

This chapter is composed of four parts. Part 1 defines education and considers its value as well as the way it can threaten the status quo, and finally, justice in the distribution and allocation of resources for education. Part 2 is a brief record of the unscientific and unjust use of the IQ test and a history of the century-old effort to uncover the hidden role of the environment—including at home and in-school education—in intellectual development and school achievement. Part 3 examines the national education programs of the past two decades, contrasts them with reforms that the United States needs to enact to overcome injustice; and indicates the possible roles of psychologists, other social scientists, and educators in such endeavors. Part 4 answers the question: Are these changes achievable?

PART 1: DEFINITIONS

In this part the following are defined: *education*, as understood in this chapter; the value of education; the threat that education can pose to the status quo; and *equity*, contrasted with *equality*, within the framework of distributive justice.

Education

The word *education* conjures up a mental picture of a classroom, a teacher and about 25 or 30 students. That picture—that is, school as synonymous with education—is vastly incomplete. Education, both in this chapter and in life, begins at birth and a child's future physical and mental health and intellectual development are strongly influenced by circumstance in the lives of the future parents, starting even before conception. The association between the education and social class of the parents and the future education of their child is high. The health of the mother before and during pregnancy, the circumstances of the conception, and the attitude of the expectant mother about the forthcoming infant are strongly related (Johnson et al., 2006). Although the child's future is by no means ordained before it is an embryo, its likely future, barring early and strong intervention, is foreshadowed at that time.

The life of the fetus is a crucial period in human development. Science writer Paul (2010) provides the scientific evidence for the view reflected in her book's title, *Origins: The Nine Months before Birth Shape the Rest of Our Lives.* She explores the emerging science of fetal origins, involving genes and the environment. The environment is not just a passive enclosure. Both in its internal and external aspects, it is an active participant.

If education is equated with schooling starting with kindergarten, then we have to wonder how to account for the five years of intellectual growth and knowledge acquisition prior to that time. During the period from birth to age five, some children experience enormous advances in cognitive development and knowledge acquisition, while others much less. The degree of progress experienced by children is related to the social class and education of parents, as illustrated later in a discussion of the studies by Hart and Risley (1995) showing the vast differences in opportunity for vocabulary development by age three. Here it is worth noting Barnett's (2010) findings about preschool and social class: fewer than half the children in poverty attend public preschool programs, even at age four. In the choice of preschools, the education, sophistication, and wealth of parents give them a substantial advantage in making decisions that impact the quality of education their children will receive prior to kindergarten.

In any event, the inevitable conclusion is that the education of the child begins at birth, and that any national, state, or local political entity that fails to take that into account is likely to fail. The broadened definition of education—that it begins at birth—highlights the crucial role of parent education during pregnancy and the early years of their children's lives—particularly to compensate for social class differences in opportunities for intellectual development and education.

To illustrate this crucial point about social class differences in opportunities for intellectual development and early education, consider the life situations of two women, each pregnant for two months, each of the same race and ethnic group. For illustrative purposes, I present poignant examples and by no means wish to imply these cases are completely representative of their respective social classes.

June, 15, a daughter of an unemployed mother of three, sees no future in school as she looks around her community for role models. She has plans to drop out. When she becomes pregnant, she has poor nutritional habits, in part due to living in poverty; is unaware of the availability and need for prenatal care; and sees no prospect of being able to find a job or afford preschool for her child. She has not seen a physician. In contrast, Julie, 25, a recent MBA graduate from Harvard, is the daughter of wealthy parents, and is married to a successful lawyer. Together, they look forward to the child's birth. Julie, who has seen her obstetrician, decorated the nursery in their spacious home, covered the walls with framed pictures of fairy-tale characters, and filled the shelves with picture books. She has arranged to register the child at the leading nursery school, preschool, and private elementary school. These two babies will be born into two distinctly different worlds, with distinctly different opportunities for all-round development, including cognitive development. Julie's child's education will have earned her a first-five-year equivalent of a PhD degree, while June's will be the equivalent of a school dropout. Political leaders who believe they can close that vast chasm simply by making schools, principals, and teachers accountable are naively expecting miracles.

Value

Education is valued for two different, although overlapping, reasons. First is its practical value: educational achievement is associated with income, status, and social class. Parents of modest means generally consider it important enough to work extra hours and sacrifice personal needs if necessary to be able to afford sending a teenager to postsecondary education. Wealthy parents hire educated, bilingual nannies, register their children in the best nursery and preschools and private schools at birth, and contribute to Ivy League and other favored universities to give their children admissions advantages. They consult experts on preschool admissions and tutors to prepare their children for admissions interviews and tests.

Education has another value that, in terms of intellectual and humanistic development, makes it precious. Education can be liberating, freeing humans from blind faith and superstition, opening their minds in the tradition of the Renaissance and the Age of Enlightenment. Such education promotes critical thinking and creativity, enriching the lives of those fortunate enough to have experienced these liberating effects. In this way, individuals recapitulate in their own lives the greatest of advances of civilization, the scientific mind, like Newton's, and the humanistic mind, like Shakespeare's.

The value of education to individuals is indisputable. The same may be said about its value to a vibrant democratic society. Many nations, the United States among them, have been loath to spend more than a bare minimum for the education of those who are either not needed in the economy or can be used even with bare literacy.

Threat

During the Middle Ages in Europe, only the nobility (political and religious) were educated. Millions of peasants were illiterate and ignorant. Changes in western Europe sparked by the Reformation led to the age of reason, whose protagonists were philosophers like Spinoza and Locke, physicists like Newton, and authors like Voltaire who challenged the superstition and intolerance fostered by state and church. This paved the ways to the Industrial Revolution, which created a dilemma for rulers: the machines that were radically changing society and bringing peasants into sprawling and unruly cities required literate workers who had a basic knowledge of mathematics. How can such lowly workers, formerly illiterate peasants, be given schooling so restricted that it would not open up the floodgates to outrage over the oppression, poverty, and exhausting workdays they were enduring, and perhaps even to rebellion? That contradiction is well illustrated by the words of the King of Prussia's Minister of Education, Alfenstein, who declared:

> The primary schools have only to work to the end that the common people . . . may be intelligent in regard to all matters within the narrow sphere to which God has called them . . . may learn to read and write, reckon and sing, may love their rulers and their fatherland, be contented with their social status and peaceably and happy in their lot . . . I do not think the principles enunciated will raise the common people out of the sphere designated for them by God and Society. (Stern, 1965, p. 107)

In the 19th century in southern states, teaching slaves to write, which would promote the threat of shared opposition to slavery, was a crime. Four centuries after Newton's contributions to fledgling science and three centuries after Darwin, some states in the United States chose to teach creationism along with evolution. Without ascribing intent, the national law, No Child Left Behind, emphasizes reading, science, and mathematics—essential to many skilled and some semi-skilled occupations. The heavy concentration on achievement testing in those favored subjects and holding teachers accountable for the results gives them a powerful incentive to devote most class time to those three subjects—leading to an underemphasis on the other liberating and humanizing subjects of literature, history, the social sciences, and the arts (Darling-Hammond, 2010). To those who regard an informed and enlightened citizenry vital to a well-functioning democratic society, any restrictions on learning are to be avoided.

Distributive Justice

In the situation that exists in the United States, and to varying degrees worldwide, the enormous inequalities in student achievement cannot be remedied by providing even equal resources to those who have been deprived for decades and even centuries. To achieve equality, they require an equitable, in contrast with equal, allocation of resources. A child near starvation needs more nourishment than a well-fed one. Equity, that is, fairness or justice, is difficult to determine, whereas need is less debatable. It could be said that equity requires the satisfaction of need. Bridging the gap in academic achievement between the poor and the upper classes requires an unequal distribution of resources, an equitable distribution, in order to achieve a greater measure of equality, opportunity, and achievement. Deutsch (1985) examines the concept of distributive justice in detail.

PART 2: HEREDITY AND ENVIRONMENT ON A BALANCED SCALE

This part of the chapter reviews the history of the contentious IQ debate, revealing deep-seated theoretical differences with their profound practical implications. Are low-achieving students the victims of heredity, in which case education would be of little help, or are they victims of a poor environment, in which case education would help? That question has plagued education and psychology for more than a century.

Heredity and environment do not exist in isolation; they interact with each other. Clearly, children of high, inherited intelligence are better able than others to use and exploit their environment, thus expanding their knowledge. Children with a favorable environment, such as wealthy, educated parents, are able to maximize their inherited cognitive aptitudes, for example, by the aid of tutors, travel that expands their horizons, and association with stimulating classmates (Brulles & Winebrenner, 2011; Sapon-Slavin, 2007).

Intelligence is one of psychology's major areas of research, and the IQ test is one of psychology's most widely known products. The high status of the intelligence test is shown by the recognition accorded to it when an issue of *Science*, the publication of the American Association for the Advancement of Science, included IQ tests among the 20 discoveries that "changed our lives" during the prior hundred years (Hammond, 1984). The brief history of the test's use, presented later, reveals how, in "changing our lives," this major product of psychology, in fact, innocently contributed to social injustice.

Binet: The Cultivation of Intelligence

Alfred Binet is known as the father of intelligence tests. He, with Theodore Simon, at the request of the minister of education in Paris early in the 20th century, developed the Binet-Simon Intelligence Scale. Its purpose was to identify children deficient in age-appropriate knowledge so that they could be given supplemental instruction to help overcome the backwardness. A few years later, when Binet learned that American psychologists were using his test for a diametrically opposite purpose, namely, to give children a score that was fixed and irreversible, he was outraged by the "deplorable verdict that the intelligence of an individual is a fixed quantity. . . . We must protest and act against that brutal pessimism. . . . One increases that which constitutes the intelligence of a school child, namely, the capacity to learn, to improve with instruction" (Hunt, 1961, p. 13).

Intelligence tests were used to help justify the sterilization of 70,000 Americans, most without their consent, some without their knowledge (Kamin, 1974). After World War I, American psychologists claimed that immigrants to the United States in the late 19th and early 20th centuries had lowered the intellectual level of the country and, because they propagated so frequently, had doomed the nation's future, even if the government were to terminate all future immigration. Using World War I army tests, the psychologists had come to those conclusions with the support of the eugenicists and at great cost to immigrants and their children, now marked as backward (Brigham, 1923).

Galton's Race and Class Bias

Binet's test was widely used in the United States, but from the outset, Galton (1969/1892), the pioneer of the study of individual differences, was the major theoretical influence. He introduced the concept of eugenics and coined its name. As to group differences, Galton claimed that the British aristocracy deserved its wealth and position because of its intelligence. As to populations at large, the ancient Athenians, he said, were superior to the English of his time to the same extent as the English were superior to African Americans. His judgment of the latter was based on the "half-wittedness" (Galton, 1969/1892, p. 329) of the Black servants displayed in American novels, a questionable source of objective data. Galton's class and race biases appeared early in the history of intelligence testing, particularly in their use to justify group differences, and those biases persist to the present day. Because a century after Binet there is no agreement about the meaning of the term *intelligence*, nor about the number of intelligences that humans possess, the field has been open to great variations in the nature and content of the tests, and also in the exploitation of group differences in the interest of structural violence.

The 1930s and 1940s witnessed heated exchanges between exponents of the opposing views. During that period, there was a growing recognition that the prevailing theory of human intelligence, well represented by the views of Terman (1930), that it was overwhelmingly genetic in character, was incorrect. In contrast was the theoretical position, voiced by Stoddard (1943), that intelligence was responsive to human intervention. My own observations as a counselor for the National Youth Administration, a New Deal program for unemployed youth, ages 16–21, seemed to contradict the prevailing view. Long conversations with youth, including those speaking with a Sicilian accent, a heavy Irish brogue, or a southern dialect, raised doubts about the validity of the IQ scores yielded by the paper and pencil group tests used at the time, like the Otis. Their reasoning in coping with life's problems, one of the criteria of intelligence according to Wechsler (1958), belied the results. They also belied the conclusions about immigrants drawn from the World War I army test scores.

The World War II Corrective

After World War II, Tuddenham's (1948) comparison of the intellectual performance of World War I and II soldiers on the army tests revealed no decline at all but, in fact, a statistically significant increase in performance equivalent to 12 IQ points. American adults, in this case mostly male, were "smarter" in the 1940s than those in the period around 1917–1918. This finding, coming as it did in the wake of a more open and liberal atmosphere following World War II, probably led some psychologists to revise their views about the roots of intelligence; however, it seems fair to say that in psychology, education, government, and the public at large, the genetic view held sway, with mostly lip service to the environment. In other words, the vast differences in performance between social classes, races, sexes, and ethnic groups on IQ tests, as well as the predominance of the lower classes in low-performing schools and classes, were attributed to familial genes.

This seeming attributional imbalance, which had profound educational and social justice implications, held the attention of many concerned researchers who challenged genetic determinism (e.g., Bloom, 1976; Cole, 1987; Deutsch, 1967; Hunt, 1961; Schwebel, 1968, 1974, 1986; Scribner & Cole, 1981). Students who were performing poorly on IQ tests were also in the poorest achieving schools, generally poorly equipped, and with less experienced teachers and lower per capita budgets than other schools. Many of the students were born into families below or close to the poverty level, with poorly educated parents, and others were children of immigrant parents contending with cultural and language differences. As students, these children compared unfavorably with those of financially secure families on both IQ and school achievement tests.

These poorly performing American students are to a large degree responsible for the decline of the U.S. rank in comparison with other member nations of the Organization for Economic and Cultural Development (OECD) on tests of reading, mathematics, and science literacy. Consider their disadvantages. Unlike their counterparts in other OECD member nations with whom the United States was compared, these students' families did not have the following benefits: national health insurance; paid maternity, and in some instances, paternity leave; substantial paid annual vacations; much higher unemployment insurance benefits, and for significantly longer periods of time than in the United States; free schooling from the preschool level; and much lower tuition for higher education (World Bank, 2006). All of these advantages contribute to the potential for less stress and tension and a more serene family life, conditions conducive to healthy human development and educational achievement.

Venezuela: Ministry for the Development of Human Intelligence

Two developments occurred in the final quarter of the last century, at nearly the same time, one in Venezuela, the other in New Zealand, that helped tip the scale, giving more weight to the role of the environment in intellectual growth.

In Venezuela, Alberto Machado (Ministry, 1982), a lawyer with a profound interest in facilitating mental growth, headed the new Ministry for the Development of Human Intelligence. At break-neck speed, he introduced interventions, drawn from researchers worldwide, to improve thinking in populations representing much of the life span, beginning with pregnancy and well on into adulthood. Nothing was off-limits in his nationwide campaign. He used radio and television, storefront posters, and lectures; his staff introduced programs in schools, maternity wards, factories, and military posts.

Here is a simple example of one of the many educational programs designed and implemented to alert parents to the important role they can play in making their children brighter and better students. I witnessed this scene: in a hospital in a working-class barrio, five mothers who had given birth in the prior 24 hours observed, as a sixth stood over a small table on which her infant son was lying. A nurse, trained in this form of parent education, stood opposite the mother. The infant was facing the nurse who instructed the mother to move her head close to the infant's and talk to him. The mothers laughed, and one said in ridicule: "Talk to the baby! He can't understand." The physical reactions of the other mothers and their laughter suggested they were in agreement with the outspoken one. The nurse insisted that the mother talk to him. She did, and to the obvious astonishment of the mothers, the baby turned his head in the mother's direction. As the nurse led a discussion, the mothers learned a basic principle: the importance of frequent daily communication, whether by mother or other family members, in promoting the baby's healthy development. In more general terms, they learned of the singular importance of communication and interaction in the intellectual and social development of children.

Hart and Risley (1995) underline the importance of speech in cognitive development. They found that by age three, children of professional parents have heard approximately 30 million words, whereas those of working class parents, 20 million, and the higher socioeconomic children had a much richer vocabulary. Children of unemployed African American mothers heard about 10 million by the age of three. Hart and Risley (1995) also studied the quality of the words the children heard, in particular the ratio of encouraging remarks to reprimands. For the higher socioeconomic group the ratio was six encouragement comments to one reprimand, for the working-class parents the ratio was two encouragements to one reprimand, and for the unemployed African American mothers it was two reprimands for every encouragement.

Hart and Risley's findings on encouragement and reprimands should be understood in the context of environmental and social circumstances. Regardless of race or ethnicity, one may speculate that parents living in crime and drug-infested areas may be prone to develop, or could have learned from their own parents an attitude of deterrence as a measure to protect their children from the pervasive threat of criminal or drug involvement. Also, African American mothers in interracial neighborhoods, and working-class parents in mixed-class neighborhoods, may be using control measures in their belief these will aid in their children's integration. Furthermore, the stress caused by unemployment and low income in working-class families can build to a negativism in parenting. Another possible explanation, called the Post Traumatic Slave Syndrome (DeGruy, 2005), is that generations of slave children learned to denigrate one another to avoid the negative attention of slave masters. Slaves always learned to behave in a deferential manner. In any case, although social problems appear to be a substantial contributing factor in the root of the excessive proportion of reprimands, the parents and their children could be aided by parent education.

In 1982, Venezuela hosted the First International Congress on the Development of Intelligence. The representation of many countries and UNESCO underscored the growing interest in intervention on behalf of intellectual development. A study of one of the Venezuelan programs, the teaching of thinking in the seventh grade, provided guarded validation of its effectiveness in raising performance on a variety of mental tests (Nickerson, 1986). The opportunity for completion of other program evaluations was lost when, after five years, an election brought a different political party into power, ending the activities of the Ministry for the Development of Human Intelligence. In recent years, China and South Africa have adopted, and Venezuela readopted, some of the Machado interventions for school-age children.

The Flynn Effect and the Role of the Environment

Turning now to New Zealand, in the early 1980s James Flynn, an American political scientist on the faculty of the University of Otago, began a series of studies, reported in two books (Flynn, 2008, 2009) that show the hand of the environment on intelligence. In 30 nations, including the United States, the IQ has risen a little more than three IQ points every decade for as long as IQ tests have been administered and records kept. In half a century the average national IQ in those nations rose 15 points. Since this increase cannot be attributed to evolution (50 years is less than a second in evolutionary time), responsibility for its improvement must be assigned to the environment.

Speculation abounds about the environmental stimuli for such substantial improvement. Can it be attributed to better nutrition, health care, parenting, teaching, or more education? Or, turning to the intriguing hypothesis put forth by W. T. Dickens and J. R. Flynn (Flynn, 2009), was it due to the swift scientific and technological advances in the world that demanded many more people capable of abstract thinking? Either way, it implies that society is capable of enhancing the intelligence of increasing numbers of its member.

Besides the contributions of Flynn and Machado, two psychologists helped establish the importance of the environment in intellectual development. Since the mid-1920s the works of Piaget (Gruber & Voneche, 1977; Piaget & Inhelder, 1969) and Vygotsky (Cole & Wertsch, 1996; Vygotgsky, 1978; Wertsch, 1985) have provided the nature plus nurture theory a solid base in cognitive psychology. Though their theories differ in fundamental ways, both of them allocate significant roles to environmental inputs, including the pedagogical, in the process of the individuals' own activity in developing their intelligence. Children and adolescents, in other words, are the constructors of their own intelligence; that is, others facilitate, individuals construct.

After university study, Piaget moved to Paris to teach in a school run by Binet. His observations of young children's mental processes led him to recognize that they were fundamentally different from those of older children and adults, and motivated him to study the stages of intellectual development. As children develop, they move from egocentrism to sociocentrism, in large part as a result of their interactions with older children and adults. The roles of parents, and especially teachers, are crucial in creating the environments and the interactions that foster development (Piaget, 1970; Schwebel & Raph, 1973).

Vygotsky's social-historical theory places great weight on mediated learning: this requires teachers to change their role from transmitter of knowledge to that of learning facilitator (Vygotsky, 1978). Their aim is to enable children to internalize intellectual skills en route to becoming self-learners and self-regulators in the construction of their intelligence. Vygotsky allocates extraordinary responsibility to education because learning, in his view, is the engine that drives development. Learning precedes development, the opposite to Piaget's conception.

The indispensable role of the environment is evident in the studies of more recent cognitive psychologists. Siegler (1996), for example, devotes a chapter to "How children generate new ways of thinking." New ways of thinking emerge from current interactions with the environment or from old ways of thinking that had their origins in such interactions. The central position of mediation in the intellectual development of the child underlines the importance of the social environment. Through the mediation of the mother, older sibling, or prekindergarten teacher, the child acquires the knowledge that took distant ancestors millennia to acquire; knowledge including language, literacy, and speech. The quality of mediation oftentimes determines, to a large extent, the level of the child's intellectual and social development by the age of five. Once again, social class is a major determinant of development.

The bitter IQ war of the 20th century can be illustrated by statements to the effect that the primarily genetic position continues to serve the structurally violent purposes assigned to it by Gould (1981): "invariably to find that oppressed and disadvantaged groups—races, classes, or sexes—are innately inferior and deserve their status" (pp. 24–25).

Balanced Reviews of Research

The IQ war may be tapering off as a result of a decision by the Science Directorate of the American Psychological Association to commission a group of experts on intelligence, representing diverse views to report on the accumulated knowledge. The result has been critical reviews of the findings of studies published or accepted for publication during the prior 15 years. The following are some of the findings of the second of these reports (Nisbet et al., 2012):

> Heritability of IQ varies significantly by social class . . . much has been learned about the biological underpinnings of intelligence. . . . The importance of the environment for the IQ is shown by the 12-point to the 18-point increase in IQ when children are adopted from working class to middle class homes. . . . Even when improvements in IQ produced by the most effective childhood intervention fail to persist, there can be very marked academic achievement and life outcomes . . . Sex differences in aspects of intelligence are due partly to identifiable biological factors and partly to socialization factors. . . . The IQ gap between Blacks and Whites has been reduced 0.33SD [standard deviation] in recent years. (p. 130)

These optimistic findings offer the prospect that over decades, and especially centuries, the proportion of the world's population capable of engaging in abstract thinking will continue to increase.

PART 3: WORKING TOWARD EDUCATIONAL EQUALITY

Part 3 of this chapter examines the signature educational programs of Presidents Barrack Obama, George W. Bush, and Bill Clinton. It also presents the four major components for educational reform deemed essential to overcome inequity. Then, Part 3 challenges the claim that the nation's policymakers and political leaders want to invest in reforms necessary to achieve equity.

Recent decades have been strewn with failed education programs costing billions of dollars and costly in human terms to millions of students and their families. They were given great promises that did not materialize. Worse yet, the students were victims of destructive forms of instruction. They were victims of the empty promises of three presidents who excelled in rhetoric like "No Child Left Behind," but not education. Besides, they were not generous in support of the schools. As Darling-Hammond (2010) characterized the accountability programs as "testing without investing" (p. 87), it was, and still is, reforming on the surface and on the cheap.

Three Presidents and Three National School Programs

President Clinton's Education Goals 2000 enacted by Congress in 1994 was to elevate American students to first place among the industrially advanced nations, a position it once held. The absurdity of this promise is evident when we learn it was made when American students were ranked low among the industrially advanced nations. A year after the enactment they ranked 21st in scientific literacy and 24th of 29 in scientific problem solving.

President Bush's No Child Left Behind (NCLB) program was enacted in 2002, with extraordinary emphasis as described in Part 1, on accountability through the use of tests of reading, mathematics, and science—leading unavoidably to the neglect of other subjects and giving students a decidedly unbalanced education. Through a system of stages, schools are given the opportunity to steadily increase the percentage of students who meet the standards. Failing schools can be closed, with their personnel dismissed, as has happened to some of them. By 2014 all schools must meet the standards in reading and mathematics or be replaced.

The basic weakness has cryptically been summarized, as noted earlier, in the phrase "testing without investing." Converting this to a cartoon, President Bush, wearing a red, white, and blue jockey's outfit, would be riding an exhausted, undernourished, and thirsty horse, so lacking in energy that even the whip could not stop it from falling behind the other horses. No matter what penalties are threatened school personnel, teaching children who missed out on much education in their first five years of life, or worse yet, experienced negative education in the form of an excess of reprimands—which can paralyze children psychologically—cannot compensate for the past without an enormous societal commitment and effort.

By its own standards, NCLB is a failure: At the 2014 deadline, all students are supposed to be proficient in the key subjects. Already by July 2012, thirty-two states and the District of Columbia had been granted waivers from that requirement and other such requests were under consideration.

President Obama's Race to the Top educational program involves a competition among the states, plus the District of Columbia, for awards for research and application in four categories: improving standards and assessments, improving the collection and use of data, improving teacher effectiveness, and finally achieving equity in teacher distribution and turning around struggling schools. States spend millions of dollars to prepare and file their submissions and meanwhile years of education are lost. It could be said that Race to the Top is in search for "silver bullets" to solve the educational problems: a waste of money, time, and effort, since that knowledge is available. The knowledge is available, but the will to apply it is lacking, because, for reasons discussed later, the shapers of educational policy are not prepared to pay the cost. The richest school districts spend nearly 10 times the amount per student than the poorest (Darling-Hammond, 2010).

The Charter School Movement

The mistaken belief that the chronic low achievement in American education is the fault of teachers and administrators in public schools led to the movement to start from scratch by establishing independent charter schools, publicly or privately supported, many of the latter on a for-profit basis. Failing to recognize the need for a solid social safety net, parent education, and adequately supported schools and teachers, the charters' outcomes were inevitable. In a multiple-state study, they did not fare as well in student achievement as standard public schools, all serving demographically equivalent students (Kozol, 2005).

Despite the plethora of evidence showing that the charter schools—known by their supporters as "no excuses" schools, with poverty, for instance, being no excuse—continue to fall short of expectations, avid supporters continue to laud their claimed successes. To counteract that deception, Coles (2012), former research professor in the Department of Psychiatry at the Robert Wood Johnson Medical School, analyzed the claims of the leaders of KIPP (Knowledge Is Power Program). The largest nationwide chain of charter schools, KIPP's open enrollment policy is intended to attract undeserved minority groups and to put them on track to higher education. Students attend tuition-free from 7:30 AM until 5:00 PM. Their teachers are said to be graduates of select teacher education programs who are commuted to KIPP's goals. KIPP reports fail to point out that the difference in enrollments and the higher KIPP dropout rate, especially of Black males, give KIPP an advantage in comparison with public schools. Further, the KIPP per pupil expenditure is higher than that in comparison with public schools. Coles (2012) also raised an ethical issue: in connection with the 2010 research results of a comparative study of KIPP and public school students, an investigation that KIPP leaders insisted was "independent" was in fact conducted by a researcher funded by the same organizations that fund and champion KIPP. In that KIPP study, Coles (2012) reported that the researchers did not explain how the 22 KIPP middle schools were chosen for the study, representing the 46 KIPP middle schools in operation at that time. Then, when two of the sample's middle schools were closed because of poor performance, the record of achievement of the students in those poor performing schools were excluded from the sample of students. A strong, unyielding commitment to a belief, like poverty, is no excuse and is irrelevant to intellectual development, and school achievement, can, it seems, lead to the sacrifice of accurate reporting and perhaps even ethical practices.

The first comprehensive national study of charter schools, conducted by Stanford University's Center for Research on Education Outcomes (2009), a study of 70 percent of charter schools found that only 17 percent of the students performed better than demographically similar students in public schools, and 37 percent of charter school students had poorer achievement records. The researchers concluded "in unmistakable terms," that in the aggregate, charter school students were not faring as well as their public school counterparts. Furthermore, tremendous variation in academic quality was the norm.

The Stanford Center's 2013 study of an even expanded proportion of charter schools showed considerable improvement in their students' achievement (Rich, 2013). Charter school students were faring better in 2013 than they were four years earlier, surpassing those in traditional public schools in reading gains and keeping pace in math. This very comprehensive study involved 95 percent of the 2.3 million students in charter schools.

In considering the implications of these favorable results, the following should be borne in mind. It has taken the charter school movement, with all its flexibility, about 20 years to equal and, in reading, surpass the poor performance of the traditional public schools, especially, those serving students in urban centers from families in or near the poverty level. The current level of student achievement in the charter, as well as the public schools, is deplorable, showing the effects of poverty that is too little attended, from birth onward. Besides, even the reported gains must be seen in this light: eight percent of the underperforming schools in the 2009 study of the charter schools were closed down and not included in the 2013 study. The students in those schools quite possibly returned to the traditional public schools, contributing to their lower record of performance, while also increasing class size. Already overburdened teachers in low-achieving schools were saddled with even more students in class, while losing many of the essential teacher aides as a result of the budgetary cuts. According to the Executive Office of the President (August, 2012) "since the official end of the recession in June 2009, we have lost more than 300,000 local education jobs—raising class sizes and threatening the education of our nation's children. In just the last month alone, 7,000 local education jobs—teachers, school aides, and support staff serving our children—were lost. In addition to reducing the number of teachers on their payrolls, school districts have cut pre-kindergarten and kindergarten programs, shortened the school day or school year, and have cut back on other critical education programs" (p. 3). Even just from 2008 to 2010, the average public school teacher-student ratio increased almost 5 percent, along with the termination of other personnel essential to schools serving the poor.

Social Class and Education

While the competition between charter and traditional public schools has been unfolding, important changes have been occurring. For example, studies by Reardon (2012) and Reardon and Bischoff (2011) help illuminate the current state of education for minorities and the poor. They found that although the gap in achievement between Whites and Blacks has narrowed significantly, the gap between the rich and the poor has expanded even more. One possible explanation is that more African Americans have graduated from college and are better equipped for the role of parent-teacher. Another reason may be a move to middle-class school districts as parents rose into the mid-level socioeconomic class. The studies are further evidence of the connection between economic well-being and school achievement.

Regardless of the type of school, traditional or charter, there are considerable differences in student performance among the states. Some states in the United States fare as well on the international achievement tests as the leading advanced industrialized nations. That fact reflects the enormous variation among states in such relevant variables as poverty and adult educational attainment. For example, the percentage of household poverty in New Hampshire is 5.6, and in New Jersey, 6.8. The percentages of their adult populations with a college degree or more are 32 and 34.5 percent, respectively. In Mississippi and Louisiana, by comparison with the other two states, the percentages for household poverty are 20.1 and 18.3, and for higher educational attainment are 16.9 and 21.4, respectively. One can infer from these data that many more families in the favored states can manage without a strong social safety net. Besides that, many more parents are better equipped to manage a healthy pregnancy and to provide a rich preschool education for their children.

In response to unfair criticisms of teachers, the value-added approach for evaluating the success of teachers was introduced. A fourth-grade teacher with a student reading at the first-grade level was expected to have the student raise his or her performance to the second not the fourth-grade level. This seems to be fair, but in fact, it is not. Value-added evaluation may be effective for purposes of determining how well a large group of teachers is performing, but it is invalid for use in evaluating individual teachers, as Braun (2005) of the Educational Testing Service concluded after reviewing many reports of research conducted by the Rand Corporation. Consider the many life events that could make almost any learning goals difficult to achieve: homelessness, death or serious chronic illness of a parent, parental unemployment, parental divorce or separation, death of a sibling, incarceration of a parent or sibling, a child's serious illness, and/or child physical or sexual abuse. These events are far more likely to occur to children in poor, urban schools than in the more favored school districts where both the parents and the schools are in a position to provide children with psychological or social services.

The Four Essential Components

Sweeping changes in educational policy and programs are called for in the future. The fact that the nation is in no position now to invest the many billions entailed in introducing what is necessary does not mean that cheaper, irrelevant plans, as irrelevant and destructive as, for example, NCLB, should be invoked. When the public demands quality education for all children, an effective program will contain the following four major components:

1) A social safety net that assures that all people will be adequately housed, fed, clothed, educated, and medically cared for without the onus of being on the dole. In most industrially advanced nations the safety net includes the following: a national health care program; paid maternal (in some cases, paternal as well) leave program; guaranteed paid vacations varying from two to six weeks; unemployment benefits considerably higher than in the United States, and for considerably longer periods; free or low-cost

preschool; and free or low-tuition higher education. The safety net provides the foundation of family life that gives parents a sense of security, with reduced tensions, and the opportunity to create an environment conducive to the healthy physical, social, and intellectual development of children—the kind that is characteristic of families of greater means today, a family environment conducive to curiosity and learning. These objectives, though not currently on the table, are very American, having been implicit in President Franklin D. Roosevelt's State of the Union address in 1944, known as the Second Bill of Rights.

2) Parent education, available to all parents, that begins at pregnancy, continues until the child is five, and is available, thereafter, throughout the years of schooling. Parents learn the principles of a healthy pregnancy and childbirth; cooperative parenthood whether the parents are still together or not; the critical importance of speech, conversation, and confidence-building social interactions; the value of varied experiences, including the use of available resources like libraries, parks, zoos, childcare's museums, nature in a backyard, and in nearby countrysides; books and games that are age-appropriate; and educational television programs. Parent education also marks the beginning of a close partnership between schools, teachers, in particular, and parents: a bond growing out of their mutual goal, the child's intellectual, social and physical development and success as a student.
3) Free nursery and preschool for families up to the level of the median national annual income, in settings where the experiences and instruction are attuned to the cultural and social backgrounds of the children, with teachers trained to work at the designated age level, with children—and parents—of diverse social class and cultural identities.
4) Elementary and secondary schools, with teachers trained to teach students of diverse socioeconomic classes, races, primary languages, and sexual orientations, who are adequately paid, closely supervised and coached during the first three years of service, aided by a full-time assistant to help provide individual instruction required by most of the students in low-performing schools, with class content (curriculum) suited to the population of the school, and in schools where they are welcomed by principals and teachers alike. Schools serving children of the poor receive per capita support equal to or greater than that of students in upper income school districts, in order that their schools are equally provided with libraries, computers, science, art, and music equipment, in buildings in equal repair. In these schools, parents are partners in working toward goals shared with school personnel.

Equality of opportunity, defined as an unequal distribution of resources based on need, does not begin at the age of five or three or at birth. The fact is that it should commence even before conception, in the mental and physical health and habits of the future parents. It is to be hoped that education provided by a dedicated national health program of the future, if not by the Affordable Health Care Act, will lead to physically and mentally healthier parentage.

Although all four of the major components discussed earlier are essential, they do not have to be introduced at the same time. Furthermore, until Americans demand the comprehensive changes that are needed, educators, psychologists, and other social scientists could propose and support more limited changes, always bearing in the need for a comprehensive approach. Limited objectives include: parent education during the infant's first year, intensive coaching of new teachers during their first year; an assigned teacher assistant to give individual instruction to the many children who need that, and curriculum revision appropriate to the composition of the school's population.

Providing equitable education to the many millions of students in economically depressed cities would require an enormous outlay of funds for long periods of time, perhaps for the foreseeable future. Would it pay off? That question has been answered by New Jersey's experience over a four-decade period. Four distressed urban school districts filed a complaint in 1970 claiming that New Jersey's method of allocating funds to its school districts violated the constitutional requirement that every student be given a "thorough and efficient education." In 1981 the Education Law Center in New Jersey filed a complaint on behalf of students from those districts charging that the New Jersey system was unconstitutional. That case, *Abbott v. Burke*, and 19 more, some in this century, wrought historic decisions from the New Jersey Supreme Court and made unprecedented improvements in the education of students in impoverished communities. The state was ordered to allocate funds to the urban schools equal on a per student basis to those of the well-funded schools. Furthermore, the state was required to provide all the funds needed to enable the poor school districts to give their students all of the services needed to achieve at a level of the rest of the state. The court, in other words, mandated equitable funding, enabling those urban districts to provide full-day kindergarten, half-day preschool for children ages three and four, various forms of parent education, strong support for teachers in the form of supervision and teacher aides, professional assistance in humanizing and socializing subject matter, counseling services, appropriate libraries, laboratories, digital equipment and repair, and reconstruction of school facilities as needed. Furthermore, unlike NCLB with its emphasis on schooling to prepare just for an occupation, the court required instruction in literature, art, and music, the humanizing and socializing subjects (Education Law Center, 2011–2012; Goertz & Weiss, 2009). It is noteworthy that the sweeping innovations include aspects of the solid social safety nets available in the leading industrial nations, including quality, free half-day preschool for three and four-year-old children, diverse health, counseling and remedial services, and elements of parent education.

By 1998, the urban districts received funding equal to that of the rest of the state. By 2000, the state invested heavily in a quality preschool program, and in

2003 New Jersey committed itself to a major program of teacher improvement. The payoff came quickly. By 2007 New Jersey ranked among the top five in the nation on fourth- and eighth-grade achievement tests. This is especially impressive considering the student demographics: New Jersey's including almost 60 percent African American students and 19 percent Hispanics, far higher percentages than Massachusetts, Maine, Vermont, and New Hampshire—the states leading in student achievement. Furthermore, the African American and Hispanic students scored considerably higher than their peers nationwide on fourth- and eighth-grade reading and math tests (Darling-Hammond, 2010). Although it took decades to achieve parity and great increases in funding, the early results are promising. The gains on test scores are considerably higher at the fourth compared with the eighth-grade level, a condition that may change with time but that requires close professional attention. Still, the student achievement gap between rich and poor districts persists.

Linda Darling-Hammond's Components

Linda Darling-Hammond's (2010) landmark book, *The Flat World and Education: How America's Commitment to Equity Will Determine Our Future*, provides a goldmine of information on the current state of education in America, and compared with that in nations that have surpassed the United States. And she spells out the essential reforms, summarized as follows:

- Secure housing, food, and health care, so that children can come to school ready to learn each day.
- Supportive early learning environments.
- Equitably funded schools that provide access to high-quality teaching.
- Well-prepared and well-supported teachers and leaders.
- Standardized curriculum and assessments focused on 21st-century learning goals.
- Schools organized for in-depth student and teacher learning

Why Educate the Marginalized?

The two sets of objectives, Darling-Hammond's and mine, are very much in agreement, except that hers does not focus on parent education per se. There is, however, one major point of difference unrelated to goals and methods. Her subtitle reads, "How America's Commitment to Equity Will Determine Our Future." Her meaning is that the abysmally poor education provided to children of the lower socioeconomic classes will deny America the intelligence and creativity of millions of children. She is right, and she is admirable in her concern for those children and her opposition to educational deprivation. The problem, however, is that no matter how well they are educated, the economy has no room for them. There is no economic motivation to educate everyone. Millions will remain marginalized. The American economy, operating as a system that is fueled by profit and that places profit above all other values in the practical world, does not need to have all children well educated. I present evidence supporting that contention.

In daily life, one encounters numerous examples of semi-skilled and unskilled workers in diverse settings whose jobs require little more than basic literacy, workers such as road construction laborers, fruit and vegetable pickers, fast-food restaurant employees, and cleaning personnel in offices, hospitals, and airports. There is no reason to believe that performance on such jobs is improved by a quality high school education. To be very concrete, a quality education, which would very likely improve an individual's life, will not increase the individual's efficiency in slipping a hamburger into a bun.

The following data reveal that a large minority of the working-age population is superfluous or needed only for unskilled or semi-skilled occupations. In July 2012 the unemployment rate was 8.2 percent. The average rate from 1948 to 2012 was 5.9 percent of the 145 million in the labor force. Some economists predict that the post recession's normal rate of unemployment will be greater than the past normal rate. Combining 11.1 million who are unemployed with 8.2 million who are involuntarily working part time (usually without benefits), and the 2.5 million no longer in the labor force because, while seeking jobs, they have been unsuccessful over a period of a year, the total is 21.8 million. After the recession the number of part timers will probably shrink. It is safe to say, nevertheless, that the American economy does not require the services of about 20 million people.

One of Darling-Hammond's concerns is the fear that the fact that other nations have overtaken America in school achievement threatens its leadership in science. The record shows that the United States remains at the forefront of achievement in science, at least when that is measured by the number of Nobel prizes awarded to American scientists who maintain a tremendous lead over other nations in physics, chemistry, physiology or medicine, and economics. Some change in that should be expected, considering the rise in industrialization, technology, and science in China and, to a lesser extent, in India and Brazil. However, in the foreseeable future the nation's leadership is not threatened. Furthermore, advances in science worldwide should be welcomed, particularly science devoted to improving life for the world's population.

The outlook in the United States for large infusions of resources to improve the failing schools is unfavorable. The hard economic fact is that better education will not increase profit for investors, and it is they, particularly the very rich, who shape American economic and political policy. Darling-Hammond's praiseworthy objective—quality education for all—will be achievable when human values supersede or equal those of profit. And for that to occur, psychologists, other social scientists, and educators who choose to participate in the effort to see those values concretized in America's schools, the history of change in the United States, reported in Part 4, points the way. It shows that profound change came in the past when enormous numbers of Americans coalesced in their demands for change in policy. They did that to gain Social Security in the 30s and the Voting Rights Act and Medicare and Medicaid in the 60s, among other significant legislation that impacted the lives of millions. Although the history is clear, the nation's priorities change only when the public en masse demands it clearly and persistently, so that political leaders see their status dependent on satisfying the demands. Several studies (Small, 1988; Watanabe & Milburn, 1988) suggested the validity of that principle, at least as it applied to the public's demand for the end of the Vietnam War. Those committed to putting an end to the injustice of educational deprivation must create such a mass movement.

This is more difficult than creating mass sentiment against war. Whereas the desire for peace is uniformly national, with relatively few people benefiting from investments in war-related industries, the struggle for educational reform, including an equitable distribution of funds on a per capita basis, has marked differences. National, state, and local interests are involved and regional differences are considerable. The end of a war offers the hope of reductions in military expenditure and perhaps in taxation. A vast expansion in quality of education for at least 20 percent of the nation's children poses the likelihood of an equally vast *increase* in state and local taxation. That could be avoided and offset by major cuts in federal spending, for example, a reduction in the military budget, with the savings distributed to the states and assigned to schools on the basis of need. However, such a rational arrangement would bump up against political realities. When the social-economic classes compete, the higher classes tend to win.

What Needs to Be Done?

The challenge now is to determine what studies, policy statements, organizations, and activism are essential in the long campaign ahead to gain justice through equity in education, broadly defined as beginning at birth. Questions like the following call for answers:

- To what extent do the public, education professionals, and political leaders define education as defined in this chapter, that is, beginning at birth?
- What measures need to be taken to reorient those three groups?
- How can a coalition that supports the redefinition of education and the needed reforms to initiate a just system be formed?

The current state of affairs, particularly the effects of the economic recession and the calls for austerity and "small government," have led to budget reductions, handicapping the schools even more. This does not bode well for equity in the schools in the immediate future, and highlights the need to challenge the status quo and press for the very opposite.

Here is a reasonable agenda for educators, psychologists, and other social scientists to pursue in their various roles:

- Expose as fraudulent any educational program, or proposed program, that does not take into consideration the four major components, namely, parent education, social safety net, nursery and preschool, and suitable, enhanced elementary and secondary schools budgeted in all schools at a level necessary to be equivalent to those in higher social class schools.
- Work for the adoption of the four components, not as if they represented educational or psychological gospel, but because they are the soundest application of current knowledge about parenting, intellectual development, teaching, and schooling from birth onward.
- Work for modified objectives, fully aware that an equitable system of education based on need demands all four components.
- Help create a mass movement; potentially coalescing the many parent, teacher, child welfare, civic, religious and business organizations, foundations, and labor unions, all of which have been concerned with education and the welfare of children and adolescents.
- Draw on theories, research, and tested practices of social psychology, sociology, adult education, and the public media to aid in mobilizing a long-lasting mass movement.
- Recognize the campaign for equitable educational opportunity as a long process, like those described in Part 4, and use professional knowledge to maintain morale in participants.

Questions like the following call for answers:

- Do the public, the education profession, and elected government officials at the national, state, and local levels find acceptable the definition of "education" as it is defined in this chapter, that is, beginning at birth? If not, is their attitude changed after its rationale is explained?
- What measures need to be taken to reorient the diverse stakeholders and especially the potential activists among the general public, who typically constitute the mass in protest movements?

History, as reported in Part 4, predicts that the goal of true equity by achieving the four components will not be easily nor rapidly accomplished. In the meantime supporters of educational justice can work for less ambitious objectives aware, however, that anything less than the complete objectives will be unjust and fail to achieve equality of opportunity and performance. There are no short cuts.

The more modest objectives could, as stated earlier, include one or all of the following: Parent education during pregnancy and the infant's first year; teacher supervision in the form of coaching for a full year; teacher salary increases to avoid rapid turnover; curriculum review and revision to make content relevant to the lives of the students; free preschool for all children of families earning less than double the poverty level.

Achieving these modest goals would be a major accomplishment. It would improve education from birth onward; it would boost the morale of those who worked for its fruition; and it would strengthen the movement for larger gains.

PART 4: ARE THE FOUR COMPONENTS ACHIEVABLE?

The necessary reforms seem so far beyond reach, those committed to change can be discouraged. It is helpful to take note of how Americans in the past confronted with injustices that seemed equally overwhelming and irreversible, carried on nevertheless, made small gains, then larger ones and finally succeeded in gaining their objective.

Social injustice was built into the very origins of the United States. The ringing words of the Declaration of Independence, "All men are created equal," meant at the time that all White men of property were created equal. When the Constitution was approved 13 years later, no more than a third of White men, no Black men and no women were granted the right to vote. White male farmers and artisans fought for that right well into the 19th century, so that most states, though not all, gave them the vote by the time of the Civil War. Black men had to wait until 1870, 94 years after the Declaration of Independence, to win the vote through the 15th Amendment. In the South, however, 20 twenty years after the amendment was passed, they were denied it in practice by means of poll taxes, literacy tests, and physical intimidation applied by such organizations as the Ku Klux Klan. Not until the Voting Rights Act of 1965 did all Black men and, by then, Black women, have suffrage in practice. As to women, more than 140 years passed, including 80 of intense campaigning by resolute suffragettes who were subjected to hostility and imprisonment, before the 19th amendment gave them the vote in 1920.

A century ago, child labor had the imprimatur of the U.S. Supreme Court, allowing children as young as ten, boys and girls, to work in mills and mines, six or even seven days a week for 10 to 12 hours a day. Fifteen years would pass before the court reversed its decision. This victory for humane labor practices in regard to children, and that of the Nineteenth Amendment for voting equality for women, presaged the struggles of the American people and their successes during most of the rest of the 20th century, victories that would change the face of the nation.

During the Great Depression in the 1930s, millions of organized workers, war veterans, and farmers made demands that soon took the form of legislation giving the nation Social Security, unemployment insurance, the Works Progress Administration, Civilian Conservation Corps, and National Youth Administration, which together created jobs for almost 4 million people, while improving the nation's infrastructure and broadening participation in the arts. When World War II began in Europe in 1939, the country was united and transformed itself from its weak industrial base to a mighty producer of war goods for our allies as well as the United States in the fight against fascism.

After the defeat of fascism, the floodgates of independence for colonial people opened wide, and the floodgates at home for the rights of people did the same. And so victories by the Black Liberation movements were followed by those of the Latino, the Native American, the women's, the gay and lesbian, and the physically and mentally challenged. One victory after another shattered substantial elements of the basis for the structural violence to which these people had been subjected. Together, these victories made Americans of 1990 so different in social status from those of 1950. The progress in some of these realms has continued to this day as shown by an unexpected reversal: In 2010 women constituted about 57 percent of all college graduates. Although there have been serious setbacks as well, such as the racist reaction to President Obama's election and the surge in prejudice against Mexican Americans and Muslims, the social reality of oppressed groups has improved, when compared to the not so distant past.

The Power of Mass Movements

The record shows that when the people, mobilized in powerful groups, made their demands known through the policy statements of their organizations and broadcast those demands widely, often through repeated massive demonstrations as well as on election day, they often, though not always, succeeded in electing responsive leaders. With presidents like Franklin D. Roosevelt and Lyndon B. Johnson and the favorable majorities in the Congresses they had elected, victories came in the form of legislation that gave the nation the following: Medicare, Medicaid, the Civil Rights Act of 1964, the Voting Rights Act of 1965, Head Start, the Elementary and Secondary Act (which gives large sums of federal money to states and localities), Title IX (which prohibits institutions receiving federal funds from discrimination based on gender, thereby giving women an equivalent share of funds for intercollegiate sports and spurring their participation in athletics), and the Americans with Disabilities Act (which, parallel to the Civil Rights Act of 1964, prohibits discrimination against people with disabilities). Finally, numerous states have made progress in protecting some rights of gay and lesbian individuals. Collectively, these laws made life much more secure for the vast majority of people. They were victories over social injustice.

This history suggests that chances are favorable that the United States will ultimately move in this direction by action of the public at large. The questions are how that process can be facilitated through the efforts of social scientists and educators. In the struggle to eliminate the injustice of education deprivation, research and policy formulation are essential, but not enough. Research articles in journals on the library shelves, figuratively speaking, turn yellow while their implications for change are underutilized. As American history reveals, social and political action is essential to change the consciousness of the American people and activate them to demand human rights in an egalitarian democracy.

There are plenty of examples of such activism by psychologists, other social scientists, and educators. The American Psychological Association (APA) with a membership of almost 150,000, after much effort on the part of activists, adopted the "Resolution on poverty and socioeconomic status." In 1999, six divisions of the APA, later joined by two more, formed a loose association known as the Social Justice Divisions of the American Psychological Association, and agreed to work together pursuing social justice issues both within APA governance (e.g., working together to appoint social justice–oriented individuals to APA committees; working with the Public Interest Directorate), and in terms of ongoing social justice–related research, action, and public policy.

The American Educational Research Association (AERA), with a membership of over 25, 000, had, as its theme at the 2012 annual meeting: "To know is not enough." The presidential address by Peggy McIntosh was titled "Knowing and Doing: The Transformational Journey of Using Privilege to Weaken Privilege Systems."

Some of the transformations in both the APA and the AERA had their seeds in two activist organizations, both established in 1982. Psychologists for Social Responsibility and Educators for Social Responsibility are committed to action in support of social justice and peace. It could be said about them, that "to know is not enough."

NOTES

1. I am deeply grateful to Robert Schwebel, PhD., for his extraordinary help in the final editing of this chapter.

2. Portions of this chapter were previously published in *Peace and Conflict: Journal of Peace Psychology* (Schwebel, 2011) and are reprinted here with the permission of the American Psychological Association.

REFERENCES

Barnett, A. S. (2010). Universal and targeted programs to preschool education in the United States. *International Journal of Child Care and Educational Policy, 1,* 1–12.

Bloom, B. (1976). *Human development and school learning.* New York, NY: McGraw-Hill.

Braun, H. I. (2005). *Using student progress to evaluate teachers: A primer on value-added models.* Princeton: NJ: Educational Testing Service.

Brigham, C. C. (1923). *A study of American intelligence.* Princeton, NJ: Princeton University.

Brulles, D., & Winebrenner, S. (2011). Maximizing gifted students' potential in the 21st century. *School Administrators.* Retrieved from www.aasa.org/content.aspx?17440

Center for Research on Education Outcomes. (2009). Multiple choice: Charter school performance in 16 states. Stanford, CA: Author. Retrieved from http://credo.stanford.edu/reports/MULTIPLE_CHOICE_CREDO.pdf

Cole, M., & Wertsch, J. V. (1996). *Contemporary implications of Vygotsky and Luria.* Worcester, MA: Clark University Press.

Coles, G. (1987). *The learning mystique: A critical look at learning disabilities.* New York, NY: Pantheon Books.

Coles, G. (2012, August 15). *Gerard Coles: KIPP Schools: Power over evidence.* Retrieved from http://blogs.edweek.org/teachers/living-in-dialogue/2012/08/gerald_coles_kipp_schools_powe.html

Darling-Hammond, L. (2010). *The flat world and education: How America's commitment to equity will determine our future.* New York, NY: Teachers College Press.

DeGruy, J. A. (2005). *Post traumatic slave syndrome: America's legacy of enduring injury and healing.* Oakland, CA: Uptone Press.

Deutsch, M. (1967). *Selected papers of Martin Deutsch and Associates.* New York, NY: Basic Books.

Deutsch, M. (1985). *Distributive juristic: A social-psychological perspective.* New Haven, CT: Yale University Press.

Education Law Center. (2011–2012). *The history of Abbott v. Burke.* Newark, NJ: Author.

Executive Office of the President. (2012, August). *Investing in our future: Returning teachers to the classroom.* Retrieved from http://www.whitehouse.gov/sites/default/files/Investing_in_Our_Future_Report.pdf

Flynn, J. R. (2008). *Where have all the liberals gone? Race, class, and ideals in America.* Cambridge, UK: Cambridge University Press.

Flynn, J. R. (2009) *What is intelligence? Beyond the Flynn Effect.* Cambridge, UK: Cambridge University Press.

Galton, F. (1969/1892). *Hereditary genius.* London, UK: Macmillan.

Geortz, M. E., & Weiss, M. (2009). *Assessing success in school finance litigation: The case of New Jersey.* Education, equity and the law, No. 1. New York, NY: The Campaign for Educational Equity, Teachers College, Columbia University.

Gould, S. J. (1981). *The mismeasure of man.* New York, NY: W. W. Norton.

Gruber, H., & Voneche, H. (1977). *The essential Piaget.* New York, NY: Basic Books.

Hammond, A. L. (Ed.). (1984). *Century of the sciences: Twenty discoveries that changed our lives.* American Association for the Advancement of Science Archives.

Hart, B., & Risley, T. R. (1995). *Meaningful differences in the everyday experiences of American children.* Baltimore, MD: Brookes.

Hunt, J. McV. (1961). *Intelligence and experience.* New York, NY: Ronald Press.

Johnson, K., Posner, S. F., Biermann, J., Cordero, J. F., Atrash, A. K., Parker, C. S., . . . Curtis, M. G. (April 21, 2006). *Recommendations to improve preconception health and health care.* Washington: Centers for Disease Control, 55(RR06); 1–23.

Kamin, L. (1974). *The science and politics of I.Q.* Potomac, MD: Erlbaum.

Kozol, J. (2005). *The shame of the nation.* New York, NY: Crown.

Ministry of Education, Ministry of State for the Development of Human Intelligence. (1982, October). *Development of thinking skills, First International Congress on the programs taking place in Venezuela for the development of human intelligence.* Caracas, VE: Author.

Nickerson, R. S. (1986). Project intelligence: An account and some reflections. In M. Schwebel & C. Maher (Eds.), *Facilitating cognitive development: International perspectives, programs, and practices* (pp. 83–102). New York, NY: Haworth Press.

Nisbet, R. E., Aronson, J., Blair, C., Dickens, W., Flynn, J., Halpern, D. F., Turkheimer, E. (2012). Intelligence: New findings and Theoretical developments. *American Psychologist, 67,* 2, 130–159.

Paul, A. M. (2010). *Origins: How the nine months before birth shape the rest of our lives.* New York, NY: Simon and Schuster.

Piaget, J. (1970). *The science of education and the psychology of the child.* New York, NY: Grossman.

Piaget, J., & Inhelder, B. (1962). *The psychology of the child.* New York, NY: Basic Books.

Reardon, S. (2012). The widening academic achievement between the rich and the poor. *Community Investments, 24*(2), 19–39.

Reardon, S., & Bischoff, K. (2011). Income inequality and income segregation. *American Journal of Sociology, 116*(4), 1092–1153.

Rich, M. (2013). Charter schools are improving, a study says. *New York Times,* 162, 56,178, A15.

Sapon-Slavin, M. (2007). *Widening the circle: The power of inclusive classrooms.* Boston, MA: Beacon.

Schwebel, M. (1968). *Who can be educated?* New York, NY: Grove Press.

Schwebel, M. (1974). The inevitability of ideology in psychological theory. *International Journal of Mental Health, 3,* 4–26.

Schwebel, M. (1986). Facilitating cognitive development. *Prospects, 15,* 155–173. UNESCO. Also in Arabic, Chinese, French, Russian, and Spanish.

Schwebel, M., & Raph, J. (Eds.). (1973). *Piaget in the classroom.* New York, NY: Basic Books. Also British, Dutch, French, Hebrew, Italian, Japanese, Spanish, and Swedish editions.

Scribner, S., & Cole, M. (1981). *The psychology of literacy.* Cambridge, MA: Harvard University Press.

Siegler, R. (1996). *Emerging minds: The process of change in children's thinking.* New York, NY: Oxford University Press.

Small, M. (1988). *Johnson, Nixon and the doves.* New Brunswick, NJ: Rutgers University Press.

Stern, F. R. (1965). *The politics of cultural despair: A study in the rise of Germanic ideology.* New York, NY: Doubleday.

Stoddard, G. D. (1943). *The meaning of intelligence.* New York, NY: Macmillan.

Terman, L. M. (1930). The autobiography of Lewis M. Terman. In C. Murchison (Ed.), *History of psychology in autobiography.* (Vol. 2, pp. 297–331). Worcester, MA: Clark University Press.

Tuddenham, R. D. (1948). Soldiers' intelligence in World War I and II. *American Psychologist, 3,* 54–56.

Vygotsky, L. (1978). *Mind in society: Development of higher psychological processes.* M. Cole, V. John-Steiner, S. Scribner, & E. Souberman (Eds.). Cambridge, MA: Harvard University Press.

Watanabe, P. Y, & Milburn, M. A. (1988). Activism against Armageddon: Some predictions of nuclear-related political behavior. *Political Psychology, 9*(3), 459–470.

Wechsler, D. (1958). *The measurement and appraisal of adult intelligence.* Baltimore, MD: Williams & Wilkins.

Wertsch, J. V. (1985). *Vygotsky and the social formation of mind.* Cambridge, MA: Harvard University Press.

World Bank. (2006). *Social safety nets in OECD countries.* Primer Notes no. 25. Retrieved from http://siteresources.worldbank.org/SAFETYNETSANDTRANSFERS/Resources/281945-1124119303499/SSNPrimerNote25.pdf

Part 2

Disciplines in Psychology

Chapter 7

Social Justice in Counseling and Clinical Psychology

Rebecca L. Toporek and Karen L. Suyemoto

One of the biggest challenges of engaging in social justice work in any discipline or context is that social *in*justice is so extensive, so embedded in societal structures and institutions, in group and interpersonal relationships, and even in the socialization that individuals and communities internalize to create their identities and self-images. Thus, there is much that needs to be addressed within complex intersecting systems and perspectives. This can be daunting, but this also presents (somewhat paradoxically) a possibility for multiple opportunities because there are so many ways to contribute to social justice through counseling and clinical psychology.

By social justice, we mean the equitable distribution of, and access to, all kinds of capital (Goodman et al., 2003; Vasquez, 2012). This would include goods and resources, social capital, knowledge capital, natural capital (e.g., environmental resources and health), and opportunities to develop all of the above. However, this distributive justice is not enough; we must also attend to (1) procedural justice (justice in decision making and process), (2) relational justice, including intrapersonal justice (acting in fairness to and respect of self), and (3) interpersonal justice (treating others with dignity and respect; Prilleltensky, 2012). These additional kinds of justice extend beyond resource access to include humane treatment, respect, integrity, and recognition of the value of every person's worth. A central assumption of this chapter is that distributive justice, procedural justice, and relational justice are all necessary, interrelated, and interdependent: addressing one aspect without the others results in an imbalanced system.

Although the interpersonal aspect of healing pain and promoting health is widely recognized as representative of counseling and clinical practice, the related social justice framework (e.g., relational justice and interpersonal justice) for such practice is not as widely integrated. Furthermore, although social justice affects people at the individual level, and efforts to alleviate the negative effects of injustice at the individual and interpersonal levels are certainly valuable; the promotion of social justice requires an understanding that injustice is a structural issue. In addition, a number of authors have noted that the individual level of service is inadequate to address even individual-level issues resulting from injustice given the great numbers of people in need (Prilleltensky & Nelson, 2002; Vera & Speight, 2003). Therefore, promoting social justice must encompass "actively working to change social institutions, political and economic systems, and governmental structures that perpetuate unfair practices, structures, and policies in terms of accessibility, resource distribution, and human rights" (Fouad, Gerstein & Toporek, 2006, p. 1).

Addressing structural-level concerns can be a challenge for clinical and counseling psychologists, given that these specialties have largely focused on the individual (or small group) level of intervention or service and that many clinicians have entered their professions with a desire to establish meaningful relationships with individuals over time and see change or resolution (Adams, 2007). However, individuals and systems interact and co-create each other. Individuals compose groups and systems, take action to create, maintain, challenge, or change norms and values, and create coalitions and movements to challenge injustice as well as demand and develop just policies and practices. Bronfenbrenner's (1979) ecological model, and variations thereof, reinforces that individuals are always affected by the multiple systems in which they are situated and that these systems are made up of individuals. An ecological model provides a useful framework for this chapter with a particular emphasis not on how people are nested within and influenced by varying levels of interpersonal and structural systems, but instead on how they create and influence the systems of which they are a part (see Figure 7.1). The application of the ecological model illustrates how individuals can promote social justice and intentionally design and enact research, teaching, practice, leadership, and service to change the values, understandings, policies, norms, and identities of the counseling and clinical specialties and the discipline of psychology overall in order to promote social justice.

Figure 7.1
Interactional Ecological Model. Adapted from Bronfenbrenner (1979) and Okun and Suyemoto (2012).

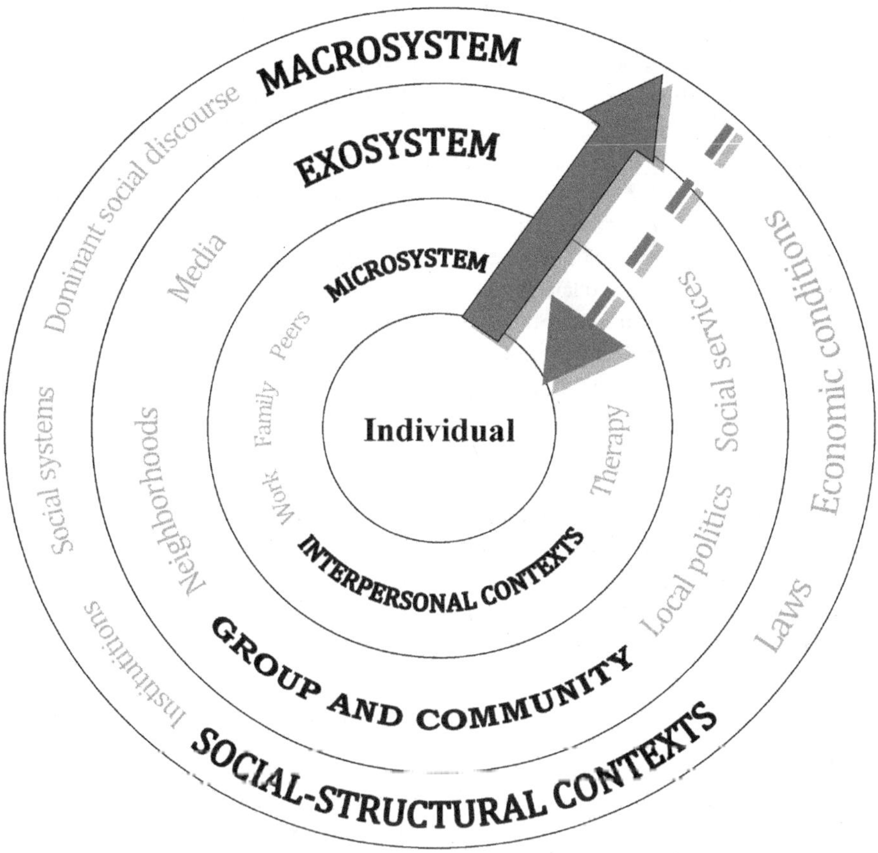

An understanding of the interactive nature of the ecological model rests on a foundation of the individual's awareness and acknowledgment of himself or herself as embedded in the structure, with worldview and actions inherently informed by his or her position in respect to systems of power and privilege. Therefore, as authors we recognize that this chapter reflects not only abstract knowledge but also our own experiences, perspectives, and positionalities, and thus feel compelled to present these positionalities as foundation.

I, Rebecca, am a White, cisgender woman, who grew up in the United States identifying as Canadian and in a family with mental health issues. Growing up, I remember often feeling displaced, an invisible outsider. I was somewhat late in beginning my self-education regarding my place as a person of racial, social class, and ascribed sexual orientation privilege within a sociopolitical structure through my professional and personal journey to develop cultural competence. As a community college counselor, and later as a counseling psychologist, I was repeatedly struck by the inadequacy of counseling theories and approaches that exclusively focused on intrapsychic conceptualizations and interventions. I committed myself to trying to understand and advocate for the role of counselors and counseling psychologists in addressing social justice and systems-level change. I believe there are significant challenges that remain in counseling psychology, perhaps somewhat obscured by the increased visibility of social justice in the profession. I am fortunate to work in a department and university that articulate social justice and multiculturalism as core values and aspirations.

I, Karen, am a multiracial Japanese European Asian American woman. My commitment to social justice is related to personal experiences with oppression based on my race, gender, and sexual orientation as well as to my family experiences, including my father's imprisonment as a teenager in the World War II Japanese American internment camps, my mother's mental illness, and the recognition of my class and educational privilege. My application of that commitment to my professional identity and activities is strongly related to the challenges I faced in graduate school (see Suyemoto, 2006) as a feminist, and as a racial and sexual minority. As a clinical psychologist with a split line appointment in psychology and Asian American studies, I am blessed by being in a clinical psychology doctoral program that embraces a social justice mission. Simultaneously, I have struggled with the relative lack of attention to social justice within the specialty of clinical psychology as a whole, and with my own identity and place as a clinical psychologist given this lack of attention.

RELATION OF COUNSELING AND CLINICAL PSYCHOLOGY TO SOCIAL JUSTICE

Within both clinical and counseling psychology, the emphasis historically has been on promoting well-being and relieving distress. Although these goals are not, in and of themselves, a reflection of social justice, promoting social justice is frequently motivated by authentic empathy leading to a desire to heal the pain and promote the health of individuals, relationships, and society within an ecological model.

This does not mean, however, that counseling and clinical psychology, as formally organized specialties, explicitly recognize this connection or embrace the promotion of social justice as part of their professional organizational identity, or that all counseling and clinical psychologists agree on this perspective. In fact, as with other areas of psychology, there is much within the history and current practices of counseling and clinical psychology that represents ways in which the specialties either have been complacent or have actively supported oppressive systemic injustice (e.g., Kivel, 2007). We acknowledge the history of injustice within these specialties, but for the purpose of this chapter, we will focus on exploring efforts toward justice, current challenges, and strategies influencing the extent to which psychologists in each specialty engage in social justice. There are also differences between counseling and clinical psychology that affect their respective positions in relation to integrating social justice into healing and health promotion as well as the extent to which they integrate social justice as part of their professional identities.

Defining Counseling and Clinical Psychology as Specialties

The Society of Counseling Psychology of the American Psychological Association (2013) defines counseling psychology in the following way:

> Counseling Psychology is a specialty within professional psychology that maintains a focus on facilitating personal and interpersonal functioning across the life span. The specialty pays particular attention to emotional, social, vocational, educational, health-related, developmental, and organizational concerns. The practice of Counseling Psychology encompasses a broad range of culturally-sensitive practices that help people improve their well-being, alleviate distress and maladjustment, resolve crises, and increase their ability to function better in their lives. With its attention to both to [*sic*] normal developmental issues and problems associated with physical, emotional, and mental disorders, the specialization holds a unique perspective in the broader practice-based areas of psychology.

The Society of Clinical Psychology of the American Psychological Association (n.d.) defines clinical psychology in the following way:

> Clinical Psychology integrates science, theory, and practice to understand, predict, and alleviate maladjustment, disability, and discomfort as well as to promote human adaptation, adjustment, and personal development. Clinical Psychology focuses on the intellectual, emotional, biological, psychological, social, and behavioral aspects of human functioning across the life span, in varying cultures, and at all socioeconomic levels. . . . The Clinical Psychologist is educated and trained to generate and integrate scientific and professional knowledge and skills so as to further psychological science, the professional practice of psychology, and human welfare. . . . Their work can range from prevention and early intervention of minor problems of adjustment to dealing with the adjustment and maladjustment of individuals whose disturbance requires them to be institutionalized.

Counseling and clinical specialties clearly have a great deal of overlap as evidenced by the previous descriptions as well as by research comparing the specialties on qualifications of graduate students admitted, training curricula, problems and populations addressed, professional activities, internship placements, and employment settings (Cobb et al., 2004; Morgan & Cohen, 2008; Norcross, 2000; Norcross, Sayette, Mayne, Karg, & Turkson, 1998).

However, this research is also consistent in identifying areas of differentiation, while noting that both specialties have considerable variability. In general, clinical psychology is more closely aligned with a medical model of understanding psychopathology, more severe psychopathology, a focus on pathology, and an emphasis on training, activities, and work placements that reflect these priorities. Counseling psychology is, generally, more closely aligned with a holistic lifespan model encompassing both health and pathology, a greater emphasis on normative human development and wellness, including career development, and an emphasis on training, activities, and placements that reflect these priorities. It is important to note that the specialties of counseling and clinical psychology have their origins in the Western world and in the United States specifically. Although there has been some development of these disciplines and engagement with social justice oriented work throughout the world, it is beyond the scope of this chapter to provide an extensive discussion of the globalization of the disciplines although we will provide examples of social justice engagement later in this chapter.

Developmental Histories: Acknowledging Social Justice Progress in Counseling and Clinical Psychology

Although there is much more work needed to transform clinical and counseling psychology to more closely represent the ideals of social justice, it is important to acknowledge the work that has formed the foundation of these fields. Both have been influenced by civil rights movements generally, and more specifically by movements aimed at rectifying injustice for mental health service consumers and groups targeted by oppression as reflected in feminist psychology, multicultural psychology, LGBT psychology, and the disability and consumer rights movements within psychology. These movements have made significant contributions, including raising consciousness about the impact of power imbalances and discrimination on mental health and therapy, creating models that value rather than denigrate cultural differences, identifying the cultural and power basis of dominant views within the field of psychology, urging psychologists to take action in the face of injustice, and recognizing the rights and strengths of recipients of mental health services (e.g., Adame & Knudson, 2008; Brown, 1992, 1997; Casas, Brady, & Ponterotto, 1983; Division 44/Committee on Lesbian, Gay, and Bisexual Concerns Joint Task Force, 2000; Enns, 1993; Guthrie, 1973; Hahn, 1985; Jones, 1990; Katz, 1985; Kearney, 1979; Melton, 1989; Middleton, Rollins, & Harley, 1999; Sue, Arredondo, & McDavis, 1992; Sue & Sue, 1977; Toldson, 1973; Williams, 1970).

The rise of community psychology has been complementary for many counseling and clinical psychologists who recognize the need to address social problems at a systemic level to address conditions that perpetuate oppression and inequity, for example, prevention and participatory action research (e.g., Evans et al., 2011; Hage & Kenny, 2009; Kenny & Romano, 2009; Smith, Rosenzweig, & Schmidt, 2010). Similarly, the rise of critical psychology has provided a forum for those psychologists who challenge the history and contemporary actions of the field of psychology as well as the specialties, particularly clinical psychology (see Walsh, 1987). Many of the founding psychologists of both community psychology and critical psychology have roots in clinical psychology (e.g., Sarason, 1976). There are also examples of important social justice work being done globally within applied psychology, such as exhumation processes in Latin America (Navarro García, Pérez-Sales, & Fernández-Liria, 2010), the effect of political violence on urban youth in Peru (Saavedra, 2010) and working with political resistance in Chiapas (Santiago Vera, 2007). However, in many cases the scholar's professional specialization is often not specified and thus it is often difficult to discern the extent that this work reflects the specialties of clinical or counseling psychology particularly and may point to a more general orientation toward social justice rather than toward specific professional psychological specialty affiliation. In addition to these general influences, the following is a selective review of several influential forces supporting social justice within each specialty.

Counseling Psychology

Many of the early advocates for institutionalizing cultural competence standards came from counseling psychology (Fouad et al., 2004; Fouad et al., 2006; Kiselica & Robinson, 2001; Sue et al., 1992). Major venues of the profession published articles recognizing civil and human rights advances and the implications for counseling psychologists (e.g., Fitzgerald, 1973; Morin, 1991) and challenged the profession to contribute to these advances (e.g., Katz, 1985; Neville & Carter, 2005). Given counseling psychology's emphasis on vocational issues, it is particularly important to recognize the contributions of Frank Parsons, who advocated for providing employment services for unemployed and underemployed workers at the turn of the century (Shullman, Celeste, & Strickland, 2006), as well as other vocationally related counseling psychologists who have worked to increase equity in employment and educational access. Important legacies also include Leona Tyler's (1972) advocacy for the consideration of social context and Carolyn Payton's (1984) charges to the American Psychological Association regarding the ethical responsibility of the organization to speak out about human rights. Some counseling psychology researchers, such as Janet Helms, have taken findings regarding bias in assessment to the courts (*Ricci et al. v. Destefano et al.*, 2009). In global terms, there are counseling psychologists who have worked collaboratively with members of communities worldwide to address human rights issues, such as political freedom for Tibet (Gerstein & Kirkpatrick, 2006), community organizing (Norsworthy & Khuankaew, 2006), and conflict resolution (Moeschberger, Ordóñez, Shankar, &

Raney, 2006). There are other numerous examples of social justice work by counseling psychologists and organizations to which we refer the reader (see Toporek, Gerstein, Fouad, Roysircar, & Israel, 2006a).

Clinical Psychology

There have been a number of contributions to social justice issues from individual researchers and scholars whose roots come from clinical psychology, although they often did not identify as a clinical psychologist in their social justice work. A brief listing of some concerns addressed include poverty (Sarason, 1978b); access to mental health for marginalized populations (Sue & Sue, 1977); bias and ethnocentric prejudice (Haaken, 1988; Sanford, 1946), violence and dehumanization (Sanford, 1971); mental health consumer rights and activism (Bassman, 2001, 2005); and the sociopolitical foundations of pathology (Marsella, 1993). George Albee (1985) made a compelling case for the need to focus on prevention of psychopathology, stating that "the prevention of psychopathology requires finding ways to redistribute social power and to increase social justice" (p. 7). Some clinical psychologists have examined the role of psychologists in social action (e.g., Hersch, 1969; Sarason, 1978a; Sanford, 1965, 1969, 1970) and challenged psychology to recognize the role of injustice and move the profession toward actively dismantling oppression rather than perpetuating it (e.g., Albee, 1998; Hare-Mustin & Marecek, 1997; Sarason, 1981).

Where Are Counseling and Clinical Psychology Now?

Individual counseling and clinical psychologists have formed entities and coalitions for social justice across disciplines and specialties. The recent handbook, *Advancing Social Justice through Clinical Practice* (Aldarondo, 2007) is an excellent example of work centered on the theme of social justice from scholars, researchers, activists, and educators across the specialties of clinical and counseling psychology as well as from social work and other disciplines.

Despite these advances and collaborative initiatives, there is much work yet to do to centralize social justice within counseling and clinical psychology's organizational identities, expectations of professional roles, training, and activities. Although this is true of both specialties, there are clear developmental differences between them in terms of their current position in relation to promoting social justice. Whereas research indicates that both clinical and counseling programs include multicultural and diversity terms in their program descriptions and recruitment materials (Morgan & Cohen, 2008), counseling psychology faculty are more likely to have research foci on gender, sexual orientation, and racial and ethnic minorities, and counseling programs have a greater number of racial and ethnic minority students (Morgan & Cohen, 2008; Norcross et al., 1998).

In addition, outcome variables such as numbers of published articles in specialty journals, divisional representation/commitment in social justice coalitions, conference sponsoring and programming, and so on, indicate that clinical psychology, as a specialty, does not prioritize social justice as much as counseling psychology does. For example, in the past decade, there have been enormous strides in counseling psychology research and conceptual publications in counseling psychology addressing social justice in prevention and clinical practice (e.g., Blustein, McWhirter, & Perry, 2005; Goodman et al., 2004; Toporek, Gerstein, Fouad, Roysircar, & Israel, 2006b; Vera & Speight, 2003). Moreover, entire issues of major publications in counseling psychology and conferences have been devoted to social justice, for example, Volumes 32(1) and 32(6) of *The Counseling Psychologist* (2004) and Volume 31(3) of *The Counseling Psychologist* (2003). The number of publications addressing social justice *or related issues* in the journals of the APA divisions of counseling and clinical psychology and in APA-published journals specifically focused on counseling or clinical psychology reveals major differences within the specialties (see Table 7.1).

Table 7.1
Social Justice Publications in Counseling and Clinical Psychology from 1992 to 2012

Journal Name	Total Number of Articles	Articles with the Specific Words "Social Justice"	Articles with "Social Justice" or Related Issues in the Title[1]
The Counseling Psychologist (TCP)[2]	577	7.1% ($n = 41$)	19.6% ($n = 113$)
Journal of Counseling Psychology (JCP)[3]	1,101	0.8% ($n = 9$)	19.4% ($n = 214$)
Clinical Psychology: Science and Practice (CPSP)[2]	428	0% ($n = 0$)	1.9% ($n = 8$)
Journal of Consulting and Clinical Psychology (JCCP)[3]	2,487	0% ($n = 0$)	6.6% ($n = 164$)

Table notes: Search results reported in this table and in text resulted from a search performed January 21, 2013. Search settings set "Expanders" (apply related words) to "on."

[1]"Social justice or related issues" searched the following words in the title only: race or racial or ethnic* (e.g., ethnicity, ethnic,) or racism or racist or "sexual orientation" or queer* or lesbian* or gay* or bisexual* or LGBT or GLBT or transgender* or homophobia or heterosexism or gender or sexism or "social class" or classism or poverty or poor or advoca* (advocacy, advocating, advocates) or activis* (e.g. activism or activist) or multicultural or divers* (e.g. diverse or diversity) or "social justice."

[2]*TCP* and *CPSP* are the official journals of Division 17and 12, respectively. These were searched within PsycInfo, including articles from 1994 (when CPSP started) to 2012 and document type was restricted to "journal article."

[3]*JCP* and *JCCP* are APA publications and were searched within PsycArticles, including articles from 1992 to 2012 with book reviews and non-article content excluded.

Organizational examples support this differential emphasis as well. Vasquez (2012) provided an overview of social justice within APA organizationally, including the meaning of social justice, relation to APA mission, history in APA, and individual as well as group exemplars. She described the establishment of the Divisions for Social Justice within APA, which was established at the first National Multicultural Summit, a member-driven conference that incorporates social justice as part of its mission. Notably, Division 17 (the Society of Counseling Psychology) is both a co-host of the summit and a member of the Divisions for Social Justice, while Division 12 (the Society of Clinical Psychology) is neither. Yet, it is still uncertain the extent to which efforts within counseling psychology are actually transformative and challenging of the dominant power systems benefitting from institutional and systemic oppression. The visibility or invisibility of social justice in professional venues does not necessarily mean that all counseling psychologists embrace social justice as part of their professional identities, or that all clinical psychologists do not.

CHALLENGES AND STRATEGIES FOR COUNSELING AND CLINICAL PSYCHOLOGISTS

There is clearly a considerable amount of work yet to be done to address the immensity of injustice. As social justice requires structural and organizational change, we begin this section with a brief overview of some of the challenges for counseling and clinical psychology overall and particularly in relation to professional identity and activities. We then explore challenges and strategies for individuals within counseling and clinical psychology seeking to promote social justice, situated within the ecological model presented earlier that emphasizes how individuals may affect systems.

Organizational-Level Challenges

Although counseling psychology has made visible strides in its attention to social justice advocacy, it should not be assumed that social justice is actually infused into the specialty in all possible ways. A challenge for the specialty is to ensure implementation and resist being placated by words rather than deed. An additional challenge for counseling psychologists is to be conscious of ways that they may communicate a sense of exclusivity with regard to social justice advocacy, implying a hierarchical better-than-thou projection in comparison to other specialties and disciplines. Albeit perhaps unintentionally, comments and implications that suggest that professionals from other specialties do not understand, care, or belong in social justice promotion undermine the goal of advancing social justice in all specialties, all disciplines, and all areas of society. Finally, a challenge for counseling psychology is to look beyond integration of social justice concepts into curriculum and training and consider fundamental ways that power structures within training programs, service delivery, and all aspects of the profession may need to be transformed as agents of change rather than serving as a "buffer zone" (Kivel, 2007, p. 134). The seduction of assuming that the profession integrates social justice can interfere with the praxis needed to ensure continuous reflexivity and action toward justice in practice, research, and training.

For clinical psychology, the current challenge is to move toward a more active embracing of social justice as part of the professional organizational identity. The trend of individual clinical psychologists committed to social justice moving away from being active in clinical psychology and instead investing in community psychology, critical psychology, or multicultural psychology, means that clinical psychology as a specialty is not challenged from within to move forward toward social justice. The result is that the specialty does not change and social justice is situated as something separate and unrelated to clinical psychology. Students entering clinical psychology with a social justice commitment are then not provided with the training necessary for social justice promotion. Instead, they have experiences of being marginalized within their specialty and see models suggesting that clinical psychologists must leave the specialty in order to enact social justice commitments. Developmentally, clinical psychology is arriving at a time in history wherein a critical mass is needed—and available—to act as a catalyst for an evolution of clinical psychology toward social justice promotion. For clinical psychologists who do have social justice commitments, this means a stronger linking of one's identity as a clinical psychologist to that commitment. This does not mean abandoning investments in community, critical, multicultural, or counseling psychology, but it does mean refraining from investing exclusively in these specialties to the detriment of clinical psychology. Clinical psychologists with social justice commitments need to bring their knowledge and skills to clinical psychology, to demand better attention to social justice promotion in training, publications, and professional identity within the specialty.

We turn now to a discussion of challenges and strategies for individuals within counseling and clinical psychology who seek to promote social justice and to contribute to their specialties' social justice actions. We have two primary premises regarding social justice counseling and clinical psychology practice. First, there is a need to work toward integrating individual and community healing with systemic transformation. Second, the role of social justice–oriented clinicians extends beyond the therapy room.

Attending to the Need for Individual and System Change for Healing

Although systems-level transformation is needed within the discipline and the society to address systemic injustice, the important role of counseling and clinical psychologists in healing individuals should not be dismissed. Addressing the pain of oppression, nurturing strengths and resilience, and empowering individuals to resist oppression for themselves and others in their communities have the potential for impact not only at the level of the individual client, but also for the client as a member of a broader community, as someone whose healing contributes to his or her capacity to contribute to social justice himself or herself. As Sloan noted:

> We can work for social justice at many points along a continuum of types of participation. We help people suffering from anxiety or depression to participate in everyday life with others. We help family members build connections with each other and engage with their communities. We support workers in their efforts to speak up for themselves and others in the face of exploitation or racism. And, at the other end of this continuum, we can foster the emergence of leaders among those who are doing well, and sustain them in self-care and in making wise and courageous choices. (personal communication, August 17, 2012)

Helping people who are suffering by providing therapy does not mean helping the individual adapt by accepting oppression; therapy that contributes to social justice reflects transformation, not amelioration (Prilleltensky & Nelson, 2002). Providing transformative services can engage some of the specialized clinical skills counseling and clinical psychologists are trained to use. The emotional and psychological pain experienced by people as a result of injustice is not relieved easily. Clinicians' ability to be present allows them to stay with the person in the moment and validate the pain from oppression, a first step toward resistance.

However, providing psychological service, whether remedial or preventative, is not necessarily synonymous with justice. Counseling and clinical psychologists may be challenged by the tendency to focus primarily on the individual's pain and relieving distress. Although this may be temporarily valuable to the person receiving the service, the extent to which it maintains the problematic system may actually increase pain through delaying or prohibiting justice. With a goal of relieving distress or improving a client's coping mechanisms, well-meaning clinicians may inadvertently facilitate the client in accepting or adapting to oppression without acknowledging or working to confront the source of the distress. Balancing systemic change may be particularly challenging when solutions at the systemic level seem abstract or even invalidating to clients struggling with deeply personal pain. There are times when the client experiencing the injustice may choose not to confront an injustice, while the counseling or clinical psychologist may believe it is in the interest of the larger cause to do so. To push clients to take action that they believe will be harmful or to act for them disempowers them and maintains a hierarchy of power. In such a case, a significant challenge is to determine what is the best action for social justice while maintaining client autonomy.

How can counseling and clinical psychologists promote not only distributive justice but also procedural and relational justice—maintaining respect for the power and context of others, and promoting a process of collaborative decision making? We believe that actively recognizing this challenge as integral to social justice promotion contributes to counseling and clinical psychologists' ability to effectively negotiate this issue. Sometimes, the solution will entail increasing clients' awareness of options and consequences for those who may choose to take systemic action. At other times, justice is best served by focusing on the individual, rather than the system, at a particular moment. Ideally, the ability to be present with individuals and to address their personal pain must be combined with an ecological understanding and social justice agenda to connect the individual and the therapy endeavor to the systemic level in a way that is emotionally and socially meaningful to the client (see, e.g., Gerber, 2007).

This balance is facilitated through principles commonly described in multicultural and feminist therapy, and integrated and articulated by Goodman et al. (2004): (1) self-examination including analysis of one's biases and positionality in relation to power; (2) sharing power within therapy relationships and emphasizing collaboration; (3) giving voice or amplifying voice by facilitating shared community narratives, recognizing the expertise of the client and community, and collaboratively disseminating these voices through scholarship and policy advocacy; (4) consciousness raising, which relates to helping clients and communities understand systems of oppression and their effects; (5) focusing on strengths such as the skills and expertise clients and communities have to affect social justice; and (6) fostering the development of tools and skills for continuing healing and social justice without the presence of the therapist or psychologist. An additional resource is Harro's (2000) cycle of liberation, portraying a core of mental health, self-acceptance, and growth and outlining a cycle of empowering self, reaching out to others, building community, taking action, and maintaining personal and structural gains. This is a model both for considering how to see therapy as capacity building for clients as social justice agents and for considering how, as a counseling or clinical psychologist, one might connect the personal with the interpersonal and with the systemic through action.

The challenge of integrating individual healing with structural transformation is a continual process, rather than a particular attitude or achievement. Thus, it brings up the second major challenge for counseling and clinical psychologists committed to social justice action: how to stay the course while advocating within systems.

STAYING THE COURSE: CENTERING COMMUNITY, WORKING POSITIONALITY, AND NEGOTIATING SYSTEMS

As noted earlier, psychologists committed to social justice may need to work from a framework that is larger than the daily lived experience of individuals. This can contribute to a feeling of disconnection from people or issues at the base of their social justice commitment. One strategy to meet this challenge is to stay close to the storied experience of the individuals within this larger framework, remembering that understanding how policies or institutions create patterns of injustice is linked to hearing the pain of clients and research participants.

Staying close to the people means resisting the challenge of a sense of self-righteousness and particularly resisting the challenge of thinking that one's own perspective is right because of one's power or position. This is even more challenging when power is earned—for example, when one has worked hard for a long time to promote social justice and so feels somewhat entitled to judge what is the best course of action. But procedural and relational justice require a collaborative process, engaging an active process of empathy and perspective taking that takes advantage of clinicians' training.

This process and the meaning of staying close to the people are inevitably influenced by one's own positionality. Awareness of one's own worldview, culture, and experiences with privilege and oppression is necessary for basic cultural competence and effective social justice work. Constant and active reflection on how one's own sociopolitical identities, privileges, and professional socialization influence values, conceptualization, interventions, and strategies help to protect against complacency and erosion of commitment. Recognition of one's own intersectionality—places where one is relatively privileged as well as relatively oppressed—helps maintain empathy for other's resistance and others' pain.

Members of dominant groups are often presented with challenges from their own socialization and ongoing pressure to be oblivious to the privilege from which they benefit. Furthermore, they may have difficulty fully understanding the pain of daily invalidation and oppression. Although people holding privileged identities may face consequences that are often less penalizing than active oppression, they may experience ostracism from their own families and communities because of their social justice advocacy. Clinicians who experience oppression due to their own marginalized status in a culturally hierarchical society are often presented with challenges related to healing from their own pain. Although taking action against oppression and facilitating others' healing processes may contribute to this personal healing, these actions may also catalyze dissonance, pain, or retraumatization, requiring ongoing work (see, e.g., Ahluwalia, 2011). Given the presence of daily aggression toward members of oppressed groups, this is an ongoing process. In addition, it is important to note that individuals reflect a complex weaving of multiple dimensions of identity, often blending both privileged and oppressed statuses and encountering aspects of all of these challenges.

For those working from outside, who do not share the statuses or experiences of oppression that are central to the social justice issue(s) being addressed, there are often specific challenges of credibility, and the need to nondefensively meet the well-grounded questions and doubts frequently presented to those with relative privilege (Hardy & Laszloffy, 2002, p. 587). However, the more difficult challenges are frequently insidious and involve societal-level structures and generational reinforcement of separation and privilege. For example, as a person often differing in socioracial, educational, and economic privilege relative to certain communities with whom I (Rebecca) collaborate, it is necessary for me to constantly examine how I may be imposing my relative privilege and how I may not hear critical voices and experiences because of my socialization.

Those who are positioned as a part of the community affected most directly by the social justice issue may find it easier to stay close to the community in some ways, but other challenges arise. Community members may have specific expectations or judgments of those who are seen as an insider, and, similar to an outsider, one must be continually aware of the impact of intersecting statuses (e.g., the meaning of being a middle-class, educated Asian American within a group of people of color). In addition to the challenges Rebecca described related to attention to imposing privilege, I (Karen) have experienced additional challenges related to working through the pain of being oppressed in similar ways as the community, negotiating my own internalized oppression, and negotiating the ways that communities may enact oppression in other areas (e.g., homophobia within the Asian American community), which is particularly difficult to encounter when one is depending on the safe space of the insider.

Because counseling and clinical psychology have originated with a Western worldview, psychologists from these disciplines who are engaged in international social justice work must be particularly cognizant of the potential for perpetuating colonization and be very deliberate in collaboration and power sharing (Horne & Mathews, 2006; Norsworthy & Khuankaew, 2006). This process is complex given the considerable disparity of resources as well as social and political capital when Western psychologists are working with international communities that are historically, economically, and politically oppressed.

Staying the course is additionally challenged by the systems and contexts within which counseling and clinical psychologists work. An additional challenge to staying the course is the circumstance of confronting unjust systems when the work is often funded or made possible by these same systems. In the practice realm, reliance on a medical model that necessitates a "sick patient" and a service provider who is paid based on individual services rendered maintains a system prioritizing individual amelioration rather than systemic transformation. Helms (2003) highlighted this in her discussion of pragmatic issues for counseling psychologists pursuing social justice and emphasized that when social justice is primarily a pro bono activity, the extent to which counseling psychologists, or other professionals, can sustain this work over time is limited. Consequently, social justice work is not validated structurally, and systems are not challenged to consider the ways in which they may be perpetuating injustice. Furthermore, individuals can only sustain pro bono work so long as they have the personal resources to do so.

In research and scholarship, similar challenges exist, as psychologists with social justice commitments must survive within structurally biased systems in order to continue their professional activities. The discipline of psychology has a particular epistemological stance, wherein knowledge based on experimental methods aimed at establishing causality and generalizability to an assumed-to-be homogeneous population is most valued. Such positivistic methods have also been criticized for their lack of attention to social justice values (e.g., Lather, 1991; Prilleltensky, 1997). In contrast, constructivist, qualitative, participatory action, and community-based research methods have been cited as highly congruent with social justice goals (Smith et al., 2010). Clinical psychology, in particular, has continued a strong commitment to a positivist and quantitative research practice that has resulted in very limited acceptance of participatory or democratic research practices. Both clinical and counseling psychologists encounter barriers to advancing social justice agendas situated within the system of publications and privileged voice; social justice–related research is more frequently published in multicultural or counseling journals rather than in what are considered more mainstream journals. This means that research focused on social justice is less likely to be read by the audiences that maintain (unintentionally or intentionally) an oppressive status quo within the discipline.

Furthermore, university tenure committees, grant reviewers, and journal editors in the discipline who adhere to a positivist view of science may not see the methods most appropriate to social justice research as acceptable. In addition, even though counseling psychology as a specialty has increasingly honored participatory and qualitative research, Kidd and Kral (2005) note that because of the investment of time required, these methods may not provide a researcher faculty member with the number of publications required for tenure or advancement. Finally, these issues are made even more complex and burdensome if one is a member of an oppressed group, because the act of acquiescing to methods that are more oppressive in order to publish and obtain tenure is tantamount to colluding in one's own oppression.

There is a constant negotiation of advocacy for social justice balanced against the need for professional survival in order to maximize the effects of that advocacy. Furthermore, privilege is not only related to social statuses but also to access to supports and training for promoting social justice. Working positionality also means having empathy for those who may have social justice intentions but who may work within particularly hostile or oppressive systems and thus may need support to move to action. This empathy itself becomes action through developing relationships and coalitions that foster social justice and make space for training, mentoring, and supporting others who have social justice intentions and commitments.

RELATIONSHIPS AND COALITION BUILDING FOR MAINTAINING PERSONAL SANITY AND PROMOTING SOCIAL JUSTICE

A major challenge in working for social justice in any discipline or specialty is maintaining one's own health and well-being. Counseling and clinical psychologists working to develop as advocates to resist oppression related to their own identities or communities may be particularly vulnerable if professionally isolated. Confronting or coping with daily microaggressions and macroaggressions requires a tremendous amount of psychological and physical energy (Sue, 2010). Building personal relations with like-minded people is one strategy for maintaining well-being. For those resisting their own oppression, such relationships can offer a safe space for respite, where one can relax the constant vigilance and preparedness to deal with microaggressions in professional interactions. For those resisting their own oppression as well as those with relative privilege, sustaining relationships can provide a touchstone of reality: validation for experiences that others may minimize or ignore and support for emotional responses of anger, pain, frustration, and exhaustion. These relationships provide a balance of encouragement and challenge: renewal of hope by seeing change, reminders of the importance of self-care in the constant moments of struggling with feeling that one is never doing enough, as well as encouragement to continually question how one's own actions are actually promoting social justice.

Such relationships also contribute to the awareness and skills necessary to promote social justice. In developing as an ally in areas of relative privilege, these relationships are often catalysts to explore areas of injustice that may be less personally salient. For those with complex intersections of privilege and oppression, these relationships can provide an environment that validates and supports the working through the pain of one's oppression, enabling one to be vulnerable and acknowledging areas of relative privilege without threat of invalidation or hostility (Vasquez & McGraw, 2005).

Although these relationships are essential to staying the course, the challenge is knowing how to develop such relationships. Some counseling and clinical psychologists will have the gift of training in programs with mentors and peers who share their social justice commitment and will therefore have naturally developing sustaining relationships embedded in their professional development. However, many will not and may feel isolated, disconnected, and struggle to maintain their commitment to social justice or question their choice of profession and training. Although there are no easy answers, our experience suggests that getting involved in social justice initiatives and organizational service and leadership can be an effective strategy for building and sustaining relationships and gaining knowledge and skills.

This kind of involvement can seem daunting, however, particularly to graduate students or young professionals; those whose cultural styles of communication, service, or leadership are different than that commonly represented within psychological organizations; or those who feel marginalized or different within these advocacy groups (e.g., because of additional minority statuses such as being lesbian *and* a person of color, or because one is not a member of the oppressed group that brings the initiative together). This is a moment to stretch beyond one's comfort zone, to step up to a task, propose an initiative to address a need, ask for help or guidance from others to help make it a success, and trust that one has something valuable to offer. Organizational involvement is a strategy for using already established systems to access communities of people brought together because of similar social justice commitments in order to overcome the isolation that makes it so difficult to maintain these commitments within the discipline.

Reaching beyond one's own specialty or discipline is an additional strategy for building relationships and coalitions. Collaborating with others whose training focuses on systems-level interventions can help increase effectiveness toward the balance of individual- and systems-level interventions. Academic disciplines such as women's studies, ethnic studies, queer studies, and public health often have active central missions related to social justice. Community or advocacy organizations focused on serving marginalized communities outside the discipline of psychology may also have such missions.

Given the similarities of counseling and clinical psychology as well as the different strengths and opportunities that each can offer in promoting social justice, we also propose that a stronger coalition between these specialties, as organizational units (rather than individual relationships), is needed at this developmental juncture. This kind of collaboration may help to confront territoriality that may be present as well as strengthen social justice commitment and action in the discipline of psychology more broadly.

CALL TO ACTION

In sum, we suggest that the major challenge within both counseling and clinical specialties in psychology is to address resistance, collusion, or passive acceptance of injustice within these specialties as well as within the discipline of psychology and related structures (e.g., universities, health policies, service organizations). As specialties within psychology concerned with promoting mental health and healing, counseling and clinical psychology must make progress toward integrating social justice into the very meaning of the specialties.

> [U]nlike other participants in our society, mental health professionals have proclaimed a commitment not only to witness and decrease human suffering, but also to promote human values of equality and justice. And, our ability to fulfill this commitment is constantly being tested. . . . (Aldarondo, 2007, p. 5)

Social justice cannot be an add-on or simply an aspirational commitment within the specialties of counseling or clinical psychology. Without integrating social justice into the fabric of the specialties, there is a risk of confirming the view of mental health practice and research as "encompassing the use of social power and functioning as a handmaiden of the status quo" (Sue & Sue, 1999, p. 71). An ecological model of reciprocal influence emphasizes that systems—including psychological specialties—are made up of individuals. The responsibility for the values, policies, practices, and effects of these systems is therefore within each and every individual. Large-scale change, the type needed to address systemic injustice, takes time and energy, particularly given the inherent resistance both on the part of those who benefit from the current system and on the part of those who have come to ascribe to its existence. Our call to action for counseling and clinical specialties is for the individuals and organizations to consider how their actions can transform these professional specialties to contribute to social justice. It is critical to take up the call, to act, individually, systemically, and as a community devoted to health and justice.

Authors note: The authors wish to thank Fanny Ng for her help with the ecological model figure (Figure 7.1).

REFERENCES

Adame, A. L., & Knudson, R. M. (2008). Recovery and the good life: How psychiatric survivors are revisioning the healing process. *Journal of Humanistic Psychology, 48*(2), 142–164. doi: 10.1177/0022167807305544

Adams, E. M. (2007). Moving from contemplation to preparation: Is counseling psychology ready to embrace culturally responsive prevention? *The Counseling Psychologist, 35*(6), 840–849. doi: 10.1177/0011000007304596

Ahluwalia, M. K. (2011). Holding my breath: The experience of being Sikh after 9/11. *Traumatology, 17*(3), 41–46. doi: 10.1177/1534765611421962

Albee, G. (1985). The contributions of clinical psychology to strategies for the primary prevention of psychopathology. *Bulletin of the Hong Kong Psychological Society*, 157–23.

Albee, G. W. (1998). Fifty years of clinical psychology: Selling our soul to the devil. *Applied & Preventive Psychology, 7*(3), 189–194. doi: 10.1016/S0962-1849(05)80021-6

Aldarondo, E. (2007). Rekindling the reformist spirit in the mental health professions. In E. Aldarondo (Ed.), *Advancing social justice through clinical practice* (pp. 3–17). Mahwah, NJ: Lawrence Erlbaum Associates Publishers.

Bassman, R. (2001). Whose reality is it anyway? Consumers/survivors/ex-patients can speak for themselves. *Journal of Humanistic Psychology, 41*(4), 11–35. doi: 10.1177/0022167801414002

Bassman, R. (2005). Mental illness and the freedom to refuse treatment: Privilege or right. *Professional Psychology: Research and Practice, 36*(5), 488–497. doi: 10.1037/0735-7028.36.5.488

Blustein, D. L., McWhirter, E., & Perry, J. C. (2005). An emancipatory communitarian approach to vocational development theory, research, and practice. *The Counseling Psychologist, 33*(2), 141–179. doi: 10.1177/0011000004272268

Brown, L. S. (1992). While waiting for the revolution: The case for a lesbian feminist psychotherapy. *Feminism & Psychology, 2*(2), 239–253. doi: 10.1177/095935359222012

Brown, L. S. (1997). The private practice of subversion: Psychology as Tikkun Olam. *American Psychologist, 52*(4), 449–462. doi: 10.1037/0003-066X.52.4.449

Casas, J., Brady, S., & Ponterotto, J. G. (1983). Sexual preference biases in counseling: An information processing approach. *Journal of Counseling Psychology, 30*(2), 139–145. doi: 10.1037/0022-0167.30.2.139

Cobb, H. C., Reeve, R. E., Shealy, C. N., Norcross, J. C., Schare, M. L., Rodolfa, E. R., . . . Allen, M. (2004). Overlap among clinical, counseling, and school psychology: Implications for the profession and combined-integrated training. *Journal of Clinical Psychology, 60*(9), 939–955. doi: 10.1002/jclp.20028

Division 44 Committee on Lesbian, Gay, and Bisexual Concerns Joint Task Force on Guidelines for Psychotherapy with Lesbian, Gay, and Bisexual Clients. Guidelines for psychotherapy with lesbian, gay, and bisexual clients (2000). *American Psychologist, 55*(12), 1440–1451. doi: 10.1037/0003-066X.55.12.1440

Enns, C. Z. (1993). Twenty years of feminist counseling and therapy: From naming biases to implementing multifaceted practice. *The Counseling Psychologist, 21*(1), 3–87. doi: 10.1177/0011000093211001

Evans, S. D., Prilleltensky, O., McKenzie, A., Prilleltensky, I., Nogueras, D., Huggins, C., & Mescia, N. (2011). Promoting strengths, prevention, empowerment, and community change through organizational development: Lessons for research, theory, and practice. *Journal of Prevention & Intervention in the Community, 39*(1), 50–64. doi: 10.1080/10852352.2011.530166

Fitzgerald, L. E. (1973). Women's changing expectations: New insights, new demands. *The Counseling Psychologist, 4*(1), 90–95. doi: 10.1177/001100007300400109

Fouad, N. A., Gerstein, L. H., & Toporek, R. L. (2006). Social justice and counseling psychology in context. In R. L. Toporek, L. H. Gerstein, N. A. Fouad, G. Roysircar, & T. Israel (Eds.), *Handbook for social justice in counseling psychology: Leadership, vision, and action* (pp. 1–16). Thousand Oaks, CA: Sage Publications. doi: 10.4135/9781412976220.n1

Fouad, N. A., McPherson, R. H., Gerstein, L., Blustein, D. L., Elman, N., Helledy, K., & Metz, A. J. (2004). Houston, 2001: Context and Legacy. *The Counseling Psychologist, 32*(1), 15–77. doi: 10.1177/0011000003259943

Gerber, L. A. (2007). Social justice concerns and clinical practice. In E. Aldarondo (Ed.), *Advancing social justice through clinical practice* (pp. 43–61). Mahwah, NJ: Lawrence Erlbaum Associates Publishers.

Gerstein, L. H., & Kirkpatrick, D. (2006). Nonviolent activism: Independence for Tibet! In R. L. Toporek, L. H. Gerstein, N. A. Fouad, G. Roysircar, T. Israel (Eds.), *Handbook for social justice in counseling psychology: Leadership, vision, and action* (pp. 442–471). Thousand Oaks, CA: Sage Publications.

Goodman, L. A., Liang, B., Helms, J. E., Latta, R. E., Sparks, E., & Weintraub, S. R. (2004). Training counseling psychologists as social justice agents: Feminist and multicultural principles in action. *The Counseling Psychologist, 32*(6), 793–837. doi: 10.1177/0011000004268802

Haaken, J. (1988). Field dependence research: A historical analysis of a psychological construct. *Signs, 13*(2), 311–330. doi: 10.1086/494408

Hage, S. M., & Kenny, M. E. (2009). Promoting a social justice approach to prevention: Future directions for training, practice, and research. *The Journal of Primary Prevention, 30*(1), 75–87. doi: 10.1007/s10935-008-0165-5

Hahn, H. (1985). Disability policy and the problem of discrimination. *American Behavioral Scientist, 28*(3), 293–319. doi: 10.1177/000276485028003002

Hardy, K.V., & Laszloffy, T.A. (2002). Couple therapy using a multicultural perspective. In A. S. Gurman & N.S. Jacobson (Eds.), *Clinical Handbook of couple therapy* (3rd ed., pp. 569–593). New York: Guilford Press.

Hare-Mustin, R. T., & Marecek, J. (1997). Abnormal and clinical psychology: The politics of madness. In D. Fox, & I. Prilleltensky (Eds.), *Critical psychology: An introduction* (pp. 104–120). Thousand Oaks, CA: Sage Publications.

Harro, B. (2000). Cycle of socialization. In M. Adams, W. J. Blumenfeld, R. Castañeda, H. W. Hackman, M. L. Peters, & X. Zúñiga (Eds.), *Readings for diversity and social justice:*

An anthology on racism, anti-Semitism, sexism, heterosexuism, ableism, and classism (pp. 15–20). New York, NY: Routledge.

Helms, J. E. (2003). A pragmatic view of social justice. *The Counseling Psychologist, 31*(3), 305–313. doi: 10.1177/0011000003031003006

Hersch, C. (1969). From mental health to social action: Clinical psychology in historical perspective. *American Psychologist, 24*(10), 909–916. doi: 10.1037/h0028891

Horne, S. G., & Mathews, S. S. (2006). A social justice approach to international collaborative consultation. In R. L. Toporek, L. H. Gerstein, N. A. Fouad, G. Roysircar, & T. Israel (Eds.), *Handbook for social justice in counseling psychology: Leadership, vision, and action* (pp. 388–405). Thousand Oaks, CA: Sage Publications.

Jones, J. M. (1990). Invitational address: Who is training our ethnic minority psychologists, and are they doing it right? In G. Stricker, E. Davis-Russell, E. Bourg, E. Duran, W. Hammond, J. McHolland, . . . B. E. Vaughn (Eds.), *Toward ethnic diversification in psychology education and training* (pp. 17–34). Washington, DC: American Psychological Association. doi: 10.1037/10071-002

Katz, J. H. (1985). The sociopolitical nature of counseling. *The Counseling Psychologist, 13*(4), 615–624. doi: 10.1177/0011000085134005

Kearney, H. R. (1979). Feminist challenges to the social structure and sex roles. *Psychology of Women Quarterly, 4*(1), 16–31. doi: 10.1111/j.1471-6402.1979.tb00696.x

Kenny, M. E., & Romano, J. L. (2009). Promoting positive development and social justice through prevention: A legacy for the future. In M. E. Kenny, A. M. Horne, P. Orpinas, & L. E. Reese (Eds.), *Realizing social justice: The challenge of preventive interventions* (pp. 17–35). Washington, DC: American Psychological Association. doi: 10.1037/11870-001

Kidd, S. A., & Kral, M. J. (2005). Practicing participatory action research. *Journal of Counseling Psychology, 52*(2), 187–195. doi: 10.1037/0022-0167.52.2.187

Kiselica, M. S., & Robinson, M. (2001). Bringing advocacy counseling to life: The history, issues, and human dramas of social justice work in counseling. *Journal of Counseling & Development, 79*(4), 387–397. doi: 10.1002/j.1556-6676.2001.tb01985.x

Kivel, P. (2007). Social service or social change? In INCITE! Women of Color against Violence (Eds.), *The revolution will not be funded: Beyond the non-profit industrial complex* (pp. 129–149), Cambridge, MA: South End Press.

Lather, P. (1991). *Getting smart: Feminist research and pedagogy with/in the postmodern.* New York, NY: Routledge.

Marsella, A. J. (1993). Sociocultural foundations of psychopathology: An historical overview of concepts, events and pioneers prior to 1970. *Transcultural Psychiatric Research Review, 30*(2), 97–142. doi: 10.1177/136346159303000201

Melton, G. B. (1989). Public policy and private prejudice: Psychology and law on gay rights. *American Psychologist, 44*(6), 933–940. doi: 10.1037/0003-066X.44.6.933

Middleton, R. A., Rollins, C. W., & Harley, D. A. (1999). The historical and political context of the civil rights of persons with disabilities: A multicultural perspective for counselors. *Journal of Multicultural Counseling and Development, 27*(2), 105–120.

Moeschberger, S. L., Ordóñez, A., Shankar, J. & Raney, S. (2006). Moving from contact to change: The act of becoming aware. In R. L. Toporek, L. H. Gerstein, N. A. Fouad, G. Roysircar, & T. Israel (Eds.), *Handbook for social justice in counseling psychology: Leadership, vision, and action* (pp. 472–486). Thousand Oaks, CA: Sage Publications.

Morgan, R. D., & Cohen, L. M. (2008). Clinical and counseling psychology: Can differences be gleaned from printed recruiting materials? *Training and Education in Professional Psychology, 2*(3), 156–164. doi: 10.1037/1931-3918.2.3.156

Morin, S. F. (1991). Removing the stigma: Lesbian and gay affirmative counseling. *The Counseling Psychologist, 19*(2), 245–247. doi: 10.1177/0011000091192009

Navarro García, S., Pérez-Sales, P. & Fernández-Liria, A. (2010). Exhumation processes in fourteen Latin American countries. *Journal for Social Action in Counseling and Psychology, 2*(2), 48–83.

Neville, H. A., & Carter, R. T. (2005). Race and racism in counseling psychology research, training, and practice: A critical review, current trends, and future directions. *The Counseling Psychologist, 33*(4), 413–418.

Norcross, J. C. (2000). Clinical versus counseling psychology: What's the diff? *Eye on Psi Chi, 5*(1), 20–22.

Norcross, J. C., Sayette, M. A., Mayne, T. J., Karg, R. S., & Turkson, M. A. (1998). Selecting a doctoral program in professional psychology: Some comparisons among PhD counseling, PhD clinical, and PsyD clinical psychology programs. *Professional Psychology: Research and Practice, 29*(6), 609–614. doi: 10.1037/0735-7028.29.6.609

Norsworthy, K. L., & Khuankaew, O. (2006). Bringing social justice to international practices of counseling psychology. In R. L. Toporek, L. H. Gerstein, N. A. Fouad, G. Roysircar, & T. Israel (Eds.), *Handbook for social justice in counseling psychology: Leadership, vision, and action* (pp. 421–441). Thousand Oaks, CA: Sage Publications.

Okun, B. F., & Suyemoto, K. L. (2012). *Conceptualization and Treatment Planning for Effective Helping.* Belmont, CA: Cengage.

Payton, C. (1984). Who must do the hard things? *American Psychologist, 39,* 391–397. doi: 10.1037/0003-066X.39.4.391

Prilleltensky, I. (1997). Values, assumptions, and practices: Assessing the moral implications of psychological discourse and action. *American Psychologist, 52*(5), 517–535. doi: 10.1037/0003-066X.52.5.517

Prilleltensky, I. (2012). Wellness as fairness. *American Journal of Community Psychology, 49*(1–2), 1–21. doi: 10.1007/s10464-011-9448-8

Prilleltensky, I., & Nelson, G. (2002). *Doing psychology critically: Making a difference in diverse settings.* New York, NY: Palgrave Macmillan.

Ricci et al. v. Destefano et al., No. 07–1428 (2009, June 29). Retrieved from http://www.supremecourt.gov/search.aspx?Search=RICCI+ET+AL.+v.+DESTEFANO+ET+AL.&type=Site

Saavedra, C. (2010). *Algunas Veces el Polvo Está en Nuestros Ojos, No Afuera:* Dificultades y logros de una intervención de orientación psicoanalítica con niños en un barrio urbano-marginal de Lima, *Journal for Social Action in Counseling and Psychology, 2*(2), 124–144.

Sanford, R. (1946). Identification with the enemy: A case study of an American Quisling. *Journal of Personality, 15,* 53–58. doi: 10.1111/j.1467-6494.1946.tb01050.x

Sanford, N. (1965). Will psychologists study human problems? *American Psychologist, 20*(3), 192–202. doi: 10.1037/h0022184

Sanford, N. (1969). Research with students as action and education. *American Psychologist, 24*(5), 544–546. doi: 10.1037/h0037805

Sanford, N. (1970). Whatever happened to action research? *Journal of Social Issues, 26*(4), 3–23. doi: 10.1111/j.1540-4560.1970.tb01740.x

Sanford, N. (1971). Dehumanization and collective destructiveness. *International Journal of Group Tensions, 1*(1), 26–41.

Santiago Vera, C. (2007). La Mirada Psicosocial en un Contexto de Guerra Integral de Desgaste: Chiapas. *Journal for Social Action in Counseling and Psychology, 1*(1), 14–28.

Sarason, S. B. (1976). Community psychology, networks, and Mr. Everyman. *American Psychologist, 31*(5), 317–328. doi: 10.1037/0003-066X.31.5.317

Sarason, S. B. (1978a). The nature of problem solving in social action. *American Psychologist, 33*(4), 370–380. doi: 10.1037/0003-066X.33.4.370

Sarason, S. B. (1978b). An unsuccessful war on poverty? *American Psychologist, 33*(9), 831–839. doi: 10.1037/0003-066X.33.9.831

Sarason, S. B. (1981). An asocial psychology and a misdirected clinical psychology. *American Psychologist, 36*(8), 827–836. doi: 10.1037/0003-066X.36.8.827

Shullman, S. L., Celeste, B. L., & Strickland, T. (2006). Extending the Parsons legacy: Applications of counseling psychology in pursuit of social justice through the development of public policy. In R. L. Toporek, L. H. Gerstein, N. A. Fouad, G. Roysircar, & T. Israel (Eds.), *Handbook for social justice in counseling psychology: Leadership, vision, and action* (pp. 499–513). Thousand Oaks, CA: Sage Publications. doi: 10.4135/9781412976220.n33

Smith, L., Rosenzweig, L., & Schmidt, M. (2010). Best practices in the reporting of participatory action research: Embracing both the forest and the trees. *The Counseling Psychologist, 38*(8), 1115–1138. doi: 10.1177/0011000010376416

Society of Clinical Psychology of the American Psychological Association. (n.d.). About clinical psychology. *American Psychological Association, Division 12: Society of Clinical Psychology.* Retrieved from http://www.apa.org/divisions/div12/aboutcp.html

Society of Counseling Psychology of the American Psychological Association. (2013). What is counseling psychology. *Society of Counseling Psychology: American Psychological Association, Division 17.* Retrieved from http://www.div17.org/students_defining .html

Sue, D. (2010). *Microaggressions in everyday life: Race, gender, and sexual orientation.* Hoboken, NJ: John Wiley & Sons Inc.

Sue, D. W., Arredondo, P., & McDavis, R. J. (1992). Multicultural counseling competencies and standards: A call to the profession. *Journal of Counseling & Development, 70*(4), 477–486. doi: 10.1002/j.1556-6676.1992.tb01642.x

Sue, D. W., & Sue, D. (1977). Ethnic minorities: Failures and responsibilities of the social sciences. *Journal of Non-White Concerns in Personnel & Guidance, 5*(3), 99–106. doi: 10.1002/j.2164-4950.1977.tb00074.x

Suyemoto, K. L. (2006). Processes of emergence and connection: Interrelations of past, present, and future in journeying for *conocimiento*. *Human Architecture: Journal of the Sociology of Self-Knowledge, 4,* 339–346.

Toldson, I. L. (1973). The human potential movement and black unity: Counseling Blacks in groups. *Journal of Non-White Concerns in Personnel & Guidance, 1*(2), 69–76. doi: 10.1002/j.2164-4950.1973.tb00145.x

Toporek, R. L., Gerstein, L. H., Fouad, N. A., Roysircar, G. S., & Israel, T. (Eds.). (2006a). *Handbook for social justice in counseling psychology: Leadership, vision, and action.* Thousand Oaks, CA: Sage Publications.

Toporek, R. L., Gerstein, L. H., Fouad, N. A., Roysircar, G. S., & Israel, T. (2006b). Future directions for counseling psychology: Enhancing leadership, vision, and action in social justice. In R. L. Toporek, L. Gerstein, N. A. Fouad, G. S. Roysircar, & T. Israel (Eds.) *Handbook for social justice in counseling psychology: Leadership, vision, & action* (pp. 531–552). Thousand Oaks, CA: Sage

Tyler, L. E. (1972). Reflections on counseling psychology. *The Counseling Psychologist, 3*(4, Pt. 2), 6–11. doi: 10.1177/001100007200300403

Vasquez, H., & McGraw, S. (2005). Building relationships across privilege: Becoming an ally in the therapeutic relationship. In M. Mirkin, K. L. Suyemoto, & B. Okun (Eds.) *Psychotherapy with women: Exploring diverse contexts and identities* (pp. 64–86). New York: Guilford Press.

Vasquez, M. J. T. (2012). Psychology and social justice: Why we do what we do. *American Psychologist, 67,* 337–346. doi: 10.1037/a0029232

Vera, E. M., & Speight, S. L. (2003). Multicultural competence, social justice, and counseling psychology: Expanding our roles. *The Counseling Psychologist, 31*(3), 253–272. doi: 10.1177/0011000003031003001

Walsh, R. T. (1987). A social historical note on the formal emergence of community psychology. *American Journal of Community Psychology, 15*(5), 523–529. doi: 10.1007/BF00929906

Williams, R. L. (1970). Report to the APA Council of Representatives. *American Psychologist, 25*(5), xxvii–xxviii. doi: 10.1037/h0037753

Chapter 8

Community Psychology and Social Justice

Scot D. Evans, Adam D. Rosen, and Geoffrey Nelson

INTRODUCTION

Community psychology may be defined most simply as the applied study of the relationship between social systems and individual well-being in the community context. It is a subdiscipline of psychology that is concerned with understanding people in the context of their communities, the prevention of problems in living, the celebration of human diversity, and the pursuit of social justice through social action (Prilleltensky & Nelson, 2009). It is *community* psychology because it emphasizes a level of analysis and intervention other than the individual and their immediate interpersonal context. It is community *psychology* because it is nevertheless concerned with how people feel, think, experience, and act as they work together, resisting oppression and struggling to create a better world (Burton, Boyle, Harris, & Kagan, 2007).

It is important to note that community psychology has emerged around the world over the past 40 years, for varying purposes and in unique social, political, and cultural circumstances. The common thread in its emergence has been the recognition of inequity and injustice within social systems and the resulting negative impact on people's well-being (Dalton, Elias & Wandersman, 2006). In the United States, community psychology emerged in the 1960s to address some of the shortcomings of clinical and traditional applied psychology (Rappaport, 1977;

Sarason, 1988; Walsh, 1987). Influenced by the crisis in confidence in social institutions during this time, community psychologists began to question the value of helping individuals when so many societal structures were inimical to human welfare. Community psychologists challenged the prevailing professional and scientific norms that excluded values and social change from psychology. As community psychologists, the pioneers in the field wanted to use their skills to improve not just the well-being of individuals but of society as a whole.

COMMUNITY PSYCHOLOGY AND SOCIAL JUSTICE

Social justice as a value and an aim is baked into the vision of the Society for Community Research and Action (SCRA), Division 27 of the American Psychological Association.

> The Society for Community Research and Action will have a strong, global impact on enhancing well-being and promoting social justice for all people by fostering collaboration where there is division and empowerment where there is oppression. (Society for Community Research and Action [SCRA], 2010, para. 2)

Social Justice is also part of one of the main goals:

> To engage in action, research, and practice committed to promoting equitable distribution of resources, equal opportunity for all, non-exploitation, prevention of violence, active citizenry, liberation of oppressed peoples, greater inclusion for historically marginalized groups, and respecting all cultures. (SCRA, 2010, para. 10)

Although a concern for social justice was central to the emergence of community psychology and is currently identified as a guiding principle for the field, the terms *justice*, *social justice*, *distributive justice*, and *procedural justice* were nowhere to be found in the subject indices of some of the leading U.S. community psychology textbooks before 2002 (Fondacaro & Weinberg, 2002). In the past two decades, there have been increasing calls for the field of community psychology to be concerned with social justice and raising critical consciousness. This has established a growing expectation that community psychologists would become allies with oppressed groups in the struggle for social justice (Prilleltensky & Nelson, 1997, 2009; Rappaport, 2005).

In this chapter we will first discuss the definitions of social justice used in the field of community psychology and explore how social justice is framed through the lens of a vision of a just society and the values that drive this vision. Second, we will highlight the beliefs and assumptions pertaining to social justice in community psychology and contrast these with common beliefs and assumptions often held in traditional clinical and applied psychologies. We then discuss and provide examples of specific research and action approaches used by community psychologists to understand injustice and promote social justice. We end by reflecting on the global or international aspects of social justice in the field and highlight some future trends and implications for future social justice research and action in community psychology.

DEFINING SOCIAL JUSTICE IN COMMUNITY PSYCHOLOGY

Although social justice is espoused as a central focus in community psychology, one concern is that social justice as a concept is so commonly used that its meaning and relationship to practice is widely assumed to be self-evident (Fondacaro & Weinberg, 2002). In the past decade, however, there have been several attempts to articulate a greater level of specificity in describing this construct in order to create a framework for understanding justice within the work of community psychology. In this section we highlight a community psychology perspective on social justice that (1) distinguishes between distributive and procedural justice, (2) recognizes social justice as a multilevel construct capable of being broken down into several subtypes, and (3) locates justice within the appropriate social, historical, cultural, and political context.

Distributive and Procedural Justice

What has been generally articulated as social justice has more recently been refined into two subtypes of justice: distributive and procedural. Despite this relatively recent refinement, when discussing social justice, many are specifically referring to distributive justice. *Distributive justice* is the "fair, equitable allocation of resources, opportunities, obligations, and power in society as a whole" (Prilleltensky, 2001, p. 754). This definition reminds us that any understanding of social justice must encompass both rights and duties. Justice consists of two complimentary statements: to each (individual, family, organization, community) according to his or her needs, ability, effort, opportunities, rights and power, and from each (individual, family, organization, community) according to his or her needs, ability, obligation, duties, opportunity, and privilege (Prilleltensky & Nelson, 2009; Sandel, 2009).

Procedural justice refers to fair, transparent, inclusive, respectful, and participatory decision-making processes. Whereas distributive justice focuses on outcomes, procedural justice focuses on the process and the desire that the methods of collective decision making include fair representation, voice, and power of citizens (Dalton et al., 2006; Miller, 1999; Prilleltensky, 2012). The emphasis is on the importance of procedural fairness as a mechanism for enhancing collaboration and empowerment beyond the traditional focus on distribution of resources (Drew, Bishop, & Syme, 2002).

Social Justice as a Multilevel Construct

Both distributive and procedural dimensions of justice have different implications for promoting the well-being of individuals, groups, and communities. Prilleltensky (2012) offers a tripartite framework to elucidate the contextual nature of social justice as a multilevel construct. Although much of this work is in its nascent stages in the field, this type of analysis demonstrates how community psychologists address issues of justice across the various levels of social environments. Thus, multiple potential subtypes of justice are summarized from the micro-level of individual relationships to the meso- and macro-levels of groups and societies.

At the micro-level, distributive and procedural forms of justice are largely concerned with fairness within the sphere of individual relationships. For example, distributive justice within interpersonal interactions involves the sharing of goods and responsibilities in a given relationship. Similarly, procedural interpersonal justice relates to non-exploitive relationships characterized by dignity, respect, and shared decision-making processes (Prilleltensky, 2012). This general conception of the two dimensions of justice runs across all other levels of the current analysis.

At the meso-level of organizations and institutions, the same principles underlying the current conception of justice apply, but are translated to increasingly broader contexts. One example of distributive justice at this level would be fairness in pay at the workplace. Procedural justice considerations at this level require that people are adequately informed and have a voice in the decisions associated with organizational- and institutional-level distributions. For instance, the term *informational justice* has been used to emphasize the importance of transparent decision-making processes at the institutional level (Prilleltensky, 2012). In the absence of this particular subtype of justice, marginalization and social exclusion ensue.

At a broader, macro-level of analysis, additional considerations regarding justice exist specific to the sphere of communities and nations. In line with the other levels of analysis, distributive and procedural justice require that all individuals have equal access to economic resources and services, while also receiving equitable treatment by these social systems. These issues are particularly salient to societal dynamics involving social group affiliations (e.g., race, gender, social class) and therefore often speak to issues of equality and civil rights. Examples of systems at this level, where this type of cultural justice is an important issue of consideration, are the justice system, public education, social security, and other sociopolitical structures and services.

> At each level of analysis, from the personal to the communal, unique types of justice play significant roles. In all cases, however, we are talking about the exchange of a good or obligation (subtype of distributive justice) or the process by which the allocation is made (subtype of procedural justice). All subtypes of justice try to answer either what or how questions. (Prilleltensky, 2012, p. 8)

Social Justice in Context

Although community psychologists are starting to more clearly articulate various forms of justice across different levels of social environments, attempts to enact these concepts is not without challenge. For instance, a salient issue related to distributive justice is how to ascertain what is due a person. Prilleltensky (2012) noted that the crux of the debate lies in whether to use merit or need criteria. Applying the merit criterion implies that people should be rewarded based on effort, talents, and capacity. The need criterion calls for a distribution of resources based on what individuals require in order to experience a certain level of well-being. In light of the distinct issues characterizing these two criteria, it is important to note that these perspectives are not completely irreconcilable. Drew et al. (2002) suggest that conceptions of justice should also be located within the appropriate socio-historical cultural political milieu. In certain contexts, need ought to take precedence, whereas in others, merit should be preferred (Corning, 2011). The dynamic interrelationships among a given time, geographic place, and sociopolitical climate must be taken into account when dealing with issues of justice. Consistent with community psychology's attention to the role of context in all aspects of well-being, any understanding of social justice has to be considered relative to these shifting dimensions of social circumstances. For instance, level of inequality is one issue that is highly influenced by the aforementioned contextual influences. Under conditions of relative equality, it would be fair to apply the merit criterion and allow advantage to those who work harder or who have higher capacities. However, under conditions of inequality, like in the United States, it would seem fair to privilege need over merit (Prilleltensky, 2012). Even in contexts of high inequality, most cultures continue to privilege merit over need, thus perpetuating injustice (Barry, 2005; Ehrenreich, 2009; Fleischacker, 2004; Lakoff, 2006; Lareau & Conley 2008; Schwalbe, 2008).

SOCIAL JUSTICE VISION, VALUES, BELIEFS

Social Justice Vision

Community psychology always implies a particular vision of society: one grounded in the ideals of social justice, social inclusion, self-determination, solidarity, and collective wellness (Kagan, Burton, Duckett, Lawtham, & Siddique, 2001; Prilleltensky, 2001). This vision begins with a conception of what ought to be that is not constrained by what might be normally acceptable (Angelique & Kyle, 2002; Rappaport, 2005). Community psychologists are therefore concerned with the gap between the current state of affairs and an idealized set of societal conditions.

> We evaluate a situation as it is (interpreted through the lens of our values); the situation ethically challenges us because we find it lacking compared with our values, our standards of what ought to be; and we intervene to lessen or remove the situation's is-ought discrepancy. (Dokecki, 1996, p. 38)

Community psychology thus explores the possibilities of prefiguring a just society while also identifying what gets in the way of this vision in order to identify systems, policies, and community conditions in need of transformation (Kagan et al., 2011).

Social Justice Values

The values we use to guide action should be compatible with our vision of a good society and they should bring us closer to that desired end (Prilleltensky, 2001). For community psychologists, values are in the foreground and they guide the process of working toward a vision of a just society. As a core value in community psychology, social justice is about making the fair and equitable allocation of resources, bargaining powers, and obligations in society a top priority. It is an expectation of economic security, shelter, clothing, nutrition, access to vital health and social services for all (Nelson & Prilleltensky, 2005). Without a fair distribution of social goods, other basic values, needs, and rights cannot be fulfilled (Prilleltensky & Nelson, 2009). As procedural justice recognizes the importance of the processes associated with these distributions and individual experiences, community psychologists value democratic and fair decision-making processes. Emphases on collaboration, participation, engagement, giving voice, and empowerment are values often used to both describe the targeted outcomes and guide the activity of the field (Nelson & Prilleltensky, 2005). Thus, social justice is a "collective value" without which the prospects of personal and relational well-being remain elusive. Researchers and practitioners in community psychology have an ethical obligation to redress social injustice and to work actively to transform economic, social, cultural, and institutional arrangements that foster injustice (Angelique & Kyle, 2002). Concerns with justice and equality, political education, and social change movements reflect the value of social justice in community psychology (Albee, 1986; Prilleltensky & Nelson, 1997).

Social Justice Beliefs

A key theme in community psychology is the belief that most of the social issues community psychologists are concerned with in research and community interventions are symptoms of profound social injustice and that much preventable human suffering is intrinsically tied to injustice (Angelique & Kyle, 2002; Martín-Baró, 1994; Nelson & Prilleltensky, 2005). Community psychologists believe that in the absence of fair and inclusive processes and the equitable allocation of resources, there are dire consequences for individuals, their social relationships, and the broader society. These negative effects are felt in health, education, housing, transportation, and other areas of concern (Prilleltensky & Nelson, 2009). Therefore, community psychologists believe that in order to promote well-being, they should attend to the "causes of the causes" of problems in living: injustice (Joffe & Albee, 1991). Unless they understand and consider power, and view its unequal distribution as a central determinant of health and well-being, they will continue to shift pieces within the present configuration of injustice, without challenging injustice (Ife, 2002).

SOCIAL JUSTICE RESEARCH AND ACTION

Community psychology as a field has made explicit its commitment to social justice research and action.

> Community psychology will become a field of research and action that makes a significant difference on issues of social change by promoting social justice. . . . The field will explicitly state its commitment to social changes that promote social justice and greater inclusion for historically marginalized groups and will see that commitment manifest in the various aspects of the field's work. (SCRA website, 2010, para. 11)

In this section, we highlight some examples of social justice research and action in community psychology. First we turn the focus to one of the foundational strategies in community psychology—prevention—and utilize the example of early childhood development as a social justice approach in action. Then we discuss how research, policy advocacy, and general community psychology practice can be tools for the promotion of social justice.

Prevention and Social Justice

Prevention, as opposed to remedial treatment, is one of the foundational concepts in community psychology. In his article "Toward a Just Society," the late George Albee (1986) linked the population-focused, public health approach that underpins prevention with social justice. Albee presented research on the relationship between social class and mental illness that was extensively reviewed and theorized by Dohrenwend and Dohrenwend (1981) in community psychology. The Dohrenwends' review established what is now called a "gradient" between social class and mental illness; the higher one moves up the social class ladder, the lower the rate of mental illness. Furthermore, they presented a social stress model that accounts for this gradient; as one moves down the social class ladder, one is exposed to more noxious social conditions that give rise to mental illness. There is no threshold at which mental illness develops; rather, the relationship between class and illness is continuous. Albee then invoked two principles from Rawls's (1971) theory of justice.

> According to the first principle, each person is to have an equal right to the most extensive basic liberty compatible with a similar liberty for others. According to the second, social and economic inequalities are to be arranged

> so that they are both to the greatest advantage of the least advantaged and attached to offices and positions open to all, under conditions of fair and equal opportunity. (Albee, 1986, p. 897)

Essentially the first principle asserts that rights are universal and must be accessible to everyone, whereas the second principle calls for a reduction of inequality. Albee concluded that the task for community psychology was to make clear the relationship between "social pathology and psychopathology" and to change social structures so that they are more just (p. 897).

One Example: Early Childhood Development

As community psychology has developed prevention approaches that strive for social justice in different contexts (e.g., racism, heterosexism) (Kenny & Hage, 2009), one issue that is squarely related to social justice is early childhood development (ECD) (Social Justice in the OECD, 2011; UNICEF, 2012). First of all, the field of ECD adopts a child rights approach that all children have the right to ECD resources (Hertzman et al., 2010), including health and nutrition, child protection, social protection and welfare, and education, which is congruent with the Millennium Development Goals and the Education for All goals (Britto, Yoshikawa, & Bowler, 2011). Second, the field of ECD utilizes an ecological perspective (Siddiqui, Hertzman, Irwin, & Hertzman, 2012), recognizing that child wellness is predicated on family wellness and collective wellness, the latter of which is based on social justice in the allocation of resources and support for strong community structures (Prilleltensky, 2012; Prilleltensky, Laurendeau, Chamberland, & Peirson, 2001). Third, ECD research has shown social class gradients for various domains of child development (e.g., health, academic achievement) (Keating & Hertzman, 1999; Siddiqui et al., 2012). Moreover, these gradients have been found in both "have" and "have not" nations across the world (Hertzman et al., 2010; Siddiqui et al., 2012). Across countries, social class gradients vary in terms of how steep or flat they are. Those nations with flatter gradients, which are due to lower levels of social class inequality, have better child development outcomes (McCain, Mustard, & Shanker, 2007; Siddiqui et al., 2012). For example, Sweden, which is rich in terms of ECD and family support policies, has a relatively flat gradient and low levels of child development problems (Hertzman et al., 2010). Similarly, Cuba, a relatively poor country, also has a flat gradient and outperforms other Latin American countries in terms of children's health and academic performance, and matches that of many European countries and the United States, with its strong emphasis on universal education and health care (McCain, Mustard, & McCuaig, 2011; McCain et al., 2007; Hertzman et al., 2010). These findings about the social class gradient and child development outcomes support Prilleltensky's (2012) thesis, noted earlier, that justice leads to wellness.

Based on the principles and research aforementioned, it has been recognized that "early childhood education is therefore a key component of efforts to level the playing field" (Social justice in the OECD, 2011, p. 23), prompting Siddiqui et al. (2012) to call it a "powerful equalizer." In the past, ECD programs have tended to be targeted at children and families living in poverty. In the United States, Head Start, the Abecedarian program, the Perry Preschool program, and the Chicago Parent-Child Centers are all examples of ECD programs that have been demonstrated to have long-term positive impact and to be cost-effective (Nelson, Westhues, & Macleod, 2003). However, they are all targeted or selective interventions, as are many ECD programs. As McCain et al. (2007) observe:

> To work, programs must be universal. Vulnerable children are found in all SES groups but populations are not evenly distributed between groups. The largest numbers of children overall are found in the middle groupings. The lowest SES group has a greater percentage, but a smaller number, of vulnerable children. Conversely, children in the middle SES groups are less likely to be vulnerable, but because of the size of the group, this is where the most vulnerable children are found. Restricting programs to vulnerable children in the low SES group therefore misses the majority of children experiencing difficulties. (p. 46)

So, targeted programs, although effective, cannot flatten the social class gradient because too many vulnerable children, roughly 60% in the middle and affluent classes, are not reached (Pascal, 2009). For this reason, programs such as full-day early learning for preschool children have been proposed and implemented (Pascal, 2009). Evaluations of ECD programs outside of the United States have demonstrated that not only are such programs effective (Nores & Barnett, 2010), but that they "appeared to reduce socioeconomic inequalities, as children from less advantaged backgrounds benefited more than those from more advantaged background" (Melhuish, 2011, p. 300). Furthermore, universal ECD programs pay for themselves. For example, the province of Quebec's \$7 per day child care program led to increased participation of women in the workforce, generating \$1.05 to the province and \$.44 to the federal government for every dollar invested (Fortin, Godbout, & St. Cerny, 2012).

Rather than seeing universal and targeted programs as in opposition to one another, Offord, Kraemer, Kazdin, Jensen, and Harrington (1998) have argued that it is valuable to have both universal and targeted programs and to debate the relative mix of these two approaches. It is also important to note that there are some hybrid models in which ECD programs are offered universally in neighborhoods that have an overall low-income level. The Sure Start program, which has been widely implemented in the United Kingdom, is a good example of this approach. Positive child and family outcomes have been reported in a quasi-experimental evaluation of this program (Melhuish, Belsky, Leyland, Barnes & the National Evaluation of the Sure Start Research Team, 2008).

Thus far, we have focused on the dimension of distributive justice component of social justice. What about the component of procedural justice? Prilleltensky et al. (2001) argued that it is insufficient to think about children and their families solely as the objects of programs and the values that underlie them. One must also think about the agency of children and families in shaping the interventions that are designed by professionals and researchers to benefit them. Citizen participation and empowerment are important values in this regard. Too often, children and their parents, particularly those who are disadvantaged, have no say in social programs with a prevention focus that are constructed for them (Rappaport, 1981). This theme of procedural justice has been discussed in the literature in terms of community "ownership" and "power-sharing" (Sandler, 2007). A notable exception is the Better Beginnings, Better Futures program in Ontario, in which residents play an instrumental role in selecting, designing, implementing, and evaluating ECD programs for children and families (Peters et al., 2010).

Research

While some could argue successfully that most research in community psychology is relatively post-positivist in its epistemology and methods, there have been increasing calls for research to be transformative, participatory, and oriented toward social change (Lykes & Mallona, 2008). Many community psychologists operate from a critical-transformative stance that views research as a tool for social critique and actions that would increase the possibilities for social justice–oriented societal transformation. Researchers grounded in the critical research paradigm (Nelson & Prilleltensky, 2005) value participation and engagement in social justice efforts by the marginalized. Participatory action research (PAR) is the preferred research approach because, by incorporating the participation of those suffering, adverse social conditions constitute a source of transformation for them, not only regarding their social situations but also for them as active participants (Montero, 2009).

Prilleltensky (2008) put forth the concept of *psychopolitical validity* to urge community psychologists to put power issues and social justice at the forefront of research and action. He uses the term *epistemic psychopolitical validity* to suggest that research should help elucidate the role of power in the psychology and politics of wellness, oppression and liberation, at the personal, relational, and collective domains. When research has epistemic psychopolitical validity, it "accounts for the role of political and economic power in economic prosperity and in creation of social justice institutions" (Prilleltensky, 2008, p. 121).

Transformative psychopolitical validity exists when our social interventions go beyond amelioration to promote structural change. "Transformational validity derives from the potential of our actions to promote personal, relational, and collective wellness by reducing power inequalities and increasing political action"

(Prilleltensky, 2008, p. 130). In practice, these actions might focus on interventions such as empowerment and sociopolitical development (personal level); building trust, connection, and participation in groups that support social justice (relational level); and social action to support networks of resistance (collective level). Taken together, psychopolitical validity has some similarities to Lather's (1993) notion of catalytic validity in that both are concerned with research that increases our understanding of the world in order to transform it. Community psychologists are beginning to focus research more toward understanding, exposing, and transforming power inequalities while privileging PAR approaches.

The work of community psychologist Brinton Lykes exemplifies PAR approaches to promote social justice. Lykes has been involved in PAR with local communities in Guatemala, South Africa, Northern Ireland, and the United States for over 20 years (Lykes, 2003). As part of a recent Post-Deportation Human Rights Project (PDHRP), Lykes and colleagues (Brabeck, Lykes, & Hershberg, 2011) used a PAR approach to help design collaborative spaces for bridging the rifts between citizens and noncitizens and for building shared understanding of and response to injustices that Guatemalan and Salvadoran immigrant families face. Researchers and two immigrant rights community organizations collaborated with to document the experiences of Guatemalan and Salvadoran families, contextualized the current risks to families within a socio-historical/sociopolitical and transnational framework, and worked to respond to current realities through community-based actions, policy development, and social advocacy.

Policy Advocacy

> The field will encourage and prepare individual community psychologists to be active advocates in the promotion of social policies that promote social justice. (SCRA, 2010, para. 19)

The engagement of community psychologists in public policy has been advocated since the early days of the discipline (e.g., Albee, 1959; Bennet et al. 1966; Newbrough, 1980; Sarason, 1974; Syme & Bishop, 1993). A deep understanding and involvement in policy development, implementation, and analysis are fundamental for community psychologists in order to influence the allocation of resources and promote social justice (Bishop, Vicary, Browne, & Guard, 2009; Murrell, 1984). "Community psychology is ideally placed to increase input into policy making, given its history of being multidisciplinary, and theories of empowerment, participation and social change in a domain in which social input is increasingly being sought (Bishop et al., 2009, p. 111). Community psychologists seek the development of policies that redistribute wealth and income and believe in influencing policy processes through the dissemination of relevant research findings (Nelson & Prilleltensky, 2005). Bishop and colleagues (2009) argued that the "role of the community psychologist is to deconstruct the nature of policies in their broader social context, in which the issues of government power, democracy, historical and current practices of oppression and empowerment are set against the new" (p. 115).

In his commentary on Leslea Peirson's (2005) chapter in Nelson and Prilleltensky's (2005) *Community Psychology: In Pursuit of Liberation and Well-Being*, community psychology Camil Bouchard (2005) discussed the importance of working for social justice through pushing for transformative policy change. He used the example of making policy recommendations to help align family associations and childcare services to sustain pressure on the government of Québec to invest in high-quality childcare environments for birth through age five. His report—"Un Québec fou de ses enfants" (Québec crazy about its kids, Bouchard et al., 1991) helped influence the development of progressive family policies. One such policy in Québec was the creation of a universal $7 a day childcare network providing valuable resources for parents and their children, which was implemented province-wide in 1997. This social policy initiative has led to powerful social justice outcomes.

> In just a decade, Quebec has gone from the bottom to the top on many important social indicators. From having Canada's lowest female labour participation, it now has the highest. Where Quebec women were once less likely to attend post-secondary education than their counterparts in the rest of Canada, today they dominate. At the same time, student scores on standardized test have gone from below the Canadian average to above. Despite working more, Quebec women are also having more babies, and Quebec dads are more involved in child rearing. Eighty-two percent take paid leave after the birth of their infants, compared to just 12 percent of fathers in the rest of the country. In addition, childhood programs that allow mothers to work have slashed Quebec's child poverty rates by 50 percent. Finally, in an analysis that should catch the attention of policy makers everywhere, Montreal economist Pierre Fortin revealed that the tax revenues from mothers who are able to work because of low cost children's programming pay for the entire cost of Quebec's system. (McCain et al., 2011, p. 2)

This is an excellent example of how community psychologists can work at the policy level to help create systemic changes that reduce social inequality and promote child and family wellness.

Practice

In recent years, there has been increasing attention to and interest in community psychology practice as a legitimate career path for community psychologists with a focus on understanding how change benefiting community residents might be perpetuated through community practice. Whereas earlier definitions of community psychology practice focused on strengthening the capacity of organizations, institutions, and settings to better meet the needs of their communities (Bennett et al., 1966; Chavis, 1993; Elias, 1994), more recent conceptualizations stress the need to promote well-being, social justice, economic equity, and self-determination through community practice (Foster-Fishman et al., 2006; Evans et al., 2011; Evans, Hanlin, & Prilleltensky, 2007; Kagan et al., 2011; Prilleltensky, 2005). Nelson and Prilleltensky (2005) raise the concern that most of the work of community psychologists tries to ameliorate—not transform—living conditions within the existing distribution of resources and highlight the need to distinguish between ameliorative and transformative practice.

In foregrounding the social justice aim of community psychology practice, some community psychologists have been using the term *critical community practice* to imply practice with a particular vision of society: one grounded in the ideals of social justice, social inclusion, self-determination, solidarity, and collective wellness (Butcher, 2007; Evans et al., 2011; Kagan & Burton 2001; Prilleltensky, 2001; Weil, 1996). Critical community practice is "action based on critical theorizing, reflection, and a clear commitment to working for social justice through empowering and transformative practice" (Henderson, 2007, p. 1). Kagan et al. (2011) suggest that in pursuit of justice psychologists might, for example, "expose the ways in which authorities, established to be of service to people, wield their power and authority to effectively silence them. We might highlight inequities in how human services operate; we might work with people to secure access to the necessary supports, or work with services on a change agenda so that they function in a more inclusive and non-discriminatory way" (p. 37).

However, critical practice is conceptually and practically difficult. The task of promoting equality and social justice through community practice is challenging because most societal structures reflect and reproduce inequality (Nelson & Prilleltensky, 2005). In practice, pursuit of social justice must be balanced with other values, including individual healing, community and national reconciliation, and the realities of who continues to hold power in communities and society (Prilleltensky, 2001).

GLOBAL AND INTERNATIONAL DIMENSIONS TO SOCIAL JUSTICE

As Marsella (1998) asserted, "Human survival and well-being are now embedded in an entangled web of global, economic, political, social and environmental forces!" (p. 1282). Social problems are global and multisectorial and cannot be challenged with traditional psychological instruments, research, and practice (Nelson & Prilleltensky, 2005). There have been many calls for psychologists to become more involved in social justice issues in poor countries (Adler, 1990; Martín-Baró 1994; Sloan, 1990) and to examine the systems that maintain poverty. Although advocates claim globalization will promote equality and global economic prosperity for all, the downside of globalization is the increasing gap between the rich and poor within and between countries. Developing countries are burdened by billions of dollars of debt and are increasingly controlled by the financial institutions of the world's economic powers (Sloan, 2010). Global poverty is continuously increasing, human rights are being violated, and the environment is being destroyed. Economic exploitation and the further oppression of marginalized communities around the world are increasing (Osberg, 2008).

Given the widespread negative impacts of corporate globalization processes on communities around the world, these issues should be a central concern to community psychology. However, community psychologists to date have largely ignored the harmful consequences of globalization and macro political economy in their research and action. A recent review of articles published in the top three North American community psychology journals revealed that between 1970 and 2012, only 0.02 % or 11 of the 4,175 published articles addressed global political-economic issues (Fayter, 2012). This is strong evidence that community psychology in North America is not attending to global and international dimensions of social justice. Nelson and Lavoie (2010) envision the need for community psychologists to explore the contemporary global issues that have previously been ignored, such as global climate change and environmental preservation (Riemer, 2010) and the impacts of economic globalization (Morrow, 2004). Sloan (2010) argued that to attend more to the value of social justice and to develop transformative interventions, it is essential for community psychology to understand social justice issues like poverty in the context of corporate globalization

FUTURETRENDS AND IMPLICATIONS FOR RESEARCH AND ACTION

There are community psychologists who believe that several trends are coalescing to bring increased energy to research and action for social justice, liberation, and social transformation (Dalton et al., 2006). Others however are more critical of the current state of affairs in community psychology with regard to social justice research and action (Coimbra et al., 2012; Fayter, 2012; Prilleltensky & Nelson, 2009). Coimbra et al. (2012), for example, suggested that the field is gradually becoming endangered as a critical alternative to the disciplinary ideologies, theories, procedures, and practices of mainstream psychology and less relevant to the interests of people whose lives are most characterized by social injustice and oppression. It may be true that like many social science disciplines, community psychology has a subunit with a more critical bent that exists within a larger body that tends to be more pragmatic in its research and action. Whereas community psychology as a discipline seeks individual and community betterment, critical community psychology embeds research and action in wider movements for social justice (Kagan et al., 2011).

Attempting to influence the social justice research and practices of community psychology, critical community psychologists around the world continue to push for "the development and deployment of politically progressive community critical psychologies as contributions to the task of collectively transforming social reality to promote health, well-being and social justice" (Combria et al., 2012, p. 139). Nelson and Prilleltensky (2009) argued that social justice should be the centerpiece of a more critical community psychology. As such, they suggest three key themes that provide some guidance for a social justice agenda in community psychology theory, research, action, education, and training: (1) connecting the personal and political; (2) connecting constituents who are involved in, and affected by, social change; (3) connecting the micro-, meso-, and macro-levels of analysis (see Table 8.1).

Table 8.1
Key Themes for a Social Justice Agenda in Community Psychology

Activities	Connecting the Personal and Political	Connecting Micro, Meso, and Macro Contexts	Connecting Constituents
Theory	• Theoretical grounding in issues and settings • Attend to subjectivity and personal experiences of oppression • Examine the role of intrapersonal, interpersonal, and social conflict in social justice	• Interdisciplinary frameworks • Integrative theory of change • Understand interdependence of ecological levels • Address implementation of values at all levels	• Balance rights and responsibilities • Balance individual and collective issues
Research and Action	• Commit to emancipatory research and action that utilizes participatory approaches	• Multiple levels of analysis and intervention • Community-based case studies on effects of injustice and power inequality at all levels	• Engagement of multiple stakeholders and negotiation of power differences • Sensitivity to diversity of stakeholders
Education and Training	• Recruit and accept diverse students • Attend to personal interests that might interfere with actualization of values • Promote critical consciousness	• Address issues of justice within programs • Field work and mentoring in settings that espouse social justice causes • Help students identify contradictions at all levels	• Create a welcoming, inclusive climate and sense of community within the program • Build long-term relationships with settings espousing social justice

Adapted from Nelson, G., & Prilleltensky, I. (2009). Community psychology: Reclaiming social justice. In D. R. Fox & I. Prilleltensky (Eds.), *Critical psychology: An introduction* (2nd ed., pp. 166–184). Thousand Oaks, CA: Sage.

CONCLUSION

As has been argued by internal critics of the field of community psychology, the promotion of social justice remains largely an unfulfilled promise (Chavis & Wolff, 1993; Coimbra et al., 2012; Prilleltensky & Nelson, 1997). Although community psychology is unapologetically value-explicit, we readily admit that our field does not sufficiently enact the value of social justice through its research and practice (Nelson & Prilleltensky, 2009). For a variety of reasons, the promise of a community psychology focused on social justice has been hard to keep. What will it take to bridge the gap between the espoused social justice values of community psychology and actual practices? It may be time for the "tempered radicals" within community psychology to come together to push for more congruence with social justice ideals. Meyerson and Scully (1995) describe the tempered radical as "individuals who identify with and are committed to their organizations and also to a cause, community, or ideology that is fundamentally different from, and possibly at odds with the dominant culture of their organization" (p. 586). The dominant culture of community psychology—what gets published in journals and what gets discussed at our conferences—is too often limiting our social justice contribution. We identify this shortcoming, not to undermine the contributions of our field to the promotion of social justice in psychology, but to highlight community psychology's openness and commitment to critical self-reflection. Constantly reevaluating our own work fends against complacency and promotes the ability to ensure actions align with values. We believe this to be an important mechanism through which a social justice–oriented community psychology can be realized.

In this chapter, we have provided one example, the field of ECD, in which community psychologists and others in the ECD field have explicitly focused on a social justice agenda. Whereas leveling the social class gradient for child development outcomes is no small task, we have shown how a community psychologist can act as a policy advocate to reduce injustice. The work of Camil Bouchard in the context of Quebec's childcare program provides a clear example of the type of social justice work that is needed and the powerful outcomes that can result from policy changes. We firmly believe that this type of work can be done in other domains that are of concern to community psychologists—homelessness, community mental health, the natural environment, and work with LGBTQ communities, to name a few. Community psychologists will be required to clearly position social justice as a central issue of concern and to explore concrete ways that community research and action can address issues of social justice in these various contexts. This is a tall order, and there are many political and other socially constructed obstacles to social justice, but community psychology can make a difference it commits to a social justice agenda.

REFERENCES

Adler, T. (1990). Aid agencies grappling with behavioral issues. *APA Monitor, 21*(7), 34–35.

Albee, G. W. (1959). *Mental health manpower trends.* New York, NY: Basic Books.

Albee, G. W. (1986). Toward a just society: Lessons from observations on the primary prevention of psychopathology. *American Psychologist, 41,* 891–898.

Angelique, H., & Kyle, K. (2002). Monterey declaration of critical community psychology. *The Community Psychologist, A Publication of the Society for Community Research and Action, Division 27 of the American Psychological Association, 35*(1), 35–36.

Barry, B. (2005). *Why social justice matters*. Cambridge, UK: Polity.

Bennet, C. C., Anderson, L. S., Cooper, S., Hassol, L., Klein, D. C., & Rosenblum, G. (Eds.). (1966). *Community psychology: A report of the Boston conference on the education of psychologists for community mental health*. Boston, MA: Boston University.

Bertelsmannn Foundation. (2011). *Social justice in the OECD—how do the member states compare?* Retrieved from www.bertelsmann-stiftung.de

Bishop, B. J., Vicary, D. A., Browne, A. L., & Guard, N. (2009). Public policy, participation and the third Position: The implication of engaging communities on their own terms. *American Journal of Community Psychology, 43*(1–2), 111–121.

Bouchard, C. (2005). Commentary: Disadvantaged children and families: The power of a just asymmetry. In G. Nelson & I. Prilleltensky (Eds.), *Community psychology: In pursuit of liberation and well-being* (pp. 464–466). New York, NY: Palgrave MacMillan.

Bouchard, C. et al. (1991). *Un Québec fou de ses enfants*. Rapport de Groupe de travail pour les jeunes, Québec, Direction des Communications, Ministére de la Santé et des Services Sociaux.

Brabeck, K. M., Lykes, M. B., & Hershberg, R. (2011). Framing immigration to and deportation from the United States: Guatemalan and Salvadoran families make meaning of their experiences. *Community, Work and Family, 14*(3), 275–296.

Britto, P. R., Yoshikawa, H., & Boller, K. (2011). Quality of early childhood development programs in global contexts: Rationale for investment, conceptual framework and implications for equity. *Social Policy Report, 25*(2). Retrieved from www.srcd.org/publications

Burton, M., Boyle, S., Harris, C., & Kagan, C. M. (2007). Community psychology in Britain. In S. Reich, M. Riemer, I. Prilleltensky, & M. Montero (Eds.), *International community psychology: History and theories*. The Netherlands: Kluwer Academic Press.

Butcher, H. (2007). What is critical community practice? Cases studies and analysis. In H. Butcher, S. Banks, P. Henderson, & J. Robertson (Eds.) *Critical community practice* (pp 33–49). Bristol, UK: Policy.

Chavis, D. M. (1993). A future for community psychology practice. *American Journal of Community Psychology, 21*(2), 171–183.

Chavis, D. M., & Wolff, T. (1993). *Public hearing: Community psychology's failed commitment to social change: Ten commandments for action*. Public meeting held at the biennial conference of the Society for Community Research and Action, Division 27 of APA, Williamsburg, Virginia.

Coimbra, J., Duckett, P., Fryer, D., Makkawi, I., Menezes, I., Seedat, M., & Walker, C. (2012). Rethinking community psychology: Critical insights. *The Australian Community Psychologist, 24*(2), 135–142.

Corning, P. (2011). *The fair society: The science of human nature and the pursuit of social justice*. Chicago, IL: University of Chicago.

Dalton, J. H., Elias, M. J., & Wandersman, A. (2006). *Community psychology: Linking individuals and communities* (2nd ed.). Belmont, CA: Wadsworth.

Dohrenwend, B. S., & Dohrenwend, B. P. (1981). Socioenvironmental factors, stress, and psychopathology. *American Journal of Community Psychology, 9*, 123–159.

Dokecki, P. (1996). *The tragi-comic professional: Basic considerations for ethical reflective-generative practice*. Pittsburgh, PA: Duquesne University.

Drew, N. M., Bishop, B. J., & Syme, G. (2002). Justice and local community change: Towards a substantive theory of justice. *Journal of Community Psychology, 30*(6), 623–634.

Ehrenreich, B. (2009). *Bright sided: How the relentless promotion of positive thinking has undermined America.* New York, NY: Holt and Company.

Elias, M. (1994). Capturing excellence in applied settings: A participant conceptualizer and praxis explicator role for community psychologists. *American Journal of Community Psychology, 22*(3), 293–318.

Evans, S. D., Hanlin, C. E., & Prilleltensky, I. (2007). Blending ameliorative and transformative approaches in human service organizations: A case study. *Journal of Community Psychology, 35*(3), 329–346.

Evans, S. D., Prilleltensky, O., McKenzie, A., Prilleltensky, I., Nogueras, D., Huggins, C., & Mescia, N. (2011). Promoting strengths, prevention, empowerment, and community change through organizational development: Lessons for research, theory, and practice. *Journal of Prevention & Intervention in the Community, 39*(1), 50–64.

Fayter, R. (2012). Community psychology and the global political economy: A Content analysis of literature on neo-liberalism, capitalism and corporate globalization. (Unpublished Manuscript). Wilfrid Laurier University, Waterloo, Ontario.

Fleischacker, S. (2004). *A short history of distributive justice.* Cambridge, MA: Harvard University.

Fondacaro, M. R., & Weinberg, D. (2002). Concepts of social justice in community psychology: Toward a social ecological epistemology. *American Journal of Community Psychology, 30*(4), 473–492.

Fortin, P., Godbout, L., & St. Cerny, S. (2012). *Impact of Quebec's universal low fee childcare program on female labour force participation, domestic income, and government budgets.* Working paper 2012/02, Université de Sherbrooke: Sherbrooke, Quebec. Retrieved from http://www.usherbrooke.ca/chaire-fiscalite/fileadmin/sites/chaire-fiscalite/documents/Cahiers-de-recherche/Etude_femmes_ANGLAIS.pdf

Foster-Fishman, P. G., Fitzgerald, K., Brandell, C., Nowell, B., Chavis, D., & Egeren, L. A. V. (2006). Mobilizing residents for action: The role of small wins and strategic supports. *American Journal of Community Psychology, 38*(3–4), 143–152.

Henderson, P. (2007). Introduction. In H. Butcher, S. Banks, P. Henderson, & J. Robertson (Eds.) *Critical community practice* (pp 1–13). Bristol, UK: Policy.

Hertzman, C., et al. (2010). Bucking the gradient: Tackling inequalities through early child development. *BMJ Open.* Retrieved from www.bmjopen.bmj.com

Ife, J. (2002). *Community development: Community-based alternatives in an age of globalisation* (2nd ed.). Frenchs Forest, Australia: Pearson Education Australia.

Joffe, J. M. & Albee, G. W. (Eds.). (1981). *Prevention through political action and social change.* Hanover, NH: University Press of New England.

Kagan, C., Burton, M., Duckett, P., Lawthom, R., & Siddiquee, A. (2011). *Critical Community Psychology* (1st ed.). West Sussex, UK: Wiley-Blackwell.

Keating, D. P., & Hertzman, C. (Eds.). (1999). *Developmental health and the wealth of nations: Social, biological, and educational dynamics.* New York, NY: Guilford.

Kenny, M. E., & Hage, S. M. (2009). The next frontier: Prevention as an instrument of social justice. *Journal of Primary Prevention, 30,* 1–10.

Lakoff, G. (2006). *Thinking points.* New York, NY: Farrar, Straus and Giroux.

Lareau, A., & Conley, D. (Eds.). (2008). *Social class: How does it work?* New York, NY: Russell Sage Foundation.

Lather, P. (1993). Fertile obsession: Validity after post-structuralism. *Sociological Quarterly, 34,* 673–693.

Lykes, M. B. (2003). Developing an activist liberatory community psychology: One step at a time. *The Community Psychologist, 36*(4), 39–42.

Lykes, M. B., & Mallona, A. (2008). Towards transformational liberation: Participatory action research and activist praxis. In P. Reason & H. Bradbury (Eds.), *The SAGE Handbook of Action Research II.* London: SAGE Publications Ltd., pp. 260–292.

Marsella, A. J. (1998). Toward a global-community psychology: Meeting the needs of a changing world. *American Psychologist,* 53, 1282–1291.

Martín-Baró, I. (1994). *Writings for a liberation psychology* (A. Aron & S. Corne, Eds.), Cambridge, MA: Harvard University.

McCain, M. N., Mustard, J. F., & McCuaig, K. (2011). *Early years study 3: Making decisions, taking action.* Toronto, ON: Margaret & Wallace McCain Family Foundation. Retrieved from www.earlyyearsstudy.ca

McCain, M. N., Mustard, J. F., & Shanker, S. (2007). *Early years study 2: Putting science into action.* Toronto, ON: Council for Early Child Development. Retrieved from http://earlylearning.ubc.ca/documents/40/

Melhuish, E. C. (2011). Preschool matters. *Science, 333,* 299–300.

Melhuish, E. C., Belsky, J., Leyland, A. H., Barnes, J., & the National Evaluation of the Sure Start Research Team. (2008). Effects of fully-established Sure Start local programmes on 3-year old children and their families living in England: A quasi-experimental observational study. *Lancet, 372,* 1641–1647.

Meyerson, D. E., & Scully, M. A. (1995). Tempered radicalism and the politics of ambivalence and change. *Organization Science, 6*(5), 585–600.

Miller, D. (1999). *Principles of social justice.* Cambridge, MA: Harvard University Press.

Montero, M. (2009). Methods for liberation: Critical consciousness in action. In M Montero & C. Sonn (Eds.), *Psychology of liberation: Theory and applications* (pp. 73–92). New York, NY: Springer.

Morrow, M. (2004). Mental health reform, economic globalization, and the practice of citizenship. *Canadian Journal of Community Mental Health, 23,* 39–50.

Murrell, S. A. (1984). The social policy process and community psychology training. *American Journal of Community Psychology, 12*(2), 185–191.

Nelson, G., & Lavoie, F. (2010). Contributions of Canadian community psychology. *Canadian Psychology, 51*(2), 79–88.

Nelson, G., & Prilleltensky, I. (2005). *Community psychology: In pursuit of liberation and well-being.* New York, NY: Palgrave Macmillan.

Nelson, G., & Prilleltensky, I. (2009). Community psychology: Reclaiming social justice. In D. R. Fox & I. Prilleltensky (Eds.), *Critical psychology: An introduction* (2nd ed., pp. 166–184). Thousand Oaks, CA: Sage.

Nelson, G., Westhues, A., & Macleod, J. (2003). A meta-analysis of longitudinal research on preschool prevention programs for children. *Prevention and Treatment, 6,* 1–35. Retrieved from http://journals.apa.org/prevention/volume6/toc-dec18-03.html

Newbrough, J. R. (1980). Community psychology and the public interest. *American Journal of Community Psychology, 8,* 1–17.

Nores, M., & Barnett, S. W. (2010). Benefits of early childhood interventions across the world: (Under) Investing in the very young. *Economics of Education Review, 29,* 271–282.

Offord, D. R., Kraemer, H. C., Kazdin, A. E., Jensen, P. S., & Harrington, R. (1998). Lowering the burden of suffering from child psychiatric disorder: Trade-offs among clinical, targeted, and universal interventions. *Journal of the American Academy of Child and Adolescent Psychiatry, 37,* 686–694.

Osberg, L. (2008). *A quarter century of economic inequality in Canada: 1981–2006.* Ottawa, ON: Canadian Centre for Policy Alternatives.

Pascal, C. (2009). *With our best future in mind: Implementing early learning in Ontario.* Toronto, ON: Queen's Printer. Retrieved from www.ontario.ca/earlylearning

Peirson, L. (2005). Disadvantaged children and families. In G. Nelson & I. Prilleltensky (Eds.), *Community psychology: In pursuit of liberation and well-being* (pp. 448–486). New York, NY: Palgrave Macmillan.

Peters, R. DeV., Bradshaw, A. J., Petrunka, K., Nelson, G., Herry, Y., Craig, W., . . . Rossiter, M. (2010). The "Better Beginnings, Better Futures" ecological, community-based early childhood prevention project: Findings from grade 3 to grade 9. *Monographs of the Society for Research in Child Development, 75*(3), 1–176.

Prilleltensky, I. (2001). Value-based praxis in community psychology: Moving toward social justice and social action. *American Journal of Community Psychology, 29*(5), 747–778.

Prilleltensky, I. (2005). Promoting well-being: Time for a paradigm shift in health and human services. *Scandinavian Journal of Public Health, 33*(66 suppl), 53–60.

Prilleltensky, I. (2008). The role of power in wellness, oppression, and liberation: The promise of psychopolitical validity. *Journal of Community Psychology, 36*(2), 116–136.

Prilleltensky, I. (2012). Wellness as fairness. *American Journal of Community Psychology, 49,* 1–21.

Prilleltensky, I., Laurendeau, M. C., Chamberland, C., & Peirson, L. (2001). Vision and values for child and family wellness. In I. Prilleltensky, G. Nelson, & L. Peirson (Eds.), *Promoting family wellness and preventing child maltreatment: Fundamentals for thinking and action* (pp. 124–173). Toronto, ON: University of Toronto Press.

Prilleltensky, I., & Nelson, G. (1997). Community psychology: Reclaiming social justice. In D. Fox & I. Prilleltensky (Eds.), *Critical psychology: An introduction* (pp. 166–184). London, UK: Sage.

Prilleltensky, I., & Nelson, G. (2009). Community psychology: Reclaiming social justice. In D. R. Fox & I. Prilleltensky (Eds.), *Critical psychology: An introduction* (2nd ed., pp. 166–184). Thousand Oaks, CA: Sage.

Rappaport, J. (1977). *Community psychology: Values, research & action.* New York, NY: Holt, Rinehart, Winston.

Rappaport, J. (1981). In praise of paradox: A social policy of empowerment over prevention. *American Journal of Community Psychology, 9,* 1–25.

Rappaport, J. (2005). Community psychology is (thank god) more than science. *American Journal of Community Psychology, 35*(3/4), 231–238

Rawls, J. (1971). *A theory of justice.* Cambridge, MA: Harvard University Press.

Riemer, M. (2010). Community psychology, the natural environment, and global climate change.

Sandel, M. (2009). *Justice: What's the right thing to do.* New York, NY: Farrar, Straus and Giroux.

Sandler, J. (2007). Community-based practices: Integrating dissemination theory with critical theories of power and justice. *American Journal of Community Psychology, 40,* 272–289.

Sarason, S. B. (1974). *The psychological sense of community: Perspectives for community psychology.* San Francisco, CA: Jossey-Bass.

Sarason, S. B. (1988). *The psychological sense of community: Prospects for a community psychology*. San Francisco, CA: Brookline Books.

Schwalbe, M. (2008). *Rigging the game: How inequality is reproduced in everyday life*. New York, NY: Oxford University.

Siddiqui, A., Hertzman, E., Irwin, L. G., & Hertzman, C. (2012). Early child development: A powerful equalizer. In J. H. Lee & R. Sadana (Eds.), *Improving equity in health by addressing social determinants* (pp. 115–141). Geneva, CH: World Health Organization, The Commission on Social Determinants of Health Knowledge Networks. Retrieved from http://www.who.int/social_determinants/en/

Sloan, T. S. (1990). Psychology for the Third World? *Journal of Social Issues, 46*(3), 1–20.

Sloan, T. (2010). Globalization, poverty, and social justice. In G. Nelson & I. Prilleltensky (Eds.), *Community psychology: In pursuit of liberation and well-being* (2nd ed., pp. 331–352). Basingstoke, UK: Palgrave Macmillan.

Society for Community Research and Action [SCRA]. (2010). About SCRA. Retrieved from http://www.scra27.org/about.

Syme, G. J., & Bishop, B. J. (1993). Public psychology: Planning a role for psychology. *Australian Psychologist, 28,* 45–51.

United Nations Children's Fund (UNICEF). (2012). *Inequities in early childhood development—what the data say.* New York, NY: Author.

Walsh, R. (1987). A social historical note on the formal emergence of community psychology. *American Journal of Community Psychology, 15,* 523–529.

Weil, M. O. (1996). Community building: Building community practice. *Social Work, 41*(5), 481–499.

Chapter 9

Social Justice in Industrial-Organizational and Consulting Psychology

Rodney L. Lowman

This handbook and this chapter are long overdue. The uses to which one puts psychological knowledge—society's best, most valuable, and most reliable professional asset—are not a new area of concern. But the explicit focus on social justice as a value that all areas of psychology should strive to attain is particularly apt for these "best and worst of times" when technological and social advances have never been more radically disruptive nor have been disparities in income, physical and mental health, and education, among others. The central question is whether Industrial-Organizational (I-O) psychologists can (or should) use their professional expertise to advance the social good or to simply further a narrow focus, including their own interests and those of specific clients. If I-O psychologists do embrace a social justice agenda, what does that mean and are the actions simply an altruistic action or ethically mandated? And, if ethically mandated, by what and whose standards? Are these ethical standards universally accepted or culturally dependent? And do the codes of ethical conduct of psychologists vary by country in the extent to which social justice is expected?

THE MANY FLAVORS OF PSYCHOLOGY

Psychology is a vast and growing field with few aspects of human or infrahuman behavior not found in some form within the purview of its research and practice. In some larger domains, such as mental health–related aspects of psychology, the relevance of a social justice agenda may seem obvious. After all, are not those with mental health problems themselves a minority such that when psychologists are helping to ameliorate their needs, they are focusing on social justice? Even in this area of psychology, however, there are many questions about how psychologists apply their professional expertise. These include whether psychologists (as researchers and as practitioners) should increase their efforts, for example, to be more concerned with the needs of the seriously mentally ill versus of those with lesser degrees of impairment, and whether the theories, methods, and research apply across races, genders, sexual orientations, and cultures.

In the case of I-O and Consulting Psychology (CP), the focus of this chapter, the issues associated with social justice are perhaps more complex than are those in many other areas of applied psychology. These fields typically use their expertise to help make organizations and leaders more effective. They are often instigators in translating important science-based knowledge about these topics to practice and they are experts in applying their theories and science to real-world issues. However, those hiring such experts and paying the bills for psychological consultants are usually people in management (not individual employees or labor unions) and it is their issues, therefore, that often take priority. Business values and those of psychologists do not necessarily overlap (see Lefkowitz & Lowman, 2010), though neither are they inherently antagonistic. An I-O or consulting psychologist with an explicit and prominent social justice agenda, however, may soon be one without clients or employment. Therefore, it is particularly relevant in this chapter first to consider the concept of a social justice agenda as a multifaceted one wherein its applications are not always obvious.

WHAT IS SOCIAL JUSTICE?

There is not one definition of social justice. The term had its origins in the Catholic religion and has been variously defined and promoted over the years often by religious leaders or liberal politicians (see, e.g., Zajda, Majhanovich, & Rust, 2007). Barry (1989) noted, "In Plato's time as in ours the central issue in any theory of justice is the defensibility of unequal relations among people" (p. 3). Barry goes on to cite inequalities in political power, social standing, and economic resources as some of the areas in which those "unequal relations" can exist.

Social justice definitions often emphasize, with a fair amount of consensus across experts and people in general, the assurance of basic human rights being accorded to all members of groups in society, procedural justice within legal systems, and in the use of force by those legally authorized to do so. With less likelihood of universal consensus, social justice can also be used to reference the quality of opportunity, health, and education people receive, and the definition of a minimum baseline below which the inequality of outcome that is inherent in any society should not fall (see, e.g., Adams, Bell, & Griffin, 2007). Often including a safety net, social justice is also concerned with establishing the minimal conditions of food, shelter, and education that even the poorest may be assured of in any particular society. Thus, social justice can address issues of inequality of both input and output (what people are given and what their results are.) This cannot be standardized in monetary terms since the costs of minimal care are much higher in developed than developing countries (see Cawagas, 2013).

Social justice also increasingly addresses the differences between the "haves" and the "have nots," and the discrepancies between those who have amassed wealth at the highest levels and those at the lowest (see Norton & Ariely, 2011). All societies historically and currently have an inequality of results, and few would argue that this is intrinsically problematic. After all, efforts to create idealized societies that have emphasized above all equality of results while ignoring the effort-outcome connection have rarely created societies characterized by creativity, increases in overall wealth, or corruption-free governments (Eberstadt, 1988; Dăian & Manova, 2012). However, the rules and laws of the prevalent capitalistic systems have resulted in the aggregation of the bulk of wealth in the hands of a tiny minority (e.g., Kawachi, Kennedy, & Wilkinson, 1999). As Ortiz and Cummins (2011) put it, "Both income distribution accounting models offer strikingly similar results . . . we inhabit a planet in which the top quintile controls more than 80 percent of global income contrasted by a paltry percentage point for those at the bottom" (p. 10). And when the economic elites can control not just their own considerable resources but also the rules of many games (e.g., health care accessibility, decision making about personal health care issues, who gets elected to public office, and what subjects are emphasized in, and which are removed from, school curricula), the system is imbalanced in a way that ultimately is dysfunctional for the society as a whole, even the elites. We also know that being female and poor (Lund et al., 2011; Patel, Araya, de Lima, Ludermir, & Todd, 1999) is associated with higher rates of mental disorders. Addressing mental health problems in such settings will increase economic well-being (Lund et al., 2011) but lessening poverty can also lower mental disorders.

THE WORK DOMAIN OF I-O AND CONSULTING PSYCHOLOGISTS

There are those politicians who argue that the best way to lessen poverty is by creating a thriving economy with jobs for all who want them and are qualified, and that capitalism is the best route to that outcome. As U.S. president Ronald Reagan was famously quoted as saying (in words that could be mouthed today by many politicians whose views have not wavered from this perspective), "Entrepreneurs and their small enterprises are responsible for almost all the economic growth in the United States" (Reagan, 1988, para. 8).

Such beliefs often belie the economic realities of those in the bottom rungs of society and show little compassion or understanding for the plight of those born into poverty, ill health, and/or limited intellectual resources. Still I-O and consulting psychologists need not apologize for striving to help make work organizations more effective. A well-functioning economy that offers diverse employment opportunities to those at all levels of the economic spectrum, and the rigors of creating competitive organizations for an economy that is intransigently now global (see Lowman, 2013a), should not be underestimated. Nor should the rigor of the science represented in I-O and CP be trivialized. Whether in addressing job satisfaction, occupational health, work motivation, organizational climate and culture, organizational conflict, individual group and organizational assessment, to name just a few areas, psychology has been blessed with enormous advances in knowledge that is often directly related to practice regarding work.

PERSONNEL SELECTION AND SOCIAL JUSTICE

Applied psychologists in areas such as I-O and CP generally practice their profession with the nonclinical applications of psychology (see, e.g., Lowman, 2002). Their clients are often organizations and individuals in the context of their work lives. Some such psychologists also focus on the intersection of work and nonwork (e.g., Cleveland & Colella, 2010), issues of retirement (e.g., Beehr, 1986), and unemployment (e.g., Paul & Moser, 2009). However, such foci are the exceptions and not the norm (Brief, 2000), and the modal I-O or consulting psychologist works with or for organizational clients, managers and executives, in situations wherein the client is often the organization itself, and the intended outcome is to increase the organization's well-being.

Notably, I-O psychology practice guidelines do not force practitioners to address socially relevant issues. However, I-O/consulting psychologists involved in test design and selection and helping increasingly diverse workplaces to function effectively are square in the middle of many of the major social issues of the day. Still, two factors combine to distinguish how such psychologists address these issues. First, I-O and consulting psychologists, as a matter of ethics and purpose (not to mention survival), must address the goals and needs of their clients and employers. Second, the science of I-O psychology, in particular, considers issues from the perspective of evidence that sometimes includes findings that are not necessarily supportive of a social justice agenda. Indeed, when the organization is the client, psychologists are often concerned with assisting in changes that make the organization more effective but not necessarily with improving the circumstances of the individuals or groups of individuals within the organization. Yet, applied psychologists working in this area face complex ethical dilemmas in personnel selection work if the context for evaluating outcomes is extended to social justice criteria, such as whether selection recommendations or decisions are balanced across race, genders, age, and physical ability.

Although there are many organizations that tout a diversity agenda, probably few large employers would be willing to sustain this goal at the expense of the quality of the employee hired. Indeed, many rich employers bifurcate between their core business purposes and social causes by addressing the latter through their not-for-profit foundations. And, though there may be I-O psychologists who espouse an explicit diversity agenda to client organizations, they have largely not made their efforts (or their outcomes of such advocacy efforts) publicly known, and it is probably more likely that I-O/consulting psychologists are not aggressive in advocating for such an agenda.

Although I believe psychologists whose clients are organizations should address social justice concerns, I argue that there are significant limits as to I-O and consulting psychologists' ability and opportunity to change corporate policies. These psychologists typically do not set the rules by which their expertise will be used and rarely are they in positions of power within the organization wherein they can dictate policy (even if they wanted to do so).

The wishes of employers and organizational clients thus provide one set of parameters for I-O and CP work but there are others. Science and research findings provide important parameters as well. I-O and CP are highly wedded to the scientist-practitioner model—arguably more so than most other applied psychology disciplines. This provides both a balance to what I-O and consulting psychologists can be asked or ordered to do by those in organizational power (few such psychologists would practice outside the bounds of scientific findings and knowledge) and a knowledge base that must be taken into account when responding to organizational goals. Additionally, there are numerous laws (e.g., Age Discrimination Act, Americans with Disabilities Act, The Equal Pay Act of 1963, Title VII of the Civil Rights Acts of 1964 of 1991; see Landy, Guttman, & Outtz, 2010) and standards governing the practice of I-O psychology. Some of these include the *Uniform Guidelines on Employee Selection Procedures* (41CFR60-3; 1978); *Standards for Educational and Psychological Testing,* jointly published by the American Educational Research Association, American Psychological Association, and the National Council on Measurement in Education (1999); and SIOP's *Principles for the Validation and Use of Personnel Selection Procedures* (Society for Industrial-Organizational Psychology, 2003; see also Jeanneret & Zedeck, 2010). These guidelines, rules, or laws can dictate what employers and I-O psychologists may and may not do concerning issues involving the hiring of minorities, women, and older workers in the United States.

Race Matters

To take just one important and highly relevant example of the science side of the discipline as it relates to personnel selection, I-O psychologists have done some of the pioneering work in the area of racial differences in employment selection (see, e.g., Hunter, Schmidt, & Hunter, 1979). A number of studies including an early and influential study (Schmidt, Berner, & Hunter, 1973) have evaluated the question about whether employment tests are differentially valid for both majority and protected classes in the United States and whether they have adverse impact. With few exceptions, when meta-analyses of studies in this area are conducted (see, e.g., Hunter et al., 1979; Schmidt, 1988; Schmidt & Hunter, 2004), employment tests have not exhibited differential validity such that the tests were valid for some but not for other protected classes of applicants. (Some more recent studies have found small differences in validity coefficients; see, e.g., Aguinis, Culpepper, & Pierce, 2011; Berry, Clark, & McLcure, 2011). Nevertheless, the results of employment testing do differ by race such that the regression lines depicting the relationship between employment tests (predictors) and outcomes (job-related performance criteria) have the same slope but are parallel with the lines for most minority groups being lower than those for the majority group. This is called adverse impact. (An exception is that Asian Americans usually score, on average, higher than Caucasians; see Kao & Thompson, 2003).

The question of *why* these average group differences exist and persist is complex, controversial, and without expert consensual resolution at this time. There are a number of different theories put forth for such differences. Roberson and Block (2002) identified the following models that have been put forward to account for the differences: internal trait model, bias and discrimination, response to discrimination model, and the organizational context model.

Generally, the nature of the tests themselves has not shown to be the primary cause of adverse impact to the extent that cognitive ability is an important part of the tests and also required to be successful on the job (see Sackett, Schmidt, Ellingson, & Kabin, 2001; Schmidt, 1988).

That said, test-taking orientation may matter. For example, evidence that suggests that stereotype threat (Steele & Aronson, 1995) may cause underperformance among some individuals on some "high stakes" tests has been presented. Stated overly simply, stereotype threat is the theory that test-taking presented as associated with characteristics in which a person may feel inferior or inadequate (e.g., "intelligence") results in underperformance on the test. There is some suggestion that stereotype threat may in part play a role for some individuals and groups (see Steele & Aronson, 1995) but a number of issues that must be considered in evaluating this research have also been raised (see Sackett, Borneman, & Connelly, 2008, 2009; Sackett, Hardison, & Cullen, 2004). Finally, validity coefficients have two sides of the correlation: predictors and criteria. There may also be differential ratings of performance in which race of the person being rated plays a factor (see Kraiger & Ford, 1985).

Underlying some of the arguments about such differences is the concept of traits (i.e., relatively fixed characteristics). If cognitive abilities are heavily fixed, it might be interpreted to imply that this accounts for most observed differences. Yet we know that cognitive abilities can be changed. The Flynn effect (Flynn, 1987), for example, suggests that performance on cognitive abilities can change over time at least when considered at a societal or group level. This suggests a much more optimistic view about the need to address those factors responsible for change, assuming that the minimization of racial differences is a desired outcome (which a social justice perspective would support). Overall, I suggest that, from the perspective of social justice, I-O and CP have not always placed enough emphasis on the theories accounting for why there is adverse impact focusing more on the important pragmatic questions of productivity and job performance rather than on either looking at less cognitively laden tests or helping employers work on how better to improve adverse impact. (See also the important discussions by Lefkowitz, 2003, 2005; Lefkowitz & Lowman, 2010.)

There are many technical issues that also affect adverse impact in employee selection. For example, when cut scores are drawn at a particular point in the distribution using a "top down" procedure, such that those with the highest scores are hired before those with lower scores, more Asian Americans and Whites will usually be selected compared with Blacks and Latinos when the cut score on the predictor measure is drawn at a fixed point for all groups. This approach is consistent with the science of the I-O psychology research literature and with the typical goal of employers to hire the most qualified people (i.e., those scoring highest) from their pool of applicants. The ethical obligation of the I-O psychologist arguably ends there—helping the organization hire the best and to assure that the validity of the test inferences are defensible in the event of an Equal Employment Opportunity Commission (EEOC) or other challenge. By using a well-validated predictor and appropriate criterion measures, the psychologist has also protected the organization from EEOC challenges when, predictably, these measures have adverse impact.

The I-O psychologist is not, I argue, behaving unethically by helping an organization find the most qualified applicants for employment. In fact, the rules promulgated by the EEOC's *Uniform Guidelines* (1978; see also McDaniel, Kepes, & Banks, 2011) in the United States do not stipulate that a particular number of people from different racial (or age, or gender) groups be hired or that the rates of persons accepted and rejected be equal across all groups. Rather, they require that when there is adverse impact (roughly, when a selection procedure results in hiring less than 4/5 of those in a protected category, then the employer must be able to show that there is validity for the measures used. Of course, the EEOC and other such groups would object if the employer's measures were not job-related or predictors were chosen that maximized adverse impact when other, equally valid measures were available.

This could be the end of the story unless the employer wants to assure diversity in the hiring decisions or the I-O/consulting psychologist wanted to advance a diversity agenda in the organization. Then there may be many things the company can do, even in the face of adverse impact with a validated measure both to minimize the differential selection rates and to maximize the positive benefits of a diverse workplace, particularly if the psychologist takes a proactive or advocacy role. Of course, this is not the ethical responsibility of the psychologist whose role is to maximize the client's desired outcomes. Or, is it?

Balancing Organizational and Social Justice Goals

If social justice is not, as I will argue (with the notable exception of the ethics code of the Canadian Psychological Association [2000]), necessarily a mandated ethical requirement under many psychology ethics codes (see, e.g., the American Psychological Association, 2002; British Psychological Society, 2011; the International Union of Psychological Science, 2008; the Japanese Psychological Association, undated; the Professional Board for Psychology Health

Professions Council of South Africa, undated), are there reasons to address such issues anyway? Increasingly I believe, the evidence suggests the affirmative. Increasing diversity in teams, for example, has been shown to increase, not decrease, performance (see, e.g., Edwards, Colling, & Ferner, 2007; Elron, 1998). Bear, Rahman, and Post (2010) similarly found that board diversity and increased gender diversity was associated with greater social responsibility and the reputation of the firm. Rodrigo and Arenas (2008) reported that organizations having a social justice agenda had greater identification with the organization and a greater sense of the importance of their work in the context of a larger purpose.

Unfortunately, the process of balancing concern with group differences in selection procedures in order to minimize adverse impact without sacrificing validity and organizational effectiveness outcomes is not a simple task. Johnson and Oswald (2010) identified a number of issues involved in combining privacy, confidentiality, and self-determination factors that have more and less adverse impact in terms of their combined effect on organizational effectiveness. One ongoing challenge is that the best predictors of job performance have generally been shown to be cognitive abilities (see Ones, Dilchert, Viswesvaran, & Salgado, 2010; Sackett, Borneman, & Connelly, 2008, 2009), but cognitive measures may have the most adverse impact on diversity. Thus, as some organizational leaders believe, organizations wishing to promote increased diversity and social justice may have to do so at the expense of organizational outcomes. Of course, the I-O or consulting psychologist is not likely to be the decision maker as to how, if at all, to balance these concerns.

I have offered racial differences in selection rates as just one example of the issues involved with social justice. I could have named many others, including gender. Although there is very little adverse impact between men and women on measures of cognitive ability, in the case of physical abilities required for physically demanding jobs like firefighters there is considerable adverse impact that affects the ability of women to obtain such jobs. Conceptually, however, it is the same issue except that the predictors are physical rather than cognitive abilities.

Social Justice Opportunity: Employee Selection

If measures are designed in a scientifically defensible way, are clearly associated with the outcome criteria (typically, job performance), and are to predict and have the highest predictor-criterion relationships compared to alternatives that may have less adverse impact, what is the problem with I-O and consulting psychologists just doing their job? I argue that this question speaks to the heart of an ethical challenge inherent in doing this kind of work. On the one hand, psychologists have an ethical responsibility to meet the needs of their clients, including organizations. APA Ethics (enforceable) Standard 3.11 applies:

> Standard 3.11 Psychological Services Delivered to or Through Organizations (a) Psychologists delivering services to or through organizations provide information beforehand to clients and when appropriate those directly

> affected by the services about (1) the nature and objectives of the services, (2) the intended recipients, (3) which of the individuals are clients, (4) the relationship the psychologist will have with each person and the organization, (5) the probable uses of services provided and information obtained, (6) who will have access to the information, and (7) limits of confidentiality. As soon as feasible, they provide information about the results and conclusions to appropriate persons. (APA, 2002 p. 1066)

Additionally, psychologists have an obligation to do no harm to their organizational clients, just as they would to their individual ones.

> **APA Ethics Standard 3.04 Avoiding Harm:** Psychologists take reasonable steps to avoid harming their clients/patients, students, supervisees, research participants, organizational clients, and others with whom they work, and to minimize harm where it is foreseeable and unavoidable. (APA, 2002, p. 1066)

Thus, an I-O/consulting psychologist with a social justice agenda working with an organizational client that explicitly wanted only top-down, best qualified hires would not be getting the services its representatives contracted for if selection procedures with less adverse impact but lower relationships between the predictors and organizational outcomes were substituted for the most predictive measures. And if the selection methodology were scientifically defensible, and more valid than alternatives with less adverse impact, psychologists would not be meeting their client's needs by implementing alternative methodologies. Arguably, the company might be experiencing harm by hiring less qualified applicants.

What's A Psychologist to Do?

I argue that those psychologists governed by the APA's (2002) Ethics Code may not have an ethical obligation to pursue a social justice agenda except as it relates to not doing harm, engaging in discriminatory behavior, or assuring competence in working with particular populations. Social justice is further an ill-defined, perhaps overly inclusive term that does not have universal meanings that can be reduced to a "thou shalt" or "thou shalt not" set of behavioral standards.

That said, for those psychologists working with organizations who do care about such issues and who do consider it a goal of their calling to help improve the human condition, then they need to take on such issues as they fall within their sphere of work. Sticking with the personnel selection example, there are many cogent arguments that psychologists could make about why diversity in hiring may matter more than getting the "best" candidates. Here are some examples:

(1) *Diversity matters.* Few work forces in the United States in particular and globally can afford to not have a diverse work force. As I have noted

elsewhere (e.g., Lowman, 2013b), those organizations that do not know how to manage diversity will be at a disadvantage. Additionally, there is evidence that students, if not employees, prefer learning and working in diverse environments (Whitla et al., 2003) and having a diverse group of employees is more likely to mirror the customer and population base.

(2) *Consider the outcome criteria.* Much of the personnel selection outcome criteria includes subjective ratings of job performance conducted over a rather short period of time (e.g., job performance within a year or less after hire). As our understanding of criteria important on the job expands, it becomes clear that job performance alone as an outcome measure needs to be broadened to include such factors as organizational citizenship behavior (OCB; Dorsey, Cortina, & Luchman, 2010), personality characteristics (e.g., Kaiser & Hogan, 2010), and fit with the particular organization. Broadening the outcome criteria opens up other possibilities for predictors including some that have less impact.

(3) *Study what happens to new hires once they are in the organization.* Having the "most qualified" hires does not mean that such employees will stay in the organization. Longer-term criteria can help consider how selected employees fare time. Work performance can also be influenced by how employees are treated once they are selected.

(4) *Consider combining across predictors to assemble composite of predictors.* Hattrup, Rock, and Scalia (1997) and Sackett and Roth (1996) showed that alternative predictor combinations and varying the criteria used resulted in less adverse impact.

In sum, psychologists are often the major source of technical experts in work organizations. They are uniquely positioned to help organizations think through issues of selection in a way that combines concern for outcomes on job performance and the creation of a diverse environment.

CHALLENGING DISPARITIES: INCOME

The case of personnel selection is only one area in which the applications of social justice are complex and not obvious as to the behavioral mandates they make upon the psychologist. To take another example of opportunities to promote social justice in organizational contexts, the issues of discrepancies between the "haves" and "have nots" present the opportunity for I-O and consulting psychologists to consider such issues on their own organizational turf. Mishel and Sabadish (2012) have provided evidence that the financial remuneration of CEOs and those in the top 1% of incomes have increased disproportionally. As was discussed at the beginning of this chapter, this is part of a larger trend toward accumulation of great wealth among fewer and fewer people. The three richest people in the world, for example, have more financial assets than the lowest 48 nations combined. Between

2002 and 2007 income of the top 1% grew 10 times faster than the income of the bottom 90% (Johnston, 2007). Mishel and Sabadish (2012) noted that when "applying a measure of CEO compensation that include[d] the value of stock options granted to an executive, the CEO-to-worker compensation ratio was 18.3-to-1 in 1965, peaked at 411.3-to-1 in 2000, and sits at 209.4-to-1 in 2011" (n.p.).

As with their personnel selection efforts, consulting and I-O psychologists are unlikely to be the decision makers in deciding whether the ratio between the highest- and lowest-paid employees are too far apart. However, they have the opportunity to help management consider such issues by articulating them, to design surveys that may address areas of job satisfaction, including satisfaction with pay, and to be a persistent voice for broadening the values that employers consider in policy development. They can volunteer to serve on influential committees in the organization and use their research knowledge and ability to research questions to provide examples of how other companies are handling similar issues and the impact of income disparities on employees.

In the 2012 U.S. presidential election David Gergen, an advisor to four presidents and television commentator, noted President Obama's failure in his first term to create a sustained narrative for the many positive things he had achieved in his term. He noted the idea that skilled politicians create a clothesline on which all the clothes of individual achievements are hung and they constantly take every opportunity they can to narrate, contextualize, and provide sense making to their views. Similarly, psychologists who want to make a difference with an issue as complex as income disparity need to become spokespersons first for a larger narrative about doing the right thing by employees, about increasing the diversity of their hires and promotions while maintaining employee quality and performance, and about considering work-life balance issues and the needs of their aging work force. By focusing on quiet advocacy—often by just being the one to raise the issues when no one else does—the psychologist can create credibility and integrity. All battles will never be won but there are far worse things than incremental change.

Other Roles for I-O and Consulting Psychologists in Social Justice Agenda: Helping Organizations Include Social Justice Issues in Their Evaluation Parameters

Psychologists are often involved in constructing outcome measures and attitude surveys. In such roles, they can introduce outcome parameters that may not have occurred to others. Job satisfaction is a common construct measured by psychologists in the industry, and a well-developed survey can help identify both causes and consequences of such a variable as well as the impact on organizational effectiveness criteria. A balanced score card can help the organization see how it is doing on various social justice issues, for example, women versus men in managerial positions, racial distribution of employees, outcome measures for employees in remote (e.g., international) locations, turnover, and many others.

Contextualizing the Issues

I do not expect senior managers necessarily to be vocal spokespersons for social justice agendas, especially when there are compelling issues of organizational management to be fixed. I would not expect psychologists to use the words *social justice* in working with organizational clients. By understanding those issues the organizations do care about, and speaking to those issues, I/O and consulting psychologists can help focus decision makers' attention on social justice issues in a way that can potentially sustain itself over time. Managers are notoriously goal-driven. Once a social justice issue has turned from the question of why organizations should care about it at all, it is likely, if accepted as a valued outcome, to be attached to staff, resources, and goals. A company deciding that to be competitive in a diverse environment it needs diversity in its workforce may be motivated to track its efforts and outcomes over time. And managers do not like to miss their targeted goals.

Psychologists' Roles in Helping to Create Ethical Organizations

It is an obvious fact but one that needs to be made explicitly: the ethics codes of behavior promulgated by psychologists create behavioral and aspirational standards just for psychologists. Managers do not have professional codes of ethics except those related to specialty areas such as accounting. Because psychologists have such responsibilities, if not predispositions (see Aguinis, 2011), they may become spokespersons in organizations for their ethical obligations and educate managers and others about why such codes matter. Psychologists can therefore be the eyes, ears, and voices for concern with ethical issues and help key stakeholders think about what is and is not ethical in their particular context.

Increasingly, however, it is the corporations that are identifying the practical value of corporate social responsibility agendas. Business strategy increasingly embraces the virtues of "going green" (see, e.g., Hussain, 1999; Lowman, 2013) and advocacy for corporate social responsibility (Porter & Kramer, 2011; Spear, 2006). Thompson and MacMillan (2010) identified a number of businesslike principles that could be applied to social entrepreneurship. Psychologists may not be the leaders in all these efforts, but they can certainly contribute to positive ethical environments in corporations and other employers.

Executive Assessments

I-O and consulting psychologists are often called on to conduct individual-level assessments. We are now able reliably to measure not just cognitive and personality characteristics but also values and rule out criteria such narcissism and sociopathy (see, e.g., Hogan & Hogan, 2001). Choosing executives who are good fits with the values of the organization and who see it as important to advance socially minded agendas while also meeting organizational objectives provides greater likelihood over time that a social justice agenda can be sustained over time.

HELPING TO CREATE ETHICAL ORGANIZATIONAL CLIMATES

Conclusion and Moral of the Story

Although I am certainly in favor of I-O and consulting psychologists addressing and contributing to social justice issues, I believe the nuances of having a social justice agenda should not be overlooked. By the nature of their work, they are obliged to serve the best interests of their clients, which often are organizations and not individuals. They are also obliged to meet the legal parameters associated with their work. But simply because they are not ethically obligated to always consider social justice issues, this does not mean that psychologists cannot choose to apply their competencies to this cause.

I will end on a personal note. I trained in both I-O and clinical psychology at a major university. Not once in any of my training did any professor or colleague speak about a social justice agenda being a responsibility—ethical or otherwise. I have attended more psychology conferences than I care to remember but at almost none of these was the term *social justice* ever mentioned except when I said them. Still, I believe that I-O and consulting psychologists are a mostly untapped potential for furthering social justice in the world. They understand organizations, and they can speak the language of organizations. They understand the concerns of productivity and organizational effectiveness demands in a highly competitive environment. According to most professional ethical codes, there is no obligation—ethically or otherwise—to be a blind advocate for social justice but neither are the issues irrelevant to their day-to-day work or their values as psychologists. By helping major organizational stakeholders take into account the role of selection in the context of a diverse world of applicants, increasing their awareness of the costs and consequences of a work environment perceived to be unethical, and quietly helping leaders understand the divisive consequences of exaggerated discrepancies in rewards to those at the top versus at lower levels in the organizational hierarchy, consulting and I-O psychologists can begin to create a more socially just world. The stakes are not trivial. As Feagin, 2001 (p. 16) put it:

> For many millennia human beings have been tool-makers, yet in just a few decades we have created economies and technologies—such as polluting industries, fossil fuel consuming engines, and nuclear weapons—that may well threaten the survival of our species and of our living planet itself. It seems likely that the fate of our planet and its many species will be decided within the next few generations by just one of its species. As moral beings, we need to ask insistently: What would alternatives to our self destructive societies look like? And how do we get there?

REFERENCES

Adams, M., Bell, L. A., & Griffin, P. (2007). *Teaching for diversity and social justice* (2nd ed.). New York, NY: Routledge Taylor & Francis.

Aguinis, H. (2011). Organizational responsibility: Doing good and doing well. In S. Zedeck (Ed.), *APA handbook of industrial and organizational psychology* (Vol. 3, pp. 855–879). Washington, DC: American Psychological Association.

Aguinis, H., Culpepper, S. A., & Pierce, C. A. (2010). Revival of test bias research in preemployment testing. *Journal of Applied Psychology, 95,* 648–680. doi: 10.1037/a0018714

American Educational Research Association, American Psychological Association, and National Council on Measurement in Education. (1999). *Standards for educational and psychological testing.* Washington, DC: Authors.

American Psychological Association. (2002). Ethical principles of psychologists and code of conduct. (2002). *American Psychologist, 57*(12), 1060–1073. doi:10.1037/0003-066X.57.12.1060

American Psychological Association. (2003). Guidelines on multicultural, education, training, research, practice, and organizational change for psychologists. *American Psychologist, 58,* 377–402.

Barry, B. M. (1989). *Theories of justice. A treatise on social justice* (Vol. 1). Berkeley, CA: University of California Press.

Bear, S., Rahman, N., & Post, C. (2010). The impact of board diversity and gender composition on corporate social responsibility and firm reputation. *Journal of Business Ethics, 97,* 207–221. doi:10.1007/s10551-010-0505-2

Beehr, T. A. (1986). The process of retirement: A review and recommendation for future investigation. *Personnel Psychology, 39,* 31–55.

Berry, C. M., Clark, M. A., & McClure, T. K. (2011, September). Racial/ethnic differences in the criterion-related validity of cognitive ability tests: A qualitative and quantitative review. *Journal of Applied Psychology, 96,* 881–906. doi: 10.1037/a0023222

Brief, A. P. (2000). Still servants of power. *Journal of Management Inquiry, 9,* 342–351.

British Psychological Society. (2011). *Code of ethics and conduct. Guidance published by the Ethics Committee of the British Psychological Society.* London, UK: British Psychological Society. Retrieved from http://www.bps.org.uk/sites/default/files/documents/code_of_ethics_and_conduct.pdf

Canadian Psychological Association. (2000). *Canadian code of ethics for psychologists.* Ottawa, Canada: Author.

Cawagas, V. (2013). Bringing gender into multicultural and international competencies: Strategies, and challenges. In R. L. Lowman (Ed.), *Internationalizing multiculturalism: Expanding professional competencies in a globalized world* (pp. 57–81). Washington, DC: American Psychological Association.

Cleveland, J. H., & Colella, A. (2010). Criterion validity and criterion deficiency. What we measure well and what we ignore. In J. L. Farr & N. Tippins (Eds.), *Handbook of employee selection* (pp. 551–567). New York, NY: Psychology Press (Taylor & Francis).

Code of Ethics of Psychologists of the Federation of Psychologists of the Argentine Republic (Fe.P.R.A.). (1991). Retrieved from: http://www.iupsys.net/images/resources/ethics/Argentina_translation_to_english.pdf

Dăian, M., & Manova, K. B. (2012). *The veil of communism: An analysis of lifespan, GDP per capita, human capital, and agricultural productivity in Eastern Europe.* Unpublished Paper, Department of Economics, Stanford University.

Dorsey, D. W., Cortina, J. M., & Luchman, J. (2010). Adaptive and citizenship-related behaviors at work. In J. L. Farr & N. Tippins (Eds.), *Handbook of employee selection* (pp. 571–590). New York, NY: Psychology Press (Taylor & Francis).

Eberstadt, N. (2008). *The poverty of communism*. Piscataway, NJ: Transaction Publishers, Rutgers University.

Edwards, T., Colling, T., & Ferner, A. (2007). Conceptual approaches to the transfer of employment practices in multinational companies: An integrated approach. *Human Resource Management Journal, 17,* 201–217.

Elron, E. (1998). Top management teams within multinational corporations: Effects of cultural heterogeneity. *The Leadership Quarterly, 8,* 393–412.

Feagin, J. (2001). Social justice and sociology: Agendas for the twenty-first century. *American Sociological Review, 66,* 1–20.

Flynn, J. R. (1987). Massive IQ gains in 14 nations: What IQ tests really measure. *Psychological Bulletin, 101,* 171–191. doi: 10.1037/0033-2909.101.2.171

Hattrup, K., Rock, J., & Scalia, C. (1997). The effects of varying conceptualizations of job performance on adverse impact, minority hiring, and predicted performance. *Journal of Applied Psychology, 82,* 656–664.

Hogan, R., & Hogan, J. (2001). Assessing leadership: A view from the dark side. *International Journal of Selection and Assessment, 9*(1–2), 40–51. doi:10.1111/1468-2389.00162

Hunter, J. E., Schmidt, F. L., & Hunter, R. (1979). Differential validity of employment tests by race: A comprehensive review and analysis. *Psychological Bulletin, 86,* 721–735.

Hussain, S. S. (1999). The ethics of "going green": The corporate social responsibility debate. *Business Strategy and the Environment, 8,* 203–210.

International Union of Psychological Science. (2008). Universal declaration of ethical principles for psychologists (unpaginated). Retrieved from: http://iupsys.net/index.php/ethics/declaration

The Japanese Psychological Association. (undated). Ethical principles of psychologists. Retrieved from: http://www.psych.or.jp/english/ethical.html

Jeanneret, P. R., & Zedeck, S. (2010). Professional guidelines/standards. In J. L. Farr & N. Tippins (Eds.), *Handbook of employee selection* (pp. 593–625). New York, NY: Psychology Press (Taylor & Francis).

Johnson, J. W., & Oswald, F. L. (2010). Test administration and the use of test scores. In J. L. Farr & N. T. Tippins (Eds.), *Handbook of employee selection* (pp. 151–169). New York, NY: Psychology Press (Taylor & Francis).

Johnston, D. C. (2007, March 29). Income gap is widening, study shows. Business Section, New York *Times,* [unpaginated]. Retrieved from http://www.nytimes.com/2007/03/29/business/29tax.html?ex=1332820800&en=fb472e72466c34c8&ei=5088&partner=rssnyt&emc=rss&_r=0

Kaiser, R. B., & Hogan, R. (2010). How to (and how not to) assess the integrity of managers. *Consulting Psychology Journal: Practice and Research, 62,* 216–234.

Kao, G. & Thompson, J. S. (2003). Racial and ethnic stratification in educational achievement and attainment. *Annual Review of Sociology, 29,* 417–442.

Kawachi, I., Kennedy, B. P., & Wilkinson, R. G. (Eds.). (1999). *Income inequality and health* (Vol. 1). New York, NY: New Press.

Kraiger, K., & Ford, J. K. (1985). A meta-analysis of rate race effects in performance ratings. *Journal of Applied Psychology, 70*(1), 56–65. doi: 10.1037/0021-9010.70.1.56

Landy, F. J., Gutman, A., & Outtz, J. L. (2010). A sampler of legal principles in employment selection. In J. L. Farr & N. Tippins (Eds.), *Handbook of employee selection* (pp. 627–650). New York, NY: Psychology Press (Taylor & Francis).

Lefkowitz, J. (2003). *Ethics and values in industrial and organizational psychology.* New York, NY: Erlbaum (Francis & Taylor).

Lefkowtiz, J. (2005). The values of Industrial-Organizational psychology: Who are we? *The Industrial-Organizational Psychologist, 43.* Retrieved from http://www.siop.org/TIP/backissues/Oct05/03lefkowitz.aspx

Lefkowitz, J., & Lowman, R. L. (2010). Ethics of employee selection. In J. L. Farr, & N. Tippins (Eds.), *Handbook of employee selection* (pp. 571–590). New York, NY: Psychology Press (Taylor & Francis).

Lowman, R. L. (Ed.). (2013a). *Internationalizing multiculturalism: Expanding professional competencies in a globalized world.* Washington, DC: American Psychological Association.

Lowman, R. L. (2013b). Is sustainability an ethical responsibility of I-O and consulting psychologists? In Ann Hergatt Huffman & Stephanie R. Klein (Eds.), *Green Organizations: Driving Change with I-O Psychology* (pp. 34–54). New York: Psychology Press/Routledge.

Lund, C., Silva, M., Plagerson, S., Cooper, S., Chisholm, D., Das, J., . . . Patel, V. (2011). Poverty and mental disorders: Breaking the cycle in low-income and middle-income countries. *Lancet, 378*(9801), 1502–1514. doi: 10.1016/S0140-6736(11)60754-X

McDaniel, M. A., Kepes, S., & Banks, G. C. (2011). The Uniform Guidelines are a detriment to the field of personnel selection. *Industrial and Organizational Psych*ology, *4,* 494–514. doi: 10.1111/j.1754-9434.2011.01382.x

Mishel, L. & Sabadish, N. (2012, May 2). CEO pay and the top 1%How executive compensation and financial-sector pay have fueled income inequality. Washington, DC: Economic Policy Institute. Retrieved from: http://www.epi.org/publication/ib331-ceo-pay-top-1-percent/

Norton, M. I., & Ariely, D. (2011). Building a better America—One wealth quintile at a time. *Perspectives on Psychological Science, 6,* 9–12.

Ones, D. S., Dilchert, S., Viswesvaran, C., & Salgado, J. F. (2010). In J. L. Farr & N. Tippins (Eds.), *Handbook of employee selection* (pp. 255–270). New York, NY: Psychology Press (Taylor & Francis).

Ortiz, I., & Cummins, M. (2011). Global inequality: Beyond the bottom billion—A rapid review of income distribution in 141 countries. Retrieved from http://ssrn.com/abstract=1805046

Patel, V., Araya, R., de Lima, M., Ludermir, A., & Todd, C. (1999). Women, poverty and common mental disorders in four restructuring societies. *Social Science & Medicine, 49,* 1461–1471. doi: 10.1016/S0277-9536(99)00208-7

Paul, K. I., & Moser, K. (2009). Unemployment impairs mental health: Meta-analyses. *Journal of Vocational Behavior, 74,* 264–282.

Porter, M. E., & Kramer, M. R. (2011). Creating shared value. *Harvard Business Review, 89*(1/2), 62–77.

The Professional Board for Psychology Health Professions Council of South Africa. (2002). *Ethical code of professional conduct.* Retrieved from http://www.psyssa.com/aboutus/codeofconduct.asp

Reagan, R. W. (1988, May 31). *Address at Moscow State University* [speech transcript]. Miller Center, University of Virginia. Retrieved from http://millercenter.org/president/speeches/detail/3416

Roberson, L., & Block, C. J. (2001). Racioethnicity and job performance: A review and critique of theoretical perspectives on the causes of group differences. *Research in Organizational Behavior, 23,* 247–325. doi: 10.1016/S0191-3085(01)23007-X

Rodrigo, P., & Arenas, D. (2008). Do employees care about CSR programs? A typology of employees according to their attitudes. *Journal of Business Ethics, 83,* 265–283. doi: 10.1007/s10551-007-9618-7

Sackett, P. R., Borneman, M. J., & Connelly, B. S. (2008). High-stakes testing in higher education and employment: Appraising the evidence for validity and fairness. *American Psychologist, 63,* 215–227. doi: 10.1037/0003-066X.63.4.215

Sackett, P. R., Borneman, M. J., & Connelly, B. S. (2009). Responses to issues raised about validity, bias, and fairness in high-stakes testing. *American Psychologist, 64*(4), 285–287. doi:10.1037/a0015473

Sackett, P. R., Hardison, C. M., & Cullen, M. J. (2004). On interpreting stereotype threat as accounting for African American-White differences on cognitive tests. *American Psychologist, 59,* 7–13. doi: 10.1037/0003-066X.59.1.7

Sackett, P. R., & Roth, L. (1996). Multi-stage selection strategies: A Monte Carlo investigation of effects on performance and minority hiring. *Personnel Psychology, 49*(3), 549–557.

Sackett, P. R., Schmitt, N., Ellingson, J. E., & Kabin, M. B. (2001). High-stakes testing in employment, credentialing, and higher education: Prospects in a post-affirmative-action world. *American Psychologist, 56,* 302–318. doi: 10.1037/0003-066X.56.4.302

Schmidt, F. L. (1988). The problem of group differences in ability test scores in employment section. *Journal of Vocational Behavior, 33,* 272–292.

Schmidt, F. L., Berner, J. G., & Hunter, J. E. (1973). Racial differences in validity of employment tests: Reality or illusion? *Journal of Applied Psychology, 58,* 5–9. doi: 10.1037/h0035408

Schmidt, F. L., & Hunter, J. (2004). General mental ability in the world of work: Occupational attainment and job performance. *Journal of Personality and Social Psychology*, 86, 162–173. doi:10.1037/0022-3514.86.1.162

Society for Industrial-Organizational Psychology. (2003). *Principles for the validation and use of personnel selection procedures* (4th ed.) Retrieved from http://www.siop.org/_Principles/principles.pdf

Spear, R. (2006). Social entrepreneurship: a different model? *International Journal of Social Economics, 33*(5/6), 399–410.

Steele, C. M., & Aronson, J. (1995). Stereotype threat and the intellectual test performance of African Americans. *Journal of Personality and Social Psychology, 69,* 797–811. doi: 10.1037/0022-3514.69.5.797

Thompson, J. D., & MacMillan, I. C. (2010). Making social ventures work. *Harvard Business Review, 88*(9), 66–73.

Uniform Guidelines on Employee Selection Procedures (41CFR60-3) (1978). Retrieved from http://www.gpo.gov/fdsys/pkg/CFR-2010-title29-vol4/pdf/CFR-2010-title29-vol4-part1607.pdf

Whitla, D. K., Orfield, G., Silen, W., Teperow, C., Howard, C., & Reede, J. (2003). Educational benefits of diversity in medical school: A survey of students. *Academic Medicine, 78,* 460–466.

Zajda, J., Majhanovich, S. & Rust, V. (2007). *Introduction: Education and social justice. International Review of Education, 52,* 9–22.

Chapter 10

School Psychology and Social Justice

David Shriberg

Education is a social process. . . . Education is growth. . . . Education is not preparation for life, education is life itself.

—John Dewey

In this chapter I argue that school psychologists have a very strong—and unique—opportunity to engage in activities and practices consistent with a social justice framework. As professionals with particular expertise in working with children and families, school psychologists bring to the table a depth of foundational knowledge in child development, learning and motivational theory, and contemporary prevention models. As applied practitioners, school psychologists possess pertinent training and experience in areas such as mental health and academic assessment, observation, consultation and intervention, crisis response, and family-school-community collaboration.

According to U.S. Department of Education statistics, there are approximately 50 million children enrolled in U.S. public schools, a number expected to rise to approximately 53 million by the 2021–2022 academic year (U.S. Department of Education, 2013). Although the number of hours spent in school per week and the number of school days per year varies from state to state and from country to country, using conservative estimates of an average 6.5 hour school day over 180 days, the typical preK–12 student in the United States spends approximately

1,170 hours per year in school. Although compelling arguments can be made for social justice advocacy with and on behalf of persons of all ages, it is my belief that from a prevention standpoint social justice efforts geared toward children can have particularly powerful effects across society both in the short and in the long run. As the psychologists who typically have the most direct access to children in schools, school psychologists have an extraordinary opportunity to engage in prevention and advocacy work that supports social justice.

In this chapter, I explore the role of school psychologists vis-à-vis social justice. Following an overview of the relationship between education and social justice, and of psychology's relative lack of engagement in education, I provide a detailed discussion of what school psychologists do and how school psychologists can leverage their role as agents of social justice.

HISTORICAL CONTEXT

Social justice is both a process and a goal (Bell, 2013). If the goal of social justice is "full and equal participation of all groups in a society that is mutually shaped to meet their needs" (Bell, 2013, p. 21), then education stands as a primary entryway (or, conversely, a potential barrier) from which social justice can be achieved. Within the United States, in conjunction with the Emancipation Proclamation, President Abraham Lincoln understood that the education of former slaves in integrated schools was key to improving race relations and to providing freed Blacks with access to societal opportunities (Kearns Goodwin, 2005). How the fate of Reconstruction, and the history of social justice and education in the United States specifically—not to mention race relations more generally—might have been dramatically different if President Lincoln had not been assassinated in 1865, shortly before the Civil War would come to a close!

However, U.S. society would never come to know what Reconstruction might have looked like led by the guiding and generous hand of President Lincoln. Instead, as has been well documented, instead of integration came segregation. Although segregation and Jim Crow policies created much social injustice across all spheres, it was not a coincidence that schools were targeted as the focus to advance desegregation in what became the case of the 20th century, the seminal *Brown v. Board of Education of Topeka* (1954) court case. According to Thurgood Marshall's biographer Juan Williams (1998), although there was a strong legal rationale for selecting schools as the area to contest segregation laws nationally, the close relationship between segregated schools and racial inequality was well understood by segregationists and advocates of racial justice alike. In particular, as the child of both a teacher and of a very bright man who had no access to education, and as someone who had experienced many barriers to his own education due to segregation, Marshall had a strong personal interest in schools. At a time when psychological research was not well established or accepted, Marshall advocated including and featuring the then largely unknown research of Kenneth and

Mamie Clark that showed that when presented with White and Black dolls, Black children almost always stated that the White dolls were prettier, smarter, and better at everything they did than the Black dolls. Indeed, Marshall's personal experiences in talking with young Black girls and boys about their future reportedly resonated with these findings (Williams, 1998). As such, the Clark research played a pivotal role in the case, specifically cited in the Supreme Court decision as persuasive evidence, the first time psychological research played such a pivotal role in major national court case (Benjamin & Crouse, 2002).

As the Clark studies highlight, psychological knowledge has the potential to positively benefit schools in a way that supports social justice. Indeed, this potential benefit has been understood for a long time. As noted by Sarason (2001), among the small group of individuals who formed the American Psychological Association (APA) in the late 1800s were four—John Dewey, G. Stanley Hall, William James, and Lightner Witmer—who were very interested in schools. For example, in his 1899 presidential address, Dewey (1900) called for an intermediary to bring psychological knowledge to teachers. He pointed out that the vast majority of teachers and schools would benefit from a stronger knowledge of child development. Noting that many schools teach children and design school structures on the faulty assumption that techniques that would be most appropriate for adults also apply equally effectively to children, he presaged a common role of modern school psychologists by stating:

> How profound a revolution in the position and service of textbook and teacher, and in methods of instruction depending therefrom, would be effected by a sincere recognition of the psychological identity of child and adult in these respects can with difficulty be realized. Here again it is not enough that the educational commanders should be aware of the correct educational psychology. . . . It may be true, it is true, we are told, that some should take hold of psychological methods and conclusions, and organize them with reference to the assistance which they may give to the cause of education. But this is not the work of the teacher. It belongs to the general educational theorist: the middleman between the psychologist and the educational practitioner. He should put the matter into such shape that the teacher may take the net results in the form of advice and rules for action. (Dewey, 1900, p. 109)

Similarly, as noted by Fagan (1996), Lightner Witmer—considered the "father" of school psychology—made a call for psychological experts in schools in 1907. Like Sarason, Witmer and Dewey both had direct experiences in K–12 school settings, experiences that helped them understand and appreciate the important roles that schools play in children's lives and in their development. However, as Sarason notes in numerous writings, most notably his 2001 treatise *American Psychology and Schools: A Critique*, psychology has largely ignored education, to the detriment of children, society, education, and psychology. Sarason states that the reasons for this disconnect stem primarily from the effects of the decisions made at the seminal Boulder Conference in 1947. First, psychology has privileged research over practice. Second, basic research has been prioritized over applied research. Finally, rather than align with educational settings, psychology has chosen to align itself with medical models that view illnesses as residing within the individual and seeks to "solve" problems one person at a time (Sarason, 2001). In an invited address to the National Association of School Psychologists in 1996, Sarason commented on his mind-set as a participant in the Boulder Conference by stating, "All I knew really clearly was if you are engaged in the repair business, you never got to the point of prevention. If anything has been demonstrated in the post-World War II period, it is that" (Sarason, 1997). The importance of moving away from a disease model of psychopathology and toward public health models based around prevention and wellness that recognize the societal context in which psychology is practiced has been promoted by many social justice advocates in psychology (e.g., Albee, 1986; Prilleltensky, 2012).

Although today organizations such as the APA openly embrace the language of social justice in policy, as noted by recent APA president Melba Vasquez, there have been times in psychology's history where the practices endorsed by the profession were clearly harmful and unjust (Vazquez, 2012). There is also a history of psychology, either by accident or by design, being largely absent in social justice discussions and achievements related to education in the United States. For example, despite the prominence of the *Brown v. Board of Education* case nationally and despite this being the first major case in which psychological research (the Clark and Clark studies) was specifically cited as a factor in the decision, Benjamin and Crouse (2002) note that there is no evidence in the APA Board minutes from 1952 through 1956 that the *Brown* case was mentioned, and no evidence that either the case or Kenneth Clark himself was afforded any particular extra attention or commendation by APA until several decades later. Within school psychology, perhaps the most consequential major conference in the field's history, the Thayer Conference, was held in 1954, attracting virtually all of the field's major thinkers. Despite this conference occurring in very close proximity in time to the *Brown v. Board of Education decision*, Fagan (2005) notes that this case is not referenced in the comprehensive record of the proceedings.

Psychology's general lack of interest in schools and school psychology's general lack of explicit connection to social justice frameworks at the discipline level until the past decade likely have resulted in many missed opportunities to advance social justice (Shriberg, Song, Miranda, & Radliff, 2012). However, as evidenced by this volume, although there remains much work to be done, in the 21st century, leading organizations representing psychology and education are more apt to see the connection among education, psychology, and social justice. For example, in 1990 the APA created an Educational Directorate. A perusal of statements endorsed by APA and the National Association of School Psychology (NASP) in recent years reveals a gamut of topics that relate to social justice, including but not limited to taking clear stances on controversial issues such as supporting the human and educational rights of gay, lesbian, and bisexual students (DeLeon, 1993). Additionally, both APA and NASP have position statements calling on the United States to ratify the United Nations Conventions on the Rights of the Child (APA, 2001; NASP, 2012).

INTRODUCTION TO SCHOOL PSYCHOLOGY

School psychology sits at the intersection of education and applied psychology. This position has many benefits as it relates to social justice. As Gutkin and Song (2012) remind us, all adults begin as children. As such, from a developmental and prevention perspective, if one is aiming to achieve a just society, it makes sense to focus on children. If one is focusing on children, schools represent a critical opportunity at the logical locus of ecologically responsive prevention activities in support of social justice. As individuals with broad training in learning theory, child development, mental health, behavioral, and academic prevention and intervention techniques at the individual and systemic levels (NASP, 2010), school psychologists are in an ideal position to support social justice.

Although the field of school psychology has a deep connection with the origins of modern applied psychology, by virtue of the vast majority of practitioners working in the school settings (and thus subject to educational laws and credentialing procedures), school psychologists practice in ways and within certain contexts that are quite different from most other psychologists. This section provides a brief overview of the major roles and functions of school psychologists.

Entry into the Field

In my experience as a practitioner and as a school psychology faculty member for many years, the common denominator between virtually all individuals entering school psychology is a desire to make a positive difference with children. Whereas until a few decades ago the majority of school psychology graduate students were former teachers (in some states, a teaching credential was required for certification as a school psychologist), in modern school psychology many students entering school psychology are psychology majors who "discovered" school psychology in some indirect way. My personal experience is a common one. As an undergraduate major in human development and family studies, I knew that I wanted to go into psychology and that I wanted to work with children. At the time, even though I had been working with children (and, in some cases, working directly in schools) I was not aware of school psychology, so I applied and was accepted into a doctoral program in clinical psychology. When I started in the clinical program, it was fairly clear early on that this was not a good fit, but it was not until I had a clinical rotation in a school that I became aware of school psychology and realized that this was the better fit for me. In my case, it was the realization that, rather than work with individual or small groups of children in an office detached from their direct reality, I could instead work with many children at once in one of their primary ecologies—schools—that made the difference. In addition to meeting children in their ecology, I liked the possibilities of working collaboratively with children, families, schools, and communities, and serving in a preventive and facilitative role. I also enjoyed that school psychologists typically are generalists and often serve as the first mental health professionals who children experience.

I mention my personal story not because it is particularly noteworthy, but because it is reflective of an "aha!" experience that many school psychologists have had. Whether the school psychologist began as a psychologically oriented person with a bent toward working in schools or as an educator at heart with a passion also for psychology, school psychologists invariably transverse psychology and education, start with a desire to work with children, and are attracted to schools as the location from which they can have the greatest impact.

Whereas most school psychologists enjoy working with schools, from a social justice perspective, what school psychologists in the United States—and across the world—also invariably come to realize is that, in order to be effective, they need to effectively navigate the educational *system*. In this sense, the role of the school psychologist is unique from other applied fields in psychology in that school psychologists are dealing primarily with educational law and practices, not health care law and trends. As such, the history of school psychology has closely reflected the history and reality of modern education.

Although the term *social justice* is relatively new to school psychology, much of the field's history and efforts relates to events and topics with strong social justice connections (Gutkin & Song, 2012; Nastasi, 2008; Shriberg, 2009). In particular, although the term *school psychologist* has been in use for approximately 100 years (Fagan, 2005), the field experienced rapid growth beginning in the early 1970s because of the special education rights movement in the 1960s. Whereas racial segregation ceased to become law in 1954, until the passage of PL 94-142 in 1975 (Education for All Handicapped Children Act; currently, Individuals with Disabilities Education Act), children with special needs legally could be educationally segregated or excluded from public schools (Prasse, 2008). The passage of this law was the beginning of the special education system, as it is known today, whereby all students in the United States are entitled to a free and appropriate public education in the least restrictive environment possible. One of the effects of the passage of this law was a markedly increased demand for psychologists who could conduct the psychological evaluations required for special education eligibility. Into this void stepped school psychologists. Largely due to this dynamic, the number of school psychologists in the United States skyrocketed from an estimated 5,000 in 1970 to an estimated 10,000 in 1980, an estimated 22,000 in 1990 (Fagan, 2008), up to the most recently cited figure of 35,400 (Charvat, 2008).

This growth has not come without its tradeoffs. Whereas school psychologists have the training and, typically, a strong desire to engage in a wide range of professional tasks from the systemic to the individual level, covering diverse areas such as academic, behavioral, mental health, and crisis response, due to the legacy of PL 94-142, many school psychologists have been hired specifically to do special education evaluations. Even if they are not hired as part of a school's special education department, many educational administrators either are not aware of or do not value the full range of expertise held by school psychologists (Gilman & Gabriel, 2004).

School psychology is a field in which practitioners have a deep and varied toolbox from which to draw. In the most recent version of NASP's (2010) Professional Standards, 10 domains of practice are articulated: (1) data-based decision making; (2) consultation and collaboration; (3) intervention and instructional support to develop academic skills; (4) intervention and mental health services to develop social and life skills; (5) school-wide practices to support learning; (6) preventative and responsive services; (7) family-school collaboration services; (8) diversity in development and learning; (9) research and program evaluation; and (10) legal, ethical, and professional practice. In a typical day, a school psychologists might move from observing a kindergarten classroom for the purpose of providing instructional feedback to the teacher, to a crisis meeting with the family of an eighth grader who is at risk of suicide, to leading academic and mental health screenings with the entire fourth grade, to providing consultation to the school's principal on leading the school's antibullying initiative. One of the adults killed in the Sandy Hook tragedy was Mary Sherlach, a school psychologist who apparently was meeting with the school's principal when the gunman entered the school, and she rushed to protect the children when she heard gunshots. School psychologists across the world grieved this loss, not only because she was one of them, but also because the description of her role in the school and her actions in a time of crisis were so familiar.

Despite the range and depth of the skillset of the modern school psychologist, in many cases school psychologists are still viewed primarily as reactive special education evaluators who are called into a situation only after a child is viewed as potentially having a disability. This kind of reactive "wait to fail" approach is not the role that most school psychologists prefer (Gilman & Gabriel, 2004) and is a role that works against social justice. Layered on top of the guild challenges faced by many school psychologists is the general state of public education as it relates to social justice. Although, of course, there are many outstanding, well-resourced schools, there are many schools that, for various reasons, do not provide an educational experience to their students that reflect common definitions of social justice. Viewed from an international perspective, the social justice challenge becomes even larger as large swathes of the world's population (particularly girls) do not have access to adequate schooling. Although a full discussion of social justice challenges facing schools goes beyond the scope of this chapter, within the

United States, two primary challenges are inequities in school funding and institutionalized discriminatory practices.

In the United States, public school funding is not equalized, but rather is based on a formula combining local, state, and federal revenues. For the vast majority of school districts, the majority of their funding comes from local tax revenues, which results in significant discrepancies due to dramatic differences in local wealth from community to community (Kozol, 1991). As a result, it is often the case that schools with the greatest need for psychological support have the least resources. For school psychologists, this often translates to a choice between being a full-time school psychologist at a more affluent school and serving multiple schools of various sizes in less affluent areas. In general, the poorer the student-to-school psychologist ratio, and the more schools a school psychologist serves, the less opportunity a school psychologist has to engage in primary prevention and other systemic initiatives. Additionally, the less time a school psychologist has in a school, the less opportunity there is to develop important and supportive relationships with students, families, school personnel, and community members, and, as such, the less opportunity there is to be an effective agent of social justice.

Additionally, although there are numerous pockets of inspiration and innovation, U.S. public schools, like most other large organizations, are notoriously resistant to change (Noell & Gansel, 2008). Thus, school psychologists with an inclination toward social justice have to learn how to bring about successful and sustainable change within the context of a large organization that does not easily change. As described in the next section, school psychologists have identified challenging institutional power as a particularly salient social justice topic (e.g., Williams & Crockett, 2012). As such, school psychology scholarship on topics related to social justice and institutional power (e.g., racial discrimination in school discipline policies and practices; Fenning et al., 2010; combating bullying and homophobia in schools; Swearer, Espelage, Villaincourt, & Hymel, 2010) typically frame their suggested action steps within the context of the culture and power structures associated with public schools.

SCHOOL PSYCHOLOGISTS AS AGENTS OF SOCIAL JUSTICE

In considering social justice, many school psychologists are in the thorns of a dilemma. On one hand, by law, by training, and by desire, school psychologists view their professional role as working to help all children in schools; unfortunately, it does not take very long in any educational setting to observe areas of injustice (e.g., class, race, and gender biases in academic expectations and behavioral sanctions) germane to this charge. On the other hand, in order to achieve socially just ends, school psychologists typically must do so within the context of public education structures—structures that are notoriously difficult to change. Within this context, there is the additional tension between the field's historical connection with special education (which may be the reason why the school hired the school psychologist in the first place) and the training and attitude of most practitioners, which typically strongly encourages a view of practice that deemphasizes reactive special education assessment and diagnosis and instead prioritizes primary and secondary prevention. How then can school psychologists stuck in this conundrum move out of their traditional "sort and place" (Fagan, 2008) role into positions where they can support social justice by utilizing the full scope of their personal and professional skillset? This is the core challenge for many school psychologists as it relates to social justice.

One way to solve this dilemma is to develop clearer models of what "socially just school psychology practice" might look like (Speight & Vera, 2009). To date, there have been two empirical studies where school psychologists were asked to provide their opinions on social justice. The first is a Delphi study of cultural diversity experts in school psychology conducted by Shriberg et al. (2008). In this study, these cultural diversity experts most strongly endorsed a definition of social justice centered on the idea of "protecting the rights and opportunities for all." In terms of identifying priority social justice topics, experts in this study nearly universally spoke to the importance of challenging institutional power structures via advocacy, most typically advocacy directly related to elements of cultural diversity (e.g., race and socioeconomic status). Similarly, when asked to identify key social justice action strategies, experts emphasized the importance of knowledge (e.g., knowledge of best practices and the law) and action (e.g., advocacy to support children and families). Finally, when asked to identify topics that impact social justice in school psychology, either positively or negatively, respondents identified "lack of diversity in the field" and "allocation of resources" as the most notable barriers, and "equity of placement/services" as both a notable opportunity and barrier.

In a follow-up study of 1,000 randomly selected NASP members conducted by Shriberg, Wynne, Briggs, Bartucci, and Lombardo (2011), respondents provided a definition of social justice essentially identical to the definition provided by the cultural diversity experts. Additionally, 94% of respondents indicated that considerations of institutional power in schools were salient to social justice and school psychology. Respondents rated *promoting best practices in school psychology, conducting culturally fair assessments,* and *advocating for the rights of children and families* as the most realistic actions practitioners can take support social justice. In addition, significant age differences were evident, with younger/early career (age and years of experience in the field were significantly correlated at $p < .001$) respondents appearing to be both more apt to report exposure to social justice concepts and also less willing to take personal risks to pursue social justice aims than older (mid and late career) respondents.

Taken together, these studies suggest both a willingness and weariness to engage in social justice issues, with younger respondents, perhaps not surprisingly, seeming less willing to take personal risks. This finding is very consistent with the results of a study of graduate students (including school psychology graduate students), conducted by McCabe and Rubinson (2008), in which participants reported some attitudes seemingly consistent with social justice ideas, but these attitudes, particularly as they relate to intervening in support of GLBTQ students who are harassed in school, frequently did not translate to advocacy behaviors, particularly when participants stated that they worked in settings where their advocacy and support would not be viewed favorably by persons in power. In a chapter on social justice advocacy for school psychologists, Briggs (2012) highlights nearly this exact dynamic, reminding the reader that the younger the school psychologist, the more likely it is that others in the school have more authority and expertise.

In considering school psychologists as agents of social justice, public health frameworks are nearly universally recommended (Briggs, 2012, Gutkin & Song, 2012; Nastasi, 2008; Rogers & O'Bryon, 2008; Speight & Vera, 2009). Most commonly, these models combine critical self-reflection, critical reflection of the field of school psychology, critical reflection (or praxis, as described by Friere, 1970) of the world around us, and a commitment to action toward socially just ends. Rogers and O'Bryon (2008) believe that social justice advocacy requires "a rethinking of our social responsibilities and a rechanneling of some of our professional energies, expertise, and actions from the familiar role as advocate into the reformulated role as social justice advocate" (p. 495). Commenting on ways that school psychology research can advance social justice, Nastasi (2008) highlights the potential of action research as a way for the field to develop more locally responsive and meaningful interventions and ideas. Speight and Vera (2009), commenting on school psychology's potential as social justice agents, call upon the field to, among other things, critically examine its own history. While commending school psychology for its recent attention to social justice, they write:

> What seems somewhat underdeveloped, however, is a critical self-examination of the ways that the practice of school psychology historically and currently has contributed to educational inequities experienced by many students and communities. Specifically, school psychology would be called upon to first identify the systems, policies, and practices that are sources of inequities within educational systems. This potentially painful self-examination would uncover the indirect, direct, and inadvertent ways that school psychology has supported the status quo and colluded with oppression. (pp. 86–87)

In a comprehensive chapter focused on social justice advocacy, Briggs (2012) suggests that school psychologists engaging in social justice advocacy should be asking themselves the following questions:

1. *Am I engaging in critical self-reflection?*
2. *Am I listening to the perspectives of others?*

3. *Am I always critically evaluating or questioning laws, policies, systems, and practices?*
4. *Am I using data to identify social injustice and monitor the impact of advocacy efforts?*
5. *Am I developing alliances and working with them?*
6. *Am I simply doing things on behalf of others because it is easier or am I empowering others?*

Shriberg (2009), in describing a social justice agenda for school psychologists, articulates the following steps: establish a language, develop and embed priorities, connect social justice and research-based practice, establish networks, and exhibit courage. Over the past several years, the field of school psychology has begun to follow this path. For example, in 2007, NASP established a Social Justice Interest Group, and in 2010, Division 16 (School Psychology) of APA initiated a Workgroup on Social Justice and Children's Rights. Both of these groups have produced several written products (e.g., an international curriculum on social justice and children's rights has been created by the Division 16 workgroup in collaboration with the International School Psychology Association and the Tulane University Child Rights Team. See http://www.cred-pro.org/group/internationalschoolpsychologycurriculum for this curriculum) and have advocated successfully for changes in the field. For example, in 2010, NASP incorporated social justice language into its practice model, based in part on feedback and lobbying efforts of members of the NASP social justice interest group. Through these efforts and others, supportive networks of school psychologists who are committed to social justice are being enhanced. Most recently, the first book on school psychology and social justice (Shriberg et al., 2012) has been published. The edited book has 25 contributors, bringing varied voices into the discussion.

Moving forward, as social justice scholarship continues to be refined and expanded, and as social justice networks continue to be developed, the challenge will be to translate these gains to practice in a maximally effective and efficient way. Although there is, of course, no easy answer as to what "socially just practice" looks like, the ongoing commitment of the field to social justice, as both an aspiration and a practice, along with the subsequent development of scholarship and professional networks in support of social justice, holds promise for school psychologists to leverage their expertise and location in schools toward socially just ends. Dewey's and Witmer's beliefs that schools would benefit from the presence of psychological experts ring as true today as it did over 100 years ago. School psychologists who embrace a social justice orientation—an orientation that values critical self-reflection, critical reflection of the world around them, and a commitment to action—are in an advantageous position to fill this void as advocates of social justice.

REFERENCES

Albee, G. W. (1986). Towards a just society: Lessons from observations on the primary prevention of psychopathology. *American Psychologist, 41,* 891–898.

American Psychological Association. (2001). *APA resolution on UN Convention on the Rights of the Child and the convention's optional protocols.* Washington, DC: Author. Retrieved from http://www.apa.org/about/policy/rights-child-2001.aspx

Bell, L. A. (2013). Theoretical foundations. In M. Adams, W. J. Blumenfeld, C. Castañeda, H. W. Hackman, M. L. Peters, & X. Zúñiga (Eds.), *Readings for diversity and social justice* (3rd ed., pp. 21–26). New York, NY: Routledge.

Benjamin, Jr., L. T., & Crouse, E. M. (2002). The American Psychological Association's response to *Brown v. Board of Education*: The case of Kenneth B. Clark. *American Psychologist, 57,* 38–50.

Briggs, A. (2012). The school psychologist as advocate. In D. Shriberg, S. Y. Song, A. H. Miranda, & K. M. Radliff (Eds.), *School psychology and social justice: Conceptual foundations and tools for practice* (pp. 294–310). New York, NY: Routledge.

Charvat, J. (2008, September). *Estimates of the school psychology workforce.* Report prepared for the National Association of School Psychologists. Retrieved from http://www.nasponline.org/advocacy/SP_Workforce_Estimates_9.08.pdf

DeLeon, P. H. (1993). Proceedings of the American Psychological Association, Incorporated, for the year 1992; Minutes of the Annual Meeting of the Council of Representatives August 13 and 16, 1992, and February 26–28, 1993, Washington, DC. *American Psychologist, 48,* 745–788.

Dewey, J. (1900). Psychology and social practice. *Psychological Bulletin, VII,* 105–124.

Fagan, T. K. (1996). Witmer's contributions to school psychological services. *American Psychologist, 51,* 241–243. Retrieved from http://www.apa.org/pubs/journals/amp/index.aspx

Fagan, T. K. (2005). Literary history of the term "school psychologist" revisited. *School Psychology Review, 34,* 432–434. Retrieved from http://www.nasponline.org/publications/spr/index.aspx

Fagan, T. K. (2008). Trends in the history of school psychology in the United States. In A. Thomas & J. Grimes (Eds.), *Best practices in school psychology-V* (pp. 2069–2085). Bethesda, MD: National Association of School Psychologists.

Fenning, P. McArdle, L., Wilson, R., Horwitz, A., Morello, T., Golomb, S. . . . Morello, M. (2010). Schoolwide discipline policies: An analysis of the past, present and future. In J. E., Warnick, K. Warnick, & A. Laffoon (Eds.), *Educational policy and practice: The good, the bad, and the pseudoscience: Educational Theory and Policy.* (Vol. 1, pp. 67–82). New York, NY: Nova Science.

Friere, P. (1970). *Pedagogy of the oppressed.* New York, NY: Herder and Herder.

Gilman, R., & Gabriel, S. (2004). Perceptions of school psychological services by education professionals: Results from a multi-state survey pilot study. *School Psychology Review, 33,* 271–286. Retrieved from http://www.nasponline.org/publications/spr/index.aspx

Gutkin, T. B., & Song, S. Y. (2012). Social justice in school psychology: A historical perspective. In D. Shriberg, S. Y. Song, A. H. Miranda, & K. M. Radliff (Eds.), *School psychology and social justice: Conceptual foundations and tools for practice* (pp. 15–28). New York, NY: Routledge.

Kearns Goodwin, D. (2005). *Team of rivals: The political genius of Abraham Lincoln*. New York, NY: Simon & Schuster.

Kozol, J. (1991). *Savage inequalities: Children in America's schools*. New York, NY: Crown.

McCabe, P., & Rubinson, F. (2008). Committing to social justice: The behavioral intention of school psychology and education trainees to advocate for lesbian, gay, bisexual, and transgendered youth. *School Psychology Review, 37*, 469–486. Retrieved from http://www.nasponline.org/publications/spr/index.aspx

Nastasi, B. K. (2008). Social justice and school psychology. *School Psychology Review, 37*, 487–492. Retrieved from http://www.nasponline.org/publications/spr/index.aspx

National Association of School Psychologists. (2010). *Model for comprehensive and integrate school psychological services*. Bethesda, MD: Author. Retrieved from http://www.nasponline.org/standards/2010standards/2_PracticeModel.pdf

National Association of School Psychologists. (2012). *Child rights* [Position statement]. Bethesda, MD: Author. Retrieved from http://www.nasponline.org/about_nasp/positionpapers/ChildRights.pdf

Noell, G. H., & Gansle, K. A. (2009). Moving from good ideas in educational systems change to sustainable program implementation: Coming to terms with some of the realities. *Psychology in the Schools, 46*, 78–88.

Prasse, D. P. (2008). Best practices in school psychology and the law. In A. Thomas & J. Grimes (Eds.), *Best practices in school psychology-V* (pp. 1903–1920). Bethesda, MD: National Association of School Psychologists.

Prilleltensky, I. (2012). Wellness as fairness. *American Journal of Community Psychology, 49*, 1–21.

Rogers, M. R., & O'Bryon, E. C. (2008). Advocating for social justice: The context for change in school psychology. *School Psychology Review, 37*, 493–498. Retrieved from http://www.nasponline.org/publications/spr/index.aspx

Sarason, S. B. (1997). NASP Distinguished Lecture Series: What should we do about school reform? *School Psychology Review, 26*, 104–110. Retrieved from http://www.nasponline.org/publications/spr/index.aspx

Sarason, S. B. (2001). *American psychology and schools: A critique*. New York, NY: Teachers College.

Shriberg, D. (2009). Social justice and school mental health: Evolution and implications for practice. In J. M. Jones (Ed.), *The psychology of multiculturalism in schools: A primer for practice, training, and research* (pp. 49–66). Bethesda, MD: National Association of School Psychologists.

Shriberg, D., Bonner, M., Sarr, B., Walker, A., Hyland, M., & Chester, C. (2008). Social justice through a school psychology lens: Definitions and applications. *School Psychology Review, 37*, 453–468. Retrieved from http://www.nasponline.org/publications/spr/index.aspx

Shriberg, D., Song, S. Y., Miranda, A. H., & Radliff, K. M. (2012). *School psychology and social justice: Conceptual foundations and tools for practice*. New York, NY: Routledge.

Shriberg, D., Wynne, M. E., Bartucci, G., Briggs, A., & Lombardo, A. (2011). School psychologists' perspectives on social justice. *School Psychology Forum: Research in Practice, 5*(2), 37–53. Retrieved from http://www.nasponline.org/publications/spf/index.aspx

Speight, S. L., & Vera, E. M. (2009). The challenge of social justice for school psychology. *Journal of Educational & Psychological Consultation, 19*, 82–92.

Swearer, S. M., Espelage, D. L., Vaillancourt, T., & Hymel, S. (2010). What can be done about school bullying: Linking research to educational practice. *Educational Researcher, 39,* 38–47.

U.S. Department of Education (2013). *Table A-3-1. Actual and projected public school enrollment in grades prekindergarten (preK) through 12, by grade level and region; selected school years 1970–71 through 2021–22.* Retrieved from http://nces.ed.gov/programs/coe/tables/table-enl-1.asp

Vasquez, M. J. (2012). Psychology and social justice: Why we do what we do. *American Psychologist, 67,* 337–346.

Williams, J. (1998). *Thurgood Marshall: American revolutionary.* New York, NY: Random House.

Williams, S., & Crockett, D. P. (2012). Institutional barriers: Poverty and education. In D. Shriberg, S. Y. Song, A. H. Miranda, & K. M. Radliff (Eds.), *School psychology and social justice: Conceptual foundations and implications for practice* (pp. 137–154). New York, NY: Routledge.

Chapter 11

Conclusion

Chad V. Johnson, Harris L. Friedman, Jeannette Diaz, Zeno Franco, and Bonnie K. Nastasi

Our goal for the *Praeger Handbook of Social Justice and Psychology* was to provide an overview of many major topics and approaches used across the field of psychology involving the promotion of justice and elimination of oppression, both in the United States and abroad, as well as to introduce a new series with that focus. We realized at the outset that covering every such topic and approach would be impossible within even a three-volume *Handbook*, so we planned to build upon this in future volumes. In this conclusion, we outline some of the major themes and lessons we learned from gathering material for the *Handbook's* chapters, as well as highlight directions for future work, especially for social justice research and applications grounded in psychology. We also want to draw readers' attention to the appendices where we have included additional discussions on social justice, featuring a presentation on international ethical codes used in psychology by Rodney L. Lowman and a personal reflection on one psychologist's career of dealing with various social justice dilemmas by Harris Friedman. Moreover, we have included a sample of recommended readings in social justice and psychology for those interested in expanding their mastery of the important areas covered here, noting this limited sample, like the *Handbook* itself, is a starting place that falls short of being comprehensive. Finally, we have included appendices listing some resources for the interface of social justice and psychology for those interested in becoming more informed, and hopefully more involved, in social justice work around the globe.

MAJOR THEMES AND LESSONS LEARNED

There are three central themes that run through the chapters in the first volume of this three-volume *Handbook*. The first focuses on the inherently psychological nature of social justice. This theme reflects the importance of subjectivity, as well as objective scientific perspectives, for a critical understanding of both social justice processes and outcomes. Especially important is the need for an understanding of the psychological foundations for social justice, including phenomena such as empathy, reflexivity, intersectionality, empowerment, false consciousness, and critical awareness—to name just a few. The psychological understanding of social justice is also reflected in an explication of how social injustice, in its many expressions, impacts psychosocial well-being within individuals across various populations. The chapters have also emphasized a developmental perspective, looking across the life span, as well as considering the historical and cultural context of social justice concerns. The second theme reflected in these chapters is that of foundational knowledge, addressing basic information on the material and psychological conditions of marginalized groups throughout the world that is needed to appreciate many aspects of the social justice. This second focus folds into the third theme, that of informed action. This theme is reflected through the description and amplification of methods, such as participatory action research, critical pedagogy, and strategic advocacy, as useful tools for effective social justice praxis within psychology. The context for informed action is repeatedly shown through systems, human and more broadly ecological, that demonstrate the embedded and interconnected nature of individuals and communities within larger systems of oppression and/or empowerment, as the case may be.

Throughout the second volume of the *Handbook*, a primary theme is the importance of using multiple levels of analysis (ranging from individual to organizational to societal and even to global) from a systems perspective, and the corresponding need to both nuance interventions within and across these levels by spanning the boundaries between them. While systems theory is nothing new, the level of sophistication required to meaningfully tackle social justice problems and to create transformative change will increasingly require psychologists to work in multidisciplinary and/or transdisciplinary teams, and to think across conventional boundaries defined by disciplines. Clinical/counseling psychologists in particular are trained to play multiple roles in helping people—part psychological care provider, part social worker, part researcher and statistician, part organizational consultant, and so forth. However, too often psychologists operate within their own disciplinary, and even subdisciplinary, silos. In addition, too little actual attention within these two major psychological subspecialties is focused upon *prevention* rather than *treatment*, which indicates a sorely needed change to fulfill an overall vision of building a socially just society, rather than just picking up the pieces after damage has occurred. To accomplish this goal, enhanced skills needed for clinical/-counseling applications include better use of large-scale data analyzed across multilevels and other forms of more integrative research (e.g., crossing subdisciplinary boundaries, such as through incorporating approaches from areas such as political psychology, and crossing transdisciplinary boundaries by incorporating approaches from sociologists and economists). In addition, it is important to encourage approaches for gathering first-person data, especially from those whose voices have been traditionally marginalized, so all have a seat at the table. Combined, these skills can lead toward more sophisticated and effective psychological practice through multidisciplinary and/or transdisciplinary teams. This also needs to go beyond practice, as psychologists must continue to, and increase their involvement with, work at the level of public policy where systemic decisions are made, as well as learn to play lead roles in teams, as it is often the nuanced psychological view of individual and interpersonal behavior that "opens the eyes" of nonpsychologists as to why expensive, large-scale interventions often fall short of their goals or simply fail. Psychologists interested in social justice cannot continue to be segregated within a singular discipline and expect to effectively contribute to making meaningful progress toward greater social justice.

The last volume in this *Handbook* has a strong focus on the systems that influence children and youth (e.g., family, school, and community), as the young constitute a vulnerable population particularly subject to social injustice. An overarching theme is the critical role of adults (including parents, teachers, community members, policymakers, and psychologists) in ensuring social justice within society for such vulnerable groups. In addition, the chapters in the volume highlight the interconnectedness of various systems (e.g., child ecology and professional psychology) for addressing social justice issues, such the interconnection between social justice and child rights (as articulated in the UN Convention on the Rights of the Child, 1989). This final volume in the *Handbook* also focused on some of the subdisciplines of applied psychology (e.g., industrial/organizational and consulting, clinical and counseling, community, and school) that address social justice. A major theme for the section on applied psychology in this volume is the diversity across the subdisciplines regarding the integrations of social justice values and actions. Across all the chapters, authors stressed the critical role of psychology in advancing our understanding of social justice and providing direction for action to promote justice.

FUTURE RESEARCH

Following from these main themes, a critical arena for future research is that of further delineating the relationship between psychological processes and social justice. One especially fundamental concern regards the role of ideology (i.e., as governed by human values among which there can be no objective basis for consensus) versus using scientific criteria in the definition, empirical study, and application of social justice. From such a vantage, many basic conceptual questions can be asked. What is the relationship between empathy and the elimination of oppression, and can specific psychological techniques (e.g., mindfulness) make an impact on improving the world by increasing empathy? What is the relationship between power and social justice, both theoretically and empirically, and we note that those who study social justice tend to see power in inherently oppressive ways from ideological perspectives, rather than studying it in more dispassionate scientific ways as a basic dimension of human social life that has to be dealt with as a given? Considering that psychology is a learned discipline, what is the role of globalized education (or "mis-education") in the perpetuation of social injustice? How does the professionalization of psychology enhance or detract from the capacity for psychologists to be advocates, as well as researchers and practitioners? How does inequality impact the psychological well-being, if at all, of the wealthy? How do our own political and social privileges as psychologists impact our effectiveness in working with marginalized groups? How can psychological settings, such as classrooms or workshop, serve to foster a nonpartisan vision of social justice? What is the relationship between economic systems of resource distribution and social justice across the life span? Psychology needs to explore each of these, and many more, questions to advance societies understanding of social justice and the best practices for achieving it in respectful, empowering, and collaborative ways.

While psychology often focuses on social injustice, we believe a deeper exploration of the positive aspects of social justice is also vital to driving forward research and interventions. The idea of human dignity comes up throughout many of the chapters, but it is clear that psychologists' understanding of what dignity means, especially to those who are marginalized, is nascent. Psychology's definitions, philosophical, and operational understanding of dignity within the context of psychology must be robust and driven from the perspectives of those it seeks to serve. Moreover, the role of concepts such as mercy and "radical inclusion" are an important aspect, but often unstated subtext, of the discussion of human dignity. Exploration of what such ideas imply for social justice interventions and the professional practices of psychology warrant deeper consideration. Furthermore, the discussion of social justice within the domain of environmental sustainability points out ways in which the language and thought of other disciplines may change how people think—is it possible to re-language and reconceptualize this domain as, for example, "interpersonal sustainability"—reflecting the importance of creating equitable relationships as a fundamental, while also repackaging social justice for a broader audience that might not otherwise be amenable to it?

Across the chapters in this *Handbook*, several additional themes for future directions emerged. First, psychological research can play a critical role in helping to understand the personal, interpersonal, and social-cultural mechanisms that contribute to social injustice. Second, applied researchers can help to develop effective approaches for preventing social injustice, promoting social justice, and protecting individuals and group from injustices. The complexity of the phenomenon of social justice requires collaborative efforts across the different areas of psychology, for example, clinical, community, counseling, developmental, organizational, school, and social. Furthermore, critical to our work in social justice are the perspectives and experiences of individuals and groups (including children) who are perpetrators and victims of social injustice, as well as those who advocate for social justice. Representing these perspectives requires innovative research methodology within all domains of research—quantitative, qualitative, and mixed-methods approaches.

In addition, as human culture continues to evolve, many gaps in our knowledge need to be addressed. Greater cross-cultural studies, as well as studies of our close nonhuman relatives (e.g., bonobos and cetaceans), offer much promise to expand our concepts of social justice. We face a brave new world that portends grave challenges that humans have never faced before. The many ethical concerns related to medical advancements, such as genetic engineering that may literally reengineer what it means to be human, loom in the near future, along with life extension and other changes that are mind-boggling in their implications. At the same time, external transitions, such as those posed by global climate change and its accompanying major demographic shifts, are all highly salient to the interface of psychology and social justice. These types of trends suggest that this area is becoming increasingly crucial for humanity's adaptation and maybe even for survival.

FUTURE DIRECTIONS FOR SOCIAL JUSTICE AND PSYCHOLOGY

We believe the future of social justice and psychology must be a dialogical one, both at the level of theory and of practice. Psychologists must be able to engage with the theoretical goals of psychology writ large in order to foster a nomothetic and ideographic understanding of human beings that explicitly contextualizes human experience within an ecological/systems framework. A dialogical framework may mean that social justice–oriented psychologists make peace with the fact that not all psychologists will embrace the belief that psychology, as a science, must "do" something other than "study" its "subject." Conversely, basic research-focused psychologists must, eventually, also be able to understand that the context of human development and existence (i.e., individual and group capacity to access resources) directly impacts the material and subjective elements of human development—spiritually, cognitively, and biologically. The future of social justice and psychology lies in our capacity to live with difference, to remain uncomfortable in the face of injustice, and to be able to reflexively engage in informed action, not because of a belief in humanities' collective capacity to reach a utopian existence, but because to do otherwise leaves psychologists falling short of their personal and professional responsibilities—whether as teachers, researchers, or clinical or community practitioners.

As practitioners, it is easy to get caught up in the immediacy of the personal suffering of clients, the poor decisions they make, and trying to correct debilitating patterns of behavior. While social justice advocates talk about structural and institutional problems that lead to harmful outcomes for clients or communities in the abstract, it is often much more difficult to understand and work with clients to act on those barriers in meaningful ways. At once this suggests that more robust training is needed for clinical/counseling/community psychologists in particular, but also that subdisciplines like behavioral epidemiology should be more routinely integrated into undergraduate and graduate psychology research course offerings. In a very real way, the ideas advanced here around *ethics as praxis* extend to the most mundane, bureaucratic aspects of our lives as psychologists and educators. In this instance, course or curriculum development and selection is a method for having an enormous impact on societal outcomes, if psychology educators do not overlook these opportunities.

Moreover, psychologists must maintain vigilance around unintended consequences of the interventions designed to address social justice, especially given the complexity and interwoven nature of these efforts. For example, efforts to rebalance power between those in a lower-status organization and those in a higher-status organization may be the ultimate goal but, if the application of pressure is too great or the methods used are reflective of the oppressive practices they oppose, those potential allies able to create transformative change at the higher-status organizational levels may be personally injured or marginalized—resulting in just another form of injustice. These considerations also suggest that a form of "meta-supervision" might also be useful, a time for psychologists to episodically reflect with other seasoned professionals about the impact that they are having as individual practitioners and as social change agents. Indeed, psychologists would likely benefit from a regular practice of reflection examining assumptions and practices regarding social justice activities as to how they may unwittingly reflect oppressive practices or serve to maintain the status quo despite their well-meaning social justice efforts. For example, does happiness research and intervention found within positive psychology and elsewhere contribute to increasing people's happiness and contentment, but also pose a shadow rendering people less likely to use their unhappiness and discontentment as fuel for opposing injustice in their lives and communities? In other words, does psychology's role in making people (or psychotherapy clients) happy unintentionally contribute to a form of social control for maintaining an oppressive status quo? Ultimately, eliminating the "rules that hurt" and replacing these structures with processes that support human dignity are not simply nice sentiments. These ideas are fundamentally bound to global intellectual productivity, mutual economic advancement, and the realization of our full potential as a set of diverse, yet profoundly interlinked, peoples and societies.

The chapters in this *Handbook* addressed future directions for psychology in social justice efforts that extend beyond psychological research. Advancing the work of psychology in social justice requires that psychologists examine the philosophical and ethical foundations of psychology, as well as activities related to professional development, practice, and policy. First, the extent to which social justice is reflected in the collective values and ethics of the psychologists warrants attention. For example, do the professional ethics of major psychology organizations sufficiently address social justice issues? Second, psychology educators need to ensure that all future psychologists are prepared to address social justice in their teaching, practice, advocacy work, and research. For example, to what extent do training programs integrate social justice as a foundational principle for psychological work? Third, applied psychologists are in a unique position to directly address the role of social justice in service provision to clients and to identify and work with organizations and communities to address social injustice. For example, how do organizational psychologists help corporate clients to promote social justice for its employees and consumers? Fourth, the complexity of social injustice requires collective action among psychologists and with other stakeholders. Thus, how should psychology training prepare psychologists in political and social advocacy? How do educators ensure that psychologists can engage in effective collaborations? Moreover, how do social justice advocates ensure that psychology includes the voices of its stakeholders in research and action at individual and collective levels? Answers to these questions and more will need to be examined to ensure that psychology continues to advance fairness, safety, and opportunity for all citizens of the world—and not just for the privileged few.

Afterword

Marc Pilisuk

In the three volumes of this collection, these chapters have demonstrated diverse examples of how scholars dig, many more deeply than heretofore, into the pervasive consequences of injustice and how psychology's yet modest knowledge of human beings can be applied to improving society. This handbook takes us through a myriad of illustrations applying what psychology knows regarding some basic issues in the socialization of a generation of people who combine empathy, a critical stance toward what they hear, and commitment to advocacy. It includes views of how psychologists empower those displaced and traumatized by war, by impoverishment, and by decimation of their habitat and culture. Its illustrations suggest themes of environmental justice; the remaining examples of patriarchy; racial inequalities; the rights of elders, children, the disabled, and the incarcerated. Beyond this, it walks readers through the dangers of seeing oneself as an enlightened elite who knows what is best for others but from a vantage point that may fail to see one's own stakes and limitations.

What can readers take away from this voyage? Most people do not have to be told that they live in an unjust world. Modern media have made gross inequality a visible phenomenon in which the images of a shriveled homeless person lying on the street or wasting in a refugee camp are as much in view as the depictions of the affluent. The core of an elite upper crust, emboldened by the laws, institutions, and media monopolies they have created, grows in power and wealth, while the restless many are simultaneously looking beyond the bounds of a plantation mentality that prevents them from knowing that they have a voice—and from using it. Institutionalized injustice has long drowned the voices of the natural world and the voice of caring often associated with the feminine and with the spiritual spheres of culture—even as such silencing comes increasingly to threaten the dignity and even the continuity of life.

Humans have not been swept by fate into the current state of injustice; they have *progressed* there just as they have created the forms of work, education, consumption, and tools of violence. Collectively, humanity has created a social order and the selves that occupy it. For better or for worse, scholars of human behavior have developed models of thought, sometimes by intense inquiry, into the nature of how humans behave and how they make sense of things.

For the most part psychology and its related social sciences have looked at humans with insufficient attention to the effects of injustice or to the capacities to change it. As a result, those most active in explaining its roots have not typically called upon the social sciences as a force for transforming either the institutions or the ideas that contribute to so much human suffering. Of course, there have been exceptions. Some among our community of scholars have stepped forward from the pack and have been redirecting their scholarship, their practice, and their hearts to where they may do the most good. This book includes some profound efforts in this regard. In several instances the depth of critical inquiry goes into how psychology conceptualizes the contexts of injustice.

An underlying root of so many forms of contemporary injustice is the workings of global capitalism, its values, and its polarization of resources. With this understanding we can see the relationship between the injustice inflicted upon factory workers in Bangladesh and the wipeout of livable wages and community resources in developed nations. Advocates can use this insight to appreciate the revolving door assuring that governments exist primarily to protect and subsidize corporate wealth. Knowing the work of this systemic underlying power can help change agents link policies of austerity, shown to accelerate rates of depression and suicide, to the continued flow of resources from ordinary people to the top. In the emerging corporate state, observers are able to connect global and domestic surveillance, the use of drones, stop-and-frisk policies, and criminalization of immigrants and of whistle-blowers to the elaborate labyrinth of professional lobbyists. But does mention of this context of global corporate capitalism help? Or does it create an excuse for inaction? Or is there a way that it can be incorporated in action?

Another area of context comes in the analysis of how perceptions of injustice are formed. Are there modes of thought, perhaps overlearned and difficult to change, that require scapegoats, enemies, and retribution? I recall one example that might be appreciated by fans of attribution theory. In 1967 after my involvement in creating the first ever Teach-in Ann Arbor, I found myself teaching at Purdue where I was called upon to debate the Vietnam War with a popular head of the Political Science Department. During my turn I read aloud what I described as the North Vietnamese plan for a takeover of South Vietnam. I then asked him whether the practices described, including waterboarding, creating friendly spy units within families, and targeting for assassination those unalterably opposed to the takeover, were so reprehensible that American lives should be sacrificed to oppose it. He responded that this was absolute tyranny and that we should be proud to fight and die in opposition. I then explained that what I had read was from the American pacification program. Without embarrassment, he dismissed this as an example of a liberal trick and went on to denounce communists. Did the verbal presentation matter? People are all able to conceive of framing issues in ways that might find more acceptability. But would such framing have had an effect in the civil rights movement without the massive demonstrations and the fervor of hope overcoming fear?

Conscious constructed conceptions of the way things should be are a relatively recent addition to evolution. Do psychologists slight the preverbal forces of life and the indigenous traditions that sought to learn from them? As psychologists expand their scholarship to include the theme of justice, do they also risk the drain of energies into a game for which the master cannot be beaten because he can change the rules at will? Do scholars, entering the competitive marketplace for ideas, drift too far from our primordial roots?

Do social justice psychologists place too much faith upon revolutionary changes in the way people think and undervalue the importance of a revolution in how they feel? Do psychologists risk losing the ability to take personal risks, and to scream out at the sea of injustice? And are they ready to take risks that follow from their own inquiry? James Luther Adams, a professor of ethics at Harvard Divinity School who had barely escaped from the Nazi Gestapo to the United States, issued a warning letter. Adams recalled the fascist message in Germany finding biblical support for labeling opponents—homosexuals, Jews, and non-Aryans—as satanic demons who had to be crushed. His analysis was that the great universities and the major media of the United States were, like those in Germany in the 1930s, self-absorbed and would be easily compromised by their close relationship with government and corporations. If they could be given a slice of the pie, research contracts, and access to higher circles, they would prove to be complacent and would not deal with the most fundamental moral questions that unrestrained government and corporate power would present. Scholars would lack the spine to fight if the cost was to their prestige and comfort (Pilisuk, 2008).

I raise this because these three volumes help to make us serious contenders in the arena of understanding injustice. It is my belief that the study of injustice does have a role in changing it. Two directions that will involve risk and will demand spine appear to be critical.

There is surely more work to do in uncovering the web of a destructive system, understanding how the strings of injustice are pulled, and precisely by whom. There is also more to explore in building a movement in which an ethos of creative, nonviolence inspires participatory involvement in building global democracy, including efforts toward sustainability in local projects and cooperative institutions in which working people and consumers come to replace some existing structures. But our takeaway reminder from all of the revealing illustrations and analyses of this book is that injustice is not destiny. Transformative social change is possible and scholars of the human condition do have a significant part to play.

REFERENCE

Pilisuk, M. (with Rountree, J. A.) (2008). *Who benefits from global violence and war: Uncovering a destructive system.* Santa Barbara, CA: Praeger.

Appendix A

Some Ethics Resources for Social Justice Issues in Psychology

Rodney L. Lowman

Ethics codes for psychologists are one major source for understanding what they are expected or mandated to do.

THE AMERICAN PSYCHOLOGICAL ASSOCIATION'S CODE OF ETHICS

The Ethical Principles of Psychologists and Code of Conduct (APA, 2002), widely viewed as a model for psychological ethics in other countries, is both a collection of behavioral prescriptions ("thou shalt" and "thou shalt not") and an aspirational statement identifying what psychologists, beyond doing no harm, should positively be attempting to achieve in this world. Although the APA code identifies aspects of behavior that could be considered to be consistent with a social justice agenda, the code is also an enforceable set of behavioral standards and expectations that can be used as the basis for actions to be taken against psychologists for not behaving in a manner that is consistent with its prescriptions. Since ethical violations can cause professional practice licenses to be revoked or, in states that have criminalized certain aspects of sexual behavior, people to go to prison, the enforceable ethical standards are more focused on minimally acceptable standards of the professions then they are the ones that might reflect broad social objectives. Left to the aspirational principles are the larger-picture, context-setting goals of the profession. Even there, however, there is not much in the APA ethic's code explicitly on social justice (see Vasquez, 2012).

THE U.S. APPROACH

In reviewing the APA code, there are, I argue, few enforceable ethics standards that mandate psychologists to endorse or act on a social justice agenda in their work as psychologists except in a narrow range of behaviors, such as not discriminating. And, when considering the aspirational (nonenforceable) principles, there would not appear much that is directly relevant to the concept of social justice as it is typically defined.

There are five generic principles in the APA ethics code. The first of these principles concerns beneficence and nonmaleficence. It states:

Principle A: Beneficence and Nonmaleficence

> Psychologists strive to benefit those with whom they work and take care to do no harm. In their professional actions, psychologists seek to safeguard the welfare and rights of those with whom they interact professionally and other affected persons, and the welfare of animal subjects of research. When conflicts occur among psychologists' obligations or concerns, they attempt to resolve these conflicts in a responsible fashion that avoids or minimizes harm. Because psychologists' scientific and professional judgments and actions may affect the lives of others, they are alert to and guard against personal, financial, social, organizational, or political factors that might lead to misuse of their influence. Psychologists strive to be aware of the possible effect of their own physical and mental health on their ability to help those with whom they work. (Ethical principles, 2002, p. 1062)

The admonition of Principle A is basically to do good and avoid doing harm and to avoid situations that entail conflicts of interest or at least to manage such situations as they arise. The focus is on "those with whom they work," presumably clients, students, and research participants. For I-O or consulting psychologists, the clients may be organizations. I find little in this principle that describes a proactive ethical obligation to address society's ills or to help assure that the needs of the weakest and poorest in society are addressed.

The next principle, Principle B: Fidelity and Responsibility, arguably comes closer to social justice issues. The ethical principle states:

Principle B: Fidelity and Responsibility

> Psychologists establish relationships of trust with those with whom they work. They are aware of their professional and scientific responsibilities to society and to the specific communities in which they work. Psychologists uphold professional standards of conduct, clarify their professional roles and obligations, accept appropriate responsibility for their behavior, and seek to manage conflicts of interest that could lead to exploitation or harm. Psychologists consult with, refer to, or cooperate with other professionals and institutions to the extent needed to serve the best interests of those with

> whom they work. They are concerned about the ethical compliance of their colleagues' scientific and professional conduct. Psychologists strive to contribute a portion of their professional time for little or no compensation or personal advantage. (Ethical principles, 2002, p. 1062)

"Professional and scientific responsibilities to society and to the specific communities in which they work" might be interpreted to mean concerns with social justice and an ethical obligation to use their expertise to make them better. However, there is little specificity in these aspirational duties, and they could be interpreted in many different ways. For example, a consulting psychologist who helped to make a for-profit organization better (more efficient, more profitable) could be considered to have made a positive contribution to the society and community at issue.

The next principle, Principle C: Integrity, concerns integrity, here, essentially honesty and prudence. It states:

> **Principle C: Integrity**
>
> Psychologists seek to promote accuracy, honesty, and truthfulness in the science, teaching, and practice of psychology. In these activities psychologists do not steal, cheat, or engage in fraud, subterfuge, or intentional misrepresentation of fact. Psychologists strive to keep their promises and to avoid unwise or unclear commitments. In situations in which deception may be ethically justifiable to maximize benefits and minimize harm, psychologists have a serious obligation to consider the need for, the possible consequences of, and their responsibility to correct any resulting mistrust or other harmful effects that arise from the use of such techniques. (Ethical principles, 2002, p. 1062)

Of course, not stealing and not lying are desirable behavior (as is being honest, the positive side of that behavior). However, that sets a minimal standard, or floor, that is unlikely to address higher-order ethical expectations.

Principle D: Justice, presumably, is where we would expect to find a principle addressing social justice issues. It states:

> **Principle D: Justice**
>
> Psychologists recognize that fairness and justice entitle all persons to access to and benefit from the contributions of psychology and to equal quality in the processes, procedures, and services being conducted by psychologists. Psychologists exercise reasonable judgment and take precautions to ensure that their potential biases, the boundaries of their competence, and the limitations of their expertise do not lead to or condone unjust practices. (Ethical principles, 2002, pp. 1062–1063)

Alas, there is very little here addressing social justice issues except for the issue of access to psychologists' services. There is a positive obligation not to allow bias or limited competence to create or condone "unjust practices" but the nature of the construct of "injustice" remains undefined. That there is no real ethical obligation articulated in Principle D does not apparently obligate psychologists to address societal concerns. The focus is more on equality in treatment of individuals and access to service, which is part of social justice, but in practice the only ethical mandate on that dimension is to donate some part of one's professional services. The principle does not appear to establish a social justice agenda.

Finally, Principle E: Respect for People's Rights and Dignity addresses issues of psychologists' needs to respect peoples' rights and dignity. It states:

> **Principle E: Respect for People's Rights and Dignity**
>
> Psychologists respect the dignity and worth of all people, and the rights of individuals to privacy, confidentiality, and self determination. Psychologists are aware that special safeguards may be necessary to protect the rights and welfare of persons or communities whose vulnerabilities impair autonomous decision making. Psychologists are aware of and respect cultural, individual, and role differences, including those based on age, gender, gender identity, race, ethnicity, culture, national origin, religion, sexual orientation, disability, language, and socioeconomic status and consider these factors when working with members of such groups. Psychologists try to eliminate the effect on their work of biases based on those factors, and they do not knowingly participate in or condone activities of others based upon such prejudices. (Ethical principles, 2002, p. 1063)

Here the aspirational principle explicitly recognizes the groups toward which psychologists are not to have biases. Though requiring psychologists to respect the dignity and worth of all, the "rights of all" are articulated only to be "privacy, confidentiality, and self determination" and these are in the context of psychologists' work.

THE CANADIAN APPROACH

Not all ethical codes of psychologists are as indirect about introducing a social justice agenda as in the APA code, although most seem to be (see, e.g., the British Psychological Society's 2011 Code of Ethics and Conduct). A different take on social justice is found, for example, in the Canadian Psychological Association's (CPA, 2000) code of ethics. This code includes four broad overarching standards that include Principle I: Respect for the Dignity of Persons. Principle II: Responsible Caring, Principle III: Integrity in Relationships, and Principle IV: Responsibility to Society. Principle IV explicitly identifies a broader ethical obligation of psychologists inherent in a social contract. It states: "By virtue of this social contract, psychologists have a higher duty of care to members of society than the general duty of care that all members of society have to each other" (CPA, 2000, p. 2). "Society" is defined in the Canadian code "in the broad sense of a group of persons living as members of one or more human communities, rather than in the limited sense of state or government" (CPA, 2000, p. 28).

This code goes on to say:

> Psychology functions as a discipline within the context of human society. Psychologists, both in their work and as private citizens, have responsibilities to the societies in which they live and work, such as the neighbourhood or city, and to the welfare of all human beings in those societies. Two of the legitimate expectations of psychology as a science and a profession are that it will increase knowledge and that it will conduct its affairs in such ways that it will promote the welfare of all human beings" (CPA, 2000, p. 28).
>
> IV.22 Speak out, in a manner consistent with the four principles of this *Code*, if they possess expert knowledge that bears on important societal issues being studied or discussed. (p. 31)

Canada, of course, is not the United States and comes from more of a British tradition of social welfare perspectives rather than the strongly individualistic American tradition. Thus, it might be surprising to those familiar with APA's Code (2002) to find in the CPA Ethic Code's "extended responsibilities" an enforceable standard that states: "IV.30 Encourage others, in a manner consistent with this *Code*, to exercise responsibility to society" (CPA, 2000, p. 32).

All that said, in the CPA code, the four overarching principles are prioritized and Principle IV, arguably the one most relevant to social justice issues, has the lowest priority when there is conflict between it and any of the other three. In discussing this prioritization, the code states: "The dignity and well-being of a person should not be sacrificed to a vision of the greater good of society, and greater weight must be given to respect and responsible caring for the person" (CPA, 2000, p. 2) and this advice is well taken. A grandiose vision of responsibilities to society cannot take the place of the psychologist's primary obligation to perform psychological duties competently and ethically.

A SAMPLING OF OTHER ETHICS STANDARDS OF PSYCHOLOGISTS

Are the ethical codes of psychologists in other parts of the world more specific as to their expectations of psychologists as far as social justice is concerned? Here is a sampling of excerpts from the ethics codes of psychologists around the world.

Japan

The Japanese Psychological Association (undated), in a very short code, states the following:

> Awareness of responsibility and self-study. As professional psychologists, JPA members shall be aware that their research, studies, and practical activities in the field of psychology may have effects on society and the individuals that it comprises. Furthermore, members shall, through their activities, aim to improve people's welfare and happiness. (n.p.)

South Africa

The Professional Board for Psychology, Health Professions Council of South Africa (2002). (2002) code of ethics states:

> The Professional Board for Psychology (hereinafter referred to as the Board) has the statutory mandate of protecting the public where it concerns the conduct of psychologists and of guiding the profession of psychology in terms of education, training and professional conduct. This Ethical Code of Professional Conduct (hereinafter referred to as the Code), informed by international best practices and South African law, especially relevant sections of the Constitution of the Republic of South Africa, is intended to regulate the professional conduct of psychologists in all domains of their professional work.

This ethics code, which in many ways appears to be a clone of the APA's ethics code, does have some unique features arguably relating to social justice. For example, its Standard 3.1.1 states:

> Psychologists shall recognize the inalienable human right to bodily and psychological integrity, including security in and control over her body and person, and the right not to be subjected to any procedure or experiment without her informed consent, which shall be in a language that is easily understood by her. (The Professional Board for Psychology, Health Professions Council of South Africa, 2002, n.p.)

Standard 9.3.2 of this code states:

> 9.3.2 When engaged in teaching or training, psychologists . . . shall ensure that . . . [students, supervisees and trainees'] constitutional rights are upheld. (n.p.)

This reference to constitutional rights in South Africa is also reflected by the values statement of the Psychological Society of South Africa whose values statement includes the following:

HUMAN RIGHTS ORIENTATED: We commit to a Human Rights culture informed by the Universal declaration of Human Rights aligned to the Bill of Rights. We strive to ensure that our Members, Council, the Executive and staff are treated with dignity, equity and fairness.

SOCIAL RELEVANCE: We encourage a multiplicity of opinions and seek way to incorporate the voices and experiences of all communities and avenues of psychology. (Psychological Society of South Africa, 2002, n.p.)

Argentina

Argentina is a country long troubled by human rights violations punctuated by periods of improvement in policies and enforcement of human rights. The ethics code for Argentinian psychologists does include some references to social justice issues: social justice expectation. The Code of Ethics of Psychologists of the Federation of Psychologists of the Argentine Republic (Fe.P.R.A., 1991) in its preamble is one of the most explicit about identifying a social justice agenda:

[Psychologists] . . . will promote for human beings and for the society to which they belong and participate, the full currency of human rights, the defense of the democratic system and the permanent search for liberty and social justice and human dignity as fundamental values that will translate into a critical individual and supportive society.

Will understand the psychic well-being as one of the fundamental Human Rights and will operate in agreement with the social ideal of promoting equality, at the highest possible level, and with the only limitations imposed by ethics and science.

Will understand that it is the responsibility of every psychologist to aspire to reach personally, and to promote in their colleagues a responsible, lucid and committed attitude in front of humans and their circumstances. http://www.iupsys.net/images/resources/ethics/Argentina_translation_to_english.pdf

UNIVERSAL DECLARATION OF ETHICAL PRINCIPLES FOR PSYCHOLOGISTS

Finally, I note the *Universal Declaration of Ethical Principles for Psychologists* (International Union of Psychological Science, 2008) that has been adopted by the International Union of Psychological Science, the International Association of Applied Psychology, and the International Association for Cross Cultural Psychology. None of these bodies have enforcement power except, perhaps, in connection with removing members from the respective organizations, but as efforts to internationalize ethics their work is worth noting.

> The Universal Declaration describes those ethical principles that are based on shared human values. It reaffirms the commitment of the psychology community to help build a better world where peace, freedom, responsibility, justice, humanity, and morality prevail. The description of each principle is followed by the presentation of a list of values that are related to the principle. These lists of values highlight ethical concepts that are valuable for promoting each ethical principle . . .
>
> . . . Psychologists accept as fundamental the Principle of Respect for the Dignity of Persons and Peoples. In so doing, they accept the following related values:
>
> a) respect for the unique worth and inherent dignity of all human beings; . . .
> g) fairness and justice in the treatment of persons and peoples.
>
> (International Union of Psychological Science, 2008, n.p.)

Summarizing these statements, which may be representative of the more social justice–oriented codes of ethics, the concern with the greater good of humanity, concern with human rights, and assuring that basic human needs are met and rights protected, at best these expectations are aspirational for psychologists around the world. Because psychological ethics are primarily deontological and because standards that are enforceable tend to be those involving the direct practice of psychology, there is little mandated expectation in current ethics codes of psychologists to directly promote social justice.

CONCLUSION

Summarizing, from the perspective of the APA Ethics Code (2002), the prescribed and proscribed behaviors of psychologists, I argue, are not overly concerned with social justice except in the manner of providing services in a fair and nondiscriminatory way. Thus, arguably, a mandate to take on the broader issues of society may not derive from the APA code.

Non-U.S. codes of ethics for psychologists may therefore provide useful guidance.

Indeed, most countries that have professional associations of psychologists have ethics codes. Many of these are based on the APA code or can be interpreted as covering similar issues. However, there are some codes, especially the CPA's, that are much more explicit in their coverage of social justice issues. Those concerned with social justice issues in international contexts are advised to at least sample international ethics codes.

REFERENCES

American Psychological Association. (2002). Ethical principles of psychologists and code of conduct. *American Psychologist, 57,* 1060–1073. doi: 10.1037/0003-066X.57.12.1060

Canadian Psychological Association. (2000*). Canadian code of ethics for psychologists.* Ottawa, Canada: Author.

Code of Ethics of Psychologists of the Federation of Psychologists of the Argentine Republic (Fe.P.R.A.). (1991). Retrieved from http://www.iupsys.net/images/resources/ethics/Argentina_translation_to_english.pdf

International Union of Psychological Science. (2008). *Universal declaration of ethical principles for psychologists* (n.p.). Retrieved from http://iupsys.net/index.php/ethics/declaration

The Japanese Psychological Association (undated). Ethical principles of psychologists. Retrieved from http://www.psych.or.jp/english/ethical.html

The Professional Board for Psychology, Health Professions Council of South Africa (2002). Ethical code of professional conduct. Retrieved from http://www.google.com/url?sa=t&rct=j&q=&esrc=s&source=web&cd=2&ved=0CDMQFjAB&url=http%3A%2F%2Fweb.uct.ac.za%2Fdepts%2Fpsychology%2Fresources%2FEthicsCode.doc&ei=AY7PUfnoHJTi8gS5IFY&usg=AFQjCNGIUh0mshBvJFruir2WGqMwgX0SDQ&sig2=6g63PfUYwQqdqv6NNt2F4Q&bvm=bv.48572450,d.eWU

Vasquez, M. (2012). Social justice and psychology: Why we do what we do? *American Psychologist, 67*(5), 337–346.

Appendix B

Reconciling Social Justice Dilemmas through Being a "Psychopreneur" and Advocate: Personal Reflections on Professional Cooperation, Competition, and Conflict

Harris L. Friedman[1]

Professional psychologists, regardless of their areas of practice, unavoidably deal with social justice dilemmas, whether knowingly or not. To qualify as a social justice dilemma, both a social justice issue and a dilemma must be present. Social justice occurs only in relationships and refers to values, such as in terms of how something is evaluated as fair or unfair based on some human standards. A natural catastrophe does not necessarily involve social justice (e.g., if everyone in a community dies in an earthquake, this act of nature hits all equally without regard to social justice in the community). However, if there is differential suffering (e.g., if mostly the poor die in an earthquake due to living in substandard housing), social justice may be at play. Of course, one's (referring to an individual or a collection of people) perception of social justice may be contraindicated by another's perception, as the same facts may be evaluated differently, depending on relative perspective. If the poor killed disproportionately in an earthquake are seen by the survivors as deserving their fate (e.g., for being too lazy to build proper housing), then the act of nature may be seen as just. Social justice involves complex evaluations that are difficult to reduce to any simple understanding, such as a rigid categorization scheme or branding snippet. Perhaps a contribution of the present handbook is providing a complex vantage based on many perspectives from which social justice, as applicable to psychology, can be examined. In this way, the full gamut of its chapters, taken together as a whole (including its internal contradictions), could provide one of its best definitional approaches.

The dilemma aspect of social justice can be defined a little more easily than social justice. Dilemmas involve choices among alternative courses of action in which the stakes are high and there are no objectively right solutions. In other words, solutions to dilemmas are radically relativistic and usually vexing; otherwise these would not be dilemmas. I have worked on different types of dilemmas as an applied psychologist and researcher including, most recently, cultural and moral dilemmas, both of which often involve social justice themes. In the case of cultural dilemmas, my colleagues and I (e.g., Friedman et al., 2013) have been conducting research with U.S. warfighters who had been deployed in cross-cultural combat settings. Using focus groups, we harvested scenarios composed of difficult choices without clear solutions, all of which these warfighters had actually faced. For example, one scenario reflecting a salient cultural dilemma involves warfighters entering an Afghan village to search for hidden weapons. In this dilemma, the village elders offer to share a hookah pipe, likely containing hashish, with the warfighters. To the elders, this is a gesture of friendship and a precursor for relationship building that could lead to cooperation. For a warfighter to reject this offer of hospitality would be considered beyond rude by the locals, and could result in conflict with dire consequences, such as loss of lives of U.S. warfighters and local people. For the warfighters to accept the offer, however, would be violating U.S. military laws and could result in severe punishments, up to court martial leading to lengthy prison sentences. Clearly there are no singularly right answers to such a dilemma, as each choice has highly value-laden implications with serious consequences. Our data showed that the U.S. warfighters varied considerably in their responses, ranging from agreeing to smoke in order to find the hidden weapons to refusing to smoke and even turning over to the authorities for prosecution of anyone who agreed to smoke. This is not just a theoretical dilemma, as many of the warfighters studied actually faced this same dilemma during combat deployments, and both extremes were reported as having happened. The lack of consensus supports that this is a valid dilemma, rather than a mere situational judgment problem involving better or worse choices.

In another research, one of my doctoral students and I explored moral dilemmas related to religion (Needham & Friedman, 2012). There is a large psychological research literature that concludes religious conservatives (including Christian, Islamic, and Jewish fundamentalists) are less complex in their moral decision making than people from more liberal religious traditions. The literature has been primarily based on using hypothetical dilemmas, such as the following: a trolley is careening out of control down a hill, but there is a switch that can be pulled to keep it from slamming into, and killing, a crowd of people by diverting it into where only one person is standing. To pull the switch would save many lives, but actively take one life; conversely to do nothing would be to passively let many die. In making such a difficult choice, religious liberals tend to select pulling the switch, even though it actively murders one individual; in contrast, religious conservatives tend to select doing nothing, letting what they tend to be believe as "God's will be done" rather than actively violating the religious law to not murder. The conclusion that religious liberals are somehow morally superior by being more cognitively complex in their reasoning is based on their tendency to accept a utilitarian view that it is best to save many while sacrificing one. In contrast, religious conservatives, who are portrayed as more cognitively simple (and subtly denigrated as immature, concrete, and black-and-white thinkers) for rejecting a utilitarian view, instead tend to embrace the biblical view that the life of one and of many is equal from the perspective of God. My student and I placed this to a scientific test and found that religious conservatives we studied, who were highly educated Evangelical Christians, answered moral dilemmas we posed as expected from previous studies (e.g., they would not pull the trolley switch), but we also found that, when we carefully examined their reasoning, they were no less cognitively complex when approaching these dilemmas than were comparable religious liberals. The salient difference was that the religious conservatives were operating under different values relating to right and wrong, which revealed a liberal bias in a major strand of psychological research that had claimed to be value free.

Practicing psychologists of all kinds face social justice dilemmas that cannot be reduced into any simplistic framework with clearly right or wrong answers. Yet psychologists are called upon to act in the world, often with high-stakes consequences. I explore this theme here through a personal narrative about some of the social justice dilemmas I have faced within my own career as a psychologist and self-proclaimed advocate for social justice. Such narrative reflections are increasingly accepted as legitimate data within psychology (McAdams, 2008), and I note that other psychologists have explored social justice issues in their own lives using narrative methods (e.g., Ahmed, Wilson, Henriksen, & Jones, 2011). I write from a first-person perspective, and it is important to note that I have the benefit of hindsight, as well as the freedom to spin the story as I like. I also admit from the outset that the tale is undoubtedly slanted by my own values, as I use my own career as an autobiographical case study of the one I know best. This chapter is explicitly personal and idiographic, so it is not meant to be an objective overview of anything. Consequently, I forewarn readers that this is basically an opinion piece that is tucked away in the handbook's appendix for a reason, rather than presented as a scholarly chapter vetted within an academic tome. To begin, I explore the myth of scientific objectivity in psychology, after which I introduce how I view being a professional, followed by two concepts I have found useful in understanding social justice dilemmas, namely a continuum ranging from cooperation to competition to conflict and the notion of *psychopreneurship*, a term I explain later. I then present a few examples of how I dealt with some social justice dilemmas, and conclude with some thoughts about transpersonal psychology as an approach to science in relationship to social justice.

THE MYTH OF SCIENTIFIC OBJECTIVITY IN PSYCHOLOGY

The very decision to become a psychologist implies valuing certain types of knowing and acting. Once entering the field, psychologists unavoidably assert their values in terms of what they professionally pursue, whether for applied or research purposes, what methods they choose to employ, how they interpret the meaning of whatever they do, and so forth. Although psychology is mainly understood as a science, it is a *human science* that is quite different from scientific fields that focus on more inert objects, such as chemicals. Psychologists study and work with embodied beings who are inextricably socially intertwined with others within historical and cultural contexts. Not only are the subjects of psychological study and intervention sentient (humans or, sometimes, other species), but so are the psychologists. Just as the complexity of consciousness involves being aware of being aware, the co-consciousness of social life, being aware of others who are aware of their awareness and vice versa ad infinitum, leads to increasingly greater levels of reciprocal complexity. In this regard, as with all humans, psychologists simply cannot avoid social justice dilemmas any more than they can avoid gravity. Psychologists who think they can limit their pursuits to some objective scientific practice devoid of all values are simply mistaken, as even that attempt paradoxically would be embedded with a framework of values from which there is no exit. This reflects one of the major profound discoveries of modernity, Gödel's incompleteness theorem: all systems, whether mathematical or otherwise, rest on assumptions that cannot be explained fully within the very system upon which they rest (see Goldstein, 2006). I conclude that science, behind which psychologists often believe they can rationalize their many value-laden decisions, provides no refuge from subjectivity.

In this regard, context is crucial. All humans are "thrown" (Heideger, 2010/1927) into a world not-of-their-own making, while carrying baggage (cultural and historical, as well as biological and otherwise), and once in the world unavoidably face choices within limited opportunity structures enmeshed in values. This sticky-slippery stuff that makes human life so ineffable, and that resists complete scientific reduction, is nowhere more evident than in issues specifically related to social justice, and all human concerns have their social justice implications, if one looks deep enough. As an example of how values may be obfuscated in science, a colleague and I (Friedman & Robbins, 2012) recently criticized an attempt to mischaracterize the largest social science intervention and research project ever (i.e., *Comprehensive Soldier Fitness;* CSF) as being based solely on science and somehow value-free. In our paper, we pointed out the shadow-side of CSF, a project that ostensibly aims at doing good by attempting to increase the resiliency of warfighters, but ignores many possible iatrogenic implications. On the surface, it seems straightforward enough that training soldiers to be less stressed by combat is a good thing, but one possible unanticipated consequence is that this program could also make soldiers less upset by atrocities—and therefore more likely to commit them during war. As an alternative to reducing stress in warfighters by making them more resilient this way, perhaps training could instead emphasize empathy with the suffering of potential victims to reduce the likelihood of war atrocities, even if soldiers might themselves feel more suffering for involvement with causing so-called collateral damage. In other words, the stress of atrocities inures to both victims and the victimizers, and there may be need for a balance between minimizing damage to both potential victimizers and their victims. In research I am conducting in Zimbabwe, focused on rehabilitating former child soldiers by attempting to reintegrate them back into communities, the cost of being on either end of atrocities, as victimizer as well as victim, is evident (Machinga & Friedman, in press). To blindly claim scientific neutrality for such psychological interventions ignores latent underlying values and unintended consequences. Couching programs such as this under narrowly construed portrayals of psychology as a so-called objective science do not abnegate the crucial role of these underlying values, as exemplified by CSF's subtle privileging the welfare of soldiers over that of potential innocent victims under the guise of scientific neutrality.

CSF poses a basic social justice dilemma involving whether psychologists should design and implement programs that benefit one group, in this case by possibly increasing resiliency in soldiers, despite that it might possibly increase the likelihood of soldiers being more destructive toward the innocent. This is one of many social justice dilemmas that lead me to question on what basis anyone can act in the world with integrity, as people never fully know the ultimate outcome of their actions. In Indian psychology (Friedman, MacDonald, & Kumar, 2004), this is the problem of karma, and only enlightened beings supposedly can act without producing karma. For those of us who are not yet enlightened (see Johnson & Friedman, 2008), dilemmas have by definition no correct solution: they are problems that cannot be solved with any singularly right or wrong answers but, instead, are composed of choices among options that are always fraught with unknown short- and long-term costs as well as benefits, and the calculus of weighing these eludes any simple formulae due to the many looming, and intertwined, uncertainties. Simply put, if there is a clear good or bad choice, there is no dilemma, as any rational player would choose the good and reject the bad choice. Without clear knowledge of good and bad in any ultimate sense, people nevertheless are forced to act in order to exist, and this evidences the nonrationality of values that guide actions and frame social justice.

Many psychologists attracted to the area of social justice seem to suffer from the smugness of thinking they know the best solution for many vexing social justice dilemmas, similar to how previous research evaluated utilitarian decision making as better than biblical decision making, despite that there is no way to determine better or worse in this situation except through asserting arbitrary values (Needham & Friedman, 2012). A major danger of those who concern themselves about social justice issues within psychology involves assuming one's own worldview, including its accompanying values, is superior to alternate possibilities. Perhaps all people, even if only secretly, hold this perspective, but it seems stronger to me in those attracted to the area of social justice study and practice. For the most part, this area overall seems to suffer from a liberal bias, which is widely recognized as prevalent within psychology as a field, so it is essential to be self-critical, yet not so encumbered by criticalness as to cause paralysis. There is a real danger in tyranny, from any value position, by those who think they know the singularly best way to navigate social justice dilemmas, especially if the rigidity in their own beliefs results in imposing their views on others. Again, social justice dilemmas are always ambiguous and equivocal, as they depend on values that are culturally, historically, and otherwise relative, and hence can never be fully objective. To illustrate this point, I share a teaching story from the C'han Buddhist tradition, which I paraphrase from memory as it comes from an oral tradition. A young man from a poor Chinese village finds a horse in the forest, and everybody in the village is envious of him, as no one else has a horse. When the villagers tell his father how lucky the man is, the father replies, "maybe so, maybe not." Soon thereafter, the horse throws the young man and runs off, causing the young man to be crippled so that no young women in the village any longer show interest in him. The villagers tell his father how unlucky the man is, and the father replies, "maybe so, maybe not." Then a powerful warlord comes to the village and conscripts all, except the one crippled, young men to fight in a deadly war in which few would likely survive. Consequently, the crippled young man became quite popular with the village women and had many children, as he was the only young man left in the village. The villagers tell his father how lucky the man is, and again the father replies, "maybe so, maybe not." This illustrates how limited anyone's vision can be in seeing the consequences of events. From a social justice perspective, for example, was the violence stemming from discrimination and poverty that preceded the infamous 1965 Los Angeles Watts ghetto riots a good thing, as it undeniably preceded significant positive social change—or was it a bad thing due to the specific damage it caused to lives and property?

These types of social justice questions greatly trouble me, as I am called upon to act in the world within which I have been thrown and can never fully understand. However, as I look at many of my professional colleagues within psychology, I find few who acknowledge suffering over such concerns. Rather, as I know I am generalizing without data beyond my own personal experience here, most seem fixated on their daily survival issues, such as what the future of professional psychology holds for them—and that is increasingly uncertain (see American Psychological Association, 2012). There is little doubt that the economic reality of the profession is now causing considerable stress to many psychologists, and I think most would likely agree that it is becoming increasingly difficult to just earn a living commensurate with the sacrifices of becoming a psychologist, let alone to be concerned with the many social justice dilemmas in the profession. Clinical and counseling practices, the traditional mainstay of professional psychology, are now challenged to the point of breaking by the overwhelming and perverse incentives, such as of so-called managed care, which restricts access to psychological services in order to maximize corporate profits while duplicitously trying to preserve the illusion that somehow costs are being controlled for the benefit of all. Similarly, school psychologists operate in a climate of increasingly tight funding and other restrictions of needed psychological services. Together these psychological specialties constitute the majority of practicing psychologists. Organizational and forensic psychologists seem to have somewhat escaped these problems, at least for the moment (Clay, 2009; Novotney, 2011), as corporations and the legal system operate with greater impunity from the current, and seemingly growing, limitations endemic within institutional settings focused on helping (as opposed to maximizing profits or enforcing laws). Even academic psychologists are feeling the pinch of retrenchment in psychology departments with the drying-up of tenure-track positions and tightening of grant funding. Surely the field is challenged on just about all fronts (Friedman, 1996), and it is my experience that it is increasingly common for psychologists to question their choice of career path. In this moment within the profession's development, inordinate numbers of my colleagues seem caught in just keeping their heads financially above water, despite whatever original noble aspirations, including intellectual curiosity and/or desire to help others, led them to follow the path of psychology. When I raise issues related to social justice, as I have occasionally in professional circles, I tend to be dismissed as an annoying gadfly, and rebuffed with arguments that my interest in social justice would be nice in some ideal world, but psychologists primarily have to earn a living. The most stressed-out groups seem to be the newest-minted psychologists, often coming out of school with a doctorate and saddled with huge debts. Student loans, commonly in excess of a hundred-thousand dollars that are exempt from any relief (e.g., cannot be erased by bankruptcy), have to be repaid while facing employment prospects with low starting salaries, comparable to those with only bachelor's degrees in many other professions. With such debts to service after years of arduous graduate studies, and dim prospects for recouping them before retirement age, it is not surprising that the system of producing new psychologists frequently squelches the idealism that likely drew many to the field initially. Applied psychologists focus on serving their immediate and distal clients, including corporations whose motivations may be quite removed from any social justice concerns, whereas academic psychologists focus on whatever specific areas they might be teaching or investigating in trying to carve out a tenure niche and/or chasing the next grant opportunity without serious regard for the long-term consequences of their decisions. In this climate, social justice concerns just do not tend to arise, which is one reason for the existence of this handbook, namely to serve as a reminder of the importance of social justice. Although nearly all psychologists are continually exposed to the study of ethics at various stages of their careers, such as in graduate courses required to enter the field, postdoctoral level training needed to obtain licensure (as practitioners) and/or to use Institutional Review Boards (as researchers), few seem to really grasp the profound social justice implications that relate to all phases of professional life as a psychologist.

ENVISIONING THE PROFESSION OF PSYCHOLOGY[2]

Psychology is widely acknowledged as being a profession, but what does that mean and how does that relate to social justice? The common understanding of what constitutes a profession usually includes two criteria, competence acquired through extensive training and high levels of remuneration. In contrast, work performed by an amateur implies that it might be of lesser quality or performed less efficiently when compared to professional work, and that it might be provided without compensation.

The term *profession* also has a deeper meaning. A profession is different from an occupation, which can be said to merely be a role more or less passively occupied. A profession is more similar to a *vocation*, a term whose etymology relates to a calling in which a voice was literally heard, presumably from a sacred source, steering one into a purposeful lifework. As compelling as such a calling might be, the term profession implies even more: it is such a call profoundly answered. The answer is with a *professing*, a verbalized commitment to accept the calling, implicitly containing a focus not just toward pecuniary or other self-serving goals but, rather, toward upholding the larger good. I am reminded of the teaching story of three people who were building a church. When asked what they were doing, the first replied, "I'm laying down bricks and mortar." The second stated, "I am earning an honorable living to support myself and my family." The third, however, answered, "I am building a great cathedral to serve my community and honor the sacred." To be a professional requires more than to just play an occupational role or even to make an honorable living.

A professional was originally seen as one who can be trusted to act in the best interests of those served, not in the self-interest of the professional. In England, the original professionals were the clergy, and the ranks of those considered professionals soon expanded to include physicians and lawyers, all of whom were differentiated from members of guilds who were thought more self-serving (Perkin, n.d.). The label of being a professional "is cherished because it suggests special social, moral, and political status" (Welie, 2004, p. 529). Professionals, through their privileged positions, are granted special dispensations, such as a monopoly on providing certain services in which high fees are charged (e.g., licenses to practice psychology). This is no mere gift that inures without cost to professionals, however, since it is also expected that professionals will uphold their side of the bargain and not just narrowly serve their own interests.

The use of the term professional has changed from its original meanings, however. It has exploded to encompass a plethora of occupations that do not necessarily meet lofty standards. These days, people working in skilled trades, such as plumbers, and in specialized areas of business, such as real estate, call themselves professionals, showing how language can evolve. This has led to some disconnects between the original use of the term and what it means in contemporary times, specifically since the goals of trades and businesses are often at odds with idealistic professional goals.

This tension between the profession and the business of psychology is thus a source of considerable strain in contemporary times. When I attended psychology graduate school in the early 1970s, the emphasis was so thoroughly placed on noble professional ideals that this tension seldom seemed to arise, as the business aspects of psychology were clearly placed secondary. With the implicit social bargain, granting boons to psychological professionals in exchange for their complementary social tithe, appearing ruptured to many, it seems that more psychologists than ever are now viewing their profession in less lofty ways. Many sell out to the greed of corporate taskmasters, while many others are dissatisfied to the point of leaving the field. In such a climate, social justice concerns are too often placed on a back burner.

In this regard, I share an example of a social justice dilemma with which I had to contend involving the profession of psychology. Professional organizations often are more concerned with protecting the vested interests of their own constituents than the public, emblematic of the tension between the business and profession of psychology. As one example of this, a few years ago my state professional organization (i.e., the Florida Psychological Association; FPA) opposed expanding the use of the protected title *psychotherapist* to include master's-level advanced registered nurse practitioners specializing in mental health. Although there was a clear need for this group to share in such protection, such as the right to maintain patient confidentiality that comes with this title under Florida law, the FPA opposed this expansion based on the supposedly limited training held by nurses. These nurses, however, disproportionately served poor clients that psychologist tended to ignore, and denying them this title protection constituted a social justice dilemma. I considered this professional stance an example of "turf guarding," rather than as a sincere attempt to uphold high professional standards, and I responded to this by publicly opposing the FPA's position, such as by arguing that the American Academy of Psychotherapy has long recognized appropriately trained nurses as fully qualified psychotherapists. Although it is expected that a profession will promote a decent livelihood for its members, I considered it especially grievous to oppose the nursing profession on an issue involved access to care of the poor, which would have been reduced by prohibiting qualified nurses from gaining the advantages of using this privileged title. At the time, I was a volunteer lobbyist on behalf of FPA to my state legislative representative, and I also considered this turf-guarding to be inviting retaliation from one of psychology's closest professional allies, nurses. Coincidentally, my state representative happened to have been a nurse in her earlier career, so I really did not want to advocate against nurses to her! When I could not persuade FPA to drop this agenda, I resolved this social justice dilemma for me by avoidance, resigning as a lobbying psychologist. It was sad to see both valuable groups of professionals squander opportunities to cooperate or at least compete and, instead, polarize their efforts into conflict to the detriment of all in an area related to delivery of needed psychological services. This failure represented a case of social injustice as the underserved public, as well as both professional sides, lost out on important opportunities. For advocating on this particular social justice dilemma against the interests of my own profession, I also lost considerable social capital as an influential psychologist in Florida.

RECONCILING DILEMMAS: FROM COOPERATION TO COMPETITION TO CONFLICT[3]

In order to understand social justice dilemmas such as between different professions, there are many conceptual tools that can be helpful. Part of adapting to social life, for both individuals and groups, is the pursuit of goals, which may converge or diverge in varying degrees. Social psychologists (e.g., Deutsch, Coleman, & Marcus, 2006) and scholars from related disciplines (e.g., sociology, such as Denis & Kalekin-Fishman, 2009) have long identified the continuum from cooperation to competition to conflict as a key concept for understanding social interactions in relationship to goals and how to obtain them. I used this continuum to discuss interprofessional relations between psychologists and nurses in the previous example, and this concept has been used to analyze interactions within specific types of professions (e.g., lawyers; Gilson & Mnookin, 1991), within various business networks (e.g., Bengtsson & Kock, 1999), as well as across different types of interacting professionals (e.g., Makaram, 1995; Peters, 1995). However, I could find no previously published use of this concept specifically to understand interactions among practicing psychologists, or how psychologists might interrelate with other professionals or the wider community. As psychologists always practice within a professional culture that involves interactions among psychologists, as well as with other people, clarifying the dynamics of cooperation, competition, and conflict may provide a useful tool for pursuing social justice.

Cooperation refers to interactions in which not only are goals shared, but in which there is room to share the distributed fruits of goal attainment. It thus can be economically rational for individuals or groups to interact together in pursuing a common goal, if all would benefit from its attainment. Furthermore, without some degree of cooperation, social life in general would be impossible and humans would not survive. Psychologists and other professionals can cooperate when they promote a common good, such as increasing a community's awareness of the need for mental health services to treat depression by jointly sponsoring a free depression screening at a hospital through which all participating professionals may potentially benefit. This would be a so-called *win-win* scenario for the participating professionals. In addition, to the extent that the community and other stakeholders would benefit, this could be seen as a *win-win-win*.

Competition, on the other hand, involves a limited struggle among individuals or groups for the same goal, but one in which all cannot win (or win equally) in sharing the distributed fruits of attaining the goal. Competition is not necessarily bad, as it is a human universal that can be adaptive, such as by tending to stimulate efficiency and innovativeness. Psychologists and other mental health professionals may engage in pure competition when two or more seek a mutually exclusive, but valued by all parties, opportunity, such as a sole provider contract for performing all depression screenings within a hospital. In such a circumstance, when only one contract may be awarded, this would be a so-called *win-lose* scenario. However, competition involves a spirit of adhering to agreed-upon rules, such as sharing courtesy and respect—and competitors can maintain collegiality and do not have to seek to destroy each other. There are also competitive situations in which there are possibilities to partially win and partially lose in varying proportions. Psychologists and other mental health professionals may engage in such limited competition when two or more seek a valued opportunity that has rewards that might be shared to some, but not a fully equal, extent, such as participating in a free depression screening in order for individual practitioners to market their individual services to the public. They could all be cooperating in terms of attending the event together, but all competing in terms of trying to garner as many referrals as possible for themselves, thus placing them into a competitive stance somewhere between the poles of cooperation and pure competition, a so-called *mixed-motive* scenario that is neither clearly win-win or win-lose.

Then there is *conflict*, a form of struggle that leads to not only a possible winner and loser as in competition, but possibly a grave attempt by one or more parties to destroy another. It does not necessarily imply violence, as there can be nonviolent forms of destruction (e.g., limiting the conflict to the economic sphere by conflicting parties trying to put each other out of business), but it does destroy collegiality. With conflict, there not only can be a clear winner and loser as in pure competition, but sometimes it can devolve into *lose-lose* scenarios in which all get destroyed in the process. It thus can be economically irrational for individuals or groups to be in conflict, namely if it hurts all. In addition, conflict is almost always mean-spirited in some ways, such as in the frequent denigration of the other by one or more of the conflicting parties. As an aside, I believe sometimes conflict is necessary, as in so-called just wars, and I think conflict can also on occasion be a useful tool for solving social justice dilemmas, as I illustrate later. I note, however, that some psychologists active in the social justice area embrace a value stance that war is never just, and even that conflict of any sort should be shunned, regardless of the stakes or consequences. I see this ideological stance as a valid position, as there are no absolute bases for judging right or wrong in such value-laden contexts, but ironically (because such an ideological stance is usually seen as liberal) this is similar to the position religious conservatives tend to take in refusing to murder someone, even if it would save more lives (Needham & Friedman, 2012).

Understanding these nuances of cooperation, competition, and conflict can help psychologists better understand their relationship to the community of psychologists, to other professionals, and to the larger ecological context of humans and the physical environment. I find these concepts particularly useful for understanding social justice dilemmas, as they allow for ways to not rigidly bifurcate the world into extreme of cooperation versus conflict by introducing the middle-ground of varying degree of competition. In terms of an application example, some psychologists may naively operate under cooperative assumptions with colleagues who actually may be operating under alternative assumptions of competition or even of conflict. This could lead to unpleasant outcomes, as anyone attempting to be cooperative with others who are, in fact, not cooperative, especially if the ones not cooperating are feigning cooperation, will likely suffer. Alternatively, psychologists may cynically operate under assumptions involving only competing and conflicting relationships, while ignoring that others may in fact be open to cooperating, which could lead to lost opportunities for achieving cooperation that could benefit all. Although I have often been able to intentionally forge win-win cooperative agreements in many professional relationships, which I value most when possible, both with psychologists and other colleagues, sometimes these attempts have failed—and there is much that can be learned from such failures.

As an example, I share a breakdown that started with a competition that I hoped to change to cooperation, but that instead degraded into conflict. This involved an interpersonal rivalry between me and another psychologist. We were both competing for a lucrative contract to provide professional services within a large rehabilitation hospital. It was competitive because only one of us would be selected. I ultimately received the contract, but this other psychologist had a specialization that I did not possess (e.g., he was a skilled neuropsychologist and, as a general clinical psychologist, I am competent only in performing basic neuropsychological screenings), and neuropsychology was a skill needed to fulfill part of the contract terms. However, I had other valued skills making up for the deficit, resulting in the award being given to me. My original intent was to hire a third-party consulting neuropsychologist to provide the specialized skill I lacked but, in the spirit of transforming what had been competition to cooperation, I decided after I won the bid to offer a large share of this contract to my competitor, rather than to take the whole contract for myself. In other words, I tried to turn a win-lose competitive situation into a win-win cooperative situation. However, this boomeranged into conflict, as my competitor used my offer as a basis for appealing the entire award, arguing to the decision makers that he was better able to provide the services than I was. He presented the fact that I had asked for him to be a consultant as evidence of my lack of the needed neuropsychological competence to perform the required contractual duties.

Fortunately the decision makers did not change their minds, and my former competitor's (who was now in conflict with me) appeal was lost. I simply hired another neuropsychologist to consult with me, and avoided dealing professionally with this former competitor again. In essence, a competitive situation that I had tried to change into win-win cooperation instead became one of conflict in which a former competitor unsuccessfully attempted to flip the win to his side. Luckily the decision maker did not get disgusted with both of us and turn it into a lose-lose scenario, which easily could have happened. This illustrates how seeking a more socially just solution, by trying to move from competition toward cooperation, backfired.

Although many psychologists involved in social justice have biases against employing conflict, I think this can also be necessary for dealing with some social justice dilemmas. Of course, I prefer cooperating and competing, but sometimes as an advocate one has to take a strong stand against injustice (e.g., I believe that wars to stop genocide are justified). Consequently, I share an example in which I used conflict, namely "whistle-blowing," as a form of social justice advocacy.

I was consulting as a clinical psychologist with a private-for-profit prison corporation that had taken over a large state contract to provide behavioral health services within several facilities. I had worked with the previous prison contractor, and my contract had rolled over to the new contractor, which evidently cared little for both the welfare of inmates in its charge and for staff it employed, as the obvious way for it to maximize profits was to shortchange both. It was operating on a fixed-cost reimbursement, meaning it got paid the same amount regardless of the quality of its services. At first, because this corporation had taken over a previous contractor's work by offering a low bid that was accepted to save the state money, things were going smoothly with existing staff, including me, continued from the previous contract. However, gradually positions that were vacated through attrition were not filled and the situation degraded, as there were less people to do the needed work. I argued with the company that it would be in their best interest in the long run to provide the quality of service they had contracted to perform by replacing vacated positions, but my plea went nowhere, as vacated positions provided tempting revenue for its corporate coffers.

Consequently, I set out to be a whistle-blower, which is essentially a conflict role, as my goal in whistle-blowing was to shut down an abusive practice, not to find middle-ground as in competition or to seek an amicable cooperative outcome. I proceeded to covertly document this corporation's lack of performance, especially things that put inmates' lives at risk, and I cultivated a relationship with a powerful insider in the government who was motivated for his own political gain to expose corruption. Through a series of calculated maneuvers, I was able to force the government powers that were overseeing this corporation's contract to recognize the abuses, mainly through applying public pressure using the media and taking advantage of political rivalries to harness some factions against others. My conflict strategy worked, resulting in this large contract being taken from the corporation, and given, but only temporarily, to a new contractor who operated with more integrity. However, this new corporation was given a different type of contract, namely cost-reimbursement—meaning it was paid for its actual expenses plus a fixed-percentage management fee, so it had no perverse motive to deny services but, rather, had incentive to do what it was supposed to do. I was able to remain in my consulting position for another few years until, once again, this went out to bid and another contractor won a fixed-cost contract and, in line with its corporate interests, promptly deleted my consulting role before I could once more blow the whistle.

I want to emphasize, because perverse incentives in which abusive practices maximize profit are often involved in the privatization of psychological services, managed care being a salient example in which a private company profits from restricting and not from facilitating needed services, I am not taking a stance against all privatization within professional psychology. In fact, I was one of the first in

Florida to extensively use for-profit privatization within psychology to provide innovative services in ways I considered congruent with social justice aspirations, a point to which I return later. In addition, although I have seen many abuses related to privatization, I have similarly seen nonprofit and even government-run programs do dishonorable things for all sorts of motives other than profit.

LEARNING TO BECOME A SUCCESSFUL SOCIAL JUSTICE ADVOCATE

As an undergraduate and graduate student, I faced many social justice dilemmas in studying psychology, as I did in a number of part- and full-time psychology-related positions I held while a psychology student. However, after passing my doctoral qualifying exams in clinical psychology and beginning the process of dissertating, I obtained a position teaching at a small community college in Florida, which was where is where I learned, and finely honed, my skills as social justice advocate. I encountered many interesting opportunities at this college, including obtaining a grant to form an interdisciplinary Human Services Program (HSP), which I chaired (or co-chaired) for many years. The primary mission of this HSP was to train students in a variety of human services fields, not just within the single discipline of psychology. In addition, the larger mission of the school, as a community college, was to serve the community beyond the confines of the bricks-and-mortar institution. Because this college was located in a small community, there were many unmet psychological needs that would have been filled in a major community by seasoned professionals but, as a beginning psychologist, I had the privilege of being a big fish in this small pond, even before I earned my PhD. For example, I had great leeway in designing new programs and seeking grants to fund them. This arena is where I learned many social justice advocacy skills, such as conducting community needs assessments, cultivating community support through building participatory boards, evaluating programs, and learning how to obtain resources to implement innovative programs. I wrote and received numerous grants with a focus primarily on outreach to underserved populations. As one example, I was able to increase the number of students, especially minority students, enrolled in the HSP by providing educational opportunities to economically disadvantaged youth who were unlikely to have otherwise gone to college. I accomplished this through obtaining grant funding to employ them in a work-study program, which paid students full-time wages for working in part-time human service jobs (e.g., as teacher aides in special education classes) while they attended college with all their tuition and books provided free.

During this time, I also was completing a dissertation in transpersonal psychology, a field that looks at the radical interconnectedness of the self with others and the world (see Friedman & Hartelius, 2013). I chose to dissertate in this area because I believe that transpersonal psychology provides the most inclusive perspective from which to understand the world. Researching in this area was daunting, however, so I coped with my dissertation anxiety by building and running the

HSP, which allowed me to creatively work on many social justice issues while procrastinating the completion of my dissertation. Instead of being isolated from the community within the ivory tower of a university with its many academic pressures (e.g., for tenure) or being overwhelmed with a hectic clinical psychology position, working at this college gave me nearly unlimited opportunities to learn to be an advocate for social justice in the real world. After finishing my dissertation, I completed a clinical internship, became licensed as a psychologist, and began to build a private practice. In addition, I formed a private company and sought business opportunities using the same skills developed in running the HSP by seeking my own grants outside of the auspices of the college.

BECOMING A PSYCHOPRENEUR[4]

Psychopreneur is a neologism I use to refer to one who utilizes entrepreneurial approaches in delivering psychological services. I had the desire to find diverse ways to be a psychologist, and the thought of doing full-time psychotherapy and/or psychological assessments, the two activities that constitute much of traditional clinical psychology practice, lacked sustainable excitement for me. I also recognized that this type of practice would limit my income, since there are only so many hours available to directly deliver services, as well as it would limit the impact of my social justice work to those with whom I could directly work. So, when starting my private practice, I decided to restrict my direct delivery of traditional psychological services to half-time and to seek other psychological, or related, opportunities to enhance my professional satisfaction and impact on the world. Some psychologists who share this feeling have simply developed secondary careers apart from psychology, such as several I know who did quite well economically by selling real estate, but I remained focused on opportunities related to what I knew best, psychology. So I share the story of how I first "cleaned up" in the psychology business as a psychopreneur, and where this has since led me.

After being initially licensed as a psychologist in 1982 at age 34, I started a private practice and also consulted with a state *mental retardation* (the term used at the time) facility. I also continued to teach at the college, but I was biding time in my work there (i.e., fulfilling a commitment to pay-off sabbatical funding I obtained to complete my doctoral internship) while focusing my creativity elsewhere. My consulting role involved assessing clients in this facility, as well as chairing habilitation committees to guide in out-placing clients into less restrictive community settings during a time of rapid deinstitutionalization. As a consultant, I scheduled this institutional work around my newly developing psychological practice and college teaching.

In performing this consulting role, I learned that the facility was in danger of losing its federal license during this time of rapid transition, something that would have devastating financial ramifications to the institution, its staff, and its residents. There were many problems at the facility that had to be addressed to keep this important federal license, one of the least being that the workers who cleaned the facility had grown overly complacent and the facility simply did not meet standards for basic cleanliness. Many of these workers had been employed at the same janitorial jobs for decades and just were not amenable to changing their habits, in some ways being nearly as institutionalized as the facility's residents. Simply stated, despite many efforts to change these janitorial workers' productivity, it was not being done to the satisfaction of the federal inspectors. The facility's management decided that the only reasonable solution was to outsource these janitorial services, while finding other positions for these workers (e.g., transitioning them into other roles, such as program aides).

I was thinking about expanding my practice and looking for whatever opportunities might present, so I began to make some creative leaps. I recognized that I knew nothing about janitorial services and also had absolutely no interest in learning anything in this area. Nevertheless I literally *smelled* an opportunity. I recalled that a friend had shared that he had some experience with providing janitorial services, though he was currently employed in another line of work, and I sought him out to just talk about this opportunity. He assured me he had the needed skills to do the job, but that he did not possess the needed talent for obtaining a project of this magnitude, such as in writing a viable bid to provide a large service within a highly bureaucratic structure.

So, encouraged, I explored further and discovered that this opportunity was soon to be going out for bids in which there would be much competition, especially from a very large firm that provided high-quality janitorial services to similar institutions nationwide. This firm was very professionally organized, had deep pockets, and much experience in running a bottom-line profitable business. I wondered, how could I, as a psychologist completely out of my element, ever hope to compete with it? And what on earth could I be thinking to even want to get into this business, perceived by many as low status and dirty (which it undeniably was), when I was a new doctoral-level professional? My wife and many of my friends concluded I was over the edge from postdissertation and postlicensure insanity, engaging in a flight from psychological reality. But the opportunity beckoned irresistibly and I began to ruminate on possibilities.

Then it occurred to me, an out-of-the-box solution. I had previously been a consultant in delivering job-seeking skills training for a local government agency through the college: a service intended to help chronically unemployed people successfully obtain employment. I knew that this agency had some funding to cover additional job-skills training, and I was able to arrange a potential deal to start a program in which I would train people in job-seeking skills through giving them supported employment (i.e., through their working as janitors), contingent on my receiving the contract. The agency agreed to recruit unemployed people from their eligibility lists and pay half their salary for up to six months while I trained them. Of course, these would be people that essentially no one else had wanted to hire and would present with many problems, like mental illness and alcoholism, but

I could screen and select from among those eligible. As a psychologist, I thought, who would be better in working with these troubled individuals?

This possibility solved several problems. I now had a basis for a competitive advantage over the more established janitorial companies, since I could underbid them through this salary supplement that enabled cheaper labor. I could also use my psychological skills in delivering job-seeking skills training, building off my professional strengths in an area in which I otherwise had less to offer than the competition. In addition, that the salaries were only to be supplemented for six months for each employee appeared initially to me as a problem, but soon I began to see this as a great incentive for doing meaningful social justice work, as I could train these previously unemployable people with needed job-seeking skills and then work toward outplacing them in private sector jobs within the funded six months. This employee turn-around could result in being able to have a steady stream of salary-supplemented janitors and thus keeping the competitive advantage ongoing, while I would be helping people get needed jobs. I was excited at the opportunity to apply what seemed to be an interesting synergistic approach to a business that would use my psychology background in a very challenging and productive way.

As an aside, psychologists are frequently indoctrinated with an inherent bias to play it safe. This makes sense when people's lives are at stake in delivering professional psychological services, but it does not lend to being a good business person and creative advocate for social justice, as some risk taking is absolutely needed to garner success as a psychopreneur. I had to do some real soul searching to risk going for this opportunity, especially since it required putting up considerable seed money that I had to borrow (using my house as collateral).

When I bid on the contract, the facility's management was as skeptical as my family and most of my friends had been. I was asked, what could I, as a psychologist, know about janitorial services, and why was I even interested in this? It simply made no sense to them, but I was the lowest bidder and it was difficult for the management to bypass me by awarding to a higher, though more established and admittedly more qualified, bidder. I was even accused of "low-balling" the bid, intentionally manipulating the process. The facility's federal funding was on the line and, if I did not deliver the goods, not only would I be in financial trouble, but there could be a lot of other people's well-being jeopardized. However, the government's rules stated that the janitorial contract was supposed to go to the lowest bidder and I did not back down, being confident I could deliver the service—although I did have more than a few sleepless nights of private doubt.

A compromise was worked out. I was given the contract for a small portion of the janitorial services, as a trial. The major competing large janitorial company, although it had bid significantly higher, was also given a similar—but better-paying—small contract, while the state continued to clean the rest of the facility with its own employees, waiting to see if I would fail as was expected. If I could provide the service adequately during this test period, however, the entire contract would become mine; otherwise the large company would get it all.

I did perform adequately, largely due to the tremendous help of my friend who became the working supervisor. After that, I received and ran this contract for three years, while building my private psychological practice to the half-time goal that I had set for it, after which I left the college. This janitorial contract eventually grew to involve over 50 full-time workers, including a staff of supervisors and job coaches. I really enjoyed the diverse work it involved, especially the hands-on training of employees in basic skills, such as time management and even personal grooming, needed for successful job seeking. This became a win-win-win scenario as the facility received a quality service for a bargain price, many of the janitorial employees were able to benefit, and so did I. Incidentally, after the three years, I turned the program back over to the facility, and my remaining employees became hired by the state. This has been the hallmark of many of my community interventions, namely working for a year or so to build an innovative program, running it for a while to work out the "kinks," and then transitioning it in a stable way back into the community while I withdrew to explore other opportunities.

This case study of my first effort as a psychopreneur also illustrates some basic principles that I have since followed. These involve being open to perceiving an opportunity when it presents itself, being innovative in conceptualizing how the opportunity could be utilized, including making connections between whatever psychological skills might give an advantage in pursuing the opportunity, and doing something that is not solely monetarily driven but, rather, also allows for achieving social justice goals.

Since this first psychopreneurial effort, I went on to explore many similar opportunities. Adding to the principles mentioned previously, I learned to also do more than just actively scan for opportunities, that is, how to actively make opportunities happen. For example, at this same facility I noticed that deinstitutionalized clients did not have adequate social supports in the community when they left the protection of the institution, so I proposed a case management service that I started with a small pilot program, initially employing two master's-level case managers; this later grew into another large project employing over 50 case managers and support people who served not just the then-called mentally retarded clients, but also severely emotionally disturbed children (see Friedman, 2002a). I also became more committed to doing these types of projects not just for personal gain, so I learned how to work with creating nonprofit organizations and launching them into independent existences to meet the needs of various underserved populations that psychologists were usually reluctant to help (see Friedman, 2003). In this regard, after successfully managing this case management project for over a decade, I turned it over to a nonprofit I created for that purpose.

I might mention that working through psychological-related businesses and nonprofits also allowed me to grow my private practice in a psychopreneurial way. I was able to hire psychologists and guarantee them work in these ancillary efforts while their private practice activities developed. So these types of programs became extensions of, and bolstered, my burgeoning private practice, which grew to include multiple offices and employed a number of licensed psychologists, psychology residents, and master's-level staff. In accord with my quest for diverse activities as a psychologist, I and my practice delivered psychological services in quite a range of settings, including for a mental hospital, an Indian tribe, a prison, a rehabilitation hospital, a preschool intervention program, and an alcohol and substance abuse facility, to name just a few. All of these setting involved their own unique social justice dilemmas, which I attempted to address using psychopreneurial skills. I also became particularly adept in obtaining funding for numerous social justice projects, as well as personally pursued many diverse professional consulting roles, such as providing extensive forensic services (e.g., witness preparation; Pigot & Friedman, 1998) and even international management consulting (Friedman, Glover, & Avegalio, 2002). I also particularly enjoyed mentoring many psychological residents who later obtained psychology licensure through my practice, and mentoring is something I continue to especially enjoy (e.g., see, Fracasso, Franco, MacDonald, & Friedman, 2011).

Much of the current wisdom on successful psychological practice emphasizes developing specialized practice niches, but frankly if I did the same activity every day in a specialized way, I would have been bored to tears. So I think it is important for psychologists to think more broadly, not just narrowly, about the opportunities around them—and their own capacities to provide needed services that require psychological skills applied in innovative ways. While the rewards (monetary and otherwise) of traditional psychological private practice have unfortunately decreased, there are still creative opportunities for psychologists to function as psychopreneurs, including in ways that further social justice.

SERVING YOUTH OR THE ELDERLY

As a psychopreneur, I became somewhat more successful, primarily through creating psychological programs to serve the elderly through Medicare funding. I negotiated a large contract to run the psychological services at a rehabilitation hospital that primarily served elderly clients suffering from orthopedic (e.g., hip injuries) and neurological (e.g., strokes) disorders, and I also had contracts with nearly a dozen nursing homes to provide psychological services, as well as with a memory and a pain clinic. I orchestrated this by bringing in newly graduated doctoral psychology residents (unlicensed), whom I personally supervised and mentored toward licensure. When licensed, many of them joined my practice as affiliates and, in turn, worked independently and, in some cases, supervised new residents who joined my practice. In essence, I created an expanding pyramid that took advantage of the opportunity provided by Medicare at that time to bill for psychological services with little restriction—and my practice grew quickly. Although I had private practice offices in several cities in Southwest Florida, and built a solid referral basis from which I and my affiliates worked, the real volume fueling my business model was from Medicare through serving the elderly.

In running this psychology business model, however, I became increasingly concerned that the needs of youth, especially those who were economically disadvantaged, were largely ignored in my community. Although I enjoyed working with the elderly, and their needs are undeniably very important and not to be minimized, I increasingly became bothered by how many seriously disturbed youth were not getting comparable needed psychological services. Serving the elderly through Medicare yielded about $100 per hour, while the elderly clients that I and my group served were often a captive audience residing in nursing homes and hospital settings, so most could be efficiently scheduled with little unbillable down time. Many of the neediest youth in my community, however, were covered only by Medicaid, which paid approximately half of what Medicare paid, and serving youth in volume was much more problematic in terms of logistics. I struggled with justifying to myself that my group's ample provision of services to the elderly, who overall had limited life expectancies and who were often warehoused in nursing homes and similar settings with little quality to their lives, occurred while so many very needy youth, who had long lifetimes ahead of them (i.e., if they did not get killed early in life, as youth violence in this population was endemic) were being ignored. Simply put, it was easy and lucrative to serve the elderly, but I felt drawn to serve youth as well, particularly youth without many resources, despite that this was a population presenting numerous barriers making it difficult to serve them. As an example of some of the economics, if I paid a psychology resident $40 per hour total for providing a Medicare service for the elderly that yielded $100 per billable hour, my profit would be a generous $60; however, if I paid a similar psychology resident $40 per hour total for providing a Medicaid service for youth that yielded only $50 per hour, my profit would be a mere $10. Considering the no-shows and other barriers in working with youth, this was a losing proposition that explained why no other psychologists were helping these economically disadvantaged youth in my community.

I puzzled over this as a social justice dilemma, and the psychopreneurial skills I had learned at the college kicked in—as I began to think outside the proverbial box. Accordingly, I devised a number of programs to outreach to youth where they spent their time, mainly in schools. As an example of one such program I developed and ran, there was a school with several hundred severely emotionally disturbed children, ranging from elementary to high school level. These youth were considered the worst of the worst, as they were the ones who could not make it in special education programs within regular schools and so were sequestered in this problem-filled school. Almost all of these youth were from economically disadvantaged backgrounds and most were of minority ethnicity. Many were diagnosed as psychotic and on psychotropic medications, but there was only one school counselor for everyone, so few were getting any nonmedical mental health services and none were getting regular counseling. I clearly saw the need for providing psychological services at this school and approached its principal about trying to do something innovative. Her responses reflected learned helplessness, as she recited a litany of barriers against doing anything creative. For example, the principal's first response, when I stated that I could use Medicaid to fund services, was that a few of her students did not have Medicaid and it would be unfair to serve only those with coverage—so I agreed that all would be served, while only those with Medicaid would be billed through their coverage. Of course, this reduced the already slim financial feasibility even more. Her next response was that the school was overcrowded and there was no room to accommodate mental health providers—so I asked if I could have a designated space in the parking lot to locate a portable building to be used as a counseling center, creating another cost. After much negotiation of this sort, I paid to move a portable to the parking lot, staffed it with a full-time psychology resident (both as project manager and as clinician), three master's-level mental health providers, a bachelor's-level mental health technician, a full-time secretary, and a part-time consulting psychiatrist, while I personally supervised the psychology resident in my role as a licensed psychologist. Consequently, the entire school received psychological services. As there was no profit in this venture when all was tallied, and there was considerable liability exposure with high risk youth (e.g., many were homicidal and/or suicidal), I decided to put this and several similar programs I created under a nonprofit corporation, which I set up as a vehicle for delivering high-risk services where my motivation was oriented toward social justice and not toward profit. In fact, I had to supplement the funding for these youth programs through profits earned by serving the elderly in my other work.

I ran this and many similar youth programs for a number of years through Medicaid, serving approximately 1,000 youth at any one time who otherwise would have received no mental health services other than medications. Unfortunately, there was a political change in the Florida governor's office and my innovations in serving youth, which were initially lauded by government officials, grew out of favor as they grew in size. They became seen by the new political powers only as a cost, despite that they were meant to reduce the even higher cost later for mental hospitalizations and prison incarceration for these youth when they grew up, rather than as a benefit. Ironically, when I started these programs I was encouraged to expand them as much as possible due to the huge unmet need I was trying to fill but, because they were so successful in scope, this became a problem to the government. In specific, these youth programs relied almost exclusively on Medicaid money, which is a match of state and federal funds. In Florida, which has a large elderly population, Medicaid primarily is used to finance nursing home services to the elderly, and this has been the single largest state expense in recent times. The programs I developed to serve youth were diverting some of this money from services for the elderly and, instead of my programs continuing to be perceived as a good thing, they increasingly were perceived negatively, and I was even openly criticized for having developed them. Ultimately, they were closed by the state, which saddened me but I found solace in the many young people they were able to help. I did get some recognition for this work from my peers by receiving the 2003 FPA's annual award for "Outstanding Contributions in the Public Interest."

CONCLUSION

Psychologists have successfully furthered many social justice causes, such as through opposing racial segregation within public education, helping abolish life sentences without parole for most juvenile offenders, presenting research supporting adoptions by nonheterosexual people, promoting reform in health care, and working in so many other valued areas (Munsey, 2011). However, little has been written about the actual process by which some practicing psychologists have actively engaged in social justice work. This account of some of the social justice dilemmas I have faced provides a personal glimpse into how I, as an autobiographical case study of one psychologist who actively cares about social justice, managed to operate in this arena. I also explored some of the complexities defining social justice, framing this in terms of social justice dilemmas that have no unequivocal right or wrong solutions but nevertheless have to be faced, outlined some conceptual principles, such as a continuum from cooperation to competition to conflict, that can be useful, and offered a model of psychopreneurship for creatively functioning as a psychologist, including showing how this can be applied to becoming a successful social justice advocate.

I also emphasized how positioning oneself as an advocate for social justice has perils for psychologists beyond just forgoing more lucrative business arrangements, as it can even lead to having one's reputation besmirched for trying to do good. Many in science criticize social justice advocacy for taking explicit value stances, which some see as outside the purview of a psychologist as a so-called objective scientist. I have challenged this notion by claiming that objectivity in science is a myth, and instead argued that psychologists unavoidably contend with social justice dilemmas as part of their professional responsibilities. I have also shared some of my successes as an advocate dealing with social justice dilemmas, as well as a few of my failures.

I want to also add that psychopreneurial skills can be more broadly applied to social justice in work outside the realm of psychology. Having learned these skills in the practice of psychology, I have greatly enjoyed applying them to domains other than psychology. As an environmental activist, for example, I have used these skills to successfully fight a number of important battles, such as stopping the placement of a coal-burning electric power-plant adjacent to a sensitive wilderness area. This is in accord with that fact that social justice cannot be meaningful in a world that cannot support life.

I want to conclude with my belief that the "larger picture" be invoked in psychological considerations of social justice. From this vantage, understanding social justice dilemmas can be approached through transpersonal psychology (see Friedman & Hartelius, 2013), especially through using the construct of self-expansiveness (Friedman, 1983) in which the boundaries between self and other, as well as self and the entire world including the cosmos as a whole, can be seen to disintegrate. When others and even the cosmos are viewed as a manifestation of one's self, and conversely oneself as a reciprocal manifestation of the cosmos, I believe one is more likely to engage in furthering social justice—as conflicting and even competing interests can dissolve toward cooperation based on principles of identification through converging of narrow self-interest with a broader Self-interest (the capitalized Self referring to a capacity to embrace one's most expansive potential, perhaps even beyond time and space). As part of my being an advocate for social justice, and my understanding of how to free creative energy to accomplish good things in the world through being a psychopreneur, I am also committed to grounding this view in a scientific approach to transpersonal psychology (Friedman, 2002b). I do not approach this work from a dispassionate or distanced perspective through science, but rather from a worldview that seriously entertains the implications of being radically interconnected with all, from the smallest subatomic particle to the cosmos as a whole and beyond. This provides a basis for linking social justice wisdom, such as the so-called Golden Rule to "do unto others as you would have them do unto you," with an understanding of the interconnectivity of self and others, and provides a solid platform from which empirical research can be conducted (e.g., see Hoot & Friedman, 2011).

I retired at the age of 50 from the private practice of clinical psychology and most consulting work, in order to primarily research, teach, and write. Although I no longer work in the so-called trenches of psychology by being directly engaged with many social justice efforts as a professional, as a scholar I now actively strive to encourage an expanded worldview in others related to what transpersonal psychology can offer. My involvement goes beyond scientific research to also include leadership roles in this area, such as promoting transpersonal psychology by serving as the senior editor of *The International Journal of Transpersonal Studies* (see transpersonalstudies.org) and being active as the president of the Board of the International Transpersonal Association (see Grof, Friedman, Lukoff, & Hartelius, 2008), an organization coordinating efforts of the various transpersonal associations throughout the globe. This work is in accord with my conviction that transpersonal psychology can provide a powerful vehicle for reconciling even the most vexing social justice dilemmas in ways that no other approach to psychology can provide. My final thoughts involve emphasizing how transpersonal psychology can be liberating at both the levels of individuals and society, as these are reciprocally important and could not exist without each other, while similarly, without the physical world that sustains all life, none of this would matter.

NOTES

1. This work constitutes a loosely written compendium of my ideas as are suitable for inclusion within an appendix rather than as a regular chapter within a scholarly work. I also am taking some of the material forming this contribution from my previous publications, especially through drawing from several short articles I wrote for the *Florida Psychologist*, which are referenced accordingly.

2. This section is a revised and expanded version of a previously published paper (Friedman, 2005).

3. This section is a revised and expanded version of a previously published paper (Friedman, 2011).

4. This section is a revised and expanded version of a previously published paper (Friedman, 2006).

REFERENCES

Ahmed, S., Wilson, K., Henriksen, R., & Jones, J. (2011). What does it mean to be a culturally-competent counselor? *Journal for Social Action in Counseling and Psychology, 3*(1), 17–28.

American Psychological Association. (2012). Perspectives on the future of professional psychology: Panelists assessed the gaps that exist between market realities and the current state of professional psychology. *APA Practice Update, March 29*, n.p. Retrieved from http://www.apapracticecentral.org/update/2012/03-29/future-psychology.aspx

Bengtsson, M., & Kock, S. (1999). Cooperation and competition in relationships between competitors in business networks. *Journal of Business & Industrial Marketing, 14*(3), 178–194.

Clay, R. (2009). Postgrad growth area: Forensic psychology: Psychologists who work in settings where psychology and the law overlap are in hot demand. *APA gradPSYCH Magazine, November*, n.p. Retrieved from http://www.apa.org/gradpsych/2009/11/postgrad.aspx

Denis, A., & Kalekin-Fishman, D. (2009). *The ISA handbook in contemporary sociology: Conflict, competition, cooperation.* Thousand Oaks, CA: SAGE.

Deutsch, M., Coleman, P., & Marcus, E. (Eds.), (2006). *The handbook of conflict resolution: Theory and practice.* San Francisco, CA: Jossey-Bass.

Fracasso, C., Franco, Z., MacDonald, D., & Friedman, H. (2011). Measuring the transpersonal: The research and mentoring contributions of Harris Friedman. *NeuroQuantology, 9*(3), 499–515.

Friedman, H. (1983). The Self-Expansiveness Level Form: A conceptualization and measurement of a transpersonal construct. *The Journal of Transpersonal Psychology, 15*, 37–50.

Friedman, H. (1996). Psychology is severely challenged as a professional field. *The Independent Practitioner, 16*, 101–102.

Friedman, H. (2002a). Case management as an extension of psychological practice. *Independent Practitioner, 22*, 191–193.

Friedman, H. (2002b). Transpersonal psychology as a scientific field. *International Journal of Transpersonal Studies, 21*, 175–187.

Friedman, H. (2003). Nonprofit organizations as a vehicle for enhancing psychological practice. *Independent Practitioner, 23*, 9–11.

Friedman, H., Glover, G., & Avegalio, F. (2002). The burdens of other people's models: A cultural perspective on the current Fiji crisis. *Harvard Asia Pacific Review, 6*, 86–90.

Friedman, H., Glover, G., Sims, E., Culhane, E., Guest, M., & Van Driel, M. (2013). Cross-cultural competence: Performance-based assessment and training. *Organizational Development Journal, 31*(2), 18–30.

Friedman, H., & Hartelius, G. (Eds.). (2013). *The Wiley-Blackwell handbook of transpersonal psychology*. Oxford, UK: Wiley-Blackwell.

Friedman, H., MacDonald, D., & Kumar, K. (2004). Cross-cultural validation of the Self-Expansiveness Level Form with an Indian sample. *Journal of Indian Psychology, March,* 44–56.

Friedman, H., & Robbins, B. (2012). The negative shadow cast by positive psychology: Contrasting views and implications of humanistic and positive psychology on resiliency. *The Humanistic Psychologist, 40,* 87–102.

Gilson, R., & Mnookin, R. (1991). Disputing through agents: Cooperation and conflict between lawyers in litigation. *Columbia Law Review, 94,* 509–66.

Goldstein, R. (2006). *Incompleteness: The roof and paradox of Kurt Gödel.* New York, NY: Norton.

Grof, S., Friedman, H., Lukoff, D., & Hartelius, G. (2008). The past and future of the International Transpersonal Association. *International Journal of Transpersonal Studies, 27,* 55–62.

Heidegger, M. (2010/1927). *Being and time* (trans. by J. Stambaugh, revised by D. Schmidt). Albany, NY: State University of New York Press: Norton.

Hoot, R., & Friedman, H. (2011). Sense of interconnectedness and pro-environmental behavior. *International Journal of Transpersonal Studies, 30*(1–2), 89–100.

Johnson, C., & Friedman, H. (2008). Enlightened or delusional? Differentiating religious, spiritual, and transpersonal experience from psychopathology. *Journal of Humanistic Psychology, 48*(4), 505–527.

Machinga, M., & Friedman, H. (in-press). Developing transpersonal resiliency: An approach to healing and reconciliation in Zimbabwe. *International Journal of Transpersonal Studies.*

Makaram, S. (1995). Interprofessional cooperation. *Medical Education, 29,* 65–69.

McAdams, D. P. (2008). Personal narratives and the life story. In O. John, R. Robins, & L. Pervin, L. (Eds.), *Handbook of personality: Theory and research* (3rd ed., pp. 241–261). New York, NY: Guilford.

Munsey, C. (2011). And social justice for all. *APA Monitor, 42*(9), 30.

Needham, J., & Friedman, H. (2012). Moral identity versus moral reasoning in religious conservatives: Do Christian Evangelical leaders really lack moral maturity? *The Humanistic Psychologist, 40,* 343–363.

Novotney, A. (2011). Psychology job forecast: Partly sunny. *APA gradPSYCH Magazine, March,* 44. Retrieved from http://www.apa.org/gradpsych/2011/03/cover-sunny.aspx

Perkin, H. (n.d.). Crisis in the professions: Ambiguities, origins, and current problems. Retrieved from thersa.org/acrobat/perkin1.pdf

Peters, H. (1995). The interaction of journalists and scientific experts: Co-operation and conflict between two professional cultures. *Media Culture Society, 17*(1), 31–48.

Pigott, M., & Friedman, H. (1998). Enhancing fact witness effectiveness. *The Trial Lawyer, 21,* 309–320.

Welie, J. (2004). Is dentistry a profession? Part 1. Professionalism defined. *Journal of Canadian Dental Association, 70* (8), 529–532.

Appendix C

Recommended Readings in Social Justice and Psychology

BOOKS

Adams, M., Bell, L., & Griffin, P. (1997). *Teaching for diversity and social justice: A sourcebook.* New York, NY: Routledge.

Adams, M., Blumenfield, W. J., Casteñeda, R., Hackman, H. W., Peters, M. L., & Zúñiga, X. (Eds.) (2010). *Readings for diversity and social justice* (2nd ed.). New York, NY: Routledge.

Aldarondo, E. (Ed.) (2007). *Advancing social justice through clinical practice.* Mahwah, NJ: Lawrence Erlbaum Associates.

Anderson, S. K., & Middleton, V. A. (2005). *Explorations in privilege, oppression, and diversity.* Belmont, CA: Brooks/Cole.

Barry, B. (2005). *Why social justice matters.* Malden, MA: Polity Press.

Bernal, G., Trimble, J., Burlew, A., & Leong, F. (Eds.) (2003). *Handbook of racial and ethnic minority psychology.* Thousand Oaks, CA: Sage.

Bieschke, K. J., Perez, R. M., & DeBord, K. A. (Eds.) (2006). *Handbook of counseling and psychotherapy with lesbian, gay, bisexual, and transgender clients* (2nd ed.). Washington, DC: APA.

Bongar, L. Beutler, L, Brown, M., Breckenridge, J., & Zimbardo, P. (Eds.) (2006). *Psychology and terrorism.* New York, NY: Oxford University Press.

Boothby, N., Strang, A., & Wessells, M. (Eds.) (2006). *A world turned upside down: Social ecological approaches to children in war zones.* Westport, CT: Kumarian.

Bullock, H. (2013). *Women and poverty: Psychology, public policy, and social justice.* West Sussex, UK: Wiley-Blackwell.

Carr, S. & Sloan, T. (Eds.) (2003). *Poverty and psychology.* New York, NY: Kluwer.

Christie, D. J., Wagner, R. V., & Winter, D. D. (2001). *Peace, conflict, and violence: Peace psychology for the 21st Century.* Upper Saddle River, NJ: Prentice-Hall.

Chung, R. C., & Bemak, F. (2011). *Social justice counseling: The next steps beyond multiculturalism.* Thousand Oaks, CA: Sage.

Crisp, R. (Ed.) (2010). *The psychology of social and cultural diversity.* West Sussex, UK: Wiley-Blackwell.

Delgado, R. (2012). *Critical race theory: An introduction* (2nd ed.). New York, NY: New York University Press.

Denzin, N. K., Lincoln, Y. S., & Smith, L. T. (2008). *Handbook of critical and indigenous methodologies.* Thousand Oaks, CA: Sage.

Deutsch, M., & Coleman, P. (2000). *The handbook of conflict resolution: Theory and practice.* San Francisco: Jossey Bass.

Esses, U. M., & Vernon, R. A. (Eds.) (2008). *Explaining the breakdown of ethnic relations: Why neighbors kill.* West Sussex, UK: Wiley-Blackwell.

Fairclough, N. (2001). *Language and power* (2nd ed). Essex, UK: Pearson Education.

Fanon, F., & Stefancic, J. (Trans.) (2004). *The wretched of the Earth.* New York, NY: Grove Press. (Originally published as *Damnés de la terre.* Paris, France, Maspero, F., Ed.).

Fine, M., Weis, L., Powell, L., & Burns, A. (Eds.) (2004). *Off-white: Readings on power, privilege, and resistance* (2nd ed). New York, NY: Routledge.

Fiske, S. T. (2011). *Envy up, scorn down: How status divides us.* New York, NY: Russell Sage Foundation.

Fox, D. Prilleltensky, I., & Austin, S. (Eds.) (2009). *Critical psychology* (2nd ed). Thousand Oaks, CA: Sage.

Freire, P. (1996). *Pedagogy of the oppressed* (rev. ed.). London, UK: Penguin.

Goodman, D. J. (2001). *Promoting diversity and social justice: Educating people from privileged groups.* Thousand Oaks, CA: Sage.

Hale, G. E. (1998). *Making whiteness: The culture of segregation in the south, 1890–1940.* New York, NY: Pantheon.

hooks, b. (1994). *Teaching to transgress: Education as the practice of freedom.* New York, NY: Routledge.

hooks, b. (2003). *Teaching community: A pedagogy of hope.* New York, NY: Routledge.

Jacobsen, M. F. (1999). *Whiteness of a different color: European immigrants and the alchemy of race.* Cambridge, MA: Harvard University Press.

Jacobsen, M. F. (2000). *Barbarian virtues: The United States encounters foreign people at home and abroad, 1876–1917.* New York, NY: Hill and Wang.

Jonas, K. J., & Morton, T. A. (Eds.) (2012). *Restoring civil societies: The psychology of intervention and engagement following crisis.* West Sussex, UK: Wiley-Blackwell.

Jost, J. T., Kay, A. C., & Thorisdottir, H. (Eds.) (2009). *Social and psychological bases of ideology and system justification.* New York, NY: Oxford University Press. [Political Psychology series].

Jost, J. T., & Sidanius, J. (Eds.) (2004). *Political psychology: Key readings.* New York, NY: Taylor & Francis.

Jun, H. (2009). *Social justice, multicultural counseling, and practice.* Thousand Oaks, CA: Sage.

Kivel, P. (2002). *Uprooting racism: How White people can work for racial justice* (rev. ed.). Gabriola Island, BC: New Society Publishers.

Krenn, M. L. (2006). *The color of empire: Race and American foreign relations.* Washington, DC: Potomac.

Lake, M. & Reynolds, H. (2008). *Drawing the global colour line: White men's countries and the international challenge of racial equality.* Cambridge, UK: Cambridge University Press.

Long, W., & Brecke, P (2003). *War and reconciliation: Reason and emotion in conflict resolution.* Cambridge, MA: MIT Press.

Lott, B. (2009). Multiculturalism and diversity: A social psychological perspective. West Sussex, UK: Wiley-Blackwell.

MacNair, R. M. (2003). *The psychology of peace: An introduction.* Westport, CT: Praeger.

Marsella, A. J., Johnson, J., Watson, P., & Gryzycinski, J. (Eds.). (2007). *Ethnocultural perspectives on disasters.* New York, NY: Springer SBM.

Mayton, D. (2009). *Nonviolence and peace psychology: Intrapersonal, interpersonal, societal, and world peace.* New York, NY: Springer.

Nelson, G., & Prilleltensky, I. (Eds.) (2010). *Community psychology: In pursuit of liberation and well-being.* New York, NY: Palgrave/Macmillan.

Normore, A. H. (Ed.) (2008). *Leadership for social justice: Promoting equity and excellence through inquiry and reflective practice.* Charlotte, NC: Information Age Publishing.

Pilisuk, M., & Rountree, J. (2007). *Who benefits from global violence and war?: Uncovering a destructive system.* Westport, CT: Greenwood/Praeger.

Pratto, F., Sidanius, J., & Levin, S. (2006). *Social dominance theory and the dynamics of intergroup relations: Taking stock and looking forward. European Review of Social Psychology, 17,* 271–320.

Prilleltensky, I., & Nelson, G. B. (2002). *Doing psychology critically: Making a difference in diverse settings.* New York, NY: Palgrave Macmillan.

Prilleltensky, I., & Prilleltensky, O. (2006). *Promoting well-being: Linking personal, organizational, and community change.* Hoboken, NJ: John Wiley & Sons.

Ratts, M. J., Toporek, R. L., & Lewis, J. A. (2010). *ACA advocacy competencies: A social justice framework for counselors.* Alexandria, VA: ACA.

Rawls, J. (1999). *A theory of justice* (rev. ed.). Boston, MA: Harvard University Press.

Reason, P., & Bradbury, H. (Eds.) (2008). *The Sage handbook of action research: Participative inquiry and practice* (2nd ed). Thousand Oaks, CA: Sage.

de Rivera, J. (Ed.) (2009). *The handbook on building cultures of peace.* New York, NY: Springer.

Roediger, D. (1991). *The wages of whiteness: Race and the making of the American working class.* London, UK: Verso.

Rothenberg, D. (2006). *The engaged spiritual life: A Buddhist approach to transforming ourselves and the world.* Boston, MA: Beacon Press.

Rothenberg, P. S. (2008). *White privilege.* New York, NY: Worth.

Rousseau, J., & Cole, G. D. H. (Trans.) (2003). *On the social contract.* Mineola, NY: Dover Publications.

Schwebel, M. (2003). *Remaking America's three school systems: Now separate and unequal.* Lanham, MD: Scarecrow Education Press.

Sen, A. (1999). *Development as freedom.* New York, NY: Random House.

Shriberg, D., Song, S. Y., Miranda, A. H., & Radliff, K. (Eds.) (2012). *School psychology and social justice: Conceptual foundations and tools for practice.* New York, NY: Routledge.

Sloan, T. (1996). *Damaged life: The crisis of the modern psyche.* London, UK: Routledge.

Sloan, T. (Ed.) (2000). *Critical psychology: Voices for change.* London, UK: Palgrave.

Smith, L. (2010). *Psychology, poverty, and the end of social exclusion: Putting our practice to work.* New York, NY: Teachers College Press.

Tatum, B. D. (1997). *"Why are all the Black kids sitting together in the cafeteria?" and other conversations about race.* New York, NY: Basic Books. (Reissued with new introduction by Basic Books, 2003).

Toporek, R. L., Gerstein, L. H., Fouad, N. A., & Roysircar-Sodowsky, G. (2006). *Handbook for social justice in counseling psychology: Leadership, vision, and action.* Thousand Oaks, CA: Sage.

Wagner, U., Tropp, L. R., Finchilescu, G., & Tredoux, C. (Eds.) (2008). *Improving intergroup relations: Building on the legacy of Thomas F. Pettigrew.* West Sussex, UK: Wiley-Blackwell.

Wise, T. (2011). *White like me: Reflections on race from a privileged son.* Berkeley, CA: Soft Skull Press.

Young, I. M. (1990). *Justice and the politics of difference.* Princeton, NJ: Princeton University.

JOURNALS

Analyses of Social Issues and Public Policy. http://www.spssi.org

Annual Review of Critical Psychology. http://www.discourseunit.com/annual-review/

Education, Citizenship, and Social Justice. http://esj.sagepub.com/

Equity and Excellence in Education. http://www.tandfonline.com/toc/ueee20/current#.UherDLxszbM

Journal for Social Action in Counseling and Psychology. http://jsacp.tumblr.com/

Journal of Poverty and Social Justice. http://www.policypress.co.uk/journals_jpsj.asp

Journal of Social Issues. http://www.spssi.org

Journal of Social Justice. http://www.transformativestudies.org/publications/journal-of-social-justice/

Patterns of Prejudice. http://www.tandfonline.com/toc/rpop20/current#.UheqK7xszbM

Peace and Conflict: The Journal of Peace Psychology. http://www.peacepsych.org/JournalofPeacePsychology.htm

Peace Review: A Journal of Social Justice. http://www.tandfonline.com/toc/cper20/current#.UhejkLxszbM

Psychology of Violence. http://www.apa.org/pubs/journals/vio/

Self and Identity. http://www.tandfonline.com/toc/psai20/current#.UheqirxszbM

Social Issues and Policy Review. http://www.spssi.org

Social Justice Research. http://www.springer.com/psychology/personality+%26+social+psychology/journal/11211

Violence against Women. http://vaw.sagepub.com/

Appendix D

Resources for Social Justice and Psychology

Lindsay Plott-Buckner

American Psychological Association (APA) and Relevant Divisions

APA Headquarters
750 First Street, NE
Washington, DC 20002-4242 USA
Telephone: 800-374-2721 or
202-336-5500
www.apa.org

Society for the Psychological
Study of Ethnic Minority Issues
(Division 45)
www.division45.org

Society for the Psychological
Study of Lesbian, Gay, Bisexual,
& Transgender Issues
(Division 44)
www.apadivision44.org

Society for the Psychological Study of
Social Issues (Division 9)
208 I Street, NE
Washington, DC 20002-4340 USA
Telephone: 877-310-7778
(toll free); 202-675-6956
www.spssi.org

Society for the Psychology of Women
(Division 35)
www.apadivisions.org/division-35;
www.fempopculture.blogspot.com
(Division 35-sponsored blog)

Society for the Study of Peace,
Conflict & Violence (Division 48)
www.peacepsych.org

Additional Associations for Psychology Professionals (U.S.-Based)

Asian American Psychological Association (AAPA)
PMB #527
5025 North Central Avenue
Phoenix, AZ 85012 USA
www.aapaonline.org

Association for Women in
Psychology
www.awpsych.org

Association of Black Psychologists
7119 Allentown Road, Suite 203
Ft. Washington, MD 20744 USA
Telephone: 301-449-3082 www.abpsi.org

National Latina/o Psychological
Association
229 E. Wisconsin Ave., Suite 800
Milwaukee, WI 53202 USA
Telephone: 414-220-9800
www.nlpa.ws

Psychologists for Social Responsibility
www.psysr.org

Radical Psychology Network (Critical Psychology)
www.radpsynet.org

Society of Indian Psychologists
(American Indian and Alaska Natives)
www.aiansip.org

Additional Associations for Psychology Professionals (Regional/International) (Visit www.apa.org for a more comprehensive list)

ASEAN Regional Union of Psychological Societies (ARUPS)
Rm 1609 Br Andrew Gonzalez Hall Counseling and Educational Psychology Department De La Salle University Manila, 1004 Philippines

Association for Child and Adolescent Mental Health (ACAMH)
St. Saviour's House, 39-41 Union Street
London, SE1 1SD UK
Telephone: +44-20-7403-7458
www.acamh.org.uk

International Association for Cross-Cultural Society
www.iaccp.org

Japanese Psychological Association
5-23-13-7F, Hongo, Bunkyo-ku Building Tamura Tokyo, 113-0033 Japan
Telephone: +81-3-3814-3953
www.psych.or.jp

Mexican Psychological Association
(Sociedad Mexicana de Psicología)
Indiana 260 Despacho 608 Col. Nápoles, C.P. 03710, Del. Benito Juárez
México City, D.F., Mexico
www.sociedadmexicanadepsicologia.org

Middle East Psychological Association
www.mepa.me

World Federation for Mental Health
Office of Promotion and Prevention:
The Sheppard & Enoch Pratt Hospital
P.O. Box 6815
Baltimore, MD 21285-6815 USA
www.wfmh.com

Human Rights, Advocacy, and Activism

American Association of People with Disabilities
(AAPD) 2013 H Street, NW, 5th Floor
Washington, DC 20006 USA
Telephone: 202-457-0046 (V/TTY)
or 800-840-8844 (toll free V/TTY)
www.aapd.com

American Association of Retired Persons
Experience Corps National Office
601 E St. NW, Washington, DC 20049 USA
Telephone: 202-434-6400
www.aarp.org

American Civil Liberties Union
125 Broad Street, 18th Floor
New York, NY 10004 www.aclu.org

Australian Human Rights Commission
GPO Box 5218
Sydney, NSW 2001
Telephone: +2-9284 9600
www.humanrights.gov.au

Childwatch International Research Network
University of Oslo, P.O. Box 1132
Blindern, Oslo, N-0317 Norway
Telephone: +47-22-85-43-50
www.childwatch.uio.no

Equal Rights Advocates (Women's Rights)
180 Howard Street, Suite 300
San Francisco, CA 94105 USA
Telephone: 415-621-0672
www.equalrights.org

Human Rights Campaign (LGBT Rights)
1640 Rhode Island Ave. NW
Washington, DC 20036-3278 USA
Telephone: 202-628-4160 or 800-777-4723
www.hrc.org

Human Rights Watch
350 Fifth Avenue, 34th floor
New York, NY 10118-3299 USA
Telephone: +1-212-290-4700
www.hrw.org

International Disability Alliance
Geneva 150 route de Ferney, PO Box 2100 CH 1211 Geneva 2, Switzerland
Telephone: +41 (0)22-788-42-73

New York 245 Park Avenue 39th Floor
New York, NY 10167 USA
Telephone: +1-212-672-1614

Madrid Fundación ONCE C/ Sebastian Herrera, 15 28012 Madrid, Spain
Telephone: +34-91-506-88-86
www.internationaldisabilityalliance.org

International Federation of Ageing
351 Christie Street
Toronto, ON, Canada M6G 3C3
Telephone: +1-416-342-1655
www.ifa-fiv.org

National Association for the Advancement of Colored People (NAACP) (Civil Rights)
4805 Mt. Hope Drive
Baltimore, MD 21215 USA
Telephone: 410-580-5777 or (877) NAACP-98 (toll-free)
www.naacp.org

National Center for Transgender Equality, The
1325 Massachusetts Ave., NW
Suite 700
Washington, DC 20005 USA
Telephone: 202-903-0112
www.transequality.org

National Council of La Raza (Hispanic American Civil Rights)
Raul Yzaguirre Building 1126
16th Street, NW, Suite 600
Washington, DC 20036-4845 USA
Telephone: 202-785-1670
www.nclr.org

Office of the United Nations High Commissioner for Human Rights (OHCHR)
Palais Wilson 52 rue des Pâquis
CH-1201 Geneva, Switzerland
Telephone: +41-22-917-9220
www.ohchr.org

Polaris Project (Anti-Trafficking Advocacy)
P.O. Box 53315
Washington, DC 20009 USA
Telephone: 202-745-1001
www.polarisproject.org

Prison Activist Resource Center (PARC)
PO Box 70447
Oakland, CA 94612 USA
Telephone: 510-893-4648
www.prisonactivist.org

Southern Poverty Law Center
400 Washington Ave.
Montgomery, AL 36104 USA
Telephone: 334-956-8200
www.splcenter.org

U.S. Commission on Civil Rights (Headquarters)
1331 Pennsylvania Ave., NW
Suite 1150
Washington, DC 20425 USA
Telephone: 202-376-7700
www.usccr.gov

Appendix E

Resources for Human Rights

Thema Bryant-Davis, Pamela A. Counts, and Anthea A. Gray

Resources for Human Trafficking

Outreach and Awareness Materials

Polaris Project
http://www.polarisproject.org/resources/outreach-and-awareness-materials

Nationwide

National Human Trafficking Resource Center
1-888-3737-888
http://www.polarisproject.org/what-we-do/national-human-trafficking-hotline/the-nhtrc/overview

Trafficking in Persons and Worker Exploitation Task Force Line
1-888-428-7581

National Center for Missing and Exploited Children (NCMEC) National Hotline
1-800-843-5678 (THE-LOST)
www.cybertipline.com

International Trafficking Lines

Llama y Vive—Serves Latin America
- Peru: 0800-2-3232
- Nicaragua: 133
- El Salvador: 911
- Costa Rica: 911
- Ecuador: 101
- Dominican Republic: 1-809-200-7393
- United States (Washington, DC Metro Area): 1-888-NO-TRATA (668–7282)

The Angel Coalition—Serves Russia and the CIS
From the Netherlands, Belgium, Germany (to Russia):
00-800-455-05 555
http://www.angelcoalition.org/
From the United States (to Russia): 1-866-800-0270
From within Russia: 8-800-200-2400

Crimestoppers/Blue Blindfold—Serves the United Kingdom
From within the UK: 0800-555-111
http://www.blueblindfold.org/
http://www.crimestoppers-uk.org/

La Strada International
Poland: + 48 22 628 9999
http://lastradainternational.org/?main=home
- The Netherlands: + 31 33 448 11 86
- Czech Republic: + 420 2 22 71 7171
- Ukraine: + 380 44 205 36 94
- Bulgaria: + 359 2 981 76 86
- Belarus: + 375 17 295 31 67

Bosnia-Hercegovina: + 1261 OR
+ 387 36 557 190
Macedonia: + 389 2 2777 070
Moldova: + 373 22 23 33 09

National Center for Victims of Crime
800-FYI-CALL (800-394-2255)
http://www.ncvc.org

Resources for Refugees

International Organizations

Immigration Customs Enforcement
http://www.ice.gov/

International Rescue Committee
http://www.rescue.org/

UN High Commission of Refugees
http://www.unrefugees.org/site/c.lfIQKSOwFqG/b.4778881/k.BE35/Home.htm

Association for Solidarity for Asylum Seekers and Migrants
http://www.asam.8k.com/

National Network for Immigrant and Refugee Rights
http://www.nnirr.org/drupal/

Refugee Council, UK
http://www.refugeecouncil.org.uk/

Norwegian Refugee Council
http://www.nrc.no/

Organization for Aid to Refugees Czech Republic
http://www.opu.cz/

U.S. Committee for Refugees and Immigrants
http://www.refugees.org/

Refugees International
Canadian Council for Refugees
http://ccrweb.ca/

Settlement Services in Australia
http://www.immi.gov.au/media/fact-sheets/98services.htm

Oxfam: Australia
https://www.oxfam.org.au/explore/emergencies/refugees/

National Organizations

International Rescue Committee: Los Angeles http://www.rescue.org/us-program/us-los-angeles-ca

Boston Center for Refugee Health and Human Rights
http://www.bcrhhr.org/

Florida Immigrant Advocacy Center
http://aijustice.org/

Refugee Development Center: Pennsylvania http://www.refugeedevelopmentcenter.org/

Health Related

LGBT Immigrant Rights Initiative
http://www.immigrantjustice.org/programs/lgbt-immigrant-rights-initiative

Refugee and Asylum Seekers Health
http://www.medact.org/ref_about_network.php

Religious and Spiritual Networks

Catholic Charities
http://www.catholiccharitiesla.org/what-we-do/assist-immigrants-and-refugees/immigration-services.html

Episcopal Migration Ministry
http://www.episcopalchurch.org/emm/

Lutheran Immigration and Refugee Services
http://lirs.org/

Refugee Immigration Ministry
http://www.r-i-m.net/

Interfaith Refugee and Immigrant Service
http://iris-la.org/

Information and Resources for Survivors of Torture

Advocates for Survivors of Torture United States (Washington, DC):
1-410-464-900
http://www.astt.org/index.html

Association for Services to Torture and Trauma Survivors
Australia:
61-8-9227-2700
http://www.asetts.org.au

Bellevue/NYU Program for Survivors of Torture United States (New York, NY):
1-212-562-8713
http://www.survivorsoftorture.org

Berlin Center for the Treatment of Torture Victims
Germany (Berlin):
030-30-39-06-0
http://www.folteropfer.de/homeen.html

Canadian Centre for Victims of Torture Canada:
1-416-363-1066
http://ccvt.org

Center for Survivors of Torture, Dallas United States (Dallas, Texas):
1-214-827-2314
http://www.cstnet.org

The St. Louis Center for Survivors of Torture and War Trauma Center for Victims of Torture United States (St. Louis, Missouri):
1-314-533-4114
http://stlcenterforsurvivors.org

The Center for Victims of Torture United States (Minnesota):
1-612-436-4840

United States Toll Free
1-877-265-8775
Kenya:
+254 (0) 205-202-114
http://www.cvt.org

Center for Victims of Torture, Nepal
977-1-4373900/4373902/4373486
http://www.cvict.org.np

Detained Torture Survivor Legal Support Network
United States:
1-410-230-2700
http://lirs.org/our-work/partnership/service-partners/detained-torture-survivor-legal-support-network/

Florida Center for Survivors of Torture
United States (Florida):
1-727-479-1800
http://gulfcoastjewishfamilyandcommunityservices.org/refugee/refugee-programs/florida-center-for-survivors-of-torture/

Freedom from Torture
England (London):
020-7697-7777
http://www.freedomfromtorture.org

Program for Torture Victims
United States (Los Angeles, California):
1-213-747-4944
http://www.ptvla.org

Survivors of Torture International
United States (San Diego, California):
(619) 278-2400
http://www.notorture.org

Groupo Tortura Nunca Mais Brazil:
21-2286-8762 & 21-2526-2491
http://www.torturanuncamais-rj.org.br

Torture Abolition and Survivor Support Coalition
United States (Washington, DC)
1-202-529-2991
http://tassc.org/blog/

Vancouver Association for Survivors against Torture
Canada (Vancouver):
604-299-3539
http://www.vast-vancouver.ca

Foundation House: The Victorian Foundation for Survivors of Torture
Australia:
03-9388-0022
http://www.foundationhouse.org.au/home/index.htm

Information and Resources for Survivors of Genocide

Foundation Rwanda
http://www.foundationrwanda.org/home.aspx

Genocide Survivors Support Network
United States (New Jersey):
1-973-752-7439
http://www.genocidesurvivorssupportnetwork.org/Survivors_Support.html

Intervention Network for Persons Affected by Organised Violence
Canada (Montreal):
1-514-282-0661
http://www.web.net/~rivo/

Rwanda Gift for Life
http://rwandagiftforlife.org

Rwanda Women Network
Rwanda:
250-252583662
http://www.rwandawomennetwork.org

Supporting Survivors of the Rwandan Genocide United Kingdom (London):
44-0-20 7617-7121
http://survivors-fund.org.uk

Yale: Rwandan Genocide Project
http://www.yale.edu/gsp/rwanda/index.html

Office of the Special Adviser on the Prevention of Genocide
http://www.un.org/en/preventgenocide/adviser/projects.shtml

Oxfam: Responsibility to Protect
https://www.oxfam.org.au/search/?q=genocide&cx=014035679944838072922%3Akzml7htxf0c&cof=FORID%3A10&ie=UTF-

Genocide in Cambodia
http://www.hmh.org/ed_Genocide_Cambodia.shtml

Project Disappeared Argentina
http://www.desaparecidos.org/arg/eng.html

End Genocide
Genocide Intervention Network
http://endgenocide.org/

Enough Project
Congo, Darfur http://www.enoughproject.org/

Genocide Watch
Congo
http://www.genocidewatch.org/

Genocide 1915
Armenia
http://www.genocide1915.info/
Armenian National Institute
Armenia http://www.armenian-genocide.org/index.html

International Criminal Tribunal for the Former Yugoslavia
Yugoslavia
http://www.icty.org/

Yale Cambodian Genocide Program
Cambodia
http://www.yale.edu/cgp/

Samsara: Survival and Recovery in Cambodia Cambodia
http://www.brunofilms.com/samsara.html

Prevent Genocide International, Guatemala
http://www.preventgenocide.org/edu/pastgenocides/guatemala/resources/
Save Darfur
Darfur http://www.savedarfur.org/content

Yale Studies on Rescuers of Genocide
http://www.yale.edu/gsp/rescue/index.html

Center for Holocaust and Genocide Studies
University of Minnesota
http://www.chgs.umn.edu/

Journal of Genocide Research
http://www.tandfonline.com/toc/cjgr20/current

Index

About the Editors and Contributors

ABOUT THE EDITORS

JEANNETTE DIAZ, PhD, is an assistant professor of psychology at the University of West Georgia. Dr. Diaz's scholarship focuses on globalization, social justice and community-based approaches to mental health with an emphasis on critical and humanistic approaches to praxis. She is involved as a community psychologist both in her local community, where she is engaged in asset-based approaches to community development, and in Haiti where she is assisting in the establishment of a community-based mental health program.

ZENO FRANCO, PhD, is assistant professor of community engagement at the Medical College of Wisconsin (MCW) in the Department of Family and Community Medicine's Center for Healthy Communities and Research. He is also faculty in MCW's NIH supported Clinical and Translational Science Institute Community Engagement group. His research focuses on improving mental health and community resilience outcomes in collaboration with veteran, Hispanic, and African American–serving organizations in the city of Milwaukee. Dr. Franco's recent publications include "Heroism: A Conceptual Analysis and Differentiation between Heroic Action and Altruism"—in *Review of General Psychology*; "The Dirty Dozen: Twelve Key Failures of the Hurricane Katrina Response & How Psychology Can Help"—in *American Psychologist*; and "Community Engagement for Translational Disaster Research: Fostering Public, Private & Responder Group Partnerships"—in the *Proceedings of the Ninth International Conference on Information Systems for Crisis Response and Management.*

HARRIS L. FRIEDMAN, PhD, is a Florida-licensed psychologist specializing in clinical psychology and organizational development/consulting. He recently retired as research professor of psychology at University of Florida, where he remains on the courtesy faculty, and he is also professor emeritus at Saybrook University. He has over 200 professional publications, mainly in the areas of clinical and organizational psychology, as well as research methodology, and he has special interest in transpersonal psychology. He is a fellow of the American Psychological

Association, and serves as senior editor of *The International Journal of Transpersonal Studies* and associate editor of *The Humanistic Psychologist.*

CHAD V. JOHNSON, PhD, is an associate professor of human relations, clinical assistant professor of psychiatry, and a project director in the Center of Applied Research for Nonprofit Organizations at the University of Oklahoma. His scholarship and clinical interests include spirituality and psychology, social justice, group psychotherapy, and humanistic/existential/transpersonal studies. He has participated in community-based participatory research projects with several organizations and community groups, such as Indian Health Care Resource Center of Tulsa, Oklahomans for Equality, the Oklahoma Center for Community and Justice, the YWCA, and the Johns Hope Franklin Center for Reconciliation. His scholarship and clinical work include social justice (e.g., LGBTQ rights, race relations), spirituality, and group psychotherapy. He serves on the editorial boards for *The Journal of Counseling Psychology* and *The International Journal for Transpersonal Psychology.* He is also a licensed psychologist and has a private psychotherapy practice in Tulsa, Oklahoma. Dr. Johnson holds a doctorate in counseling psychology from Pennsylvania State University.

BONNIE K. NASTASI, PhD, is an associate professor in the Department of Psychology at Tulane University. Dr. Nastasi's research focuses on the use of mixed-methods designs to develop and evaluate culturally appropriate assessment and intervention approaches for promoting mental health and reducing health risks, such as sexually transmitted infections (STIs) and HIV, both within the United States and internationally. She has worked in Sri Lanka since 1995 on development of school-based programs to promote psychological well-being and is currently directing a multicountry study of psychological well-being of children and adolescents with research partners in 12 countries. She has worked in India since 2001 as one of the principal investigators of an interdisciplinary public health research program to prevent STIs among married men and women living in the slums of Mumbai. She is active in the promotion of child rights and social justice within the profession of school psychology, and is an associate of the International Institute of Child Rights & Development (IICRD), Centre for Global Studies, University of Victoria, British Columbia. She directed the development of a curriculum for training school psychologists internationally on child rights, *School Psychologist as Advocate for Child Rights*, a joint effort of International School Psychology Association, IICRD, and Tulane University's School Psychology Program. Her published works include the book, *School-Based Mental Health Services: Creating Comprehensive and Culturally Specific Programs*, published by the American Psychological Association in 2004. Dr. Nastasi is immediate past-president for Division 16 (School Psychology) of the American Psychological Association. She holds a doctorate in school psychology and early childhood education from Kent State University.

ABOUT THE CONTRIBUTORS

THEMA BRYANT-DAVIS, PhD, is an associate professor of psychology at Pepperdine University and director of the Culture and Trauma Research Lab. She is a past-president of the Society for the Psychology of Women. Dr. Bryant-Davis is also a former American Psychological Association representative to the United Nations. She is author of multiple peer-reviewed articles and chapters as well as the author of the book *Thriving in the Wake of Trauma: A Multicultural Guide* and editor of the book *Surviving Sexual Violence: A Guide to Recovery and Empowerment*. Her research and clinical work focuses on cultural considerations of recovery from traumatic experiences such as sexual assault, intimate partner violence, human trafficking, and racism.

PAMELA A. COUNTS, MA, is a doctoral student in clinical psychology at Pepperdine University. She is a research assistant at Pepperdine's Culture and Trauma Lab, and a founding co-chair of the university's Asian American Psychology Student Association. Her clinical and research interests include trauma, multicultural issues, women's rights, and children and families.

SCOT D. EVANS, PhD, is an assistant professor in the Department of Educational and Psychological Studies in the School of Education and Human Development and the director of the undergraduate major in Human and Social Development. He received his PhD in community research and action at Peabody College of Vanderbilt University and has a master's degree in human development counseling also from Vanderbilt. Dr. Evans is active in researching and promoting the role of community-based human service organizations in the promotion of community well-being and social justice.

MARY A. FUKUYAMA, PhD, is a licensed psychologist and clinical professor at the University of Florida Counseling & Wellness Center, where she has worked for the past 30 years counseling students, supervising interns, teaching, and writing on multicultural topics. She is a graduate in counseling psychology from Washington State University. Her current interests include spirituality and counseling, and international initiatives such as promoting study abroad programs. She is a fellow in Division 17 (Counseling Psychology) of the American Psychological Association.

ANTHEA A. GRAY is currently a PsyD student at Pepperdine University and a student therapist at the Union Rescue Mission. She also works as a research assistant in Pepperdine's Culture and Trauma lab and is the Advisory Board secretary for the Georges Malaika Foundation, a nonprofit organization that educates Congolese girls. Gray holds an MA from Teachers College at Columbia University.

STUART N. HART, PhD, is deputy director of the International Institute for Child Rights and Development (Victoria, British Columbia) and professor emeritus,

School of Education, Indiana University Purdue University, Indianapolis. He directed the Office for the Study of the Psychological Rights of the Child for 20 years at Indiana University. He is a licensed psychologist, co-directs Child Rights Education for Professionals, was a member of the NGO Advisory Panel for the UN Study of Violence against Children, co-principal investigator of the national project to develop operational definitions for emotional maltreatment, co-chaired the development of the draft General Comment 13 (The right of the child to freedom from all forms of violence) for the UN Committee on the Rights of the Child, and was president of the National (USA) Committee for the Rights of the Child. He has written and presented extensively on children's rights and on the psychological maltreatment of children.

MARVA L. LEWIS, PhD, is associate professor in the School of Social Work with appointments in the psychology and Department of Child Psychiatry at Tulane University in New Orleans, Louisiana, and is founder and director of the Early Connections Project. Her scholarship and research focuses on infant mental health, hair combing task and African American parent-child relationships, attachment, diversity, colorism, and the historical trauma of slavery. Lewis hold a doctorate in sociocultural psychology from the University of Colorado, Boulder.

RODNEY L. LOWMAN, PhD, is currently distinguished professor at the California School of Professional Psychology at Alliant International University in San Diego, California, and president of Lowman & Richardson/Consulting Psychologists. He earned his PhD in psychology from Michigan State University with specializations in industrial-organizational and clinical psychology. He consults in areas related to career choice and change, organizational strategy, and effectiveness. He is widely published and currently serves as editor of *Consulting Psychology Journal: Practice and Research.* His most recent book is *Internationalizing Multiculturalism: Expanding Professional Competencies in a Globalized World.*

ROSA MARIA MULSER, PhD, grew up in Voels am Schlern, Italy. She attended the Pedagogical Institute in Brixen, Italy, which awarded the equivalent of a teaching degree upon graduation after which she matriculated at Innsbruck University, Austria. After two years of studying psychology in Innsbruck, she transferred to the University of New Orleans where she received a bachelor's degree in psychology in 2005. In 2006, she entered the doctoral program in school psychology at Tulane University, which awarded her a doctoral degree in school psychology in 2012. Dr. Mulser is currently working as a postdoctoral resident in psychology at a private group practice in Pennsylvania, providing psychological services to children and adolescents.

SHEREEN NASER received her bachelors of science from the University of Texas, Austin, and is currently in her final year of the school psychology doctoral program at Tulane University in New Orleans, Louisiana. While there, Ms. Naser completed a special training program in trauma psychology, and is also interested in studying school programs and systems around mental health and behavior. Underlying all of her work is Ms. Naser's strong belief that promoting and protecting child rights is the responsibility of each and every person and with the help of the Tulane Child Rights Team has worked to develop curricula to help other school psychologists learn about the promotion and protection of child rights, particularly in the school setting.

GEOFFREY NELSON, PhD, is professor of psychology at Wilfrid Laurier University, Waterloo, Ontario. He received his PhD in clinical psychology from the University of Manitoba, Canada. He has served as senior editor of the Canadian *Journal of Community Mental Health* and Chair of the Community Psychology Section of the Canadian Psychological Association. Dr. Nelson was the recipient in 1999 of the Harry MacNeill award for innovation in community mental health from the American Psychological Foundation.

MARC PILISUK, PhD, is emeritus professor in University of California and professor in Saybrook University. He is a past president of the Society for the Study of Peace, Conflict, and Violence. He was a founder of the first Teach-in and of the Psychologists for Social Responsibility. His awards for teaching, research, and action in peace, justice, and transformative change include the 2011 Howard Zinn Award from the Peace and Justice Studies Association. His most recent books are *Who Benefits from Global Violence and War: Uncovering a Destructive System* by Marc Pilisuk with Jennifer Achord Rountree (Greenwood/Praeger, 2008), *Peace Movements Worldwide* (three volumes) by Marc Pilisuk with Michael Nagler (Eds.) (Praeger/ABC-CLIO, 2011).

ADAM D. ROSEN, MA, EdM, is a counseling psychology doctoral student at the University of Miami. His research and clinical work focuses primarily on socially just psychological practice with marginalized populations. Specific areas of scholarship and applied experiences include critical psychology, multicultural counseling pedagogy, and substance abuse counseling.

MILTON SCHWEBEL, PhD, was an emeritus professor of psychology at Rutgers University in New Brunswick, New Jersey, where he served as dean of the Graduate School of Education and professor at the Graduate School of Applied and Professional Psychology, following 18 years on the faculty of New York University's School of Education; this experience was preceded by earning a BA (major in philosophy, with economics, political science, and English minors) from Union College in Schenectady, New York, an MA in human development and social sciences from the State University of New York, Albany, the PhD in counseling psychology from Columbia University, and a certificate in psychotherapy after a three-year fellowship at the Postgraduate Center for Psychotherapy in New York City. During those years he was lecturer or consultant on education, mental health, peace and social justice issues at many universities and ministries/departments of education in the United States, Europe, Asia, and the Near East, published extensively, including "Who Can Be Educated?" (1968), which challenged the prevailing, genetically determined theory of intelligence, and was the founding editor of *Peace and Conflict: Journal of Peace Psychology*, published by the American Psychological Association. He cherishes his extensive, preacademic experience with children and teenagers, most of them in or near poverty, in schools, an orphanage, the New Deal National Youth Administration, many of them immigrants or children of recent immigrants.

DAVID SHRIBERG, PhD, is an Associate Professor of school psychology at Loyola University Chicago and the Editor-Elect of *Journal of Educational and Psychological Consultation.* His research interests relate to equity issues in education broadly and the application of social justice principles to school psychology practice specifically. He is the lead editor of the recently published "School Psychology and Social Justice: Conceptual Foundations and Implications for Practice" (Shriberg, Song, Miranda, & Radliff, 2012). Shriberg received his doctorate in school/counseling psychology from Northeastern University.

CHRISTINE SIEGEL, PhD, is an associate vice president for academic affairs at Fairfield University in Fairfield, Connecticut, where she also holds tenure as an associate professor of school psychology. She received a PhD in educational psychology and statistics from the State University of New York at Albany. Siegel's areas of teaching and scholarly expertise include developmental psychology, learning theory, and psycho-educational assessment.

KAREN L. SUYEMOTO, PhD, is an associate professor in psychology and Asian American studies at the University of Massachusetts, Boston. She has conducted research and taught undergraduate and graduate classes focused on racial justice for almost 20 years. Her scholarship particularly focuses on (1) how racial and ethnic identities and experiences of discrimination are associated with development and mental health for Asian Americans; (2) how individuals and communities create and maintain meanings of race and ethnicity that contribute to or resist oppressive systems; and (3) the processes and effects of antiracist and social justice education and community interventions. Dr. Suyemoto is the past-president of the Asian American Psychological Association, the former codirector of the New England Center for Inclusive Teaching, and provides consultation and training on antiracist therapy and education.

ALLISYN L. SWIFT is currently a school psychology doctoral student at Tulane University. Ms. Swift's is a former Zero to Three national fellow and previously served as consultant and trainer for early childhood programs in New York. Her scholarship and research focuses on infant mental health and works closely with schools to develop comprehensive mental health programs that center around the unique needs of families and school communities.

REBECCA L. TOPOREK, PhD, is an associate professor and coordinator for the career and college counseling specializations in the Department of Counseling at San Francisco State University. She has written or cowritten more than 50 articles and book chapters on the topics of multicultural training, advocacy and social justice, ethics, privilege, and career counseling. In addition, she has co-edited three books and serves as co-editor and cofounder for *The Journal for Social Action in Counseling and Psychology*, the official journal of Counselors for Social Justice and Psychologists for Social Responsibility. She is a fellow of the American Psychological Association, Society of Counseling Psychology, and the American Counseling Association. She is dedicated to bringing voices forward and facilitating the next generation of counselors and psychologists to see the social responsibility inherent in their work.